Seventh Edition

Short Cases in
SURGERY

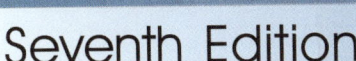

Seventh Edition

Short Cases in
SURGERY

Swaraj Kumar Bhattacharya

MS (Cal) FRCS (Edin)

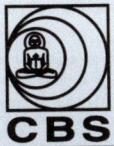

CBS

CBS Publishers & Distributors Pvt Ltd

New Delhi • Bengaluru • Chennai • Kochi • Kolkata • Mumbai
Bhopal • Bhubaneswar • Hyderabad • Jharkhand • Nagpur • Patna • Pune
• Uttarakhand • Dhaka (Bangladesh) • Kathmandu (Nepal)

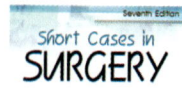

Short Cases in
SURGERY

ISBN: 978-93-88902-81-6

Copyright © Ranjana Bhattacharya

Seventh Edition: 2020

First Edition: 1978
Second Edition: 1983
Reprint: 1984
Third Edition: 1987
Reprint: 1992
Fourth Edition: 1993
Reprint: 1996, 1997, 1999, 2000, 2001, 2002
Fifth Edition: 2003
Reprint: 2004, 2005, 2006, 2008, 2009, 2010
Sixth Edition: 2012
Reprint: 2013, 2015, 2017

Published by Satish Kumar Jain and produced by Varun Jain for

CBS Publishers & Distributors Pvt Ltd

4819/XI Prahlad Street, 24 Ansari Road, Daryaganj, New Delhi 110 002, India
Ph: 011-23289259, 23266861, 23266867   Website: www.cbspd.com
Fax: 011-23243014   e-mail: delhi@cbspd.com; cbspubs@airtelmail.in

Corporate Office: 204 FIE, Industrial Area, Patparganj, Delhi 110 092
Ph: 011-49344934   Fax: 011-49344935   e-mail: publishing@cbspd.com; publicity@cbspd.com

Branches

- **Bengaluru:** Seema House 2975, 17th Cross, K.R. Road,
  Banasankari 2nd Stage, Bengaluru 560 070, Karnataka
  Ph: +91-80-26771678/79   Fax: +91-80-26771680   e-mail: bangalore@cbspd.com
- **Chennai:** 7, Subbaraya Street, Shenoy Nagar, Chennai 600 030, Tamil Nadu
  Ph: +91-44-26680620, 26681266   Fax: +91-44-42032115   e-mail: chennai@cbspd.com
- **Kochi:** 68/1534, 35, 36, Power House Road, Opposite KSEB, Kochi 682018, Kerala
  Ph: +91-484-4059061-65   Fax: +91-484-4059065   e-mail: kochi@cbspd.com
- **Kolkata:** 6/B, Ground Floor, Rameswar Shaw Road, Kolkata-700 014, West Bengal
  Ph: +91-33-22891126, 22891127, 22891128   e-mail: kolkata@cbspd.com
- **Mumbai:** 83-C, Dr E Moses Road, Worli, Mumbai-400018, Maharashtra
  Ph: +91-22-24902340/41   Fax: +91-22-24902342   e-mail: mumbai@cbspd.com

Representatives

• Bhopal	0-8319310552	• Bhubaneswar	0-9911037372	• Hyderabad	0-9885175004	• Jharkhand	0-9811541605
• Nagpur	0-9421945513	• Patna	0-9334159340	• Pune	0-9623451994	• Uttarakhand	0-9716462459
• Dhaka (Bangladesh)	01912-003485	• Kathmandu (Nepal)	977-9818742655				

Printed at:
Magic International Pvt. Ltd., Greater Noida, U.P., India

to

Late Sri Sibdas Bhattacharjee
Late Srimati Mina Bhattacharjee

My Beloved Parents

Preface to the Seventh Edition

At long last, the much awaited seventh edition of the book *Short Cases in Surgery* is being presented to the students of medicine and surgery. It is my sincere hope that the readers will find it useful both in theory and in oral examinations.

Every edition of this book has improved in text and illustrations. Fresh and updated information in the form of new contents has been added in this edition as well.

A special feature of this edition is the provision of many new images of clinical cases. I remain indebted to those surgeons and teachers in medical colleges who most kindly provided me with the same. I encourage and solicit the medical fraternity, both teachers and students in India and abroad, to send in more clinical photographs highlighting the features of, and clarifying the reasons for the diagnosis of particular cases and their treatment for the subsequent editions of this book.

Further, a few important facts are mentioned at the end of each chapter under the section 'Notes'. It will be helpful for meeting the requirements of *viva voce* examinations as well as serve as a great resource for writing short notes and tackling multiple choice questions in MS entrance examinations.

I am profoundly grateful to the members of our joint family for their inspiration. I am also thankful to my publisher, Mr SK Jain CMD and Mr YN Arjuna (Senior Vice President—Publishing, Editorial and Publicity) of CBS Publishers & Distributors Pvt Ltd, New Delhi, for their keen interest in publishing this new edition. Mr Dharmvir of the same publishing house also deserves thanks for his painstaking efforts to give the book its present shape.

I welcome constructive criticism and suggestions from the readers of this book.

Swaraj Kumar Bhattacharya

Acknowledgments

The author is happy to bring out the seventh edition of the book *Short Cases in Surgery*. Thanks to the constant help and support of the many teachers in surgery. He remains indebted to the following teachers for their help and suggestions.

- Late Dr NK Pal MS FRCS (Eng): Ex-Professor and Head of the Department, Calcutta National Medical College, Kolkata, WB; Ex-President, ASI
- Dr AK Banerjee FRCS (Eng) FRCS (Edin): Ex-Professor, Calcutta National Medical College, Kolkata, WB
- Dr DK Roy MS: Ex-Professor and Head of the Department, Calcutta Medical College, Kolkata, WB
- Dr Sudeb Saha MS FAMS: Professor and Head of the Department, NRS Medical College, Kolkata, WB
- Dr Bansari Goswami MS: Ex-Professor and Head of the Department, NRS Medical College, Kolkata, WB
- Dr Tarun Kr Chattopadhyay MS: Professor, NRS Medical College, Kolkata, WB
- Dr Diptendra Sarker MS DNB FRCS (Edin): Professor, IPGNE and R, SSKM Hospital, Kolkata, WB
- Dr Sukumar Maity MS FRCS (Edin) MCh (Paed) MNANS: Professor and Head of the Department, Calcutta Medical College, Kolkata, WB
- Dr S Tibrewal MS MRCS BNB MNAMS: Assistant Professor, NRS Medical College, Kolkata, WB
- Dr US Chatterjee MS MCh (Paed) MCh (Uro): Consultant Paediatric Surgeon and Urologist
- Dr RL Modak MS: Ex-Clinical Tutor, RG Medical College, Kolkata, WB; Ex-Surgeon, SNP Hospital, Kolkata, WB; Senior Surgeon, Ramkrishna Seva Protisthan, Kankhal, UP
- Dr Somnath Ghosh MS: Ex-Clinical Tutor, NRS Medical College, Kolkata, WB
- Dr Sugato Bandopadhyay MS MCh (Paed): Professor, KPC Medical College, Kolkata, WB
- Dr Nirjhar Bhattacharya MS FAIS: Professor, NRS Medical College and Hospital, Kolkata, WB
- Dr Samindra Basak MS FRCS DNB: Professor, Vivekananda Institute of Medical Sciences, Kolkata, WB
- Dr Sailen Paul MS: Professor, KPC Medical College, Kolkata, WB
- Dr Sandip Chakraborty MS DGO: Ex-Resident Surgeon, SNP Hospital, Kolkata, WB
- Dr Subrata Roy MD: Ex-Gynaecologist, SNP Hospital, Kolkata, WB
- Dr Abinas Roy MD: Ex-Gynaecologist, SNP Hospital, Kolkata, WB
- Dr Yogesh Salphale D Ortho
- Dr J Jaychandan MDS
- Dr Sharmistha Bhattacharya MS
- Dr Gurusaday Bhattacharya MS FRCS: Professor and Head, Department of Surgery, KPC Medical College, Kolkata, WB
- Dr Arun Anand MS

I am also grateful to the students of surgery, both undergraduate and postgraduate, whose interests have prompted the sustenance of this work through many editions.

Last, but not the least, I remain eternally grateful to my beloved wife, Smt Ranjana Bhattacharya, and my doting children, Dr Sharmistha Bhattacharya MS, and Adhraj Bhattacharya BE, without whose constant support and encouragement to publish this book would have remained a distant dream.

Swaraj Kumar Bhattacharya

Preface to the First Edition

The aim of this book is a very modest one: To help the students, who are preparing for qualifying examinations, in readily grasping the problems of surgery—the problems they have to tackle in their examinations as well as in the wider world outside the examination halls. Though no originality of the author is marshalling all the necessary pieces of information in surgery with a medical student requires to be armed with.

The features of the book are precisely as follows:

1. Most of the surgical problems which are very often posed as 'Short Cases' in examinations will be found adequately discussed here. Cases in orthopaedics have, however, been kept outside the purview of the book.
2. Each problem has been explained with arguments from all the three dimensions of medical knowledge—anatomy, physiology and pathology. Also the principles of surgical operations have been briefly laid down, wherever possible.
3. Discussion has been, whenever necessary, amply illustrated with schematic diagrams to facilitate easy and ready understanding of the subjects.
4. Precision is the hallmark of this book. While no necessary information or explanation has been left out, the subjects have been presented in a neat and pointed fashion.
5. The book provides necessary aids for ready recapitulation of the important features of problems and their solutions.

The author, however, feels obliged to point out that the book does not in any way replace the modern textbooks by authors of eminence keeping pace with the latest developments in science. The author suggests that a student should constantly consult a textbook or textbooks of his choice. This book will prove to be useful in following the treatises by noted writers.

Even a small endeavour like this has its origin in the help and assistance of many. The author is deeply indebted to all his teachers. The author mentions in particular Dr DK Roy MS, Assistant Professor in Surgery, Calcutta Medical College; Dr SP Sen MS, Assistant Professor in Surgery, North Bengal University Medical College.

The author gratefully acknowledges Dr AK Dutta, MS, Reader in Anatomy, University College of Medicine, for kindly reviewing the discussions in anatomy; and Dr AC Ganguly, MS, Associate Professor and Head, Department of Plastic Surgery, Calcutta Medical College, for suggesting improvements on the first draft on 'Cleft Lip and Cleft Palate'.

The author records his thanks to many of the fellow-professionals, both junior and senior, to the teachers and non-teaching staff of the Department of Anatomy of the Calcutta National Medical College, to Dr CR Basu, MS, MAMS, Lecturer in Anatomy, in particular, for their encouragement and cooperation.

Sri KC Pal of Nabajiban Press, Calcutta, has taken pains to print the book in a dignified form in a very short span of time and deserves sincere appreciation of the author.

The author finally gratefully acknowledges his profound debt to his parents and brothers and sisters for the constant inspiration they offered.

The author alone is responsible for the shortcomings in this piece of work. He welcomes suggestions for improvement from the readers.

Swaraj Kumar Bhattacharya

Contents

Lumps, Ulcers and Fistula/Sinus

CLINICAL EXAMINATION OF A LUMP OR SWELLING

This should be conducted in a systematic manner – history, local examination, state of local tissues, state of regional lymph nodes, and general examination of the patient.

- **History**
  - Age, sex, ethnic group, occupation.
  - Duration: *How long the lump is there?*
  - Mode of onset: *How the lump has started?*
  - Progress of the swelling: *Is the lump changing its size and surface?*
  - Painful or painless?
  - Family history.

- **Local examination**
  - *Inspection*
    - Site
    - Number
    - Shape and size
    - Colour
    - Surface and edge
    - Skin over the swelling
    - Visible pulsation
    - Impulse on coughing
  - *Palpation*
    - Local temperature
    - Tenderness
  - Site, size and shape
  - Surface and edge
  - Consistence ⎤ Solid
  - Fluctuation ⎟ or
  - Translucency ⎟ Fluid
  - Fluid thrill ⎟ or
  - Resonance ⎦ Gas
  - Compressibility ⎤ Vascular
  - Pulsatility ⎦
  - Indentation
  - Impulse on coughing: Visible or palpable?
  - Reducibility
  - Mobility
  - *Percussion*
  - *Auscultation*
- **State of local tissues**
- **State of regional lymph nodes**
- **General examination of the patient**

LUMP

A lump or swelling may arise from the skin, subcutaneous tissue, muscle, tendon, bone, nerve, lymphatics and lymph nodes, blood vessels, gland, or lie within one of the body cavities.

A lump may also arise due to protrusion of a viscus from the body cavity through a weak spot of its wall, e.g. hernia.

Causes of a lump or swelling

A. Congenital

- Present since birth, e.g. meningocele, dermoid cyst, teratoma.
- Not evident at birth but appears years later, e.g. branchial cyst, thyroglossal cyst, cystic hygroma.

B. Acquired

- Traumatic: Swelling develops immediately after a trauma, e.g. haematoma, muscular lump caused by rupture, bony projections following fracture or dislocation.
- Inflammatory: Acute or chronic.
- Neoplastic: Benign or malignant.
- Otherwise, e.g. autoimmune disease.

DIAGNOSIS OF A LUMP OR SWELLING

History

- Age, sex, ethnic origin, occupation.
- Duration: *How long the lump is there?*
  - Congenital and present since birth, e.g. meningocele, dermoid cyst, teratoma.
  - Congenital but not evident at birth and appears years later, e.g. branchial cyst, thyroglossal cyst, cystic hygroma.
  - Acquired.
- Mode of onset: *How the lump has started?*
  - The swelling may appear after trauma or develop spontaneously. A swelling may arise on some pre-existing condition, e.g. a keloid may develop over a scar; malignant melanoma may develop over a mole or birth mark.
- Progress of the swelling: *Whether the lump is changing in size or surface.*
  - Rapid enlargement may imply inflammation particularly if it is painful, whereas progressive enlargement may signify neoplasia.
- Painful or painless?
  - Painful lumps are commonly due to trauma and inflammation. Pain is absent in benign growth and in early carcinoma.

Local examination

Inspection

1. *Site:* Location of the lump and its relation to certain landmarks present in the vicinity of the lump.

   Typical position of a swelling is almost diagnostic of some lesion, e.g.
   - Postauricular dermoid behind the ear;
   - External angular dermoid at the lateral end of the eyebrow;
   - Meningocele over the back in the midline;
   - Thyroid swelling in front of the neck.

2. *Number:* Whether single, or multiple, e.g. neurofibromatosis, adiposis dolorosa, warts, naevi, secondary carcinomatous nodules, diaphyseal aclasia.

3. *Shape and size:* Whether spherical, ovoid, kidney-shaped, pyriform or irregular. The lump may be pedunculated or sessile.

4. *Surface:* Smooth (cyst), lobulated (lipoma), nodular (a mass of enlarged lymph nodes, multinodular goitre), rough and irregular (irregularity of a wart; carcinoma), red, shiny and oedematous (inflammatory lesion).

   There may be presence of a *pit or punctum* (sebaceous cyst), *peau d'orange* (due to underlying carcinoma infiltrating towards the skin, e.g. carcinoma breast), *scar* (irregular scar from injury; broad, depressed and puckered scar from suppuration; linear scar with suture marks from previous operation – *this indicates that the lump appears after operation, e.g.* incisional hernia; *recurrence of lump, e.g.* Paget's recurrent fibroid. *Tense shiny skin with overlying prominent veins* (sarcoma).

   There may be *ulcer over a swelling* (necrosis over a malignant nodule).

5. *Edge of the swelling:* Whether circumscribed or of the nature of a general bulge, i.e. without any definite margin. The edge may be sharp, rounded, regular or irregular.

   Well-defined and regular (most of the benign swellings); *well-defined and irregular* (malignant swelling infiltrating the surrounding skin); *diffuse and ill-defined* (inflammatory swellings like cellulitis, abscess).

6. *Colour:* Red or purple (inflammation, haemangioma), blue (ranula, mucous cyst), black (melanoma).

7. *Visible pulsation:* Visible expansion synchronous with each pulse beat (aneurysm, vascular growth).

8. *Visible impulse on coughing* depending on the site of the lump. When the swelling is noticed over the groin, abdomen, chest, spine or cranium: *Note cough impulse*, e.g. hernia, meningocele.

9. *Movements of the swelling on deglutition* when the swelling is situated in front of the neck – *thyroid swelling moves up on deglutition.*

10. *Note any pressure effects* when the swelling is on the limb – inspect the distal part for any pressure effect like oedema, footdrop, wristdrop from nerve palsy.

Palpation

Before starting palpation of the lesion, the patient should be asked, whether the lesion is painful and/or tender.

1. *Temperature: Examined by dorsum of the fingers.* Raised in presence of acute inflammation, cellulitis or abscess. Some vascular tumours (e.g. sarcoma) may also show raised temperature. *For examination of other features of the swelling* – examine with the palmar surfaces of the fingers.

2. *Tenderness (pain on pressure):* Present over a traumatic or inflammatory lump and is a feature of inflammation. Tenderness is also often noted over a rapidly expanding malignant lump. A swelling along the nerve is also tender, e.g. solitary neurofibroma. A swelling caused by bony fracture is also tender.

   Benign growth is painless and non-tender.

3. *Confirm the site, size and shape, surface and edge.* Edge may be well-defined or ill-defined. *In lipoma, the edge is well-defined and when pressed upon, it slips away under the examining finger (slipping sign) – this is a characteristic of lipoma.*

   Measure the size of the swelling with tape in three dimensions – length, breadth and height.

4. *Consistence:* Depends on the contents of the lump which can be composed of cells, fluid or gas. So, consistence varies from soft to bony hard – *soft* (lipoma, haemangioma), *cystic* (cyst, aneurysm and abscess), *firm* (fibroma, papilloma, goitre), *hard but yielding* (chondroma), *stony hard* (metastatic lymph nodes), or *bony hard* (osteoma, osteochondroma).

   Consistence may be uniform throughout or variable. *Variegated consistency*, i.e. some part is soft, some part firm, some part hard – suggests malignant growth.

   A *cystic swelling* feels softer at the centre than at the periphery. A *solid swelling* feels firm at the centre than at the periphery.

5. *Indentation or moulding:* Certain cysts like sebaceous cyst or dermoid cyst contain pultaceous or putty-like material and can be moulded. Such swelling when pressed upon with the tip of the finger, in contradistinction to the sign of emptying, *it stays indented.* Such sign of indentation can also be demonstrated over the palpable sigmoid colon loaded with solid faeces, in the left iliac fossa.

6. *Compressibility:* Some soft or cystic lumps are compressible. When they are squeezed, they diminish in size considerably or disappear, but reappear slowly on release of pressure. This is known as *the sign of emptying* and is a characteristic of blood-filled lesions such as haemangioma, aneurysm, arteriovenous fistula, but may also be seen in lymphangioma and narrow-necked meningocele.

   The sign of emptying in haemangioma may be accompanied by blanching, i.e. the lesion becomes colourless or pale as the blood is expressed out of the lesion. The colour returns on release of pressure.

7. *Fluctuation:* This determines the presence of fluid (or gas) in a swelling – *cystic swelling.* This clinical sign can be elicited in a non-tense cystic swelling where an impulse transmitted to the finger or fingers of one hand on one side of the swelling by

sudden pressure exerted with the finger or fingers of the other hand on the other side of the swelling and vice versa. *Fluctuation implies transmitted impulse in two planes at right angles to each other. So, fluctuation should be elicited in both directions, at right angles to each other*, as fleshy muscle in the thigh can be fluctuant across but not in longitudinal direction.

Fluctuation is positive in cystic swellings like hydrocele, cystic hygroma, meningocele, bursa, etc.

For small swellings (<2 cm) do the Paget's test. Test for fluctuation in a small lump is elicited by watching two of the examining fingertips on the lump moving apart when a third finger is used to press on the lump.

Pseudo or false fluctuation is felt in a large soft swelling but without any fluid content, e.g. lipoma.

Cross fluctuation is the fluctuation between two separate swellings but communicating with each other, e.g. *compound palmar ganglion in the wrist* above and below the flexor retinaculum; *psoas abscess pointing to the thigh* above and below the inguinal ligament; *deep plunging ranula in the floor of the mouth* extending to submental region.

8. *Transillumination:* Once the swelling is found to be cystic, *test for translucency* in order to determine the nature of the fluid in the cyst – clear or otherwise. *Cystic swelling containing clear fluid* (e.g. hydrocele, meningocele, lymphangioma, cystic hygroma, ranula, bursa, etc.) *will trans-illuminate with pointed light provided the covering skin is thin.*

Hydrocele due to filaria, haematocele, though cystic, will not transilluminate.

Spermatocele, lipoma poorly trans-illuminate.

Note

Brilliantly transilluminable swellings

- Cystic hygroma
- Congenital hydrocele

- Epididymal cyst
- Ranula
- Meningocele with thin skin cover.

Note

For any scrotal swelling transillumination test is a must. Any scrotal swelling when felt hard and transillumination is negative: consider testicular tumour and proceed accordingly.

Spermatocele, filarial hydrocele and lipoma – very poorly transilluminate.

9. *Pulsatility:* A swelling may pulsate synchronous with each pulse beat of the patient.

The pulsation may be *expansile pulsation* where the swelling expands in all directions as well as it pulsates, e.g. *aneurysm, vascular malformation, arteriovenous fistula.*

This pulsation of the swelling may be *transmitted pulsation* where the swelling does not increase in size but is merely raised with each throb of the underlying artery, e.g. *a pancreatic mass* situated in front of the abdominal aorta, a *carotid body tumour* at the bifurcation of the common carotid artery.

A carotid body tumour may have rich blood supply and may exhibit expansile as well as transmitted pulsation. Some other tumour like telangiectatic type of osteogenic sarcoma have a rich blood supply to show expansile pulsation.

In case of an aneurysm, pressure over the main artery proximal to the swelling results in diminution in the size of the swelling as well as pulsation.

Note

- Carotid body tumour – hard and may show transmitted pulsation.
- Carotid aneurysm – soft and usually shows expansile and transmitted pulsation.

10. *Reducibility:* It indicates that a swelling can be emptied by squeezing, but the swelling does not return spontaneously on release of pressure (cf. compressibility) – reappearance of the swelling requires an additional force,

e.g. straining or coughing, or the effect of gravity. *A classic example is hernia.*

11. *Impulse on coughing:* This is present in those swellings which are soft or cystic and *are likely to be in continuity with the interior of one of the body cavities,* i.e. abdomen (external hernias, iliopsoas and lumber abscesses), chest (e.g. empyema necessitatis), spine and cranium (e.g. meningocele). *The impulse on coughing is usually both visible and palpable and when present, say cough impulse is positive.*

12. *Thrill on palpation:* This is commonly found in an arteriovenous fistula. A thrill may also be present in toxic goitre.

13. *Mobility of the lump:* To know the depth, i.e. anatomical plane, the lump is situated and its relations to the surrounding structures, i.e. to skin, subcutaneous tissue, fascia, muscle, tendon, bone, vessels and nerves. *The mobility of a lump depends on its site of origin as well as on its tethering and fixation to the surrounding tissues.* A lump may be attached, adherent or fixed to the skin, subcutaneous tissue, deep fascia, muscle, tendon, bone, vessels or nerves.

(a) *Fixity to the skin:* A lesion arising from the skin, e.g. papilloma, wart, mole, sebaceous cyst, keloid, epithelioma etc., moves with the movement of the skin.

Swelling deeper to the skin: Try to pinch the skin over the swelling at various places or try to move the skin over the swelling by sliding movement after fixing the swelling.

• Lipoma – skin can be pinched suggesting the swelling is not fixed to the skin.
• Malignant breast lump – skin cannot be pinched or slid over the swelling as the swelling is fixed to the skin. *Even if skin can be pinched over the swelling, move the skin or the swelling* – the skin can be seen puckered as seen in early carcinoma of breast when the swelling is said to be tethered to the skin. *Tethering is indirect fixity to the skin* and is due to fixity of fibrous septae

due to infiltration, e.g. infiltration of Cooper's ligament in carcinoma breast.

(b) *Subcutaneous lump* is free from the skin and moves freely over the contracted muscle. *Contraction of the underlying muscle and fascia makes a subcutaneous lump more prominent and easily palpable.*

(c) *Fixity to the deep fascia only* is difficult to demonstrate. *A lump beneath the deep investing fascia of the neck becomes less palpable by pressing the chin on the opposite side of the swelling against the examiner's hand.*

(d) *Fixity to the muscle:* A lump may be attached to a muscle, or incorporated in the muscle or situated underneath the muscle.

When the muscle is relaxed, the lump may be easily palpable and freely movable across the long axis of the muscle.

When the muscle is contracted, the swelling may change its character:
• The swelling may become prominent, as when it lies above the muscle.
• The swelling may remain unaltered, as when it is incorporated in the muscle.
• The swelling may diminish in size or impalpable, as when it lies under the muscle.

Mobility of the lump over the relaxed and contracted muscle – a lump which is adherent to the muscle becomes immobile when the muscle contracts.

(e) *Fixity to the tendon:* A swelling in connection with the tendon of a muscle *becomes fixed* when the concerned muscle is contracted against resistance. A swelling in connection with a tendon *also moves with the tendon* on movement of the concerned muscle.

(f) *Fixity to the bone:* Swelling in connection with the bone cannot be moved apart from the bone, e.g. jaw tumour, exostosis.

(g) *Fixity to the vessels and nerves:* A lump in connection with a vessel or nerve can be moved across (i.e. at right angles to their axes) but not along the direction of their axes.

Percussion

To differentiate *gaseous* swelling from *fluid* or *solid* swellings, *the first being resonant, the latter two are dull.* Tympanic or resonant in enterocele or pharyngocele. In a small swelling percussion is not done.

Auscultation

All pulsatile swellings should be auscultated with a stethoscope for any bruit or murmur. It may be systolic, diastolic or continuous murmur. *A continuous buzzing sound, known as machinery murmur or bruit* is audible over an arteriovenous fistula.

Bruit is also heard over a very vascular lesion, e.g. thyrotoxic goitre.

State of the local tissues

1. *Presence of induration:* Induration implies thickening and firmness of the surrounding tissues and is due to inflammatory oedema or infiltrating neoplasia. The indurated area may be indented or depressed on pressure, or hard. It may be tender.
2. There may be ecchymoses, pigmentation, metastatic nodules, prominent vessels.
3. If the swelling is overlying a bone – *feel for bony indentation or erosion deep to the margin of the swelling,* e.g. dermoid cyst, meningocele.
4. If the swelling is on the limb –
   (i) Look for oedema, dilatation of veins due to pressure over the vein.
   (ii) Palpate the distal pulse for any pressure over the artery.
   (iii) Look for wasting of muscles, paresis or paraplegia, footdrop, wristdrop due to pressure over the nerve.
5. Examine the neighbouring joints, above and below the swelling to note whether there is impairment of joint movements.

State of the regional lymph nodes

- The draining lymph nodes must always be palpated for involvement in presence of inflammatory or malignant lesion.
- The head and neck drain to the cervical nodes.
- The skin, muscles and bones of the limbs and trunk drain to the axillary and inguinal nodes.
- The intra-abdominal structures and testes drain to the pre- and para-aortic nodes.
- The penis drains into the inguinal nodes.

General examination

Look for any systemic effects produced by infection, trauma or malignancy.

Is there similar swelling elsewhere, e.g. neurofibromatosis, diaphyseal aclasia?

In case of suspected malignant growth, a search should be made for secondary deposits elsewhere, e.g. *neck, axillae and groins* for enlarged lymph nodes; *abdomen* for enlarged, hard and nodular liver, mass due to enlarged nodes, ascites; *chest* for pleural effusion or consolidation.

DIAGNOSIS OF A CYSTIC SWELLING

1. **Site:** Most of the congenital cystic swellings have a typical location as follows:
   - *Branchial cyst* – anterior triangle of the neck, partly covered by upper one-third of sternomastoid.
   - *Dermoid cyst* – along the planes of fusion, such as midline of the body, e.g. at the root of the nose; on the scalp, e.g. pterion, asterion (postauricular dermoid), on the inner or outer angles of the eye (angular dermoid).
   - *Meningocele* – in the new born along the midline of the back, commonly at lumbosacral region.
   - *Ganglion* – on the dorsum of the hand.
2. **Shape:** Majority of cystic swellings are round and oval. Exceptions are:
   - *Subhyoid bursitis* – transverse oval cystic swelling in the midline of the neck.
   - *Thyroglossal cyst* – vertical oval cystic swelling in the midline of the neck.

- *Sebaceous cyst, dermoid cyst* – globular or hemispherical swelling.
3. **Surface:** Most cystic swellings in the skin and subcutaneous tissue have smooth surface.
4. **Consistence:** Cystic or firm to hard. *Fluctuation is positive in all cystic swellings. Fluctuation is to be elicited in two directions right angle to each other.*
   - *Soft cystic swelling* – meningocele, thyroglossal cyst, cystic hygroma, aneurysm.
   - *Tense cystic swelling* – hydrocele, ganglion. A tense ganglion may feel hard.
   - *Soft cystic at the centre with firm thickened periphery* – cold abscess.
   - *Putty or tooth paste* – sebaceous cyst, dermoid – the swelling is usually indented by a finger tip.
5. **Signs of compressibility:** The swelling may disappear completely or partially on application of pressure, but reappears on release of pressure, e.g. aneurysm, haemangioma, lymphangioma, meningocele.
6. **Pulsations:** Expansile or transmitted.
   - *Expansile pulsation* – aneurysm.
   - *Transmitted pulsation* –
     (i) When a swelling lies over a vessel, e.g. pseudopancreatic cyst in front of abdominal aorta;
     (ii) When an artery is pushed by a structure underneath, e.g. subclavian artery over the cervical rib.
7. **Transillumination:**
   - *Positive* with cysts containing clear fluid, e.g. hydrocele, meningocele, cystic hygroma.
   - *Negative* with cysts containing thick or opaque fluid, e.g. hydrocele due to filaria, haematocele.

Note

Causes of pulsatile bone tumour

1. Osteoclastoma
2. Angiocarcinoma
3. Angioendothelioma of bone
4. Aneurysmal bone cyst
5. Metastases from renal cell carcinoma and thyroid carcinoma

ULCERS

An ulcer is a persistent breach in continuity of the surface epithelium – the skin or mucous membrane – due to microscopic death of tissue. This is due to gradual necrosis of the surface tissue which results in the formation of *a sore or ulcer*. The dead tissue, which becomes separated from the living tissue during the process of necrosis, is termed as **slough** which covers the floor. *The base of the ulcer* may be necrotic, granulating or malignant.

Parts of an ulcer

Parts of an ulcer are:

1. Margin
2. Edge – various types of edges of the ulcer usually help to identify the definite ulcer type
3. Floor
4. Base – on which the ulcer rests

Examination of an ulcer

For quick examination of an ulcer, the following points must be noted:

- Note the site, size, edge, margin, floor, base and surrounding tissues.
- Note for pigmentation (venous ulcer), dark, thin and shiny surface (ischaemic), adjacent oedematous area (spreading ulcer), adjacent scar (Marjolin's ulcer), adjacent bony thickening.
- Look for fixity of the ulcer to the underlying structures – check the movements of the ulcer
- Probing of the adjacent ulcer margins for depth and any associated sinus.
- Examine the arterial pulses – arterial ulcer
- Examine for varicose veins – venous ulcer
- Examine for sensation – neuropathic ulcer
- Examine for nerve thickening – Hansen's disease
- Examine the regional lymph nodes –
  (a) Enlarged due to infection – firm in feel and may be tender
  (b) Enlarged due to malignancy (secondary) – hard in feel and non-tender
- Movements of the adjacent joints
- Note the following predisposing causes: diabetes, atherosclerosis/hypertension, venous

insufficiency, neuropathy – both sensory and motor supply, syphilis, tuberculosis and history of trauma.

Pathological classification of ulcer

On pathological basis ulcers are classified as:

- Non-specific
- Specific
- Malignant

Non-specific ulcers

1. *Mechanical*
   - Traumatic – due to mechanical, physical or chemical injury, e.g. dental ulcer (caused by sharp tooth or ill-fitting dentures), pressure sores (caused by prolonged pressure, e.g. by splints or plasters, or prolonged bed rest).
   - Physical – burns and scalds, electric burn, X-ray burn.
   - Chemical – caused by acids or alkalis.
2. *Infective:* Due to secondary infection of wounds by non-specific pyogenic organisms like *Staphylococcus* or *Streptococcus* (pyogenic ulcer, Bairnsdale ulcer).
3. *Trophic or nutritional* (Greek *Trophe* = nutrition) – *due to an impairment of the nutrition of tissues* which depends upon adequate blood supply and nerve supply, e.g. diabetic ulcer (atherosclerosis and/or neuropathy).
   - Vascular insufficiency: *Usually causes painful ulcers.*
     - *Poor arterial supply:* Burger's disease, Raynaud's disease, arteriosclerosis.
     - *Venous stasis:* Varicose ulcer over medial gaiter area proximal to the medial malleolus; venous ulcer in post-phlebitic limb.
   - Neuropathic: *Usually causes painless ulcer.* Ulceration is due to sensory impairment or anaesthesia, e.g. tabes dorsalis, syringomyelia, leprosy, diabetes, spina bifida, peripheral nerve injury. *Neuropathic ulcers are often called perforating ulcers.*
4. *Tropical ulcer:* Develops in the legs and feet of the people living in tropical countries by *Vincent's organism* (bacteroides fusiformis) in a small abrasion. Ulcers are common in poor people with malnutrition, anaemia and avitaminosis.
5. *Bazin ulcer* (associated with erythrocyanoid frigida)*:* Tender erythema with induration of subcutaneous tissue usually over the calves followed by ulceration in neglected cases – *due to cutaneous tuberculosis.* Common in women.
6. *Leprosy ulcer:* Chronic, non-healing, *painless skin patch or ulcer due to loss of sensation. Common in tuberculoid leprosy.* Common on the hands and feet – more common at the metatarsal heads. May be associated with footdrop or claw hands. *There may be painless thickening* of ulnar nerve palpable behind the medial epicondyle or common peroneal nerve palpable over the fibular neck (due to sub-cutaneous position).

   In *lepromatous leprosy* – sensation is present.
7. *Cryopathic ulcer:* Due to chilblains and frostbite.
8. *Martorell's ulcer:* Hypertensive ulcer seen in calf region – *punched out ulcer.*

Note

Decubitus ulcer/pressure sore/bedsore is an example of trophic ulcers which are painless and punched out ulcers.

Specific ulcers

Due to specific infections.

1. *Tubercular ulcer* – undermined edge; a probe can be easily insinuated between the edge and the floor of the ulcer.
2. *Syphilitic ulcer* – punched out deep edge with wash leather slough in the floor and with deep indurated base.
3. *Soft chancres* – painless genital ulcer formed during the primary stage of syphilis – at this stage syphilis is highly contagious.
4. *Leprosy* – caused by *Mycobacterium leprae* – in addition to ulcer there will be *nerve thickening.*

5. *Actinomycotic ulcer*
6. *Meleney's ulcer* – postoperative, progressive bacterial gangrene, common in immuno-compromised individuals – *rapidly spreading ulcer involving a large area.*
7. *Bairnsdale or Buruli ulcer* caused by *Myco-bacterium ulcerans – a painless ulcer on the skin.*

Malignant ulcers

1. Rodent ulcer or basal cell carcinoma – raised and beaded edge
2. Epithelioma or carcinomatous ulcer – raised and everted edge
3. Malignant melanoma
4. Any malignant growth fungating through skin.
5. Marjolin ulcer – squamous cell carcinoma which arises on chronic benign ulcer or scar.

CLINICAL EXAMINATION OF AN ULCER

This should be conducted in a systematic manner – history, local examination, examination of regional nodes, general examination.

History

The following points to be enquired.
1. Age, sex, ethnic origin and occupation
2. Mode of onset
   How has the ulcer developed?
   • Following trauma – traumatic ulcer.
     OR
   • Spontaneously:
     · Over a nodule or lump, e.g. tuberculous lymphadenitis or abscess, gumma, or rapidly growing malignant growth;
     · Over unhealthy skin, e.g. a varicose ulcer, an irritable patch of dermatitis;
     · Over a corn or callus, e.g. perforating or trophic ulcer;
     · Over a scar, e.g. Marjolin's ulcer.
   • *Has the ulcer developed after sexual contact, e.g. chancre or chancroid?*
     · *Chancre* – painless genital ulcer commonly found during primary stage of syphilis.
     · *Chancroid* – a venereal infection causing painless ulceration of the lymph nodes in the groin.

3. Duration
   How long is the ulcer present there?
   • Short in acute ulcer; long in chronic ulcer.
   • Chronic burrowing ulcer caused by micro-aerophilic streptococci.
   • Incubation period in venereal ulcer: *3 to 4 weeks* in case of Hunterian chancre (syphilis) and *3 to 4 days* in case of chancroid (soft sore).

4. Painful or painless
   Is the ulcer painful?
   • Inflammatory ulcers are painful.
   • Tuberculous ulcers are mildly painful.
   • Malignant ulcers are absolutely painless unless they, in late stage, infiltrate the adjacent structures supplied by the nerve endings.
   • Syphilitic ulcers and trophic ulcers resulting from nerve diseases (tabes dorsalis, syringomyelia, transverse myelitis, peripheral neuritis) are painless.

5. Progress of the ulcer
   Is it changing in size or surface?
   • Healing or non-healing.

6. Nature of discharge
   • Serum, pus, or blood.

7. Past history
   • *Note the following predisposing causes:* diabetes, atherosclerosis, venous insufficiency, neuropathy – both sensory and/or motor supply, history of trauma, tuberculosis, syphilis and history of exposure.

Local examination

Inspection followed by palpation:
• Site
• Number, size and shape
• Different parts of the ulcer–
  · Margin
  · Edge
  · Floor
• Base
• Discharge
• Tenderness, friability or bleeding
• Movements of the ulcer – fixity of the ulcer to the underlying structures

Site

This is often typical, e.g. *rodent ulcer* on the upper part of the face; *tuberculous ulcer* on the neck; *trophic ulcer* over the weight-bearing area, e.g. over the heel, over the sacrum or other bony point in a bed-ridden patient; *ischaemic ulcer* over the dorsum of the foot and toes; *varicose ulcer* on the medial side of the lower half of the leg.

The three common types of lower limb ulcer – *venous, arterial* and *neuropathic* ulcers *have specific site predilection.*

Number, shape and size

- *Number:* Single or multiple, i.e. similar ulcers elsewhere in the body, e.g. pressure sores.
- *Shape:* The ulcer may be round, oval, irregular, or serpiginous.
- *Size:* Measure the size in cm in two directions.

Different parts of an ulcer

(Figs 1.1 and 1.2)

Margin

Margin of the ulcer is the border or 'transitional zone' of skin around the ulcer, i.e. *it is the line demarcating the ulcer from the intact skin.* Three types of margins are encountered:

1. *Healing ulcer margin:* Shows typical bluish line of growing epithelium which is squamous without cornification.
   Margin of a healing ulcer shows three zones:
   (i) Outer – white
   (ii) Intermediate – blue
   (iii) Inner – red
2. *Spreading ulcer:*
   (i) Irregular in malignant ulcer, e.g. basal cell carcinoma
   (ii) Red, inflamed and irregular margin with inflamed surrounding tissue in infective ulcer.

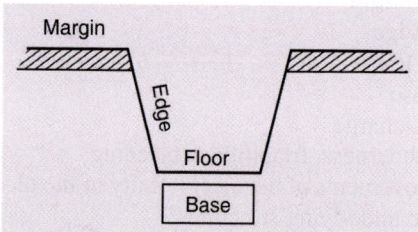

Fig. 1.1: Parts of an ulcer. Edge of the ulcer connects the floor of the ulcer to the margin.

3. *Chronic non-healing ulcer:* Shows marked fibrosis with thick white skin margin without the blue line of growing epithelium.

Edge

Edge of the ulcer is the mode of union between the floor and the margin of the ulcer, and it has thickness in three dimensions. It can be inspected as well as palpated.

Edge is often characteristic of the underlying pathology:

1. *Slopping edge:* A healing non-specific ulcer, venous ulcer.
2. *Punched out edge:* Trophic ulcer. The tissue destruction is equal in all planes from skin to bone, so the ulcer becomes deep *with a vertical edge as if the tissues have been punched out.*
3. *Undermined edge:* In a *tubercular ulcer,* the tissue destruction is more in the subcutaneous plane than in the skin, so that the skin overhangs at the edge – flask-shaped ulcer. *This can be well demonstrated by passing a probe under the margin. This is termed as undermined edge.*

   Undermined edge is also noted in ulcer due to *pressure necrosis* particularly over the buttocks and in carbuncles.

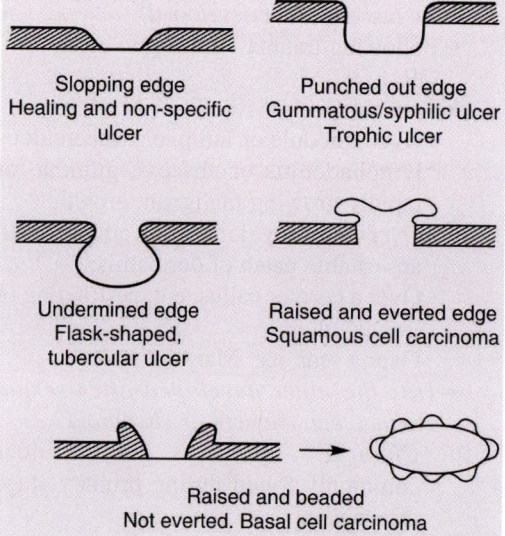

Fig. 1.2: Various types of edges of the ulcer.

Undermined burrowing ulcer may be associated with the formation of burrowing cutaneous fissures and sinus tracks that open at the distant sites (*Maloney's burrowing ulcer*) and is caused by microaerophilic non-haemolytic streptococci and aerobic haemolytic streptococci.

4. *Raised edge: Rodent ulcer.* The ulcer edge is raised and rolled but not everted. This is a slow growing malignancy. There may be nodules on the raised edge of the ulcer – *beaded appearance.*

5. *Raised and everted edge: Epithelioma.* In a malignant ulcer, the malignant tissue grows very fast and overhangs the skin margin. The ulcer itself is raised above the skin margin. The ulcer edge is raised and also overhangs the margin of the ulcer towards the surrounding skin – *raised and everted margin.*

Floor

This is exposed surface of the ulcer, i.e. *the part which can be seen within the edge of the ulcer.* This may show:

• *Pink or red and granular granulation tissue.* No slough is present. There may be small amount of serous discharge, e.g. healing ulcer.

• *Pale, flat and smooth granulation tissue* which does not bleed easily on touch, e.g. chronic or slowly non-healing ulcer.

• *Areas of unhealthy granulation tissue and areas of slough*, e.g. spreading or infective ulcer. *Slough is the necrotic soft tissue which has not yet separated from the living tissue*, e.g. infected bedsores.

• *Hypertrophic granulation tissue* where epithelialisation is not completed in time and thus shows hypertrophic granulation tissue. The exuberant granulation tissue rises above the skin surface. This is termed as *sprouting flesh* and is accompanied by excessive sero-sanguineous discharge. *Sprouting granulation tissue also delays wound healing*, e.g. a larger sized ulcer of some duration.

• *Watery or apple jelly granulation tissue*, e.g. tuberculous ulcer.

• *Wash leather slough*, e.g. a gummatous ulcer.
• Malignant tissue.
• *Relationship of the floor to the surface.*
   (i) Floor below the surface level – non-malignant ulcer.
   (ii) Floor above the surface level, i.e. raised from the surface – malignant ulcer.
• *Look for fixity of the ulcer to the underlying structures* – check the movements of the ulcer over the base.

Discharge

This may be small or profuse. The type of discharge may be typical, e.g.

• *Purulent discharge* – indicates active infection.
• *Bloody opalescent discharge* – typical of *Streptococcus* infection.
• *Yellowish and creamy discharge* – *Staphylococcus* infection.
• *Greenish discharge* suggests infection with *Pseudomonas pyocyanea. Pseudomonas* infection is commonly hospital acquired.
• *Watery discharge* – typical of tuberculosis.
• *Sulphur granules* – typical of actinomycotic ulcer.
• *Bloody discharge* – from healthy granulation tissue in a healing ulcer or a malignant ulcer.
• *Serous discharge* – from healing or malignant ulcer.

Base

This signifies the area on which the ulcer rests. *The base is to be palpated through the floor of the ulcer* for:

• Mild induration due to fibrosis may be felt in any chronic ulcer.
• Marked induration is almost diagnostic of malignant ulcer.
   Hunterian chancre also shows marked induration at the base.
• Mobility of the ulcer over the underlying structures – *reduced mobility implies* fixity to the underlying structures, muscle or bone. Malignant ulcer has reduced mobility. Varicose ulcer is also usually attached to the tibia.
   If the ulcer is small, try to pinch it up and palpate the base between two fingers.

Tenderness

Arterial ulcers, tuberculous ulcer, soft chancres – usually painful and tender.

Friability

Too much friability is often diagnostic of malignancy.

Bleeding on touch

Suggestive of malignancy. May also be noted in presence of healthy granulation tissue.

Examination of the surrounding area

This may show important features.

(i) If the ulcer is infected and spreading due to cellulitis, surrounding skin appears shiny, red and oedematous with tenderness.
(ii) Dark pigmentation and eczema in a varicose ulcer.
(iii) Multiple scars and puckering of the skin, sinuses surrounding the ulcer: Suggestive of tubercular ulcer.
(iv) Matted nodes surrounding the tubercular ulcer.
(v) Melanotic halo in malignant melanoma.
(vi) Satellite nodules within 5 cm proximal to malignant melanoma.
(vii) A chronic ulcer within a large scar suggests Marjolin's ulcer.

Examination of the regional lymph nodes

The absence or presence and the consistence of the nodes may often indicate the type of the ulcer, e.g.

- Nodes are soft and tender in case of infective ulcer.
- Nodes are firm and matted and non-tender in Koch's ulcer.
- Nodes are enlarged, hard and even fixed in case of carcinomatous ulcer.
- *Nodes are not enlarged* in case of rodent ulcer unless secondarily infected.
- *Inguinal nodes draining a syphilitic chancre of the penis are firm and 'shotty'.*

When the regional nodes are palpable, then palpate the next higher groups of lymph nodes in a malignant ulcer.

General examination

1. *Examination for debility and malnutrition* – anaemia, diabetes, cardiac failure, etc., which delays ulcer healing. *Ulcer refuses to granulate or heal if Hb% is less than 10 gm% and serum albumin is less than 3 gm%.*
2. *Examination for impairment of circulation:*
   - *Look for arterial pulsation: Arterial ulcer. Absence of arterial pulsation* – arteriosclerosis, Burger's disease, Raynaud's disease, diabetes – since *poor blood supply* may result in ischaemic ulcers and delayed healing.
   - *Look for varicose veins: Venous ulcer. Varicosity of veins* in presence of varicose ulcer. Also test for deep vein thrombosis and *calf muscle tenderness.*
3. *Neuropathic ulcer. Examination for neurological deficits – both sensory and motor supply*, e.g. diabetes, tabes dorsalis, spina bifida, peripheral neuritis, leprosy may give rise to ulceration *because of anaesthesia of the part* – neuropathic ulcer.
   Look for nerve thickening – Hansen's disease.
4. *Examine the joint movements active and passive*, close to the ulcer. Restriction of joint movements and presence of deformity indicate a painful inflammation and tendon/muscle involvement. *Varicose ulcer may cause equinus deformity of foot.*
5. *Examine abdomen* for splenomegaly in haemolytic anaemia – leg ulcers.

Pathological examination

1. *Examination of blood*
   - Hb% – anaemia; RBC – sickle cell anaemia; WBC – infection.
   - ESR: Tuberculosis, malignancy, chronic infection.
   - Sugar: *Diabetes.*
   - W.R., Kahn and VDRL tests: *Syphilis.*
2. *Examination of the discharge from the ulcer: Bacteriological examination of the discharge* – smear test and culture and sensitivity test – are often required to determine the nature of bacterial infection.

AFB study for tuberculosis.

Spirochetes are found in the discharge or scraping of a primary chancre.

3. *Biopsy for cell cytology*
   - *Wedge biopsy:* Removing a wedge from the margin of the ulcer. The central part of the ulcer is not chosen as it contains mainly necrotic material.
   - *Excision biopsy:* The whole of the ulcer including the base may be excised and examined.
4. *X-ray*
   - Of the underlying bone for periostitis and/ or osteomyelitis.
   - Chest, in tubercular or malignant ulcer spread.
5. *FNAC of lymph node* – if malignancy is suspected.

LIFE HISTORY OF AN ULCER

This consists of three stages:

1. *Stage of extension*, i.e. spreading or sloughing.
2. *Stage of transition*, i.e. preparation for healing.
3. *Stage of repair.*

Different characters of ulcers are evident in different stages.

Stage of extension

- *Floor:* Covered with exudates and sloughs. No granulation tissue.
- *Discharge:* Often purulent and even blood-stained.
- *Edge:* Sharply defined, thickened and inflamed.
- *Surrounding area:* Inflamed and oedematous.
- *Base:* Indurated and fixed.
- *Slough and small amounts of discharge* may dry to become a *scab*. A layer of dead tissue may become dehydrated and *form a dark brown or black eschar such as after a burn or ischaemic necrosis.*

Stage of transition

- *Floor:* Becomes cleaner with sloughs separating. Small, reddish areas of granulation tissue appear which link up ultimately to cover the whole surface.
- *Discharge:* Becomes serous.
- *Base:* Induration diminishing.

Stage of repair

Follows the transition stage and may either show signs of healing or characters of a callous ulcer.

(a) Signs of healing

- *Floor:* Contains smooth and even red granulation tissue covered by a single layer of epithelium. The granulation tissue is transformed into fibrous tissue which gradually contracts to form a scar.
- *Edge:* Becomes more shelving with the bluish epithelium gradually extending from the margin onto the floor of the ulcer to cover it up (at a rate of 1 mm per day).
- *Discharge:* It is merely serous, if the surface is kept at rest.
- *Surrounding skin:* It is soft, flexible and free from congestion.
- *Base:* It is free from fixity.

(b) Change to indolent or callous ulcer (chronic non-healing ulcer)

This means that the ulcer refuses to heal by itself.

- *Floor:* Covered with unhealthy pale granulation tissue with or without serous discharge.
- *Edge:* Thickened, oedematous, indurated and often discoloured. The edge may be fixed to the base or inverted which delays healing. *It requires to be freed to allow healing.*

  It does not show any tendency to heal because of callous attitude of the patient.
- *Surrounding area:* Oedematous and indurated.
- *Base:* Indurated and hard.

Note

In a malignant ulcer, the base is formed of malignant tissue. There is no formation of granulation tissue and skin ingrowth.

Clinical classification of an ulcer

1. **Spreading ulcer:** Edge of the ulcer is inflamed and oedematous. Floor is covered

with unhealthy slough without granulation tissue; purulent or offensive discharge with surrounding cellulitis around the ulcer margin. No sign of epithelialisation. Its size gradually increases due to loss of more and more epithelium.

2. **Healing ulcer:** Edge is sloping with healthy red/pink granulation tissue with thin layer of serous discharge on the floor. *On rubbing – blood oozes out.*

3. **Callous ulcer:** Floor contains pale unhealthy granulation tissue with or without serous discharge. The edge and base are also indurated and hard. The edge may be fixed to the base or inverted which delays healing. *Callous means hard and indurated.* Ulcer does not show any tendency to heal because of the callous attitude of the patient who refuses care and treatment. It continues for many months to years. *The edge fixation requires to be freed to allow healing.*

Causes of delayed healing of ulcer

1. Old age.
2. *Malnutrition:* Hypoproteinaemia, avitaminosis, anaemia.
3. Secondary infection.
4. *Diabetes mellitus* – leading to both atherosclerosis and neuropathy.
5. Neurological defects, e.g. sensory loss (leprosy) and/or motor loss.
6. Poor blood supply or arterial insufficiency, atherosclerosis.
7. Ulcer situated over bony prominences mainly due to prolonged pressure – pressure sores.
8. Excessive movements of ulcer-bearing area.
9. Callous ulcer (callous means hard or indurated).
10. Malignancy.
11. *Marjolin's ulcer:* SCC developing over a long-standing ulcer.

Note

Chronic burrowing ulcer is caused by microaerophilic streptococci.

Typical features of some common ulcers

Epithelioma (Syn. Carcinomatous ulcer; Squamous cell carcinoma of skin)

1. May occur anywhere but commonly found in lips, cheeks, tongue, breast, penis and anus.
2. Usually painless.
3. *Irregular shape with rolled out and everted edges are typical.*
4. *Regional lymph nodes enlarged and hard.*

Rodent ulcer (Syn. Basal cell carcinoma of skin)

1. Commonly found in the upper face above a line joining the angle of the mouth with the lobule of the ear.
2. Usually painless.
3. Usually circular in shape *with raised and beaded edges are typical.*
4. *Minute venules in the edge of the ulcer are characteristic.*
5. *Regional nodes are not enlarged.*
6. Spread by direct spread.

Tuberculous ulcer (Figs 1.3 A and B)

1. Usually results from bursting of caseous lymph nodes, so commonly seen on the neck.
2. Usually painful.
3. *The edge of the ulcer is thin and undermined* and frequently bluish in colour.
4. There is *pale granulation tissue at the floor with watery discharge.* The base is mildly indurated.
5. *Presence of matted lymph nodes* adjacent to the ulcer.

Syphilitic ulcer (Syn. Gummatous ulcer)

1. *Usually seen over the subcutaneous bone (e.g. tibia, ulna, sternum and skull).*
2. *Painless ulcer.*
3. *Most characteristic features are the punched out edge of the ulcer* and the presence of wet wash leather (yellowish grey) slough in the floor.
4. Lymph nodes are seldom involved unless secondarily infected.

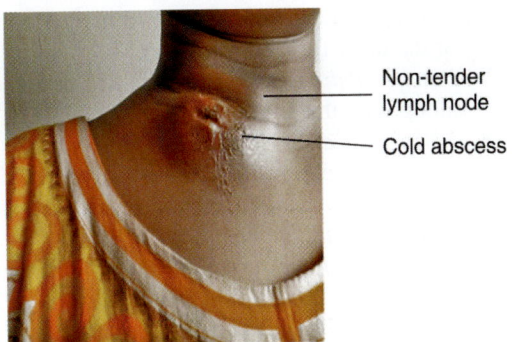

Fig. 1.3A: Tubercular lymphadenitis with two swellings—**solid** and **soft** cystic (cold abscess).

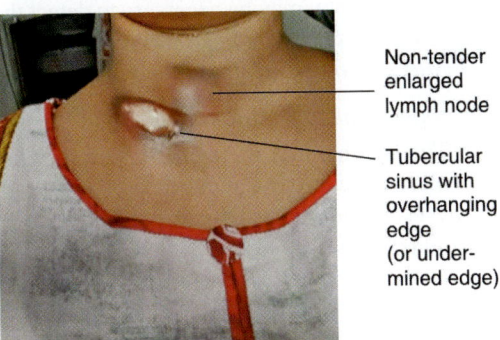

Fig. 1.3B: Tubercular sinus in the neck—right side. Same patient as in Fig. 1.3A reviewed after 3 weeks, when cold abscess turned into non-tender sinus.

Hunterian chancre (primary syphilitic sore)

1. *Usually seen over the penis, lips and tongue.*
2. *Usually appears 3 weeks after the infection from sexual exposure.*
3. *The ulcer is painless.*
4. It is usually oval in shape with a slopping edge and exudes a blood-stained discharge. The base of the ulcer is characteristically indurated that feels like a button.
5. *T. pallidum* can be demonstrated in the serous discharge.
6. The lymph nodes in the groin are enlarged, and '*shotty*', i.e. hard and small and *painless* with no tendency to soften or suppurate.
7. Extragenital chancres (lips and tongue) are frequently not indurated, and the involved lymph nodes are often considerably enlarged.

Soft chancres (Ducrey ulcer)

1. *Usually seen on the genitalia.*
2. *Usually appear within 3 days after infection following sexual exposure due to Gram –ve coccobacillus.*
3. *Painful ulcers.*
4. Present as *multiple acute painful ulcers* with oedematous edge and yellowish slough, discharging copious purulent secretion, often bleeding.
5. *Involved lymph nodes show the picture of acute lymphadenitis* with tendency towards suppuration.

Varicose ulcer

1. *Typically situated on the medial side of the lower half of the leg.*
2. It is *painless* callous ulcer.
3. The ulcer is *vertically oval in shape* with slopping or stepping edge. *It never penetrates the deep fascia.*
4. *Presence of pigmentation or eczema in the skin around the ulcer.*
5. *Presence of varicose veins in the upper part of the leg or thigh clinches the diagnosis.*
6. Ask the patient to stand and examine both long and short saphenous veins for varicosity. Also note for scattered and irregular varicosities, blowouts.
7. Varicose ulcer may cause *equinus deformity of the foot.*

Marjolin's ulcer

- It is an aggressive ulcerating squamous cell carcinoma developing on an area of previously traumatised, chronically inflamed or scarred skin, e.g. following burn or chronic venous ulcer.
- *Involvement of lymph nodes is not a feature of Marjolin's ulcer* because it develops within the scar tissue which does not have lymphatics.

Post-thrombotic ulcer

1. It *follows deep vein thrombosis* following parturition or operation.
2. *A painful ulcer*, situated on the lower leg. *The ulcer always penetrates the deep fascia.*

3. *Do the test for deep vein thrombosis: Calf muscle tenderness*, Homan's sign and Moses' sign.
   - *Homan's sign:* With the leg extended, forcible dorsiflexion of the foot causes pain in the calf muscle.
   - *Moses' sign:* With the knee flexed, squeezing the calf muscles from side to side causes pain in the calf muscles.
4. CT/MRI may be helpful to detect deep vein thrombosis.

Trophic ulcer

A trophic ulcer is due to an impairment of nutrition to the tissues – either an impairment in blood supply, i.e. *ischaemia* or an absence of properly functioning nerve supply, i.e. *anaesthesia*. So there are two types:
1. Arterial ulcer – *ischaemic*
2. Neurogenic ulcer – *neurotrophic*

Arterial ulcer (ischaemic ulcer)

1. *The ulcer is caused by inadequate blood supply to the tissues or skin*, mostly due to peripheral arterial disease resulting in poor peripheral circulation leading to ischaemic necrosis. So, mostly found in presence of atherosclerosis (commonest), Burger's disease, Raynaud's disease, diabetes.
2. Commonly seen in old people.
3. Commonly occur in those parts of the limbs which are subjected to repeated pressure and trauma. Repeated trauma and superadded infection cause destruction of the poorly vascularised skin which fails to heal because of poor arterial blood supply.
4. *Usually occur on the anterior and lateral aspects of the leg, on the toes, dorsum and sole of the foot, or the heel* (these are the parts exposed to repeated pressure or trauma). *May also occur on the finger tips and dorsum of the hand.*
5. *Painful ulcer. Moreover, a history of intermittent claudication with or without discoloration of the toes is mostly present and characteristic.*
6. Ulcers may have *punched out edges* with slough in the floor. *Very often the deep fascia*

is involved exposing the tendons in the floor of the ulcer (cf. venous ulcer).
7. *Patches of dry gangrene* may also be present along with the arterial ulcer.
8. *Peripheral arterial pulses – diminished or absent. Palpate all the related arteries of both sides to rule out arterial insufficiency.*
9. *The ischaemic limb feels cold.*
10. *Elevation of the affected limb above the heart's level causes a marked pallor of the limb within 2–3 minutes and the patient will complain of pain in this position. Lowering of the limb below the horizontal leads to cyanotic congestion.*
11. Angiography may be necessary to detect the arterial disease. *Duplex color ultrasound or MRI angio are helpful and non-invasive.*

Neurogenic ulcer (neurotrophic)

1. The mechanism of formation of such an ulcer is repeated trauma or pressure *in an area which has absent sensation, i.e. anaesthesia due to impaired nerve supply.*
2. Such ulcers are found in presence of diabetic neuritis, peripheral nerve injury, spina bifida, leprosy, tabes dorsalis, syringomyelia.
   Bedsores and perforating ulcers are also examples.
3. These ulcers are *commonly seen on the buttock and on the back of the heel when the patient is non-ambulatory; on the heel and ball of the foot when the patient is ambulatory.*
4. Ulcers may have punched out edges with slough in the floor. Very often the deep fascia is involved exposing the tendons and bones in the floor of the ulcer.
5. *Painless ulcer because of anaesthesia.*
6. The ulcer starts as a callosity under which suppuration takes place. The pus comes out from a small central hole and thus an ulcer is formed which gradually burrows silently through the deep fascia, muscles and the tendons to bones and joints. *That is why this ulcer is also called perforating ulcer.* The resultant cavity becomes filled with offensive matter. Finally, the track becomes lined with unhealthy granulation tissue or skin thus healing becomes impossible.

7. Peripheral arterial pulsations are well palpable.
8. Neurological examination will reveal diminished or absent sensation. *Test the sensation of the skin surrounding the ulcer using a sharp pin.*

Note

Commonest type of trophic ulcer – pressure/bedsore.

Diabetic ulcer

Three aetiological components are responsible for a diabetic ulcer:

1. *Impairment of peripheral circulation* leading to local ischaemia:
   - Atherosclerosis – as diabetic patients are more prone to it at an earlier age;
   - Microvascular disease.
2. *Impairment of sensation* due to peripheral neuropathy leading to trophic changes.
3. *Poor resistance of the tissues* to trauma and infection owing to the presence of sugar in the tissues.

Characteristics of ulcer are same as that of trophic ulcer.

Leprosy ulcer (Hansen's disease)

- Caused by infection with *Mycobacterium leprae*.
- Note the following.
  1. *Hypopigmented anaesthetic patches* over the limbs, back, face – due to peripheral neuropathy.
  2. Features of leonine face.
  3. *Palpate for nerve thickening:*
     - Common peroneal nerve over the lateral surface of fibular neck.
     - Tibial nerve – posteromedial to medial malleolus.
     - Ulnar nerve – posterior to medial epicondyle.
     - Greater auricular nerve – over the mastoid process behind the ear lobule.

Examine the deformity and the joint movements active and passive, close to the ulcer. Restriction of joint movements and presence of deformity indicates a painless inflammation and tendon/muscle involvement.

Note

Leprosy can be cured with 6–12 months of multidrug therapy. *Early treatment avoids disability.*

Ulcer due to chilblains

- Due to exposure to intense cold causing first blisters which then rupture to form superficial ulcer in the foot.
- This is also called perniosis.
- Due to excessive cutaneous arteriolar constriction.

Ulcer due to frostbite

- Due to exposure of a part to a wet cold below the freezing point – cold wind.
- There is arteriolar spasm, denaturation of proteins and cell destruction.
- This leads to local gangrene of the part leading to deep ulcers.

Both these conditions *are painful and common in soldiers stationed at high altitudes* (areas located in or near glaciers).

Meleney's ulcer (postoperative synergistic gangrene) (Fig. 1.4)

- It is commonly seen in postoperative wounds on the abdomen after surgery for septic peritonitis and on the chest wall following empyema drainage.
- It is due to symbiotic or synergistic haemolytic streptococci and *Staphylococcus aureus* and anaerobes leading to severe infection and often with end arteritis of the skin leading to spreading ulcer and destruction.
- It is an acute rapidly spreading ulcer with destruction of skin and subcutaneous tissue and burrowing deeper with a resultant undermined edge. The ulcer is painful and tender with a tendency to spread. There will be a central purplish zone surrounded by red inflammation initially. The purplish zone becomes gangrenous producing ulcer.
- Management:
  - Urgent blood sugar examination – if diabetes, it has to be controlled.

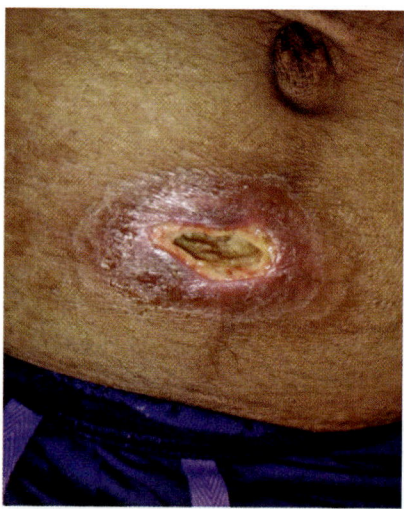

Fig. 1.4: An infected ulcer in a patient with necro-tising fascitis—Meleney's ulcer.

· Antibiotics and metrogyl infusion.
· Adequate excision of dead or necrotic tissues until it bleeds.
· Blood transfusion.
· Once healthy tissue is formed – skin grafting is considered.

Tropical ulcer
• Commonly observed in Africa, India, South America and Australia.
• It is an acute ulcerative lesion of the skin, commonly of the leg, due to infection with Vincent's organism (*Bacteroides fusiformis*) and *Borrelia vincenti*, secondary to trauma or insect bites.
• Commonly occurs in people with lower socio-economic status suffering from anaemia, vitamin deficiency and malnutrition.
• Initially abrasion, redness, papule and pustule formed with severe pain.
• This is accompanied by acute, tender lymph-adenitis.
• Eventually, pustule bursts with serosanguinous discharge with vile odour and unremitting local pain. But constitutional symptoms are minimal.
• Because of extreme tenacity of slough, the healing is delayed and ultimately a circular parchment-like, faintly pigmented scar develops.

Note

Ulcers due to extreme cold (chilblains and frostbite)
• Develop due to extreme cold – dry or wet, below the freezing point causes arteriolar spasms leading to superficial painful ulcers of the skin specially hands and feet and eventually gangrene of these areas. *These ulcers or gangrene are very painful and tender.*
• Common in soldiers stationed at high altitude – particularly in or near the glaciers.

Note

Painful ulcers
1. Arterial ulcer
2. Post-thrombotic ulcer
3. Chilblains and frostbite

Painless ulcers
1. Neuropathic ulcer
2. Venous ulcer
3. Leprosy ulcer

PRESSURE SORES (Bedsores, decubitus ulcer) (Figs 1.5 to 1.7)

• Pressure sores are *trophic ulcers* with bone at the base. These ulcers form when the soft tissues are compressed for *a prolonged period* between a bony prominence with overlying thin subcutaneous tissue and a supporting structure such as bed or wheelchair due to immobility.

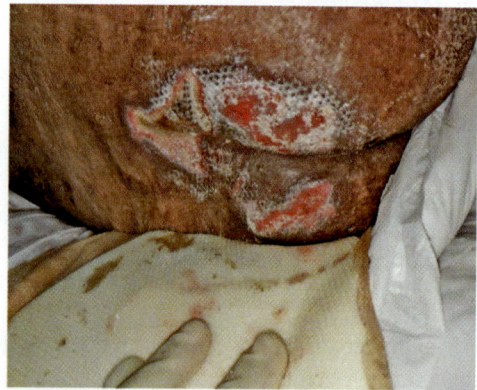

Fig. 1.5: Pressure sores over sacrum and adjacent buttocks: Skin breakdown *limited to dermis—* stage II.

- *Sites of bedsore* are occiput, heel, sacrum, ischial tuberosity and scapula.
- *Formed due to loss of sensation and diminished blood supply* following chronic persistent pressure with or without shear particularly in a debilitated patient due to poor and neglected nursing care.
- *It is a type of traumatic gangrene due to persistent pressure leading to ischaemia of the skin and subcutaneous tissue as a result of prolonged and persistent pressure against bony prominences* – in debilitated, neglected, bed-ridden or comatose patients *who are unable to move on their own.*

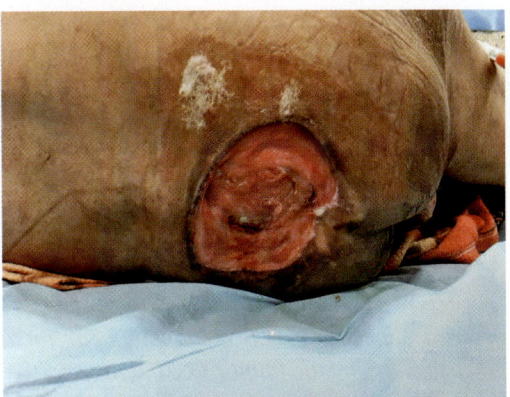

Fig. 1.6B: Same patient as in Fig. 1.6A. Bedsore over the sacrum after excision of the black eschar.

Causes of pressure sores

Following predisposing factors are responsible (mnemonics PAIM).

P	*Pressure*
A	*Anaemia*
	Anaesthesia
I	*Injury*
	Immobility
	Insufficiency of local blood supply
	Insensitivity of the wound
	Infection
M	*Moisture*

Common sites

Typically develops over the areas *subjected to constant pressure due to immobility* like sacral area, ischial tuberosity, heel, occiput, scapula,

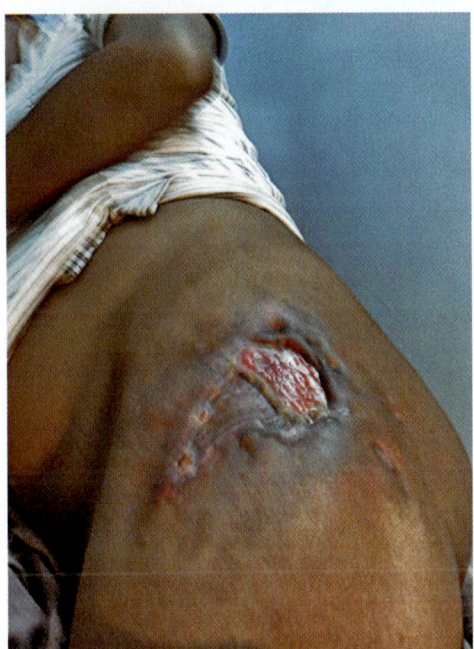

Fig. 1.7: Pressure sore stage III over the greater trochanter—left side.

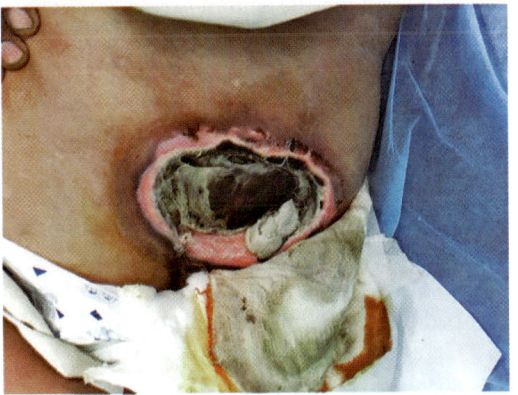

Fig. 1.6A: Bedsore with black eschar over the sacrum—stage III.

elbow *in a prolonged bed-ridden patient* where the underlying bone is covered by skin and thin subcutaneous tissue only.

Predisposing factors

1. Abrasive local injury.
2. *Prolonged and persistent pressure due to immobility:* Due to poor nursing care, patient

remains immobilised in the same position for a prolonged period leading to poor blood supply to the tissues while under pressure and results in compromised oxygenation, ischaemia, and eventual tissue necrosis leading to sores.

3. Soakage of bed sheets with loose stool, urinary leak, hot moisture causing persistent wetting of the skin.
4. Persistent folding or crease or wrinkles of bed sheets are *also responsible for local pressure in an immobile and insensitive patient causing poor blood supply to the local tissues under pressure.*
5. Other factors which accentuate the process are anaemia, malnutrition, atherosclerosis and neuropathy – *atherosclerosis* leads to poor blood supply; *neuropathy* leads to insensitivity and motor weakness leading to lack of protective reflexes.

Clinical stages of the disease

The disease may be divided into four stages with following findings:

- **Stage I:** Early non-blanchable erythema *which does not change colour on pressure (a warning sign)*, induration *without a breach in the epidermis.*
- **Stage II:** Blistering, *skin breakdown limited to dermis.* Initially a callosity may develop with or without tenderness due to constant pressure.
- **Stage III:** *Full thickness skin loss leading to ulcer/crater formation into subcutaneous tissues with overlying slough or eschar – typical bedsore.* The slough is dead tissue and appears as greyish or greyish-black in colour.
- **Stage IV:** Necrosis extending beyond the fascia, into ligaments and bones leading to osteomyelitis.

Note

Predisposing factors responsible for bedsores/pressure sores

P *Pressure:* Prolonged and persistent pressure in a bed-ridden and paraplegic patient

A *Anaemia:* Leading to poor blood supply and poor nutrition to local tissues

Anaesthesia: Leading to insensitivity of the wound due to sensory neuropathy

I *Injury:* Due to sustained or prolonged pressure
Immobility: Continuing prolonged pressure
Insufficiency of local blood supply
Insensitivity of the wound: Poor sensation of the wound
Infection

M *Moisture:* Leading to wet wound and maceration.

Avoidance and treatment of pressure sores

1. Skilled nursing care both by the nursing attendants and relatives from the beginning.
2. *Change of posture by turning the patient every 2 hours* to avoid constant pressure on one site particularly over bony points – **most important.**
3. Soft, dry and clean bed sheets to be laid in a manner that *there will be no wrinkle or folding of sheets underneath skin of the patient to avoid local erythema and induration of the skin* which is the starting point of the sore. *Avoid moisture.*
4. Specialised bed like air or water cushioned bed may be used which periodically redistributes the pressure points.
5. The skin should be kept clean and dry.
6. Finger tips pressure massage over the indurated area surrounding the ulcer is helpful.
7. Use of adhesive films over the pressure sore or wound may be helpful *to prevent soakage and maceration.*
8. Assist and encourage the patient to remain in sitting positions on the edge of the bed as many hours as possible during waking hours.
9. *Encourage for both active and passive movements and exercise of the limbs*, both in sitting and lying down positions to improve circulation and to control oedema.
10. Use of excess soft cotton or foam rubber padding over the pressure points.
11. Care of the perineum and genitalia to avoid soakage from stool, urine and sweat.
12. When the patient is able to move out of the bed even with the help of nursing staff – hot

sitz water bath with Betadine solution is helpful.

13. *Dressing of the wound*
    (a) Hot sitz bath with Betadine solution when the patient is mobile; otherwise hot fomentation of the wound before each dressing.
    (b) Cleaning of the wound with EUSOL (Edinburgh University Solution) and/or H_2O_2 to remove the slough followed by dressing of the wound with metrogyl ointment (acts on anaerobic organisms also) and sofratulle.
    (c) *If slough is excessive, desloughing and debridement are carried out.* Manual removal of slough by scissors dissection may be tried *as the slough is insensitive.*
    (d) Once slough is removed, dressing with EUSOL followed by local application of H_2O_2 (on surface application provides nascent oxygen) is tried to enhance granulation tissue formation.
    (e) Local application of metrogyl ointment is also helpful against anaerobic organism.
14. *Antibiotics:* Oral/parenteral after culture sensitivity test of pus or wound discharge should be given. Oral metrogyl tab also to be supplemented against anaerobic organism.
15. *If patient is diabetic,* insulin therapy for control of diabetes following blood sugar monitoring. Use short-acting or inter-mediate-acting insulin with modified regimen. Stop metformin and long-acting sulphonylureas and replace with insulin injections.
16. *Continuous bladder drainage may be required* to avoid spillage of urine over the bed and hence soakage of the wound. C&S of the urine may be required for antibiotic choice.
17. *Enema at regular intervals* to clean the bowel to avoid spillage of stool under the buttock.
18. *Local infrared therapy* improves local blood supply and enhances wound healing.
19. Optimise nutrition to maintain serum albumin above 2.0 g/dl.
20. *Correction of anaemia, strict control of diabetes.* Oral vasodilators to improve local blood supply may be required.
21. *Suitable reconstruction procedures after excision of the ulcer by musculocutaneous flap closure with local advancement flap* when the wound is clean and dry with healthy granulation tissue can be tried.

Note

Flap closure for pressure sores

When patient is reasonably fit, debridement of wound (removal of necrotic and scarred tissue, bursa and osteotomy) followed by flap cover are preferred.

Surgical reconstruction of pressure sores

Done preferably *by myocutaneous flaps.*

Sacral sore
- 1st choice: Gluteus maximus myocutaneous flap
- 2nd choice: Lumbosacral flap
- 3rd choice: Bilateral gluteus maximus flap

Trochanteric sore
- 1st choice: Tensor fascia lata flap
- 2nd choice: Tensor fascia lata and vastus lateralis flap
- 3rd choice: Random thigh flap

Ischial sore
- 1st choice: Gluteus maximus myocutaneous flap
- 2nd choice: Posterior thigh myocutaneous hamstring (V-Y) advancement flap

Combined ischial and trochanteric sore
- Tensor fascia lata and vastus lateralis flap

Note

Following dressing materials enhance wound healing:

1. **EUSOL** (Edinburgh University Solution): An aqueous solution of lime – a cleaning agent. Composition 12.5 gm of *bleaching powder* [$Ca(ClO)_2$] and 12.5 gm of *boric acid* in distilled water to make 1 litre of

solution. It helps to destroy the dead tissue or slough and thus inhibits bacterial and fungal growth.

2. **H$_2$O$_2$:** Another cleaning agent. In addition to destroy the slough, it also kills anaerobic organisms. It prevents capillary oozing and helps in haemostasis. It also provides nascent oxygen on exposure to the dirty or unhealthy wound to help in separation of the slough and enhance earlier coverage of the wound with healthy granulation tissue and thus early healing.

3. **Normal saline:** Cleaning agent.

4. **Metrogyl:** Local tissue application of ointment helps to destroy local anaerobic organisms.

Note

Agents used to promote growth of granulation tissue and epithelialisation

- **PDGF:** *Platelet derived growth factor. Delivered to wounds by platelets* derived from the injured capillary vessels and also produced by local fibroblasts.
- **EGF:** *Epithelial growth factor.* Stimulates proliferation of different types of cells especially fibroblasts and epithelial cells. EGF is found in skin fibroblasts.

Note

VAC therapy: Vacuum-assisted closure (negative pressure wound therapy) is being used in some centres for treatment of chronic or delayed wound healing, such as pressure sores, with good results.

DIABETIC FOOT ULCER

Diabetic patients are more prone to develop ulcers of the foot due to following reasons: *ischaemia*, *neuropathy* and *infection*.

1. **Ischaemia**
   (a) *Microangiopathy* – producing small vessels disease in the form of non-specific thickening of the basement membrane leading to slowing of circulation and tissue hypoxia.
   (b) *Macroangiopathy* – involving major vessels resulting in atherosclerosis. Both

these conditions (micro- and macro-angiopathy) result in ischaemia of the toes and foot.
- Increased glycosylated haemoglobin decreases oxygen dissociation in the local tissue.
- Increased glycosylated tissue protein also decreases the utilization of oxygen.

2. **Neuropathy:** *Dampens pain of inflammation.* Neuropathy can be distal and diffuse with a stocking-and-glove type of distribution. Loss of vibration sense and deep tendon reflexes occur early. This is followed by loss of touch, pain and temperature sensations. As a result of this, *trophic ulcers* develop which can progress and penetrate deeper layers because of insensitivity.

   Autonomic neuropathy reduces sweating causing increased dryness of the skin and thereby predisposes to infection.

3. **Resistance to infection:** Because of altered immune system, uncontrolled diabetic patients are more susceptible to infection because of diminished phagocytic activity of the leukocytes. Granulocyte mobilisation is also impaired in ketoacidosis leading to reduced chemotaxis. *Thus, the patients are susceptible to polymicrobial and fungal infections.* Infection can spread proximally to the subfascial planes.

Thus, micro- and macroangiopathy and/or neuropathy in combination with secondary infection favours the development of diabetic foot ulcers.

Ulcers may develop following a minor trauma such as thorn prick over the sole of the foot or callosity, trimming of the nail or due to shoe bite.

Presentation of diabetic foot ulcer

- *Trophic ulcers* in a diabetic patient without overt infection.
- Trophic ulcers, infection and deformities.
- Diabetic ulcers are usually found on the plantar surface of the foot over the heads or neck of the first and second metatarsals.
- Oedema is usually mild with no change in surrounding pigmentation.

Management of diabetic foot ulcer

1. Nursing care more or less the same as described under bedsore treatment.
2. Avoidance of pressure over the ulcer: Change of posture every 2 hours.
3. Early mobility with the help of attendant's support, with walker or stick.
4. *Control of oedema* by active and passive exercises of the foot and leg while on bed and active movements while mobile.
5. Lying on the bed with foot end of the bed raised by 6 inches helps to reduce oedema till the wound heals.
6. Oral diuretics also help to reduce oedema.
7. *Insulin therapy for control of diabetes.* Ensure good glycaemic control – FBS & PPBS, Hb1Ac.
8. *Antibiotics as per antibiogram* after C&S of wound discharge. In addition, metrogyl may be helpful – both orally and locally.
9. Antifungal drugs and/or ointments, if required.
10. Oral vasodilators and neurotrophic drugs may be helpful.
11. *Regular wound dressing with EUSOL and/ or H_2O_2 after warm sitz bath* followed by local betadine or metrogyl ointment application.
12. *Necrotic tissue should be judiciously debrided* and topical antimicrobials needed to control local infection. *May require repeated debridement.*
13. Removal of callus skin under aseptic control.
14. Often, resection of the underlying slough and bony prominences may improve wound healing.
15. *Improvement of circulation* – after angiogram to assess feasibility of vascular reconstruction, if required.
16. 'Custom made' microcellular rubber (MCR) shoes with moulded insoles for trophic foot ulcer without overt infection and foot deformities.
17. Often, in neglected case or delayed healing, patient may require below knee amputation – if X-ray shows periostitis or osteomyelitis of the underlying bone. MRI may be helpful to detect the level of bone involvement and the proximal neurovascular status. *Patient will be able to move around with crutches to earn his livelihood.* If patient can afford, after amputation patient can use custom-made below knee prosthesis after below knee amputation.

Note

Recent advancement for wound therapy:

- Electrical stimulation (pulsed electromagnetic field therapy)
- Ultrasound therapy (low frequency ultrasound in the kHz region)
- Use of growth factors – PDGF, FGF, VEGF
- Stem cell therapy

▌SINUSES AND FISTULAE

SINUS

A sinus (Fig. 1.8A) is an abnormal *blind tract* leading from an epithelial surface into the surrounding tissue, *so it has one opening.* The sinus is lined by either unhealthy granulation tissue or epithelium.

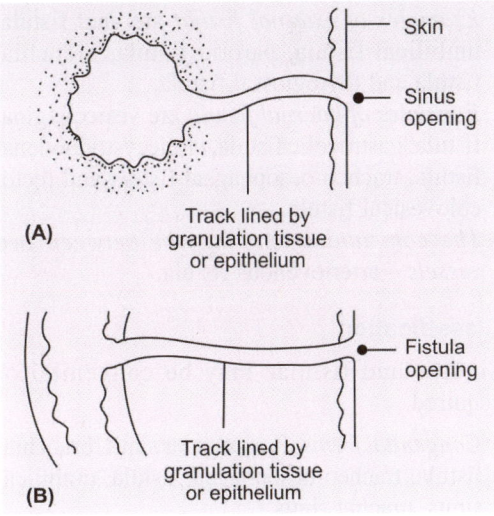

Figs 1.8 A and B: (A) Sinus; (B) Fistula.

Examples of sinus

- Congenital sinus – preauricular sinus (Fig. 1.9).
- Acquired sinus – pilonidal sinus.

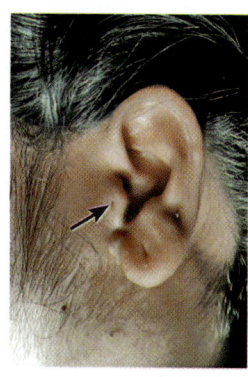

Fig. 1.9: Preauricular sinus at the base of the tragus.

• Osteomyelitic sinus discharging pus with or without bony spicules.

FISTULA

A fistula (Fig. 1.8B) is an abnormal tract between two epithelial surfaces. *So, it has two openings.*

The communication may be between a hollow viscus and the skin, termed as *external fistula*; or between two hollow viscera, termed as *internal fistula*.

The tract is lined by either granulation tissue or epithelium.

• *Examples of external fistula* are anal fistula, umbilical fistula, parotid fistula, branchial fistula and thyroglossal fistula.
• *Examples of internal fistula* are vesicovaginal fistula, gastrocolic fistula, cholecystoduodenal fistula, tracheo-oesophageal fistula and recto/colovesical fistula.
• *The communications may be between two vessels* – arteriovenous fistula.

Classification

Sinuses and fistulae may be congenital or acquired.

• *Congenital forms:* Preauricular sinus, branchial fistula, tracheo-oesophageal fistula, umbilical sinus, urachal sinus.
• *Acquired forms:* Often follow inadequate drainage of an abscess. Examples are perianal abscess bursting on the surface leading to external fistula, or opens both into the anal canal and onto the surface resulting in fistula-

in-ano. Other examples are pilonidal sinus, osteomyelitic sinus, hidradenitis suppurativa, tubercular sinus.

• Gastrojejunostomy and choledochoduodenostomy are caused by operation (iatrogenic forms).
• Acquired arteriovenous fistulas are caused by trauma or by operation (iatrogenic arteriovenous fistula for haemodialysis).

Causes of persistence of a sinus or fistula

1. Presence of a foreign body or necrotic tissue (e.g. a suture, sequestrum, a faecolith or even a worm in the depth of the wound).
2. Inadequate or non-dependent drainage.
3. Prolonged discharge of irritating materials such as urine, faeces or bile causing persisting inflammation.
4. When the tract wall becomes epithelialised.
5. Presence of dense fibrosis around the tract prevents contraction and healing.
6. Unrelieved obstruction of the lumen of the viscus or tube distal to the fistula.
7. Presence of malignant disease.
8. High output discharge (>750 ml in 24 hours).
9. Radiation induced, e.g. enteritis.
10. Distal obstruction of intestine.
11. Local infection and inflammation and sepsis.
12. Associated with specific type of chronic inflammation, e.g. tuberculosis, actinomycosis, Crohn's disease, leprosy, or carcinoma.

EXAMINATION OF A SINUS OR FISTULA

History

Duration:
• Congenital
• Acquired

Past history of:
• Tuberculosis: Tuberculous lymphadenitis followed by caseation of a lymph node, or abscess formation which had burst and discharge cheesy material.
• History of increasing swelling of the limb near a joint and then formation of an abscess which on bursting (or after operation) leaves a discharging sinus (suggestive of osteomyelitis).

- Previous anal abscess or ischiorectal abscess after inadequate drainage may lead to perianal fistula.

Local examination

1. *Number: Fistula-in-ano* may have more than one external opening particularly in presence of Crohn's disease affecting rectum and anal canal.

    Goodsall's rule for fistula-in-ano: Anal fistula with an external opening in the anterior half of anus (an imaginary transverse line dividing the anus into anterior half and posterior half) has a direct radial course to open inside the anal canal, whereas external opening in relation to posterior half of anus has a curved course to open in the midline posteriorly (Fig. 1.10).

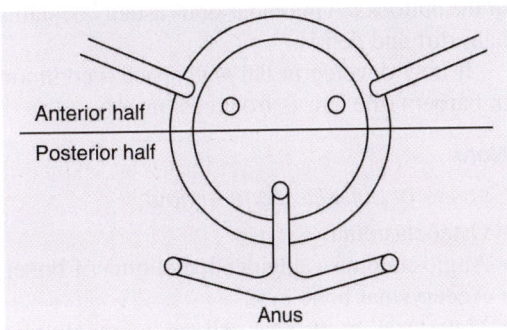

Anterior half

Posterior half

Anus

Fig. 1.10: Goodsall's rule for fistula-in-ano.

   'Watering can' perineum with multiple openings can be seen in presence of urethral stricture especially after gonococcal infection.

   Sinuses due to actinomycosis or madura mycosis are always multiple.

2. *Positions:* Specific positions are often diagnostic of specific conditions, e.g. branchial fistula, preauricular sinus, pilonidal sinus, tuberculous sinus in the neck, etc.

3. *Visible opening of a sinus or fistula:* Sprouting granulation tissue at the opening of a sinus suggests a foreign body in the depth, e.g. a sequestrum, drainage tube or bullet. The opening of a tuberculous sinus is often wide resembling an ulcer with a thin, blue and undermined edge.

4. *Character of discharge:* It may be mucus, pus, blood, sulphur granules (actinomycosis), urine, faeces, bile, etc.

5. *Surrounding skin:* Presence of a scar may indicate chronic osteomyelitis or a previously healed tuberculous lesion. There may be presence of dermatitis, pigmentation.

6. *Palpation of a sinus or fistula for following.*
   - Tenderness
   - Thickening of the wall of a sinus – thickened in a chronic sinus.
   - Mobility of the sinus or fistula over the deeper structures – osteomyelitis sinuses are often fixed to the underlying bone.
   - Nature of discharge on pressure.

7. *Examination of the draining lymph nodes* – matted lymph nodes may be found in case of tuberculous sinus.

8. *Examination with a probe:* Probing should be done cautiously without using any force. The following points are noted:
   - The direction and depth of the sinus.
   - The presence of any foreign body or a movable sequestrum in the depth of the wound.
   - Whether the probe enters a hollow viscus or a bony cavity.
   - Whether any fresh discharge comes out on withdrawal of the probe.

Note

Overzealous probing can create a false passage.

General examination

1. Examination for debility and malnutrition, anaemia, diabetes – all may cause delayed healing.

2. Examination of particular system depending on the site and cause of sinus should be performed, e.g.
   - Chest in presence of chronic empyema.
   - Rectum and anal canal in presence of perianal fistula.
   - Urethra and lower urinary tract in presence of 'watering can' perineum.
   - Bone in presence of osteomyelitis.

Special investigations

1. Examination of the discharge: *Physically* (e.g. pus, or cheesy material in tuberculosis), *chemically* (e.g. presence of urea suggests the diagnosis of a fistula of renal origin), *microscopically* (e.g. sulphur granules in actinomycosis), and *bacteriologically* (e.g. Gram stain, culture and sensitivity).
2. *X-ray examination*
   - Straight X-ray to show a foreign body or a sequestrum and bony changes in osteomyelitis.
   - *Sinogram or fistulogram:* Injection of a radio-opaque dye (lipiodol or hypaque) into a sinus or fistula will determine the course and disposition of the sinus, its relation with the hollow cavities or viscus.
3. Often methylene blue dye is injected into the fistula or sinus to stain the tract – it helps in tracing the direction or disposition of the tract and its ramifications during operation and enables total excision.
4. Biopsy from the edge of the sinus/fistula may reveal tubercular or malignant aetiology.
5. Blood sugar to rule out diabetes.
6. MRI fistulogram is the most preferred investigation to delineate complex anal fistulae to ensure total elimination of the disease.

Management of a sinus or fistula

- Correction of malnutrition, anaemia and diabetes.
- *Control of infection with antibiotics:* Specific antibiotics may require Gram stain and culture sensitivity, Leishman stain.
- Anti-Koch's therapy for tuberculosis.
- Adequate drainage and/or excision – may require radiological investigations. Methylene blue dye injection prior to operation helps in tracing the tracks.
- Sequestrectomy followed by saucerisation of the bone cavity for chronic discharging osteomyelitis.
- Removal of any foreign body.
- Adequate rest.

Note

Beware during anal fistula operation – minimal or no division of the internal sphincter muscle to prevent anal incontinence.

Note

Pilonidal sinus (*pilo* – hair; *nidus* – nest) is a small tunnel in the skin. It occurs in the cleft at the top of the buttocks. A pilonidal sinus usually contains hair, dirt and debris.

It may develop in the web space – common in barbers (the hair is from customers).

Note

Causes of pulsatile bone tumour

- Osteoclastoma.
- Angiosarcoma – angioendothelioma of bone.
- Aneurysmal bone cyst.
- Metastases from renal cell carcinoma/thyroid carcinoma.

Note

Be kind and grateful to our brave soldiers who are protecting our country and lives from the enemy at the border at high altitudes, particularly in or near the glaciers. *Be proud of them also.*

Skin and Subcutaneous Tissue

PAPILLOMA OF THE SKIN

Papilloma is a hamartoma consisting of an over-growth of all layers of skin and its appendages. It has a central core of connective tissue and blood vessels. *A cutaneous papilloma* may be derived from either the squamous or the basal cell layers.

Squamous cell papilloma

Three types are encountered:

1. *Congenital papilloma (syn. naevus verrucous):* Appears either at birth or in early life and may be single or multiple. It usually presents as a brownish warty growth.
2. *Soft papilloma:* Often seen on the eyelids, ear lobule of elderly people.
3. *Keratin horn:* A papilloma with excess keratin formation; common in elderly people (Figs 2.1 to 2.4). It is precancerous and should be excised.

Characteristic features

1. *It can occur anywhere on the body.*
2. It appears as well-defined swelling, usually pedunculated, ranging from a few milli-metres to few centimetres.
3. Surface smooth or grooved or deeply fissured, and may be associated with pigmentation or keratosis.

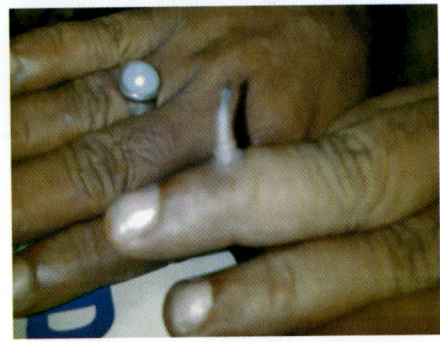

Fig. 2.1: Keratin horn dorsum of left middle finger.

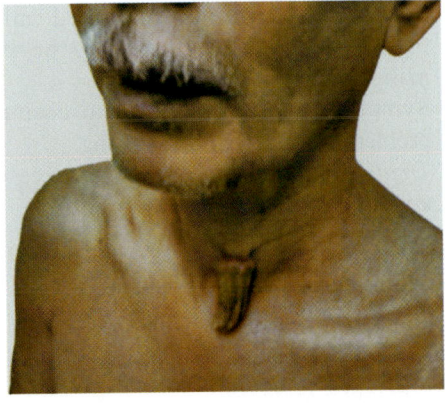

Fig. 2.2: Keratin horn arising from the front of the neck. (*Courtesy:* Dr RL Modak, MS)

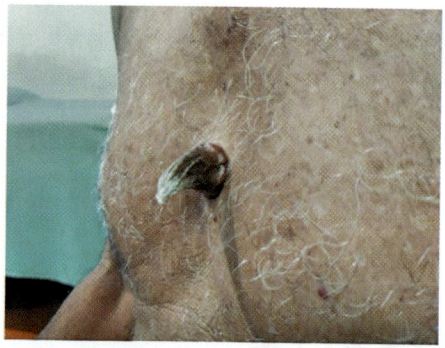

Fig. 2.3: Keratin horn anterior chest wall near xiphisternum junction.

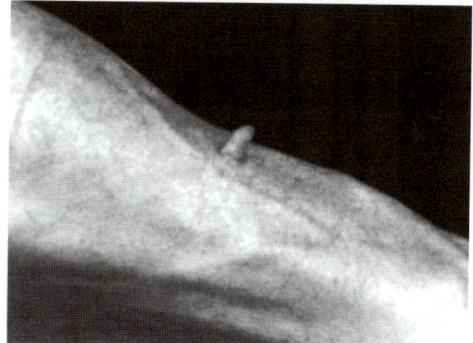

Fig. 2.4: Keratin horn on the dorsum of the forearm—just proximal to wrist.

4. *Consistence:* Solid, usually firm, but may be soft due to excess fatty component.
5. Non-invasive and non-indurated unless inflamed and ulcerated. May be premalignant.
6. Symptoms mostly give rise to cosmetic problem or can catch on clothing.
7. *Treatment:* Excision for cosmetic reasons and to prevent malignancy.

Basal cell papilloma
(*Syn.* Seborrhoeic keratosis, Senile warts)

It is due to overgrowth of the basal layers of the epidermis. It is a benign tumour.

Characteristic features

1. They usually appear as multiple lesions in the elderly people of both sexes.
2. Common in Caucasians and uncommon in Blacks and Indians.

3. They can occur in any area but most predominantly over the face and neck, and shoulders and trunk.
4. Usually the lesions look like an ovoid, verrucous, brown plaque stuck on the epidermis, and vary from few millimetres to few centimetres.
5. Surface is rough and hyperkeratotic and has a waxy look and feel.
6. Slowly growing lesion and may fall or be rubbed off.
7. May become infected and ulcerated. Malignant transformation has been recorded. *It is also considered to be a marker of visceral malignancy. When deeply pigmented, it is mistaken for a malignant melanoma.*
8. *Symptoms:* Mostly give rise to cosmetic problem or can catch on clothing.
9. *Treatment:* Removal for cosmetic reasons.
   • The lesion can be scraped with a sharp curette which leaves a flat surface which becomes covered with normal epithelium in one week.
   • Cryosurgery is also useful.

WARTS

A wart (Fig. 2.5) is a rough excrescence on the skin *due to infection with the papilloma virus of the papovavirus group.* A number of different viruses are also involved. *It is transmissible through direct or intimate contact* with inoculation through a minor abrasion.

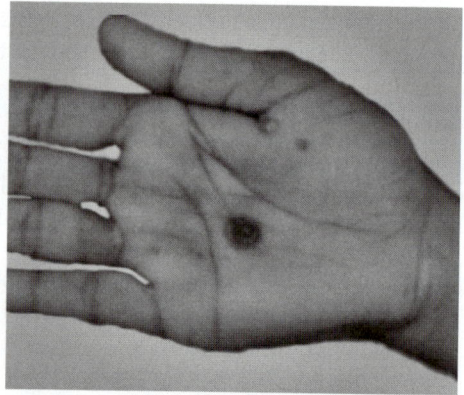

Fig. 2.5: Palmar wart.

Characteristic features

1. They occur at all ages but common in children and young adults.
2. They usually tend to occur on sites of trauma, such as the beard area, hands, fingers, genital region and feet.
3. All warts first appear as small, smooth nodules, later they may coalesce to form rough excrescence.
4. They may be pigmented, keratinised or deeply pitted with a frond-like irregular surface.
5. Warts can cause pain and irritation.
6. Plantar warts occur on the sole. They are inverted into the skin and, due to the pressure of walking are painful and tender.
7. Warts can cause cosmetic problems when on the hands. Multiple warts in the fingers may interfere with the fine movements.
8. *Venereal warts (papilloma accuminata)* are seen in the coronal sulcus or the perineum. They are multiple and moist with offensive discharge.
9. *Two-thirds of warts may disappear spontaneously.*
10. *Treatment:*
    - Curettage and diathermy
    - Repeated application of 20% podophyllin in liquid paraffin.
    - Cryosurgery – liquid nitrogen or CO_2 snow application.

CALLOSITIES

1. A callosity (Fig. 2.6) is a localised thickening of the skin due to excessive keratinisation.
2. It occurs as a protective measure at the sites of friction.
3. It appears as superficial, circumscribed, yellow white patches of hyperkeratotic material and is continuous around its margins with the normal skin.
4. It protrudes outward from the skin. *It is usually painless.*
5. *Commonly seen in the feet*, especially the inframedial aspect of the great toe, and the heel. It may also occur over the dorsal aspect

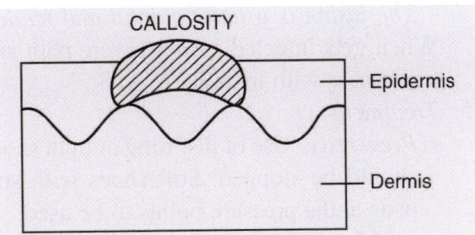

Fig. 2.6: Callosity is confined to epidermis only and usually protrudes outwards from the skin surface.

in other limb deformities particularly neuropathic. Also found in gardeners' hands and fingers of violinists.
6. Histologically there is thickening of the stratum corneum and granulosum with or without atrophy of the rete pegs.
7. Treatment is usually not required except change of footwear. *Local application of keratolytic agent like 40% salicylic acid may be helpful.*

CORN

1. A corn (Fig. 2.7) is a localised hyperkeratinisation of the skin with a hard central core over a bony projection.
2. It occurs *due to repeated external undue pressure* as seen with ill-fitting or tight shoes.
   Also common in people who walk barefooted and prone to thorn or nail prick.
3. Chiefly affects the plantar surface of toes and sole of the feet, *usually over a bony prominence.*
4. It appears as a circumscribed cone-shaped horny thickening with the base on the surface and apex pointing inwards into the dermis.

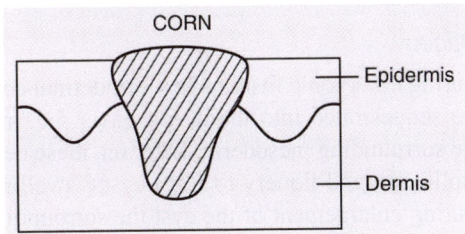

Fig. 2.7: Corn penetrates the dermis also which contains peripheral cutaneous nerves—so painful on pressure.

The lesion is usually painful and tender. When gets infected causes severe pain and tenderness with inability to walk.

5. *Treatment*
   • *Preventive:* Use of ill-fitting or tight shoes should be stopped. Soft shoes with soft pads at the pressure points to be used.
   • Local application of topical keratolytic agent, e.g. 40% salicylic acid in collodion on successive nights may be useful.
   • If conservative measures fail, excision of the corn with particular care to remove the apex of the corn is required.

One should be careful in treating corn in patients with diabetes or with a poor peripheral circulation when a secondary infection may precipitate gangrene. Peripheral pulses examination and blood sugar estimation is mandatory before operating corns particularly in elderly people.

DERMOID CYST

Syn. Epidermal cyst. Clinically four varieties of dermoid are recognised.

1. Sequestration dermoid
2. Implantation dermoid – acquired or traumatic
3. Tubulodermoid
4. Teratodermoid

SEQUESTRATION DERMOID

It is a true variety of congenital cyst arising from the entrapped primitive ectodermal cells *being buried at the line of embryonic fusion.*

Origin

During embryonic fusion a few ectodermal cells are sequestrated into the deeper layer, i.e. into the surrounding mesoderm. Later on, these cells proliferate and liquefy to form cystic swelling. During enlargement of the cyst the surrounding mesoderm can be pressed or indented giving rise to bony indentation (Fig. 2.8).

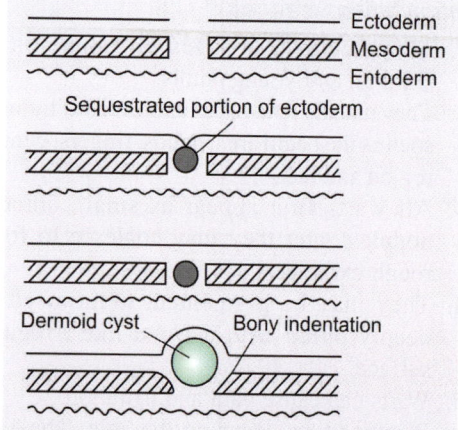

Fig. 2.8: Mode of formation of sequestration dermoid.

Sites

The planes of fusion are the usual sites of dermoid cysts, e.g.

• *At the midline of the body,* especially at the root of the neck, at the root of the nose (Fig. 2.9). *Sublingual dermoid* in the floor of the mouth due to entrapped surface ectoderm at the level of first branchial arches' fusion. It is typical midline swelling either supra- or inframylohyoid but may rarely be paramedian.
• *On the scalp:* Pterion, asterion (postauricular, Fig. 2.15), etc.

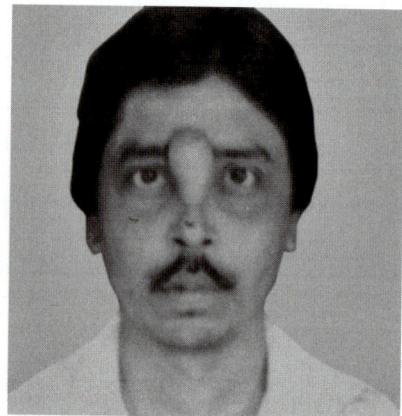

Fig. 2.9: Dermoid at the root of the nose at the frontonasal suture line.

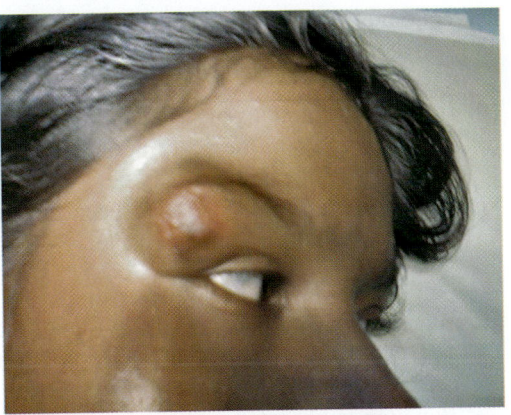

Fig. 2.10: External angular dermoid at the outer extremity of the eyebrow—zygomaticofrontal suture line.

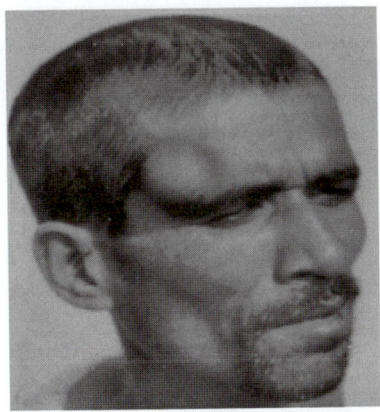

Fig. 2.12: External angular dermoid at the outer extremity of the eyebrow—zygomaticofrontal suture line.

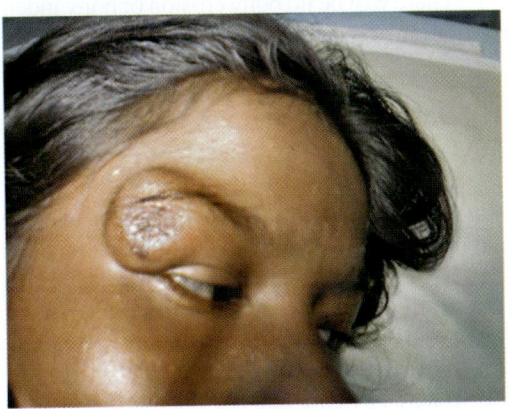

Fig. 2.11: External angular dermoid. Same patient as in Fig. 2.10. *Note indentation* over the swelling after finger tip pressure but no punctum (cf. sebaceous cyst).

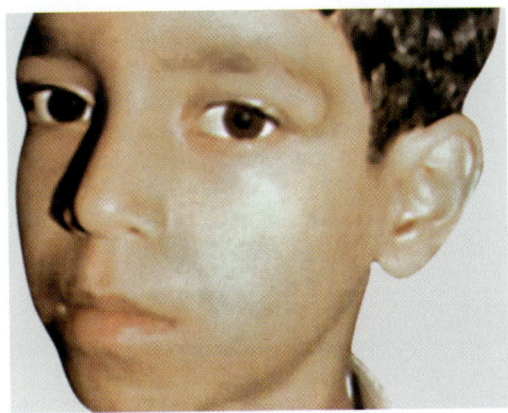

Fig. 2.13: External angular dermoid.

- At the inner or outer angles of the eye (angular dermoids) (Figs 2.10 to 2.13). *Internal angular dermoid* at the line of fusion between fronto-nasal process and maxillary process at the inner canthus of eye (Fig. 2.14). *External angular dermoid* at the outer canthus of the eye at the zygomaticofrontal suture line.
- *Pre- and postsacral dermoid.*

Pathology

- *Lining of the cyst:* Squamous epithelium with hair, hair follicles, sweat and sebaceous glands (cf. implantation dermoid).

- *Contents:* Toothpaste-like desquamated material with or without hairs. The paste is the mixture of sebum, sweat and desquamated epithelial cell debris and is usually foul-smelling.

  The cyst lies deep to the skin and not attached to the skin.

Diagnostic criteria

1. Painless lump at the common sites mentioned above.
2. *Shape and size:* Ovoid or spherical swelling varying from 1 to 2 cm in diameter.
3. *Cystic swellings:* Fluctuation positive.
4. Surface is smooth.

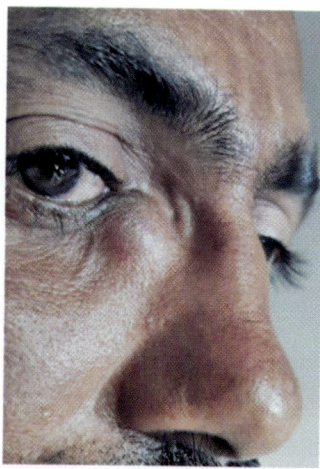

Fig. 2.14: Internal angular dermoid.

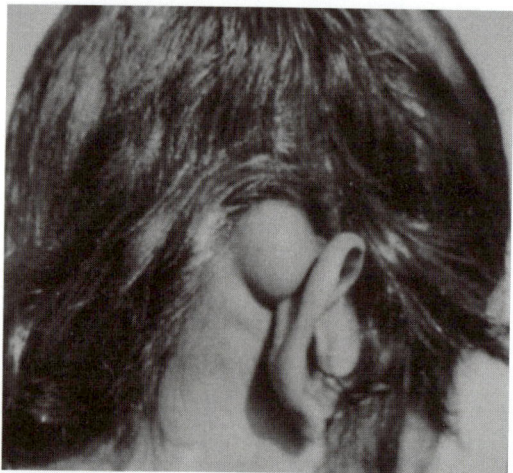

Fig. 2.15: Postauricular dermoid behind pinna (asterion).

5. Absence of punctum (cf. sebaceous cyst).
6. Skin can be pinched or lifted up (cf. sebaceous cyst).
7. Not compressible (cf. meningocele).
8. The dermoid cyst itself may indent on pressure over the surface (cf. sebaceous cyst) (Fig. 2.11).
9. *Bony indentation:* Palpate the margin of the cyst which *may reveal an indentation in the underlying bone.* Usually present when the dermoid is situated in relation to a bone. Due to enlargement in the size of the cyst, the neighbouring bone is indented which can be palpated at the base of the cyst (cf. meningocele).
10. Impulse on coughing or straining usually not present except in the scalp dermoid when an intracranial extension may be present.
11. *Transillumination:* Negative (because the content is thick) (cf. meningocele).

D/D of sequestration dermoid

1. *Sebaceous cyst:* Can occur at any site of the skin. *Punctum* is present. Dermoid cyst occurs along the lines of embryonic fusion. *Punctum is absent.*
2. *Meningocele:* Compressible. Brilliantly transilluminable.
3. *Lipoma:* Slipping sign at the edge is present. There will be no bony erosion or bony indentation

Peculiarities of scalp dermoid

1. Dermoid cyst may lie fully outside the cranial bones. No punctum is present (D/D: Sebaceous cyst).
2. It may lie completely inside the cranial bones – between the dura and the cranial bones.
3. It may be partly intracranial and partly extracranial with a connection between them (hourglass dermoid) when bony indentation may be present.
4. It may lie extracranially, but may be attached to the underlying dura by a stalk or pedicle passing through a defect in the bone.

The intracranial components may cause compression of brain and local fits.

Peculiarities of postsacral or postanal dermoid

1. It may expand within the spinal canal causing compression of cauda equina.
2. The lesion may be present at birth but usually noted in the first two years of life. Occasionally, it may appear in adulthood.

The last two varieties only may show expansile impulse on straining or coughing when they *have to be differentiated from meningocele by transillumination test* which will be positive in meningocele but negative in dermoid.

Note

Scalp dermoid and/or postanal dermoid may show expansile impulse on straining or coughing when they have to be differentiated from meningocele by transillumination test which will be positive in meningocele but negative in dermoid.

Complications

1. Infection
2. Suppuration
3. Bursting
4. Ulceration } Rare
5. Cosmetically, it looks ugly. When found in children, it causes parental distress.
6. Pressure effects on adjacent structures, particularly with intracranial or intraspinal extension.

Investigation

Scalp and postsacral dermoids should be X-rayed, particularly those showing impulse on straining or coughing. If there is an appreciable gap, the operation can be delayed till adolescence to give the bony defect an opportunity for spontaneous closure.

In the presence of persistent bony gap after adolescence, an intracranial or intraspinal extension is suspected. So, CT scan/MRI is performed to assess the extent of intracranial or intraspinal extension in scalp and postanal dermoid.

Treatment

- In the absence of bony gap as evidenced by X-ray, *simple total excision* of the cyst is performed for cosmetic reasons, to prevent complications or to relieve parental distress.
- If the age is advanced, the operation should be very carefully done, and before excising the cyst, it should be differentiated from meningocele – *transillumination is positive in meningocele*.
- *In the presence of intracranial extension as detected by CT scan*, both extracranial and intracranial parts are excised by raising an osteoplastic flap or by craniotomy. A neurosurgical intervention may be helpful.

IMPLANTATION DERMOID
(Post-traumatic dermoid)

It is an acquired cyst arising from the indriven *surface epithelium* beneath the skin following a trauma, *particularly a puncture injury*. The patient may not remember the injury.

Sites

Usually found in the areas subject to repeated trauma, e.g. in the pulps or tips of the fingers, palm and sole. So, it is common in the tailors or women with the habit of sewing (prone to needle prick); also noted in gardeners (prone to thorn prick) (Figs 2.17 to 2.19).

Pathology

- *Lining of the cyst:* Squamous epithelium but hair, hair follicles, sweat and sebaceous glands are absent (cf. sequestration dermoid). So, it is a true cyst.
- *Contents:* White greasy material which is desquamated epithelial cells with mucoid degeneration.

Diagnostic criteria

1. Spherical smooth swelling, usually 0.2 cm to 1 cm in diameter, in the areas subjected to repeated trauma.
2. The cyst feels tense and hard, sometimes stony hard. It may be painful and tender.
3. The overlying skin is often scarred.

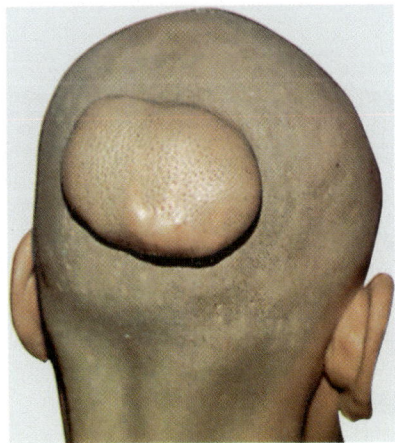

Fig. 2.16: Recurrent dermoid over the occipital region. Note the scar from previous operation.

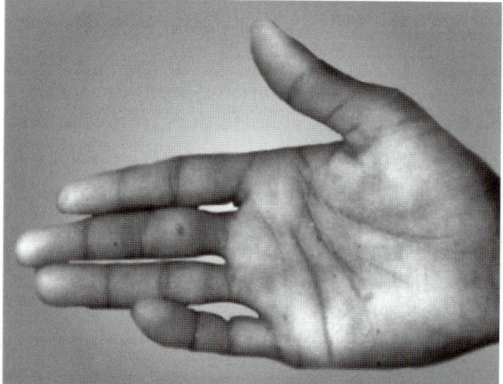

Fig. 2.17: Implanted dermoid right middle finger. Note puncture scar at the top of lump—3 months duration.

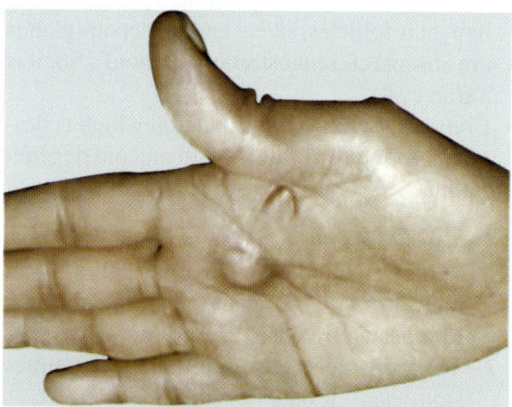

Fig. 2.18: Implanted dermoid over right palm. No puncture scar noted over the swelling.

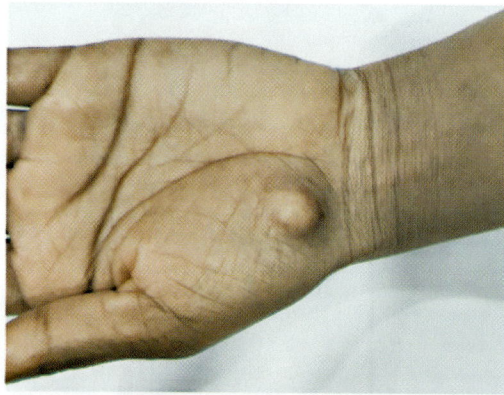

Fig. 2.19: Implanted dermoid at base of left thenar eminence.

4. The history of an old injury with or without a scar overlying the cyst is the most significant diagnostic feature.

Complications

1. The cyst on the finger or palm may interfere with the grip and touch.
2. The cyst on the sole may cause limping.
3. Infection.
4. Cosmetically looks ugly.

Treatment

Complete excision: To remove inconvenience at work, to remove pain or tenderness or for cosmetic reasons.

TUBULODERMOID

This is a cystic swelling arising from the non-obliterated portion of a congenital ectodermal duct or tube. The swelling is due to the distention caused by the accumulation of the secretion of the lining epithelium of the patent segment of the duct.

Examples

1. Thyroglossal cyst – commonest example.
2. Postanal dermoid – remnant of neuroenteric canal.
3. Ependymal cyst in the brain – remnant of neuroectoderm.

TERATOMATOUS DERMOID

This is a cystic swelling arising from the totipotent cells with ectodermal preponderance.

Common sites

1. Ovary – ovarian cyst.
2. Testis – teratoma.
3. Mediastinum ⎤ Usually appear as
4. Retroperitoneal ⎟ solid swelling
5. Presacral area ⎦ rather than cystic

Contents

Usually contains *derivatives of mesodermal elements* such as cartilage, bone, tooth, hair, and also cheesy material.

Complication

Malignant change can occur which may be carcinomatous or sarcomatous.

CERVICAL AND SUBLINGUAL DERMOID

Please refer to chapter 3 for details.

SEBACEOUS CYST

This is a *retention cyst due to accumulation of sebum resulting from obstruction to the duct of the sebaceous gland.* It is also called epidermoid cyst. (For sebaceous cysts, *see* Figs 2.20 to 2.29.)

Anatomically, sebaceous glands are situated in the dermis and their ducts open either on to the skin surface directly or open into a hair follicle. If the mouth of a sebaceous gland is blocked, the gland will get distended by its own secretions producing sebaceous cyst.

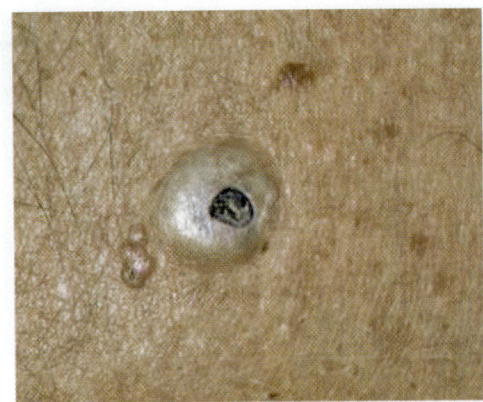

Fig. 2.20: Sebaceous cyst at the back of the trunk. Note the blue punctum which is diagnostic of such cyst.

Sites

It can occur anywhere in the body wherever sebaceous glands exist. It is an intracutaneous lesion. *Common sites* are the scalp, face, scrotum, vulva, back, shoulders, neck. They are more common in hairy areas where in cases of long duration they could result in *loss of hair on the skin surface immediately above the cyst.*

It never occurs in the palm and sole, because there are no sebaceous glands in these regions.

Pathology

- *Lining of the cyst:* Squamous epithelium as it is considered pathologically epidermoid cyst.
- *Contents:* Yellowish white poultice-like material *with an unpleasant smell.* Such material is a mixture of sebum, fat, desquamated epithelial cell debris.

Rarely, on histological section, an organism called *Demodex folliculorum* may be found, because these organisms are harboured in the wall of the sebaceous gland.

Diagnostic criteria

- Swelling in a common site as mentioned above.
- *Shape* – globular or hemispherical.
- *Size* – varies from a few millimetres to 4–5 cm.
- *Presence of bluish black spot, called punctum* indicating the site of blockage at the opening of the duct, may be noticed (Fig. 2.20).

The punctum is adherent to the cyst. *On squeezing the cyst* putty-like or cheesy sebaceous material *with an unpleasant smell* may come out through the punctum.

- *Skin cannot be lifted up* (cf. lipoma, dermoid cyst).
- *Consistence:* Cystic or tense cystic, hence *fluctuation may be positive.*
- Surface is smooth.
- Not compressible.
- Because of its putty-like consistency, *the swelling can often be indented by a finger tip pressure* (cf. dermoid cyst).
- *Transillumination:* Negative, because the content is thick.

Differential diagnosis

1. Dermoid cyst
2. Lipoma
3. Meningocele

Features of the scalp sebaceous cyst (cf. Scalp dermoid)

(a) Swelling is free from underlying structure. Sebaceous cyst moves with the movement of the scalp.
(b) Usually loss of hair is noted over the swelling.
(c) Punctum is sometimes difficult to demonstrate in the scalp sebaceous cyst (D/D: Scalp dermoid).

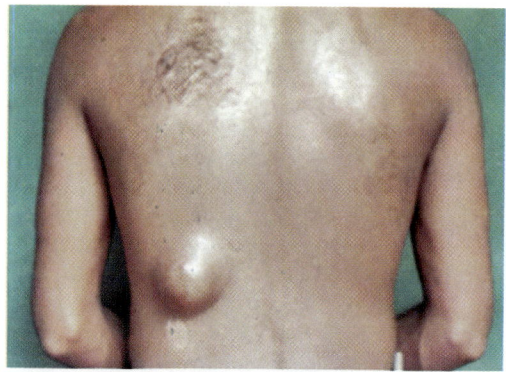

Fig. 2.21: Large sebaceous cyst on the back. Note the punctum at 12 o'clock position.

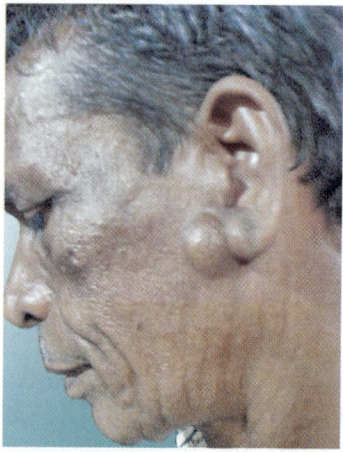

Fig. 2.22A: Sebaceous cyst in front of left ear lobule.

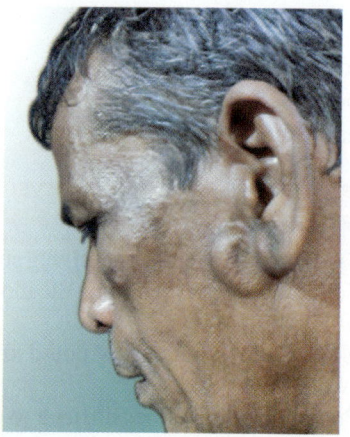

Fig. 2.22B: Same patient as in Fig. 2.22A—swelling pits on pressure.

(d) Skin is attached to the swelling (cf. dermoid).

(e) No impulse on straining or coughing (cf. meningocele).

(f) No bony indentation can be felt (cf. dermoid).

(g) But the swelling itself *can be indented by a finger tip pressure – this is diagnostic.*

Features of scrotal sebaceous cysts

Scrotal sebaceous cysts are usually multiple and when well formed they feel solid. *No punctum is usually visible.*

Complications

1. Cosmetically looks ugly.
2. *Infection and suppuration:* The cyst is commonly infected. The surface skin becomes red and inflamed. The cyst becomes tense and tender and *on squeezing the cyst, pus may be expressed through the punctum.* Repeated infection is a common phenomenon which makes the operation difficult. In the presence of infected sebaceous cyst, diabetes should be excluded in adults.
3. Ulceration.
4. Calcification

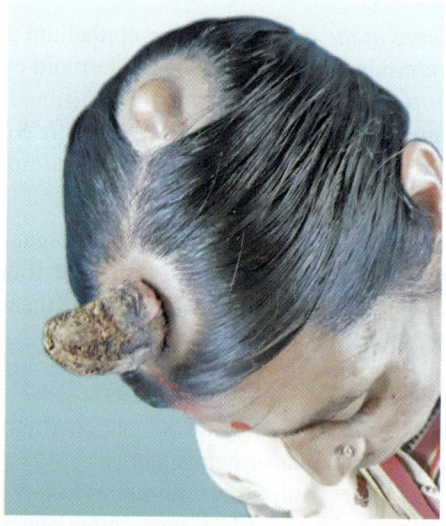

Fig. 2.23: Sebaceous horn on the anterior scalp (frontal region) and sebaceous cyst on the parieto-occipital region with discharge from punctum.

5. *Sebaceous horn:* Inspissated sebaceous materials may leak through the punctum and accumulate on the surface skin in successive layers. They get dried up and ultimately give rise to a horny projection. It should be excised along with the underlying cyst.

6. *Cock's peculiar tumour:* It is nothing but suppurating and ulcerating sebaceous cyst with excessive granulation tissue formation and looks like squamous cell carcinoma. Infection → suppuration → bursting → escape of sebaceous material and purulent material on the surface → chronic irritation leading to granulating ulcer or *a granuloma looking like a tumour.* The granuloma consists of histiocytes and foreign body giant cells (cf. epithelioma). Total excision of the tumour is advisable.

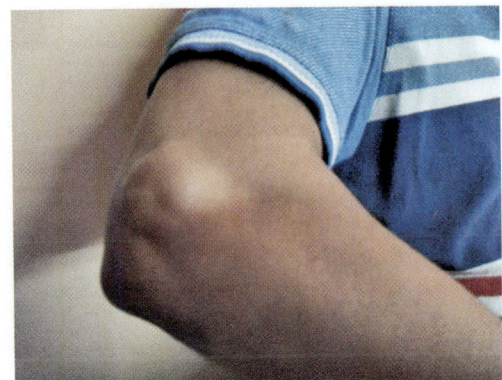

Fig. 2.25: Sebaceous cyst over lateral epicondyle of right elbow—pits on pressure.

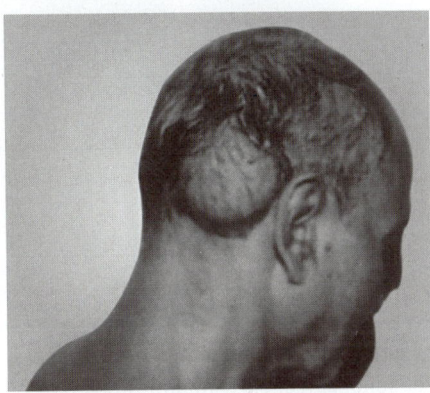

Fig. 2.26: A large sebaceous cyst of the scalp over right occipital region behind the right ear. Note the loss of hair over the surface of the swelling.

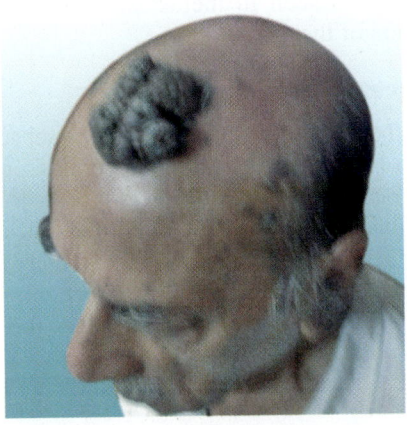

Fig. 2.24: Cock's peculiar tumour over the scalp. D/D: Melanoma due to black pigmentation. But typical history suggested cock's peculiar tumour.

7. Rarely malignancy occurs when it will be usually of basal cell carcinoma.

8. *Keratin horn:* A cutaneous horn is a type of lesion or growth that appears on the top layer of the skin. It is made up of keratin which is a protein that lies on the top layer of the skin. It is precancerous, so should be excised.

Treatment

Excision of the cyst either by dissection, or by incision and avulsion of the cyst wall under local anaesthesia.

(a) *Dissection method:* An elliptical incision is made on the skin centering the punctum. Then the cyst with overlying skin is gradually dissected from the surrounding skin and subcutaneous tissue till the entire cyst can be removed intact, otherwise recurrence is inevitable.

(b) *Incision and avulsion method:* An incision is made through the skin over the cyst. The cyst contents are squeezed out. Then the cyst wall is held with a pair of dissecting forceps and carefully avulsed out.

When sebaceous cyst is infected, preoperative antibiotic should be started. *Rule out diabetes.* When the infection subsides, excision of the cyst is performed. If infection does not subside, the

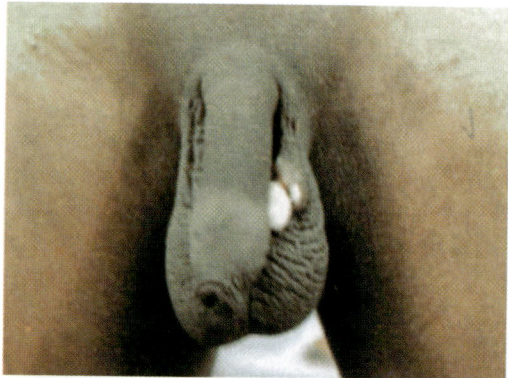

Fig. 2.27: Scrotal sebaceous cyst with calcification.

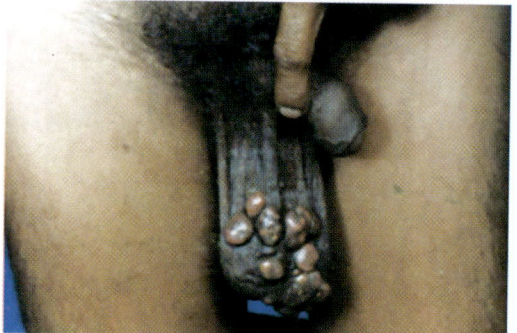

Fig. 2.28: Multiple sebaceous cysts involving the anteroinferior part of the scrotum—treated by partial excision of skin containing the cysts followed by primary suture of skin margins.

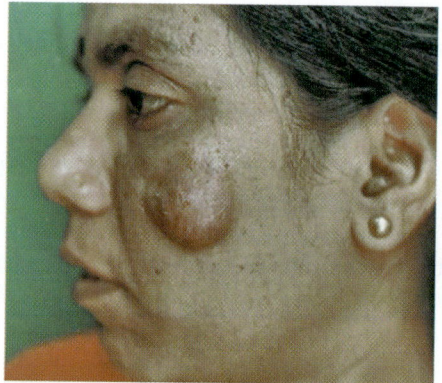

Fig. 2.29: Infected sebaceous cyst. Treated conservatively with antibiotic—the infection subsided and the swelling reduced much in size. Waiting for excision during quiescent phase. In the presence of infection, cyst removal is difficult and incomplete.

cyst should be incised and the pus and semiliquid foetid material are expelled. This is followed by dissection or avulsion of the cyst wall.

Treatment of scrotal sebaceous cyst

1. *Solitary cyst* – Total extrascapular excision of the cyst including the punctum.
2. *Multiple cysts affecting a part of the scrotum* – that part of the scrotal skin containing the sebaceous cysts should be excised.
3. *Multiple cysts scattered all over the scrotum* – the whole of the scrotal skin should be excised. The testes may have to be placed in the pocket made in the subcutaneous tissue at the medial side of the respective thigh.

Treatment of scalp sebaceous cyst

X-ray of the skull – *to rule out bony defect* that will be seen in dermoid cyst or to rule out bone destruction seen in metastasis, followed by excision of the cyst.

Sebaceous adenoma

It is a benign tumour arising from the sebaceous gland. Histologically, simple hyperplasia of the cells occurs (epiloia). *Clinically, it is a solid swelling,* may be single or multiple, occurring either in the scalp commonly in the frontal region, or in the regions of the nose and cheek, *rarely on the back.* When occurring in the scalp, this may

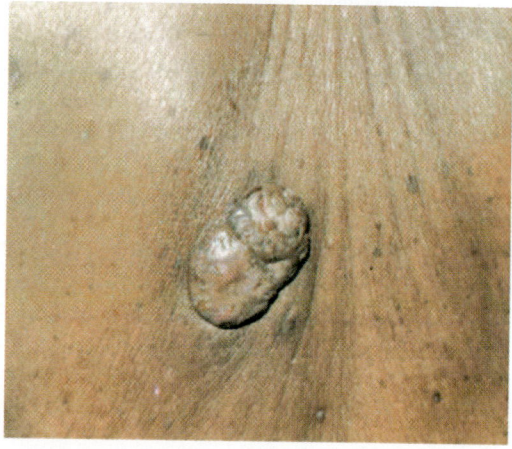

Fig. 2.30: Sebaceous adenoma arising in the skin of upper back—solid swelling, no punctum. Requires histological confirmation after excision.

be associated with some lesion in the brain, even epilepsy (tuberculous sclerosis of the brain). *When occurring on the nose, it is called rhino-phyma.*

Note

Sebaceous gland is a *holocrine variety* of exo-crine gland producing secretions by fatty degeneration of its central cells.

Exocrine glands – three varieties:

1. Holocrine: Where the whole of the cell dis-integrates and dies to liberate its secretion, e.g. sebaceous gland.
2. Apocrine: Where only the luminal part of the cell disintegrates leaving the nucleus and the basal portion from which the cell regenerates, e.g. mammary gland.
3. Merocrine: The secretion is discharged with-out any destruction of the cell. Most of the glands belong to this type.

Note

Syndrome associated with sebaceous cyst – Gardner's syndrome comprising:

- Sebaceous cyst
- Osteomas
- Intestinal polyposis

Keratin horn

A cutaneous horn is a type of lesion or growth that appears on the skin. It is made up of keratin, which is a protein that lies on the top layer of the skin. *It is precancerous, so should be excised.*

LIPOMA

It is a benign, connective tissue tumour arising from the adult fat cells (*lipocytes*). It is the commonest of all benign tumours and is composed of adipose tissue. It can occur in any situation where there is fat, hence known as *universal tumour* or *ubiquitous tumour.*

Common sites

The subcutaneous tissues over the trunk, the nape of the neck, and the limbs.

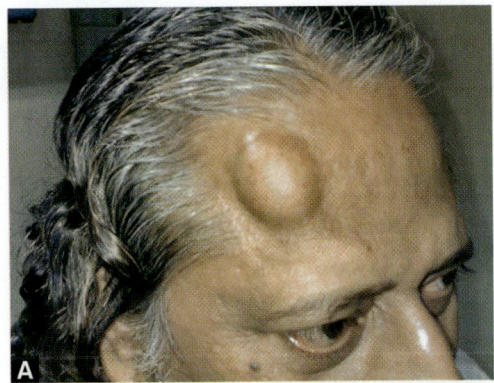
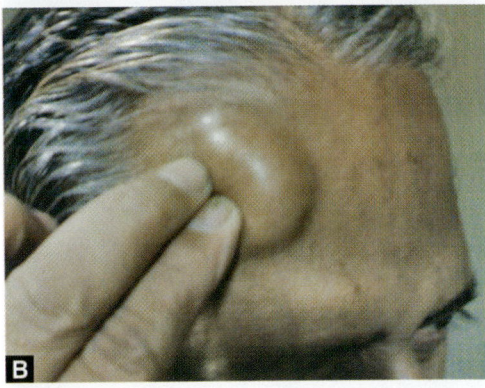

Figs 2.31 A and B: (A) Lipoma forehead; (B) Margin slipped under the fingers.

Varieties

In relation to possessing a capsule:

1. *Encapsulated variety: Commonest.* Lipoma is covered by a capsule and may occur at any site of the body. This is a *true lipoma.*
2. *Diffuse variety: Rare.* It is characterised by deposition of fat without any peripheral capsule, hence often called *pseudolipoma.* It does not possess the typical features of lipoma. Commonly found in people taking excessive alcohol, at the region of the neck which may extend to the face.

Treatment of diffuse variety of lipoma

The treatment here is nothing but to excise the excessive fat provided the patient needs that for cosmetic reasons. Profound obesity may also lead to diffuse variety of fat deposition at the region of neck, dorsal surface of arms, below the umbilicus (lower abdomen) and thighs. *Lipo-suction* is recently being used to correct these deformities with better cosmetic results *to avoid a long scar or multiple scars.*

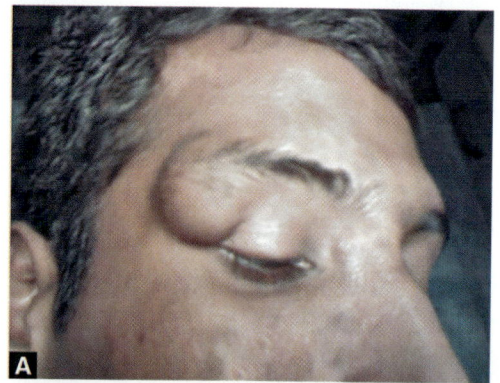

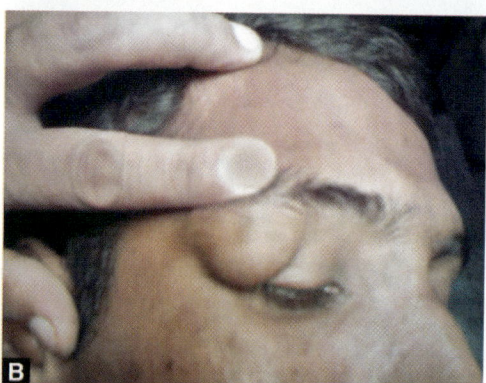

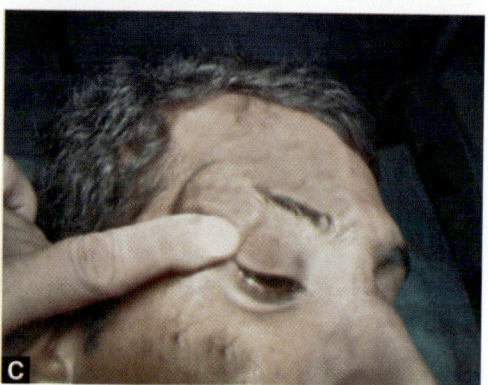

Figs 2.32 A, B and C: (A) Lump appeared to be angular dermoid on inspection; (B and C) Margins of the lump slipped under the finger. But no indentation noted on finger tip pressure. So, lipoma. D/D: Angular dermoid.

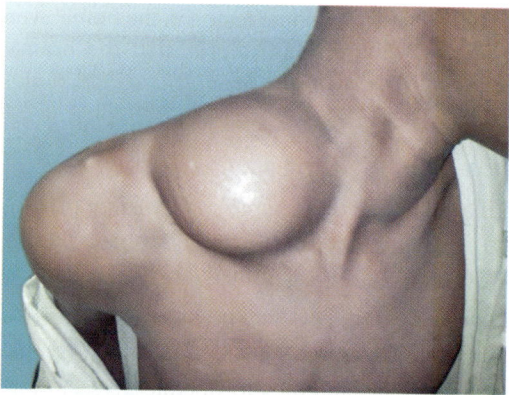

Fig. 2.33: Lipoma: Right supraclavicular region.

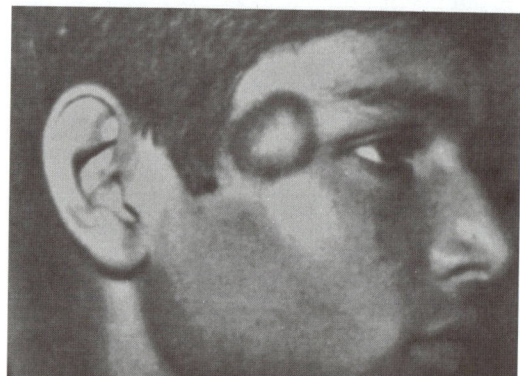

Fig. 2.34A: Lipoma. D/D: Angular dermoid.

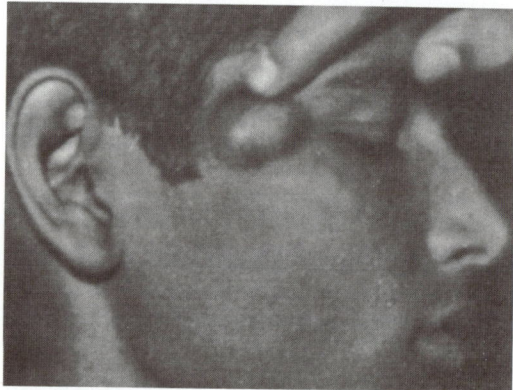

Fig. 2.34B: Same patient. On inspection—the swelling appeared to be angular dermoid. But on palpation—a soft swelling; the swelling was not smooth; *the edge of the swelling slipped under the finger.* So, the diagnosis was lipoma. Diagnosis confirmed after operation. Note: Lipoma can occur anywhere in the body.

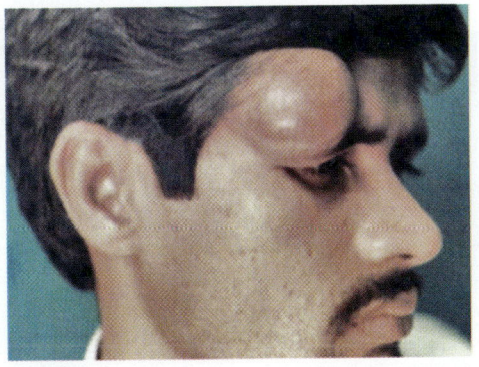

Fig. 2.35: Lipoma. Lobulated appearance and feel. *The margin slipped under the finger.* 10-year duration, gradually increasing in size. The overlying scar mark was due to application of Ayurvedic poultice. D/D: 1. Angular dermoid—but the swelling not present since birth; no bony indentation with this size of swelling. 2. Sebaceous cyst—but no punctum; no surface indentation on fingertip pressure.

Classification of lipoma

Anatomical classification

Depends on the anatomical sites.

1. Skin – subcutaneous.
2. Aponeurosis or fascia – subaponeurotic or subfascial.
3. Muscle – intermuscular.
4. Periosteum – subperiosteal.
5. Synovial membrane – subsynovial.
6. Joints – intra-articular.
7. Mucous membrane – submucous.
8. Serous – subserous (retroperitoneal).
9. Meninges – extradural or subdural (type of spinal tumour).
10. Gland – intraglandular – seen in breast, pancreas and under renal capsule.

Histological classification

Depends on the presence of other tissues in addition to adipose tissue.

1. *Fibrolipoma:* Mixture of fibrous tissue and adipose tissue.
2. *Naevolipoma:* Mixture of haemangiomatous and adipose tissues.
   Features of naevolipoma:
   • Bluish discoloration of the overlying skin.

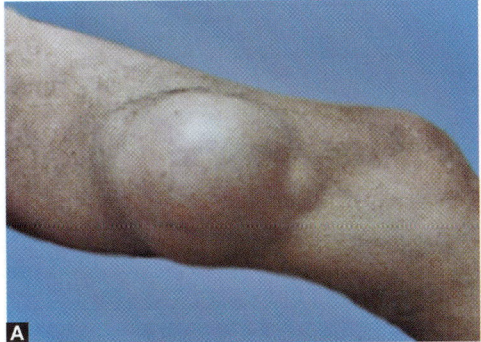

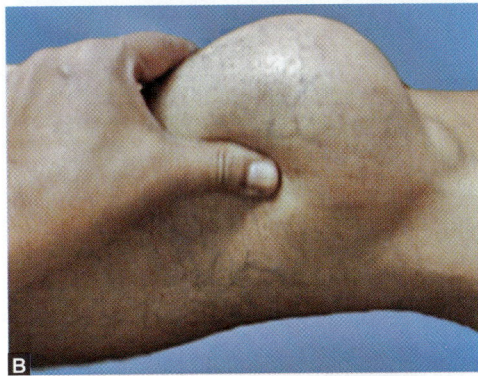

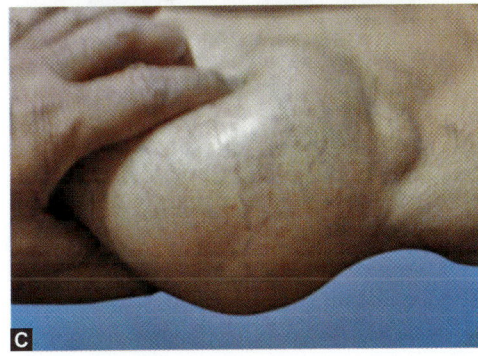

Figs 2.36 A, B and C: Lipoma on the medial side of the left thigh above the knee for nearly 10 years gradually increasing in size. Soft, solid, lobulated and *freely mobile lump both over the relaxed and contracted muscles of the thigh as the lump was over the deep fascia of thigh. Margins slipped under the finger.* (cf. Fig. 2.31 Liposarcoma)

   • Blanching.
   • Compressibility.
3. *Neurolipoma:* Mixture of nerve tissue and adipose tissue. *It is often painful.*

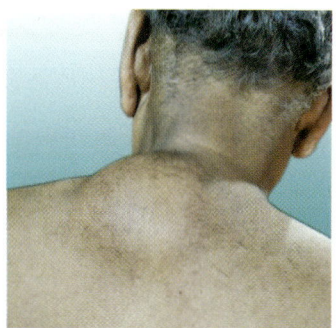

Fig. 2.37A: Lipoma over the nape of the neck. (*Courtesy:* Dr Jayprakash Rai)

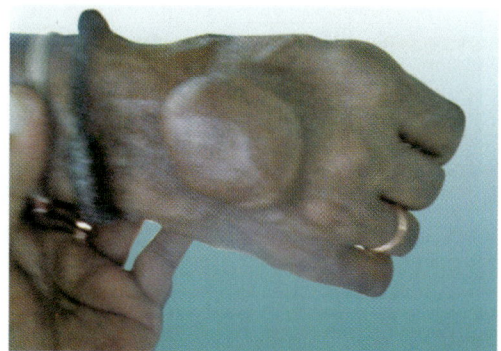

Fig. 2.38: Lipoma over the dorsum of right hand.

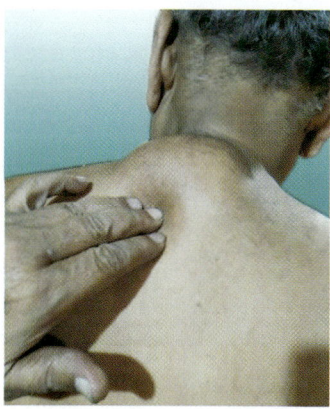

Fig. 2.37B: Same patient as in Fig. 2.37A. Slipping sign present—so lipoma. D/D: Billingate's lump—Porter's bursa.

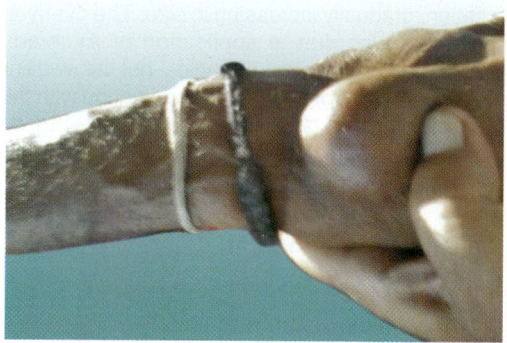

Fig. 2.39: Same patient as in Fig. 2.38. Slipping sign present.

When they are multiple with pain and tenderness, it is called *neurolipomatosis*.

When neurolipomatosis is associated with the painful, tender, diffuse or nodular deposits of fat, it is called *Dercum's disease* or *adiposis dolorosa*. Commonly found in women, particularly affecting the trunk, buttock and thighs. Usually, no capsules are formed around these fatty deposits and so, these are called false lipomas.

Clinical classification

1. Solitary ⎤ Number
2. Multiple ⎦

1. Sessile ⎤ Shape
2. Pedunculated ⎦

Pathology

On cut section lipoma appears as uniform yellow-coloured fatty tissue traversed by white fibrous

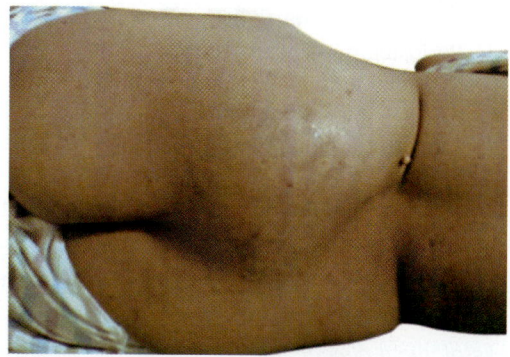

Fig. 2.40: Diffuse lipoma over the left buttock. Soft, solid, lobulated and freely mobile lump (cf. Dercum's disease). Margins slipped under the finger. D/D: Liposarcoma. (*Courtesy:* Dr Sudeb Saha, MS, FAMS)

septa of varying thickness. Occasionally, the cut surface may show patches of calcification and areas of myxomatous degeneration.

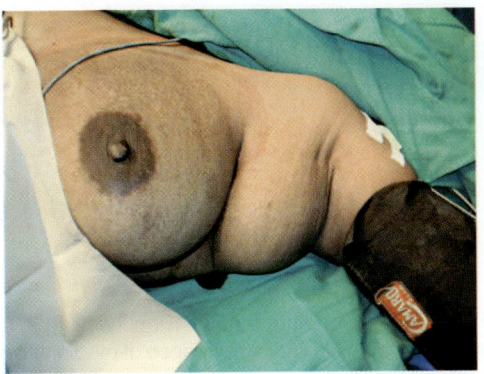

Fig. 2.41: Lipoma left axilla—soft, solid, lobulated and freely mobile lump. D/D: Accessory breast. (*Courtesy:* Dr Sudeb Saha, MS, FAMS)

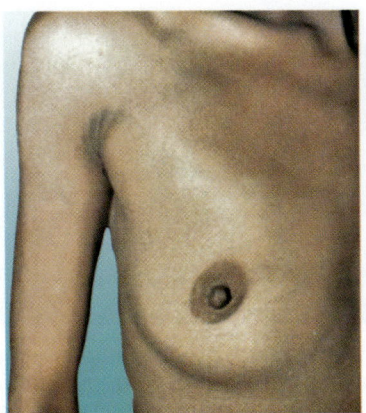

Fig. 2.42A: A soft swelling with indistinct surface lobulation noted over the right infraclavicular region. Margins were ill-defined and slipped under the finger.

SUBCUTANEOUS LIPOMA

Diagnostic criteria

1. Painless, *soft, solid swelling* occurring at the common site between the deep fascia and skin.
2. *Surface usually is smooth and lobulated.* The lobules can be seen and felt on the surface and at the edge of the lump (Fig. 2.42B).
3. Edge is well-defined and may have a series of irregular curves corresponding to each lobule.
4. Overlying skin is free and normal (cf. sebaceous cyst) but may be stretched if the tumour is large.
5. *Slipping sign* – the edge of the swelling slips under the examining finger.
6. Freely mobile on both axes. Not warm or tender.
7. Cutaneous dimples appear on the surface when the swelling is pushed away (due to fibrous strand which traverses the lipoma and is attached to the overlying skin).
8. *Fluctuation – negative*; but due to its soft consistence there may be a false sensation of fluctuation known as *pseudofluctuation.*
9. *Transillumination – negative.*
10. *Usually painless.* When painful and tender, diagnosis of neurolipoma should be considered.
11. *The classical signs of lipoma* such as slipping sign, lobulation and pseudofluctuation *are*

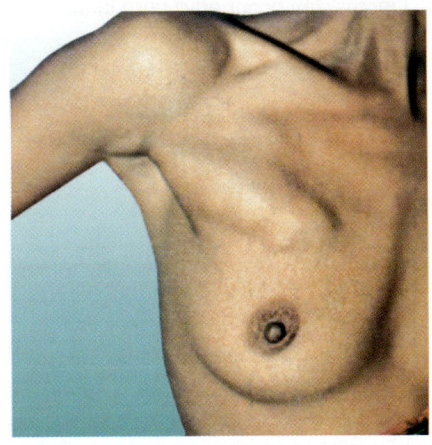

Fig. 2.42B: Same patient. Patient was asked to press on the hip—on contraction of the pectoralis major muscle, the swelling became more prominent. Note the irregular wavy margins and prominence of surface lobulation. The margins slipped under the finger—so the diagnosis was lipoma.

demonstrated in subcutaneous lipoma. Slipping sign and lobulation are not possible to demonstrate in deep lipomas.

Complications

1. Cosmetically looks ugly.
2. Fat necrosis due to repeated trauma – the lump becomes hard and painful. The overlying skin may become tethered or fixed to the underlying area of fat necrosis.

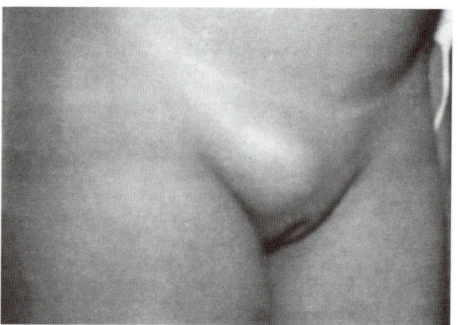

Fig. 2.43: Lipoma right inguinal region. *On inspection—the lump appeared to be inguinal hernia.* But H/O persistent swelling was present. On palpation—a soft swelling; surface was not smooth; the edge of the lump slipped under the finger; there was no cough impulse and the lump was not reducible. So, the diagnosis was lipoma which was confirmed after operation. D/D: Inguinal hernia. Note: Lipoma can occur anywhere in the body.

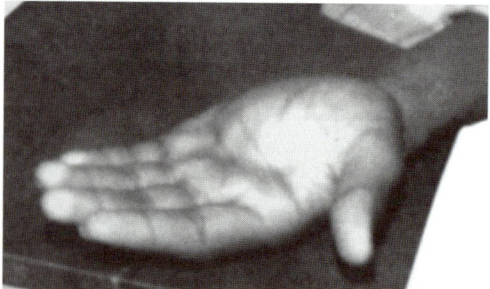

Fig. 2.45: Lipoma in the palm. Firm swelling in the proximal palm. No clinical evidence of median nerve compression (cf. carpal tunnel syndrome). D/D: Tuberculous tenosynovitis.

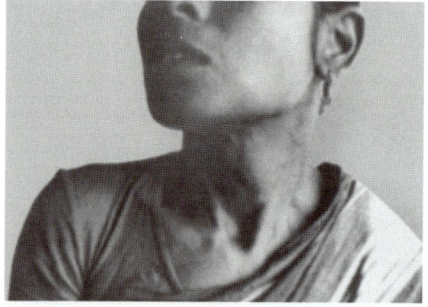

Fig. 2.44: Lipoma in the left neck anteromedial to sternomastoid muscle. On inspection—the swelling looked like left thyroid lobe enlargement. *But upward movement on swallowing was absent.* Moreover, palpation revealed soft swelling with finely lobulated surface and irregular margin. On contraction of the sternomastoid the swelling became prominent and the margin slipped under the finger. So, diagnosis was lipoma and confirmed after operation. Note: Lipoma can occur anywhere in the body.

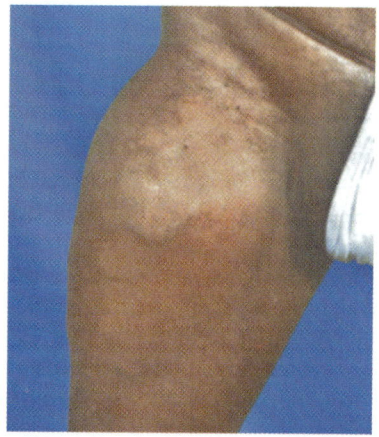

Fig. 2.46: Lipoma or liposarcoma (?). H/O soft swelling in the upper part of the right thigh for many years. The swelling suddenly started to increase in size during last six months with appearance of pain and stiffness more during walking. The lump was firm with ill-defined margins but *became hard and less mobile on contraction of the quadriceps muscle.* So, the diagnosis was liposarcoma which was confirmed after the total excision biopsy of the lump with 1 cm margin clearance. *Patient was referred for radiotherapy.* (D/D: Fibrosarcoma) (cf. Figs 2.24 and 2.25)

3. Calcification following trauma or necrosis.
4. Haemorrhage.
5. Infection.
6. Lipomatosis: Multiple contiguous lipomas may cause huge enlargement and deformity. Lipomatosis may occur in the limbs, neck, trunk and buttocks. Individual swellings within are identical to solitary lipomas.

7. Myxomatous degeneration.
8. Ulceration due to repetitive friction.
9. Presence of lipoma mechanically interferes with muscle movements.

Treatment

Excision, particularly if the lipoma is large, unsightly, or troublesome. If the lump is small,

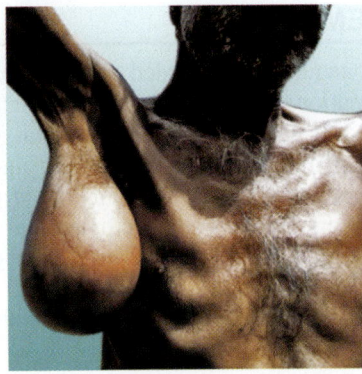

Fig. 2.47: Pedunculated lipoma—right axilla.

excision is done under local anaesthesia. Incision is made along the Langer's line, avoiding crossing a joint line and *intracapsular excision is done.*

Recently, *liposuction is performed for a big subcutaneous lipoma* for cosmetic reasons to avoid big scar.

Characteristics of other varieties of lipoma

Subfascial lipoma: Lipoma may occur beneath the palmar or plantar fascia and is often mistaken as tuberculous tenosynovitis. In the palm it can cause median nerve compression (Fig. 2.45).

Such lipomas may also occur in the areolar tissue beneath the epicranial aponeurosis of the scalp. This can erode the underlying bone and hence can be confused with a dermoid cyst.

Treatment: Early excision.

Intermuscular lipoma: Here lipoma occurs between the intermuscular fibres. Such lipoma becomes firmer on feel when the adjacent muscle contracts. It can cause mechanical interference with movement of the involved muscle. Intermuscular lipoma is mostly common in the thigh or around the shoulder. Fibrosarcoma and liposarcoma are also common in such sites and are difficult to differentiate from this condition clinically.

When the lipoma lies deep to the muscle, the lipoma will become less prominent and less mobile on contraction of the muscle.

Treatment: Early excision to exclude fibrosarcoma/liposarcoma or to prevent mechanical interference.

Subsynovial lipoma: Such lipoma occurs in the fatty pad deep to the synovial membrane. Commonly seen in the knee joint when it should be differentiated from semimembranosus bursa or Baker's cyst. May cause pain and interference in joint movements.

Subserous lipoma: Rare and found beneath the pleura or peritoneum. Retropleural lipoma may present as a benign thoracic tumour. Retroperitoneal lipoma is more common in children than adults, often presents as an abdominal mass and is confused with hydronephrosis, pancreatic cyst, or teratomatous cyst. It may attain a very large size with heterogenous surface.

Occasionally, one may find a lipomatous mass at the fundus of the sac of a femoral hernia or epigastric hernia. This is nothing but condensation of extraperitoneal fat rather than a true lipoma (*see* epigastric hernia).

Submucous lipoma: It may occur in the respiratory tract when it may cause respiratory obstruction, or in the alimentary tract when it may lead to intussusception. It may also occur in the tongue when it can lead to macroglossia.

Extradural lipoma: This is a type of spinal tumour. *Intracranial lipoma does not occur* as there is no fat in the extradural tissue inside the skull.

Intraglandular lipoma: There are three glands in which a lipoma may occur:
• the breast,
• the pancreas, and
• beneath the renal capsule.

Note

• Lipomas never turn malignant.
• *Liposarcoma arises de novo and not in a benign lesion.*
• Common sites where liposarcomas are noted:
  · Retroperitoneum
  · Mediastinum
  · Proximal thigh, buttock or back – particularly intermuscular type
  · Shoulder region

- *CT/MRI:* Confirms the lesion and *moreover delineates the relationship of the lesion with the vessels and nerves* which helps during dissection to save the vital structures.

Note

Synovial lipoma (lipoma arborescens)

Lipoma arborescens is a rare chronic intra-articular lesion characterised by diffuse replacement of synovial tissue by mature fat cells giving rise to prominent villous transformation of the synovium.

Common in knee joint particularly at the suprapatellar bursa. Involvement is usually unilateral and *may cause pain and interference of joint movements.*

HAMARTOMA

It is a tumour-like developmental malformation of various tissues of which the part or the organ is made of. It is characterised by their improper distribution with the prominence of one particular tissue.

The word 'hamartoma' means "missing the mark in spear throwing".

Characteristics of hamartomas

1. Developmental anomaly.
2. Present and often visible at birth.
3. During childhood they grow at the same rate as the surrounding tissues.
4. Enlargement continues until physiological growth ceases (i.e. on reaching adulthood).
5. Some may regress spontaneously when the tumour growth ceases, e.g. strawberry angioma.
6. May be multiple, e.g. neurofibroma.
7. Essentially a benign condition which very rarely undergoes malignant change.
8. *Different types of hamartomas* are found involving the blood vessels (haemangiomas), the peripheral nerves (neurofibroma and its variants), the intestinal tract (congenital polypi), the skin (pigmented naevus or mole), the lymphatics (lymphangioma), and in many other organs. Exostoses, lipoma, thyroglossal, branchial and dermoid cysts are also considered by some as hamartomas.

HAEMANGIOMA

A haemangioma is regarded as developmental malformation of blood vessels rather than a true tumour. It is an example of hamartoma.

It commonly occurs in the skin and sub-cutaneous tissues, but can occur in any part of the body, e.g. lip, tongue, mouth, internal organs like liver, lung, brain, intestine, etc. (*See* Figs 2.48 to 2.60.)

Haemangioma is often present since birth. *It never turns malignant.*

Types

Three types are encountered according to the nature of blood vessels involved:

1. Capillary.
2. Venous or cavernous.
3. Arterial or plexiform.

A pure form is rarely seen and an admixture of different types is common. Clinically, capillary and cavernous varieties are commonly recognised.

CAPILLARY HAEMANGIOMA

This is the one where capillaries proliferate in the superficial dermis, and *tends to occur in the head and neck region and axilla.* This includes the following varieties:

  I. Salmon pink patch
 II. Portwine stain (naevus flammeus)
III. Strawberry haemangioma
IV. Spider naevus.

I. Salmon pink patch

Characteristic features

1. Present since birth.
2. Commonly present as *pink patch over the forehead in the midline, over the occiput, upper eyelid and neck.*
3. The appearance resembles the 'stork-bites' or 'angle kisses'.
4. *Usually disappears spontaneously by the age of one year before the first birthday.*
5. Hence, no treatment is required.

II. Portwine stain (naevus flammeus)

Characteristic features

1. It is a diffuse telangiectasia or dilated blood vessels with *no swelling*, usually seen on the

face, lips and buccal mucosa. It may extend to scalp and neck. *It is a type of haemangioma occurring in the distribution of 5th cranial nerve.*

2. It takes the shape of a diffuse staining of purple or dark red discoloration *flush with the skin, which disappears on pressure.*

3. Present since birth, and it shows no tendency to progress or disappear throughout life, so may persist throughout life.

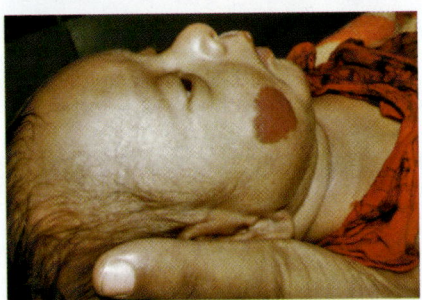

Fig. 2.48: Portwine stain over the right cheek. [*Courtesy:* Dr US Chatterjee, MS, MCh (Paed), MCh (Uro)]

Treatment

It is for removal of appearance causing disfigurement. Spontaneous regression rarely occurs by the age of 7–8 years. So, wait till that age before any intervention.

• *In a girl:* The blemish can be disguised by the skilful use of cosmetics.

• *In a boy:* Excision and skin grafting may be considered.

• Recently argon laser beam treatment is being tried for better cosmesis. It causes superficial destruction of blood vessels. But tried only after 8 years of age.

Note

Naevus flammeus may be associated with specific syndrome like Sturge-Weber, Osler-Rendu-Weber and Klippel-Trénaunay-Weber syndromes.

Sturge-Weber syndrome

Naevus flammeus is associated with a haemangioma of the ipsilateral cerebral hemisphere which may lead to Jacksonian epilepsy and mental retardation with low IQ, glaucoma with loss of vision and buphthalmos. Periodic ophthalmoscopic examination and tonometry are essential. *X-ray skull may show rail road or tram track calcification.*

Osler-Rendu-Weber syndrome

Naevus flammeus is associated with haemangioma of the gastrointestinal tract, urinary tract, liver, spleen and brain.

Klippel-Trénaunay-Weber syndrome

Naevus flammeus is associated with osteohypertrophy of the extremities and AV fistula. The extremity may be slightly enlarged to one that is grotesquely enlarged.

Note

Kasabach-Merritt syndrome: Haemangioma with thrombocytopenia *due to platelet trapping* – usually noted in infants and leads to decreased platelet counts (thrombocytopenia) and may cause life-threatening bleeding problems.

III. Strawberry haemangioma

Characteristic features

1. It is composed of immature vasoformative tissues.

2. Skin and subcutaneous tissues are often involved. Muscle and mucous membrane may also be involved. Submucous variety is prone to haemorrhage which sometimes becomes severe and alarming.

3. Presents with typical history.

   The baby is normal at birth. The lesion appears as a red mark after birth between one and three weeks of age – this red mark increases in size rapidly by the age of a few weeks to 3 months – and ultimately develops into *a strawberry-like swelling* which protrudes from the skin surface. (Strawberry is a fruit.)

   It grows with the child up to 1 year and then it ceases to grow. Then afterwards the swelling may disappear by the age of 7 or 8 years, when involution is complete.

4. Strawberry angioma can occur at any part of the body but are most seen on the head and neck.

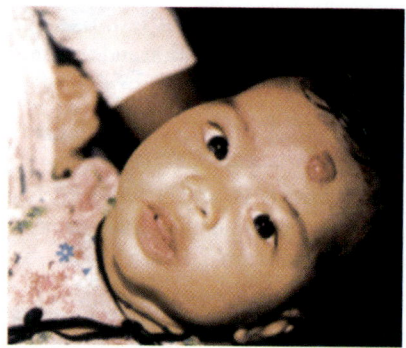

Fig. 2.49: Typical strawberry haemangioma over the forehead. Red colour swelling with nodularity—looks like strawberry fruit. Always wait and watch till 7 years of age and assure the parents for spontaneous regression or resolution.

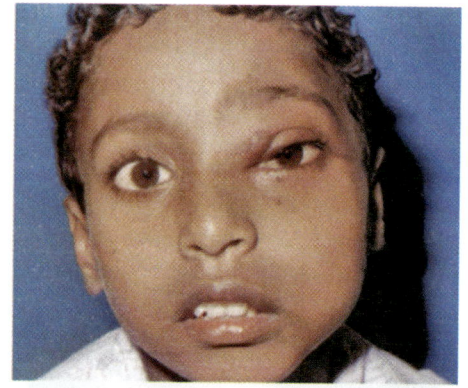

Fig. 2.52A: Capillary haemangioma upper eyelid. Look other parts of the body, e.g. oral cavity.

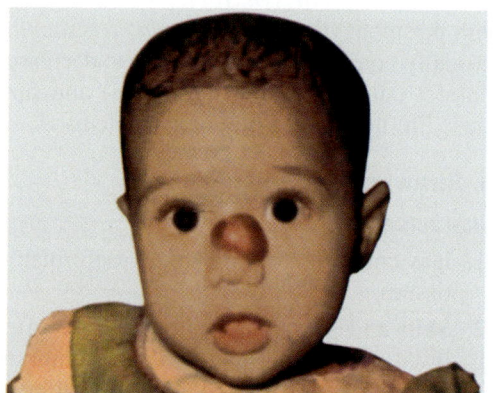

Fig. 2.50: Strawberry angioma over the nose. Usually the swelling disappears by the age of 7 or 8 years. So, better to wait up to that age for natural involution.

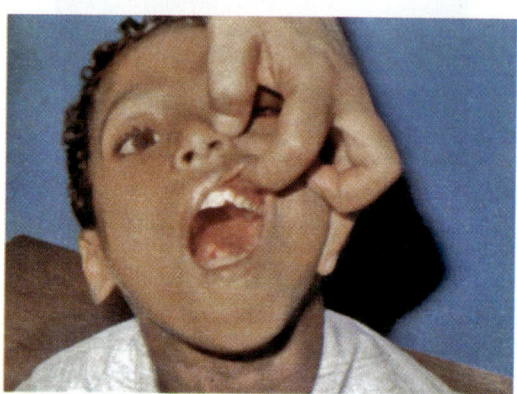

Fig. 2.52B: Same patient. Also haemangioma noted in the palate and upper gum.

5. Bright or dark red, raised, hemispherical swelling, usually 1 to 2 cm in size.

6. *The surface is irregular* and covered with smooth, pitted epithelium. There may be small areas of ulceration covered with scab. Removal of scab may cause oozing of blood.

7. The lesion is *soft and compressible; sign of emptying is present.*

8. The swelling is *not pulsatile* (cf. *aneurysm*).

Treatment

1. Strawberry angioma may resolve spontaneously. So, better to wait up to the age of 7 or 8 years for spontaneous natural involution to get a better cosmetic result.

2. The treatment is indicated when the swelling persists:

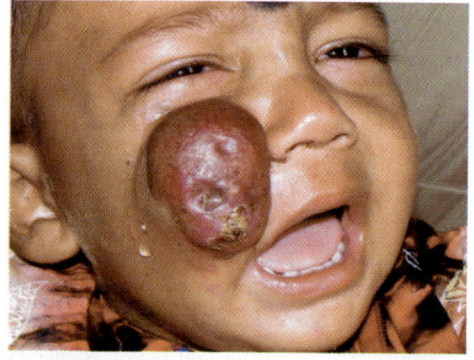

Fig. 2.51: Strawberry haemangioma on the right cheek. Note ulceration over the surface of the lesion.

(a) *Conservative:*
    (i) Application of carbon dioxide snow – cryosurgery.
    (ii) Injection of hot water, hypertonic saline, sclerosant fluid, or steroids.
    (iii) Laser ablation using carbon dioxide or Nd:YAG laser – provides best cosmetic result.
(b) *Operative:* Excision with or without skin grafting for an occasional dark purple overgrown extremity lesion.

IV. Spider naevus

1. It is an acquired condition, mostly found in association with chronic liver disease (e.g. cirrhotic liver). It may occur as an isolated lesion.
2. It has a central red spot (a small dilated skin arteriole) with numerous linear, radiating, fine blood vessels like the legs of a spider.
3. Sign of emptying is present.

Note

Spontaneous regression is seen in two varieties of capillary haemangioma:

1. Salmon patch – regresses by one year of age
2. Strawberry haemangioma – regresses by the age 7–8 years

VENOUS OR CAVERNOUS HAEMANGIOMA

Characteristic features

1. This is due to the congenital multiplicity of venous channels having varying calibre.
2. Relatively uncommon, and present since birth.
3. Usually it shows no tendency to involution. Rather it gradually increases in size and may become troublesome later.
4. It may be associated with a lipoma (naevolipoma). In some cases there may be presence of arteriovenous communications.

Common sites of cavernous haemangioma

1. Anywhere in the skin, commonly of the face, ear involving the deeper dermis and the subcutaneous tissue. Rarely on the trunk.

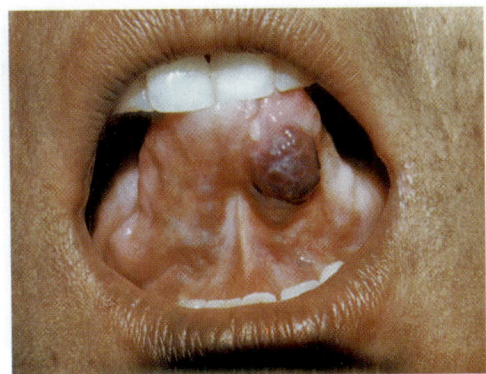

Fig. 2.53: Cavernous haemangioma undersurface of the tongue left side with bluish discoloration. Soft and compressible. Non-pulsatile. (*Courtesy:* Dr S Tibrewal, MS, MRCS, DNB, MNAMS)

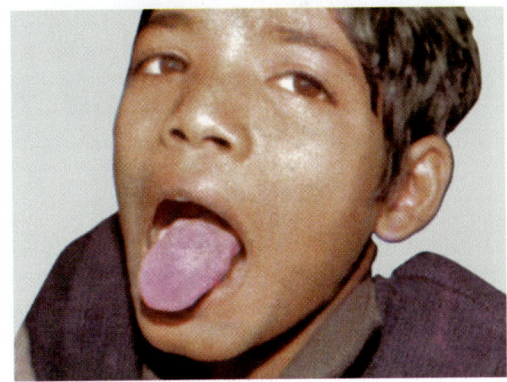

Fig. 2.54A: Cavernous haemangioma on the dorsum of the tongue at the middle—soft compressible swelling.

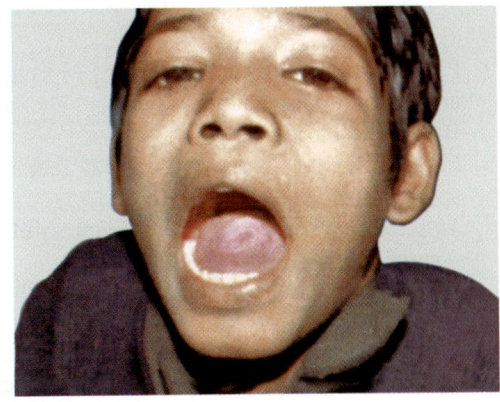

Fig. 2.54B: Same as above. Compression test positive: Sign of emptying is present.

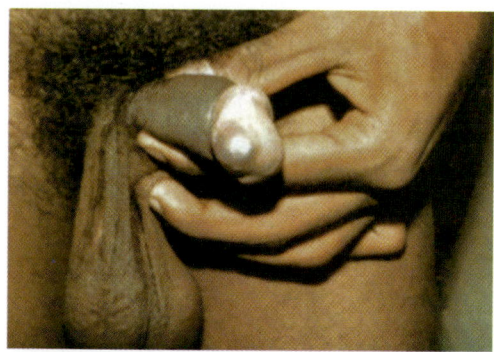

Fig. 2.55: Cavernous haemangioma at the glans penis. Soft, compressible, bluish swelling.

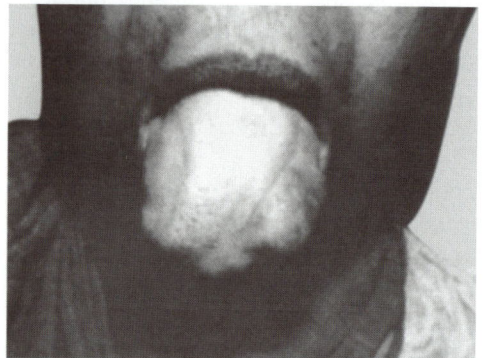

Fig. 2.56: Haemangioma of the tongue leading to macroglossia. (What are the other causes of macroglossia?—*see* Chapter 8)

2. Mucous membrane of tongue, mouth, lips.
3. Internal organs, i.e. liver, kidney, brain, etc.

Diagnostic criteria or cavernous haemangioma

1. Presents as an appreciable swelling or as an area just raised from the surface.
2. Bluish discoloration.
3. Feel – soft, fluctuant swelling. May feel as spongy masses.
4. *May be compressible*. When compressible – *emptying sign is present*.

    Compressibility may be absent over the whole area or over some part if there is associated thrombosis of underlying veins. This thrombosis may be spontaneous or due to the injection of sclerosing agent previously.

5. *Not pulsatile:* Pulsation in such a tumour indicates communication with arterial system.
6. Calcified nodules (phlebolith) can be palpated in rare cases.
7. Does not show any tendency to spontaneous involution.

ARTERIAL OR PLEXIFORM HAEMANGIOMA

This is really a type of *congenital arteriovenous fistula* due to abnormal communication between an artery and vein where the arterial blood flows towards the vein and *the veins become dilated, tortuous and thick-walled* (i.e. arterialisation of the veins).

Example is ***cirsoid aneurysm*** which is commonly found in the scalp (Fig. 2.57) – over the forehead and/or temporal region in relation to superficial temporal artery, *most common vessel involved*. Cirsoid aneurysm is also known as *racemose aneurysm*. Cirsoid means resembling a varix.

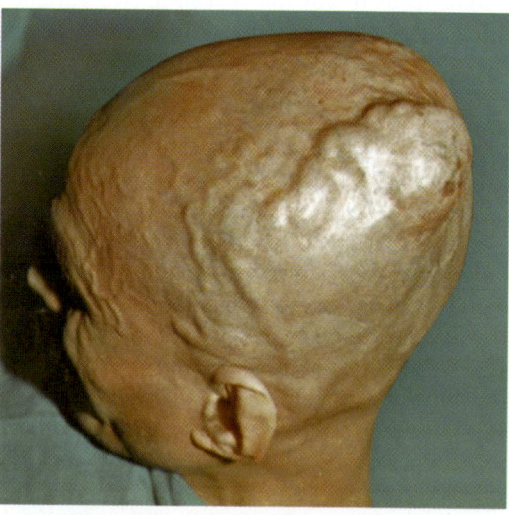

Fig. 2.57: Cirsoid aneurysm over the scalp—left temporoparietooccipital region. Note the dilated tortuous veins over the swelling and also at periphery of the lesion. *Pulsatile and compressible.* Excision of such lesion requires preliminary control and ligation of the feeding artery, e.g. superficial temporal artery and/or external carotid artery. (*Courtesy:* Dr Sudeb Saha, MS, FAMS)

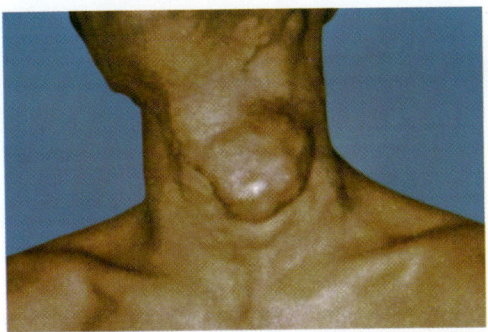

Fig. 2.58: Cirsoid aneurysm over the neck. *Soft swelling feels like a bag full of earthworms. Pulsatile and compressible. Thrill was present.*

Diagnostic criteria

1. Diffuse swelling over the part: Soft and cystic.
2. *Feels like a bag of earthworms.*
3. Swelling is pulsatile and compressible.
4. Systolic thrill and bruit are present.
5. *When in relation to bone,* X-ray may show evidence of osteoporosis or thinning out or destruction of the underlying bone.
6. Colour duplex ultrasound is helpful in diagnosing and detecting the communication between the feeding artery and the veins.

Complications of haemangioma

1. Increase in local warmth or moisture.
2. Atrophy or dystrophy of the overlying skin.
3. Skin discoloration.
4. Ulceration.
5. *Haemorrhage:* Thrombocytopenia is a rare complication and is probably due to increased mechanical destruction of platelets in the haemangioma.
6. Calcification.
7. Thrombosis.
8. Infection may lead to septicaemia.
9. Recurrence (Figs 2.59 A and B).
10. Pressure effects especially in skeletal haemangiomas: Osteoporosis or bony erosion.
11. Diffuse haemangiomatous changes in a growing limb may cause its overgrowth both in length and girth of the limb.
12. At times malignant change – haemangioendothelioma, or haemangiosarcoma.

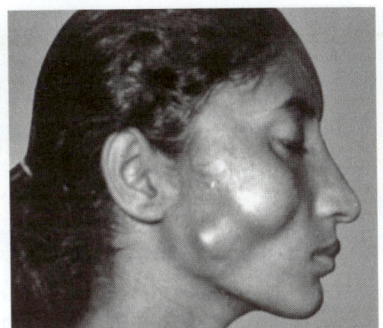

Fig. 2.59A: Swelling on the right parotid region extending to the cheek with narrowing at the middle. Both were compressible. Scar mark from previous operation noted over the lower margin of the swelling—*recurrent haemangioma.* Note: All the swellings over the parotid region are not parotid tumours.

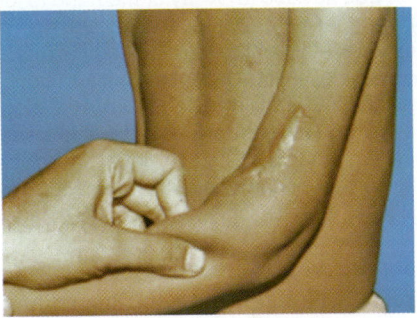

Fig. 2.59B: This patient presented with a diffuse, soft and partially compressible lump on the anterolateral aspect of the elbow extending from the lower one-third of the arm to upper one-third of the forearm. Note the hypertrophied scar from previous operation—*recurrent haemangioma.* There were also some thickened nodules palpable which were due to thrombosis of the incompletely resected veins. Signs of blanching or surface discoloration absent—because of the nodularity. D/D: Neurofibroma.

General plan of treatment of haemangioma

I. Conservative

1. Wait and watch to *expect spontaneous involution,* e.g. *in salmon patch, strawberry haemangioma.*
2. Disguise the blemish (or colour) by skilful use of cosmetics, e.g. portwine stain, particularly in girls.

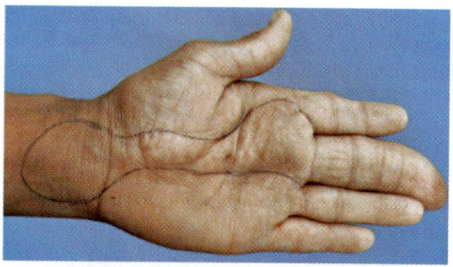

Fig. 2.60: This adult patient presented with *macro-dactyly of the left middle finger* with extended broad linear swelling over the palm which was also extended to the wrist beneath the flexor retinaculum (note the ink marking of the swelling). The swelling clinically was felt like soft spongy mass and *compressible* throughout but *not pulsatile* (cf. cirsoid aneurysm). There were no dilated veins visible over the dorsum of the hand. Cross fluctuation at the wrist was positive. Clinical diagnosis was haemangioma. Patient was advised (a) X-ray of the hand to look for bony changes, e.g. osteoporosis; and (b) colour duplex ultrasound of the hand to know exact cause of the swelling, but the patient did not turn up. Colour duplex ultrasound could be beneficial in the diagnosis of the lesion. This case will be difficult to treat; may require amputation of middle finger in addition to excision of the spongy mass. D/D: Compound palmar ganglion. (*Courtesy:* Dr RL Modak, MS)

3. *Sclerotherapy:* Injection of hot water, or sclerosing agent into the haemangioma. Sclerosing agents are hypertonic saline, hypertonic glucose, etc.
4. *Steroid therapy:* Repeated injection of hydrocortisone into the lesion.
5. Cryotherapy – using CO_2 snow.
6. Nd:YAG laser therapy.

Both are useful with a localised cavernous haemangioma in the facial or intra-oral region. Also valuable for strawberry marks or portwine stain with bleeding and infection.

Surgery is generally avoided and it is the last resort in haemangioma.

II. Surgery

1. If the lesion is localised:
   • Excision particularly by diathermy followed by skin grafting or extensive plastic procedures.
   • Sometimes excision is preceded by an injection of any sclerosing agent which will cause reduction in the size of the lesion.
2. If the lesion is extensive:
   (a) Ligation of the feeding blood vessel preceding excision of the lesion may help in decreasing the size of the cirsoid aneurysm, e.g. ligation of superficial temporal artery or rarely external carotid artery in case of cirsoid aneurysm.
   (b) Therapeutic embolisation of the feeding artery may also decrease, particularly the size of the cirsoid aneurysm.

III. Radiotherapy

Haemangioma is *radiosensitive*, but may result in disturbance of growth, necrosis of the skin, pigmentation, ulceration, haemorrhage, etc.

Radium mould sometimes helps, particularly when surgical access is difficult.

Treatment of cirsoid aneurysm

1. Ligation of the feeding artery followed by excision of the mass.
2. Therapeutic embolisation of the feeding artery followed by excision of the mass.
3. Use of Cryo or Nd:YAG laser knife to obtain a bloodless field of excision of these vascular malformations is being tried recently with good results, providing comfort to patient and surgeon.

Note

Haemangiomas occur most commonly in:
• the cervicofacial region (60%)
• the trunk (25%)
• the extremities

Note

80% of cutaneous haemangiomas are single and 20% are multiple.

Note

Local complications of sclerotherapy
• Blistering
• Necrosis
• Ulceration
• Nerve damage

Note

Parkes Weber syndrome

A complex high flow arteriovenous malformation that involves whole of a limb with symmetric enlargement – the lower limb is affected frequently. The diagnosis is confirmed by the detection of a thrill or bruit over the swelling.

Note

Maffucci syndrome

It is associated with bony exostoses and enchondromas in combination with *exophytic cutaneous venous malformation*. It presents in early to middle childhood life. *The osseous lesions appear first in the hands and feet*, then long bones of the extremities, ribs, pelvis and cranium.

GLOMANGIOMA (*Syn.* Glomus tumour)

It is a benign and circumscribed tumour arising from the 'glomus body'.

What is glomus body?

Glomus body is *a specialized arteriovenous anastomosis* in the dermis surrounded by smooth muscle cells and large pale cuboidal cells known as *glomus cells*, the whole encompassed by a network of medullated and non-medullated nerve fibrils.

Common sites

Most abundantly present in the region of nail-bed, the tips of fingers and toes, and *the palmar and plantar surfaces of the phalanges. May present in the ear.*

Function of glomus body

It regulates the temperature of the skin.

Characteristic clinical features of glomangioma

1. Blue or reddish, circumscribed swelling, rarely exceeding 1 cm in diameter situated in the common sites as mentioned above. It is a benign tumour, grows very slowly and never becomes malignant.
2. *Severe pain: The pain is burning or stabbing or lancinating in nature and radiates peripherally.* The pain may be spontaneous

or *may be caused by the slightest pressure.* The pain may be caused when the part is exposed to sudden change of temperature. *The pain is due to the pressure on the nerve endings by the dilated glomus vessels.*

3. *Two useful signs for diagnosing glomus tumour include* Hildreth sign and Love test.
   - *Hildreth sign* – disappearance of pain after application of tourniquet on the arm.
   - *Love test* – eliciting pain by applying pressure to a precise area with the tip of the pencil.

On histological section: The tumour consists of a mixture of vascular spaces, nerve tissues and muscle fibres derived from the wall of the arteriole (*angiomyoneuroma*). There may be presence of large cuboidal cells (glomus cells), each with a central dark-staining nucleus.

Differential diagnosis

1. Subungual granuloma – chronic infective granuloma from lateral nail fold.
2. Subungual melanoma.
3. Sprouting granulation tissue – due to chronic osteomyelitis of the distal phalanx.
4. Squamous papilloma.
5. Granuloma pyogenicum.

The severe pain of glomus tumour differentiates it from other lesions.

Treatment

Excision of tumour is followed by immediate, complete and permanent relief.

LYMPHANGIOMA

Lymphangiomas, like haemangiomas, are congenital in origin and due to sequestration of lymphatics that retain the ability to produce lymph. They are localised cluster of dilated lymph sacs in the skin and subcutaneous tissues *which fail to connect into the lymph system.*

The lymphangiomas are classified into three varieties:

(a) *Lymphangioma simplex or circumscriptum – capillary lymphangioma:* This superficial variety arises from the cutaneous capillary lymphatics and presents as circumscribed lesion *which appears as small blisters and slightly elevated skin patches.*

(b) *Cavernous lymphangioma:* Lymphangioma arising from the larger lymphatic channels.

(c) *Cystic lymphangioma (cystic hygroma):* Multiloculated cystic lesions composed of many cysts of varying sizes ranging from a few millimetres to a few centimetres. *It is a type of cavernous lymphangioma.*

Characteristic features

1. Developmental anomaly; so, present and often visible at birth. *90% of them can be identified by the end of first year of life.*

2. *Sites:* Usually found at the junction of limbs with the trunk and junction of neck with the trunk, i.e. around the shoulders, axillae, buttocks, groins and at the root of the neck.

3. *Size: Lymphangioma circumscriptum appears as small multiple vesicles,* whereas *cystic hygroma appears as big cystic swelling.*

4. *Colour:* Skin vesicles usually contain clear fluid and looks yellow or watery and translucent. When such vesicles contain blood they turn brown to black.

5. *Consistence:* Soft and spongy. Fluctuation can be elicited in big lesions, e.g. cystic hygroma.

6. *Transillumination:* Positive in big lesions (cystic hygroma).

7. Usually painless lesions. Occasionally, the vesicles may be rubbed with the clothes and get infected and painful.

8. Regional lymph nodes usually do not enlarge until and unless the lesion gets infected.

9. *Treatment:* Excision is the treatment of choice. It can be deferred until the child is several months old to be able to tolerate prolonged anaesthesia.

NEUROMA

Tumour of the nerve is called neuroma. Neuroma is of two varieties – *true and false* (Flowchart 2.1). True neuroma is rare.

According to the source of origin tumours of the nerves can be classified into two main groups:

1. *Tumours arising in connection with the sympathetic system – these are called true neuromas and are very rare.*

2. *Tumours arising in connection with the connective tissue of the nerve sheath – these*

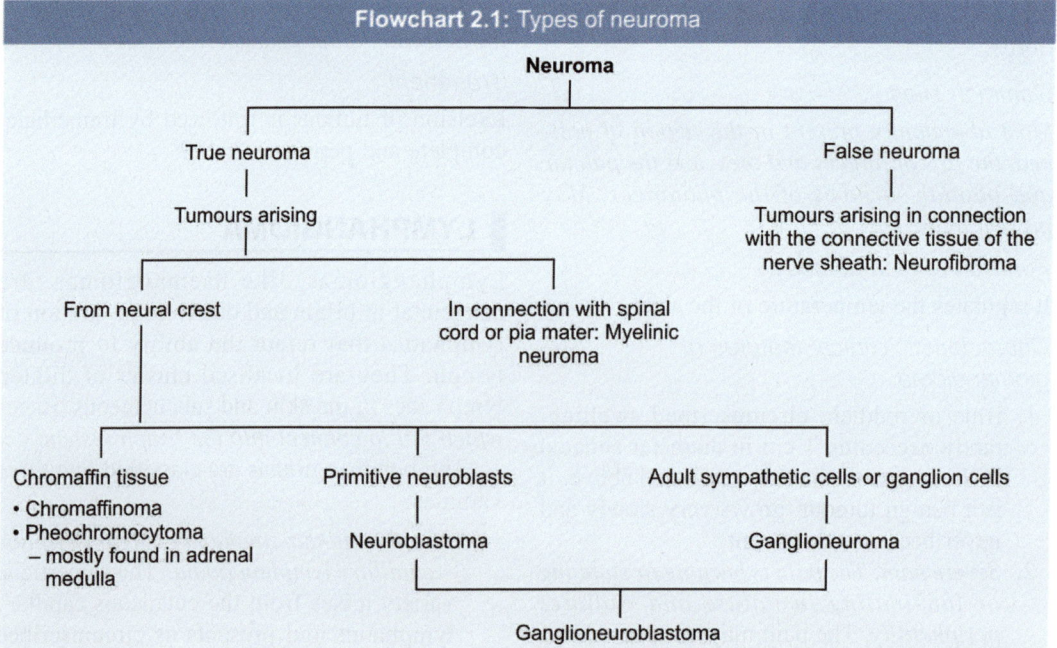

Flowchart 2.1: Types of neuroma

are called false neuromas and neurofibroma is included in these groups.

True neuromas again are of two varieties according to their development from the neural crest. The sympathetic system originates from the neural crest and develops along two lines:

(a) *Chromaffin tissue*, which is mostly found in the adrenal medulla and may give rise to tumours known as *chromaffinomas* or *pheochromocytomas*.

(b) *Primitive neuroblasts* and *adult sympathetic cells*.

Primitive neuroblasts give rise to *neuroblastomas* which have the following features:

• Here the cells are of an embryonic type, i.e. the tumours develop from unipotent cells.
• *Principally found in relation to adrenal medulla.*
• Usually occurring in infants and early childhood.
• *The tumour is usually malignant* and resembles a round-celled sarcoma.
• *Dissemination by blood is the rule.*
• Occasionally, the tumour may undergo spontaneous remission.

Adult sympathetic cells or ganglion cells give rise to *ganglioneuromas* which have the following features:

• The tumour consists of ganglion cells, non-medullated nerve fibres and fibrous tissue.
• *It arises in connection with the sympathetic cord* and hence mostly found in the retroperitoneal tissue or thorax, or in the neck (parapharyngeal mass).
• It may occur at any age.
• *Relatively benign in nature and symptomless.*

Both the neuroblastoma and ganglioneuroma are grouped together under the title 'ganglioneuroblastoma'.

Note

There is another variety of true neuroma known as *myelinic neuroma which consists of only nerve fibres*; the ganglion cells are absent. The tumour arises in connection with the spinal cord or pia mater and is very rare.

Structures developing from the neural crest

1. All the sympathochromaffin cells, i.e.
   (a) Chromaffin tissue
   (b) Primitive neuroblast
   (c) Ganglion cell or adult sympathetic cell
2. Schwann's cell
3. Suprarenal medulla
4. Probably pia mater and arachnoidea mater.

NEUROFIBROMA

Characteristic features

1. Neurofibromas are not real tumours but regarded as *hamartomas*.
2. These lesions arise *not from the nerves proper,* but *from the endoneurium which is a supporting connective tissue for the nerve fibrils or axons.* The nerve fibrils are not involved. *The epineurium and perineurium, the outer layers of the nerve sheath, remain normal.* (cf. schwannoma – derived from the Schwann's cell of the perineurium.)
3. *Majority of neurofibromas arise from the peripheral nerves* and *are present in the skin and subcutaneous tissue.*
4. These can appear at any age but *usually present in adult life.*
5. *Neurofibroma can give rise to neurodeficits, sensory and/or motor, by causing compression of the nerve fibres.*
6. These are due to an autosomal gene defect and are *transmitted as a 'Mendelian dominant'.*

Types

1. Localised neurofibroma or solitary neurofibroma.
2. Generalised neurofibromatosis or von Recklinghausen's disease.
3. Plexiform neurofibromatosis.
4. Elephantiasis neurofibromatosa.
5. Cutaneous neurofibromatosis or molluscum fibrosum.

SOLITARY NEUROFIBROMA

Pathology

1. *Occurring in connection with endoneurium.*

2. Usually found in the skin and subcutaneous tissue.
3. *Usually it grows from a peripheral nerve,* e.g. median or ulnar nerve commonly above the elbow, or *cranial nerve,* e.g. acoustic neuroma.
4. It forms an *encapsulated rounded swelling* lying alongside a nerve, often with the nerve fibres stretched over its surface. The swelling may resemble a fibroma.
5. Histologically long slender cells with elongated nuclei showing palisading arrangements are characteristic features.
6. It may undergo cystic degeneration or sarcomatous change.

Diagnostic criteria (Figs 2.61 A and B)

1. *Subcutaneous nodule:* Smooth, firm swelling in the skin and subcutaneous tissues in relation with the peripheral nerve – peripheral neurofibroma *usually pedunculated and less than 1 cm in diameter.*
2. Margins are well-defined.
3. *Mobility:* Mobile opposite to the axis of the nerve, i.e. in lateral directions.
4. Swelling sometimes becomes painful and tender.
5. There may be a history of paraesthesia or pain and/or weakness (rarely) of the muscles supplied by the nerve because of pressure of the tumour on the nerve fibres which are spread over the surface. (*So always examine the patient for the areas of sensation and for the muscle power supplied by the nerve.*)
6. It may be single or multiple and associated with other types of neurofibromatosis. (*So examine other parts of the body.*)

Differential diagnosis

1. Fibroma.
2. Lipoma.
3. Neurofibroma sometimes undergoes cystic degeneration – so to be differentiated from a cyst.
4. It often simulates enlarged lymph node – particularly when present in the neck.
5. Haemangioma – compressible lesion.

Complications

1. Neurological abnormalities such as paraesthesia and/or motor weakness in the area of nerve supply because of compression of the nerve fibril.
2. Cystic degeneration.
3. Sarcomatous change.
4. Infection.
5. Cosmetically disfiguring.

Treatment

Complete excision of neurofibroma taking care so that the nerve is not injured. *Under no circumstances partial excision is advisable as it encourages sarcomatous changes.*

Often resection of the adjacent nerves along with the neurofibroma may be required which is followed by an end-to-end suture of the divided nerve.

Indication of operation

1. Cosmetically looks ugly.
2. Painful and tender neurofibromas.
3. Producing pressure symptoms by its position, e.g. causing unbearable pain or paraesthesia, motor weakness.
4. Showing evidence of sarcomatous change.

GENERALISED NEUROFIBROMATOSIS OR VON RECKLINGHAUSEN'S DISEASE

Pathology

1. *Multiple and numerous neurofibroma,* occurring in connection with the endoneurium.
2. *This condition often runs in families.* It is inherited as an autosomal dominant disease transmitted by both sexes.
3. More common in males.
4. *It is a genetic disorder.*
5. It may diffusely involve the peripheral nerves, cranial nerves (e.g. acoustic neuroma) and/or spinal nerves (e.g. dumbbell neuroma causing paraesthesia).
6. Sarcomatous changes may occur in 5% cases.

Diagnostic criteria (Figs 2.61 A and B)

1. *Multiple nodules of varying sizes,* from a pea to an orange, are scattered all over the skin surface – face, neck, trunk, and the limbs.

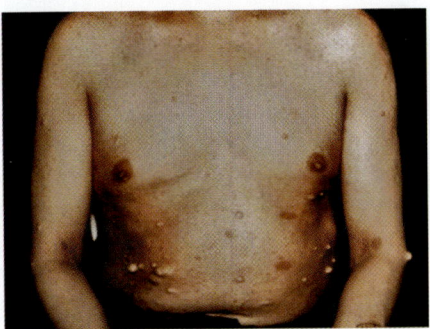

Fig. 2.61A: Multiple subcutaneous nodules over the abdomen and around both elbows—*cutaneous neurofibromatosis*. Look for cafe au lait spots also.

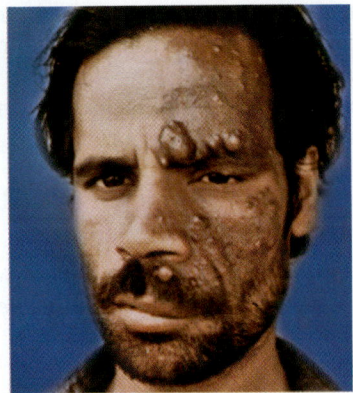

Fig. 2.62: Multiple neurofibroma of the face. Note the pigmentation of the skin (cafe au lait spot) – molluscum fibrosum). Look for lesions in any other part of the body, and any spinal deformity.

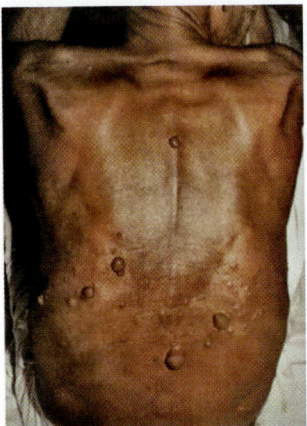

Fig. 2.61B: Multiple neurofibroma involving the back—*cutaneous neurofibromatosis*—molluscum fibrosum. The spine was straight. Examine the spine always for scoliosis or kyphosis as they are very often associated with neurofibromatosis. Look for cafe au lait spots also.

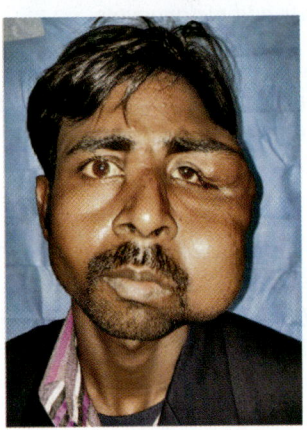

Fig. 2.63: Neurofibroma left side of face with multiple nodules and swelling.

2. The nodules vary in consistency from soft to hard and may be *sessile* or *pedunculated*. In a typical case, the body surface has a '*cobbled-stone*' appearance.

3. There may be *associated pigmentations of the skin*. These are *cafe au lait spots* – the multiple patches of pale brown pigmentation in the skin or over the swelling, look like the colour of coffee diluted with the milk. The pigment is melanin. *Freckling of skin at the arm pit or groin may also be noted.*

4. It may be associated with the *skeletal deformities* namely kyphoscoliosis, defor-mities of the limb, osteoporosis of the bone. Examine the spine and the limbs.

5. Neurological abnormalities may be rarely present. So, look for it.

6. Sarcomatous changes may occur in any of the nodules.

Treatment

The swellings are so numerous that excision of all the tumours is impossible and unwarranted.

Excision sometimes is indicated in the following conditions.

(a) When one of the lumps becomes painful and/ or tender.

(b) When one causes pressure symptoms such as neurological abnormalities commonly paraesthesia.

(c) When one causes mechanical discomfort.

(d) When one becomes large enough and unsightly.

(e) When there is suspicion of malignant change.

Neurofibroma cannot be excised without resecting a segment of the involved nerve. It should be biopsied to ensure that it is not malignant.

Note

The presence of skin pigmentation in some cases of von Recklinghausen's disease is a reminder of the *common neuroectodermal origin of nerve sheath cells and melanocytes.*

Note

Acoustic neuroma involving 8th cranial nerve – patient suffers from hearing loss, tinnitus and vertigo.

Note

Name any other disease under the name of von Recklinghausen's disease

von Recklinghausen's disease of bone: Osteitis fibrosa cystica – found in hyperparathyroidism characterised by a parathyroid adenoma, bone resorption with or without pathological fracture, recurrent renal calculi and peptic ulcer.

PLEXIFORM NEUROFIBROMATOSIS OR PACHYDERMATOCELE (Figs 2.65 and 2.66)

Characteristic features

1. There is excessive overgrowth of endo-neurium of the nerve in the subcutaneous tissue and makes the tissue look oedematous.

2. *Site: Rare condition, usually occurring in connection with the branches of the tri-geminal nerve (5th cranial nerve) in the distribution of face and scalp. It may occur in the extremities, arm or thigh along a group of nerves.*

3. There is myxofibromatous degeneration of the endoneurium of the nerve and the affected nerve becomes enormously thickened.

4. Clinically, *the overlying skin may be thickened,* oedematous, pigmented and adherent, or it may be drawn out and folded. *Sometimes the involved skin hangs down in pendulous folds.* So, the patient usually presents with a mass of soft tissue *hanging like a festoon towards the root of the neck* (pachydermatocele) which cosmetically looks ugly.

5. On palpation it resembles tortuous throm-bosed veins due to the plexiform mass of thickened nerve fibres (cf. haemangioma).

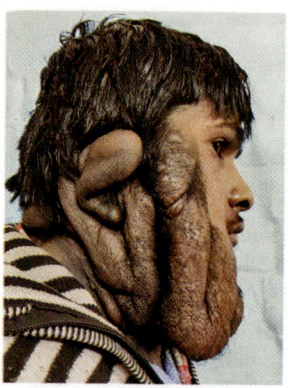

Fig. 2.64: Plexiform neurofibroma involving right side of face, neck and ear lobule—hanging like cartoon or festoon.

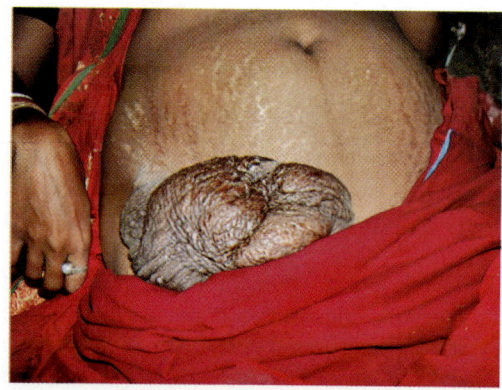

Fig. 2.65: Plexiform neurofibroma over the right groin. Note the pigmented, thickened and corrugated skin folds presented as a thickened, coiled single mass. (*Courtesy:* Dr Diptendra Sarkar, MS, FRCS, DNB)

6. It may be associated with von Reckling-hausen's disease.
7. It may undergo sarcomatous change.

Differential diagnosis

From haemangioma particularly when throm-bosed.

ELEPHANTIASIS NEUROFIBROMATOSA

Characteristic features

1. It is a severe form of plexiform neurofibro-matosis.
2. A rare and congenital condition.
3. *Limbs are common sites*, particularly the lower limb where the subcutaneous fat is replaced by fibrous tissue. When the leg is affected, the patient finds walking increasingly difficult.
4. *Clinically the skin becomes thickened, coarse and dry and looks like an elephant's leg.* The subcutaneous tissue become greatly thickened and the fat is replaced by fibrous tissue.
5. *Usually, it may be confused with the filarial elephantiasis but the lymphatics are normal.*

CUTANEOUS NEUROFIBROMATOSIS OR MOLLUSCUM FIBROSUM

Characteristic features

1. It occurs in connection with the terminal filament of cutaneous nerves.
2. The lesion appears as multiple cutaneous nodules particularly over the chest, abdomen or back.
3. The nodules are multiple, small, discrete, firm, sessile or pedunculated. *But there is no hypertrophy of the skin* (cf. plexiform variety).
4. Pigmentation of the skin may be present.

Complications of neurofibroma

1. *By its position:*
   (a) Acoustic neurofibroma.
   (b) Mediastinal syndrome when found in the mediastinum.
   (c) Dumbbell-shaped neurofibroma.

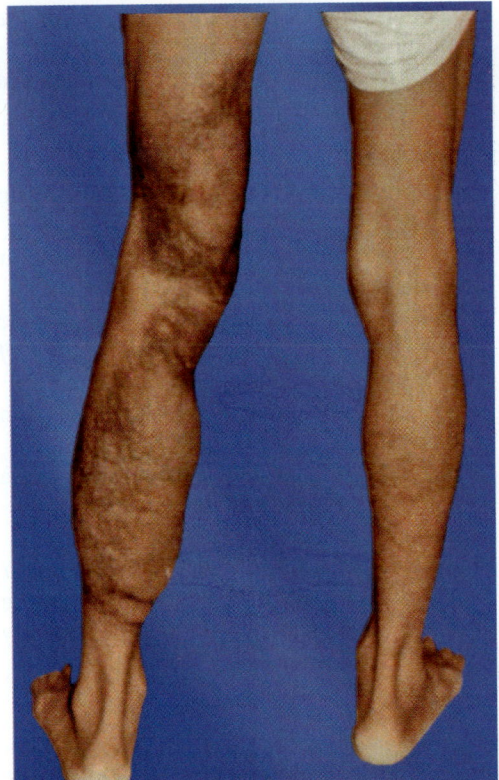

Fig. 2.66: Pachydermatocele or plexiform neuro-fibroma involving the back of the lower one-third of thigh and upper two-thirds of the leg. Look for pigmentation.

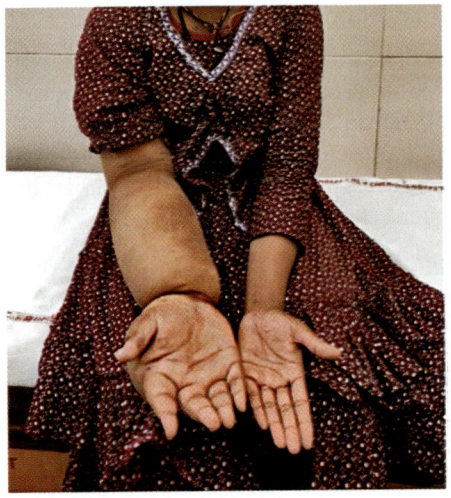

Fig. 2.67: Swelling and hypertrophy of right forearm and hand with pigmentation—neurofibroma.

(d) Abdominal neurofibroma may cause bizarre intestinal symptoms.
2. Sarcomatous change – in 5 to 10% cases.
3. Cystic degeneration.
4. Ugly deformity.

Clinical evidence of malignancy/sarcoma in a neurofibroma

1. Appearance of pain in a painless swelling.
2. Sudden increase in size.
3. Signs of paralysis or anaesthesia in the territory of the nerve distribution.
4. Evidence of increased vascularity.
5. Fixity to the surrounding structures.

RARE VARIETY OF NEUROMA

False neuroma

- Amputation neuroma – end neuroma
- Scar neuroma – lateral side neuroma

Amputation neuroma

- Also known as *stump neuroma or end neuroma*.
- Fusiform swelling occurs at the end of the divided nerve in the stump region after amputation of a limb.
- Commonly seen arising from the sciatic nerve after above knee amputation.
- It is due to outgrowth of nerve fibrils from the end of the divided nerve which becomes attached to the skin, muscle or fibrous tissue of the scar.
- This swelling consists of fibrous tissue and coiled nerve fibres. There is reparative proliferation of Schwann's cells.
- *This neuroma is painful which may be burning or electric shock-like in character. There may be tingling and numbness on pressure over the scar neuroma.*
- *Phantom limb* – patient often experiences false impression of the presence of dismembered limb and also pain in relation to the region.
- *Patient is unable to use the prosthesis because* of the severe pain or discomfort when a prosthesis is fitted over the amputation stump.

Treatment

1. *Preventive:* During amputation, *the nerves* *should be divided above the level of the proposed bone division.*
2. *Curative:* Excision of the end neuroma and refashioning of the scar.

Scar neuroma

- Pathophysiology is same as amputation neuroma.
- It is sometimes noted following chest or abdominal surgery.
- A painful nodular swelling may develop at the site of the scar – *this is due to the formation of swelling arising at the cut end of the cutaneous nerve.* Pathophysiology is same as amputation neuroma.
- The patient presents with pain and paraesthesia along the distribution of the nerve and hyper-aesthesia over the swelling.
- *Ilioinguinal nerve injury during hernia repair and saphenous nerve injury during stripping of the great saphenous vein* may be similarly involved.

Treatment

- Local injection of depo steroid with or without xylocaine sometimes helps to prevent the progress.
- But, in the presence of persistent or recurrent pain, revision of the scar with excision of the neuroma nodule is performed.

Turban tumour

Form of neurofibroma arising from the cutaneous nerves of the scalp. Multiple neurofibromas may form multiple subcutaneous swellings which when coalescing may form a massive swelling which covers the head like a wig or turban, hence, the name 'turban' tumour.

Note

Causes of turban tumour:

1. Multiple neurofibroma
2. Multiple basal cell carcinoma
3. Multiple eccrine spiradenoma

Dumbbell-shaped tumour

It arises from the dorsal nerve root (lying partly outside and partly inside the intervertebral foramen of the vertebral canal giving an appearance of dumbbell). It causes root pain and paraesthesia in the area of distribution. Spinal extension may cause cord compression and paralysis.

Schwannoma (Neurilemmoma)

1. This is a benign tumour arising from the *Schwann's cells* which lies intimately in the nerve sheath surrounding the axon.
2. It usually occurs from cutaneous nerve.
3. May be single or multiple and present as a fusiform swelling in relation with the nerves.
4. The swelling is soft, lobulated and well encapsulated and *is painless*.
5. Benign tumour and does not turn into malignancy.
6. It can also be seen in mediastinum and retroperitoneum.
7. It can be enucleated by incising the nerve sheath without sacrificing the nerve.
8. Amputation may be required for malignant schwannoma.

Acoustic neurofibroma (vestibular schwannoma)

It grows from the auditory nerve (8th cranial nerve) sheath at the internal auditory meatus.

As it arises from the 8th cranial nerve, *the first symptom is unilateral deafness (perception deafness), which is often first detected by the patient on the telephone.* There may be tinnitus, vertigo and severe headache.

Gradually the tumour enlarges and projects into cerebellopontine angle and presses upon the adjacent nerves, e.g.

(a) 7th cranial nerve – causing facial weakness.
(b) 6th cranial nerve – causing squint.
(c) 5th cranial nerve – loss of corneal reflex; there may also be either trigeminal neuralgia or trigeminal anaesthesia.

If it becomes very large, the tumour may press upon the cerebellum and brain stem, producing cerebellar signs and raised intracranial pressure. Often the disease is bilateral.

Treatment

Removal of the tumour through posterior fossa craniotomy.

Note

Sites other than skin where solitary neurofibroma can occur

(a) Dorsal nerve roots and ganglion
(b) Intracranial nerve, commonly 8th cranial nerve – *acoustic neuroma*. May arise from 5th or 9th cranial nerves rarely.
(c) Intramuscular
(d) Inside the bone

Note

Causes of elephantiasis of the limb

1. Filarial elephantiasis
2. Arteriovenous fistula
3. Nodular leprosy – elephantiasis graecorum.
4. Occlusion of previously normal lymph nodes or lymph channels by:
   (a) Surgical procedures (e.g. ilioinguinal node dissection)
   (b) Malignancy
   (c) Radiotherapy
   (d) Inflammation
5. Elephantiasis neurofibromatosa

SCAR

It is a mass of devascularised fibrous tissues and it develops *due to improper management of wound.* An abnormal scar is due to lacerations or improper surgical incisions across the tension lines which disrupt a greater number of collagen fibres leading the wound to gape. *This gape when ultimately heals may lead to several complications.* Malnutrition during the phases of healing also results in scarring.

Complications

1. *Contracture* due to thickening and shortening of collagen bundles leading to the following defects:
   (a) Deformity
   (b) Limitation of movement.
2. *Cosmetically ugly look.*
3. *Adherent scar* which may cause either:
   (a) painful movement or
   (b) some limitation of movement.
4. *Unstable scar or ulcerated scar* due to:

(a) lack of nutrition due to avascularity, and
(b) lack of rest due to repeated movement.

5. *Painful scar* due to involvement of nerve in the scar tissue – commonly found in the scar of amputation stump – *stump or scar neuroma.*
6. Hypertrophic scar.
7. Keloid.
8. Marjolin's ulcer.

Management of scar

Preventive

1. Proper incisions along the tension lines.
2. Excessive tension during the suturing of the wound edges should be avoided.
3. Proper cleansing and dressing of the wound.
4. *Infection of the wound should be avoided.*
5. Early coverage of the raw area by proper skin grafting (as in case of burn). *Ideal skin graft is split skin graft and such free graft should contain some amount of dermis.*
6. By proper positioning of the wound.
7. When the scar is near the joint, *the joint is maintained in a suitable functioning position by proper splintage.*

Curative

By operation.

Indication of operation:

1. Cosmetic (e.g. depressed scar as in small-pox).
2. If there is any complication as already mentioned.

Procedures:

The scar is excised and then the wound is covered by one of the following methods accordingly *depending on the particular site of the scar and the nature of the defect.*

1. Approximation of the edges after mobilisation of the skin margin. Excessive tension should be avoided.
2. Application of free skin graft.
3. By rotation flap.
4. By transposition of flap – the best and usual method is Z-plasty.
5. By pedicle flap.

Problems of operation:

1. The neurovascular bundle is frequently adherent to the scar tissue.

2. When the joint is deformed by the contraction of scar for a pretty long time the neurovascular bundle becomes short and contracted. So, during excision of the scar and correction of deformity, the neurovascular bundle may be injured, or may be stretched or compressed.
3. Moreover, due to prolonged deformity there is secondary contracture of the joint capsule and the surrounding healthy tissue which should be released before closure.

Note

The hypertrophic scar differs from keloid that it never gets worse after 6 months.

POST-BURN CONTRACTURE

It is a contracture of scar developing after burn and occurring usually at the junctional areas, e.g. the flexor aspects of the body involving the nearby joint.

Causes

Post-burn contracture is a sequel to improper management of burn:

(a) *In case of deep burn* involving the full thickness of skin where the subcutaneous tissue is exposed. *So, healing does not take place* by epithelialisation from the margins but occurs by fibrous tissue which when contracting leads to contracture.

(b) *In neglected cases of superficial burn* which undergo infection and ulceration, the superficial burn is converted into a deep one and *so heals by fibrosis.* This fibrous tissue gradually matures and contracts leading to contracture.

Prevention of contracture

1. Proper treatment of superficial burns.
2. Adequate splintage of the part (e.g. a limb) in extension during the process of healing – to avoid development of contracture.
3. *Prevention of infection:* In the presence of infection, the healing is delayed. Moreover, infection causes necrosis of the tissue which is then replaced by fibrosis, and thus adds to scar contracture.

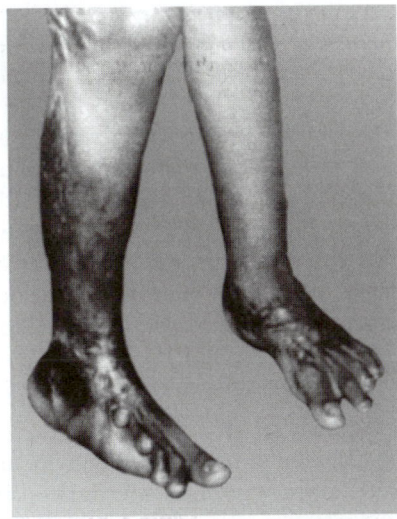

Fig. 2.68: Post-burn contracture involving the right knee, ankle and lateral three toes. There is also hypertrophic scar over the dorsum of left foot.

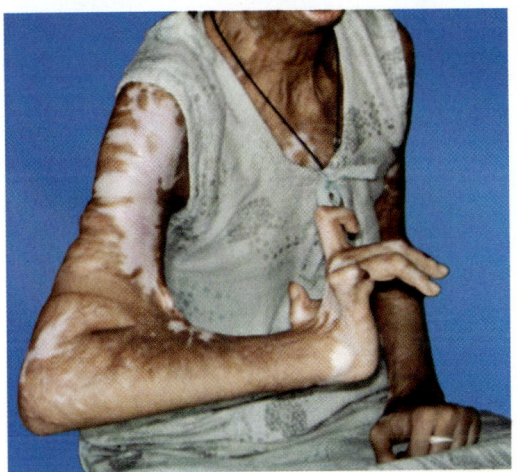

Fig. 2.69: Post-burn contracture involving neck, right axilla, right elbow, right wrist, right thumb and other fingers. Note also the hypertrophy of the scar. This type of contractures require multistage operations.

4. Application of early skin grafting: *The full thickness burn can never heal by marginal epithelialisation, so it must be skin grafted.*

Early skin grafting prevents excessive scarring and so prevents development of contractures. Moreover, early skin grafting prevents infection.

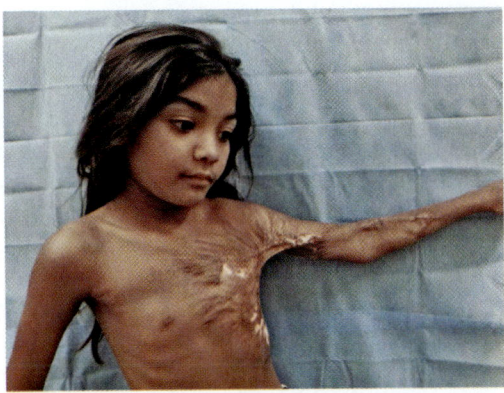

Fig. 2.70: Post-burn contracture involving the left chest wall, axilla, arm, elbow and forearm of a child.

Common sites of post-burn contracture

At the junctional areas such as:
1. Neck
2. Axilla
3. Elbow
4. Wrist
5. Groin
6. Knee
7. Ankle

Complications

1. Deformity and limitation of movement
2. False ankylosis
3. Hypertrophic scar or keloid
4. Marjolin's ulcer
5. Cosmetically ugly look
6. Scars across the joints are usually unstable, and, so, prone to trauma easily.

Treatment

Post-burn contracture should be released particularly to improve the deformity and to increase the movements of the adjacent parts at the junctional area. *May require multistage operations. Also requires postoperative splintage to maintain correction.*

Timing for release operations

The release operation is performed only after the scar tissue has matured. The scar maturation takes about 6 months to 1 year. Mature scar tissue becomes soft and supple in texture *with a whitish hue.*

Method of release

Usually by single or multiple Z-plasty at the point of maximum tension.

- *For neck scar contracture:* The fibrotic scar tissues are incised with multiple Z incisions at the point of maximum tension up to the healthy normal tissue from posterior border of one sternomastoid to the opposite sternomastoid. *Incisions should be deepened up to the strap muscles of the neck.* The neck is extended at its maximum and the raw surface should be *covered with split thickness skin graft* usually taken from the thigh. The neck is then splinted to maintain extension during the healing time.

Problem of anaesthesia in neck contracture

There may be great difficulty during endotracheal intubation which may be managed by one of the following methods.

(a) Fiberoptic bronchoscope is used to allow endotracheal intubation.
(b) Blind nasotracheal intubation.
(c) Alternatively the neck contracture is released partially under local anaesthesia to allow nasotracheal or oral intubation.

- *For contractures of axilla or limbs:* The fibrotic scar tissues are incised by single or multiple Z incisions. The scar tissues are released, the joints are manipulated till the joint deformity is corrected . *The raw surface after correction is covered with split thickness graft.* The limbs are then splinted in corrected positions.

Postoperative splinting to maintain the correction

- Neck – moulded cervical collar for 6 months.
- Axilla – abduction splint for 3–6 months.
- Elbow and knee – static extension splint (functional brace) for 3–6 months.
- Hand – keep the hand in position of function in a glass-holding position for 2–3 months.
  (i) Wrist – in 10–15° extension
  (ii) Thumb – in palmar abduction position
  (iii) Fingers – metacarpophalangeal joints at 80–90° flexion and interphalangeal joints in extension.
- Postoperative physiotherapy under supervision particularly for preventing limb contractures.

HYPERTROPHIC SCAR

A scar is defined as the residual visible mark of a wound.

A hypertrophic scar is characterised by hypertrophy or proliferation of mature fibroblast or fibrous tissue without any proliferation of blood vessels (cf. keloid). It is caused due to some extra stimulus to fibrous tissue formation during healing such as excessive tension, infection, or foreign body response to a suture or other foreign material. *Scars crossing the skin creases are particularly vulnerable to these complications, e.g. flexor surfaces of the body.*

- More common in fair-skinned individuals (cf. keloid more common in dark-skinned individuals).
- Common in female.
- Not familial.

Characteristic features

1. The scar is raised above the surface.
2. Scar surface is glossy.
3. *The hypertrophy is confined to the scar*, i.e. scar hypertrophy does not encroach areas

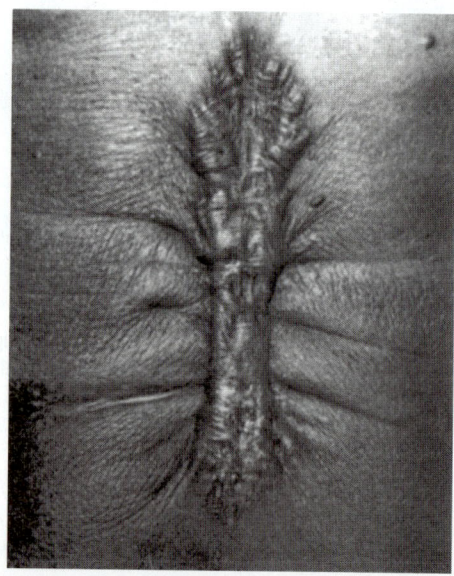

Fig. 2.71: Hypertrophied scar developing on the postoperative scar over the upper abdomen. The horizontal fissures beyond the margins of the scar are due to traction by the scar.

beyond the dimensions of the original wound (cf. keloid).

4. Common over the flexor aspects of the body which tend to be at right angles to skin creases.
5. *No claw-like processes.*
6. No sign of increased vascularity.
7. No itching, no pain or tenderness.
8. It does not spread – it will not extend to normal skin beyond the scar of the original wound.
9. The hypertrophic scar continues to enlarge for about 6 months but regresses after a year to pale, thin, stretched or flat scar tissue. *The hypertrophic scar never gets worse or spreads after 6 months* (cf. keloid). It occasionally may regress.
10. It does not recur after excision if the causative factors are eliminated.
11. Cosmetically looks ugly.
12. *Treatment:*
    • May regress with local steroid application.
    • Excision – *Ideally should be done after 6 months*. Excision of the hypertrophied scar and then closure with minimal tension either by direct suturing or Z or Y-V plasty – recurrence is uncommon.
    • Recently laser surgery with or without silicon gel cover is advocated with better cosmesis.

Note

The hypertrophic scar differs from keloid that it never gets worse after 6 months.

KELOID

Keloid is a tumour-like lesion of excessive scar tissue arising from the connective tissue elements of a scar and *grows beyond the dimensions of the original wound* (cf. hypertrophic scar). *Keloid means like a claw.*

It is characterised by disorderly proliferation of degraded collagen fibrils, immature fibroblast and immature blood vessels (cf. hypertrophic scar).

It shows no tendency to resolve.

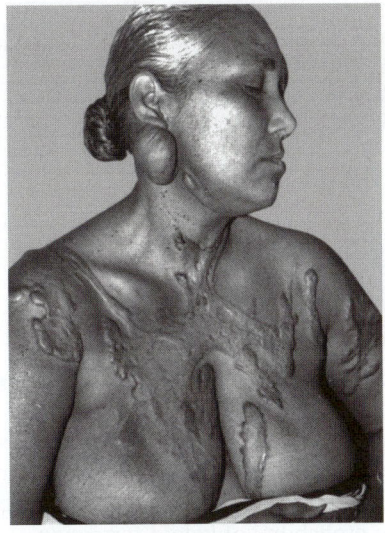

Fig. 2.72: Keloid involving the chest, neck, right shoulder and left arm. Also below and behind the right ear.

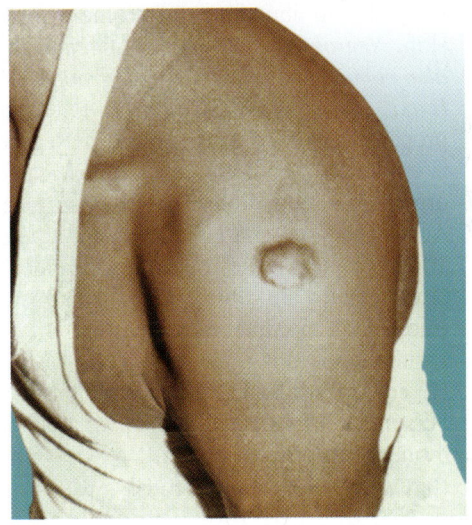

Fig. 2.73: Keloid developing on an injection site. D/D: Implanted dermoid.

Aetiology

Exact cause of keloid formation is not known. Following factors are implicated in the formation of keloid (also of hypertrophic scar).

1. Keloid forms in a scar following surgical incisions, healing burns, radiotherapy and punctured wounds such as BCG (Bacille

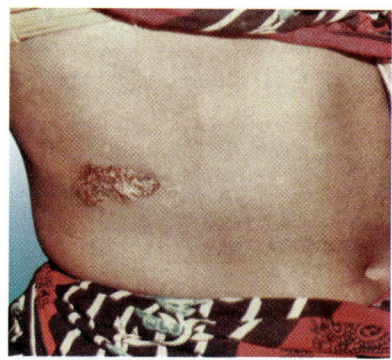

Fig. 2.74: Keloid developing over herpetic vesicles.

surrounding the base of the sebaceous and sweat glands immature fibroblasts proliferate in abundance together with the proliferation of immature collagen fibrils and immature blood vessels beyond and above the wound itself.

Due to proliferation of these cells microscopically it looks like soft fibroma, with the fibroblast disposed in parallel sheets embedded in the stroma of collagen.

Majority of the cells proliferate in claw-like processes to the surrounding tissue, hence the name keloid. Some keloids are, however, non-progressive after initial growth.

It differs from hypertrophied scar by the fact that the lesion extends well beyond the original scar and it may get worse after 6 months.

Due to the presence of plenty immature blood vessels, blanching, oozing, itching and bluish discoloration of the keloid are commonly seen.

Keloid can be considered tumour in the sense that new tissue is formed. But as there is no invasion or distant spread, *keloid is not true tumour.* However, it has a marked tendency to local recurrence after excision like a true tumour.

Types

1. According to the presence of capsule:

    (a) *Progressive:* There are claw-like processes involving the greater area with more itching, oozing and blanching. Here there is no capsule. *The word keloid means claw-like process.* A true keloid continues to get worse even after a year, and some may even progress for 5 to 10 years (cf. hypertrophic scar – which never gets worse after 6 months).

    (b) *Non-progressive:* Usually surrounded by a capsule formed by the compression of surrounding connective tissue. This variety does not grow any further than a certain limit. So, claw-like extensions are not evident.

2. According to the mode of origin:

    (a) *Acquired variety:* Developed after some sort of previous injury.

    (b) *Spontaneous variety:* This variety grows spontaneously. Patient does not give any

Calmette-Guérin) inoculation sites and pierced ears.

Incisions across the Langer's line increase the probability of keloid formation.

2. Extravasation of sebaceous material – *acne keloid.*

3. *Race:* Keloid is more common in coloured races due to abundance of pigment in the skin. *Negroes are commonly affected. It is also common in oriental racial groups. It is least common in Caucasians.* (The propensity of keloid formation in Negroes is exploited by Nilotic tribes of Africa for ornamental decoration of the body surface.)

4. *Age:* Most common in young people aged 10–40 years. They do not form in the elderly.

5. *Sex:* Females are more commonly affected (more so in multiparous women).

6. Familial diathesis.

7. Hereditary influence.

8. Persons suffering from tuberculosis are more prone to suffer from keloid.

9. Rarely regresses spontaneously.

Sites of predilection

The most common site of keloid formation is on the sternum. Keloid also occurs, in decreasing frequency, on the shoulders, neck, face, ear lobe following ear piercing, extensor surfaces of the limbs and on the trunk. *Keloid never occurs on the palms of the hands and on the soles of the feet.*

Pathology

Due to irritation of the mesenchymal cells

history of previous injury (such as pinprick, incision or burn). *This variety usually occurs in the region of the chest and is like butterfly in shape. Spontaneous variety is commonly found in coloured races.*

Diagnostic criteria

1. Common in females. More in blacks.
2. *Common over the sternum.* Other sites are upper arm, chest wall, front of lower neck.
3. The swelling is raised from the surface and freely mobile over the underlying fat.
4. Surface of the swelling is uneven or lobulated with firm thin skin cover with deep cervices in between.
5. Usually there are claw-like processes and so the keloid extends beyond the original scar both in length and in breadth (cf. hypertrophic scar).
6. *Bluish or pinkish in colour.*
7. *Blanching* is present with presence of capillaries at the edge.
8. *Patient complains of itching.* It may be painful and tender.
9. *Oozing of serosanguineous fluid* may be present.
10. Local temperature may be raised.

Differential diagnosis

Hypertrophic scar.

Complications of keloid

1. Cosmetically ugly look
2. Infection
3. Suppuration
4. Ulceration
5. Malignant change on the top of keloid is called Marjolin's ulcer. (Some authorities believe that keloid can never undergo malignancy.)
6. If formed on the flexor aspect of a joint, keloid can lead to contracture and may interfere with mobility.
7. If located in a hairy area, *there may be formation of pilonidal sinus* which then enhances the further growth of the keloid.
8. *Recurrence of keloid – tendency is very high.*

Treatment

Treatment is very difficult. Recurrence rate is very high – more than 50% in spite of different modalities and treatment.

Conservative

Usually it has no role, as the result is disappointing and it does not settle itself. *The patient should avoid scratching.* Conservative treatment includes:

1. Intrakeloidal (intralesional) injection of hydrocortisone. The most effective agent is triamcinolone. The maximum dose is given – 0.5 ml at one site. The solution can be diluted and is injected with an insulin syringe. The injection is continued while withdrawing the needle. Administration should be weekly for 4–8 weeks.
2. Intrakeloidal injection of hyaluronidase – because it might help the dispersion of, or the solution of, the fibroblasts and collagen fibrils.
3. Intrakeloidal injection of vitamin A and/or methotrexate.
4. Parenteral administration of vitamin A.
5. Deep X-ray therapy. The ideas are:
   (a) to suppress the proliferation of immature fibroblasts and collagen fibrils, and
   (b) to suppress the proliferation of immature blood vessels and thus to stop to a great extent itching and oozing.
6. Ultrasonic therapy – recently advocated for hypertrophic scar and keloid with a good result.
7. Laser therapy.
6. Topical methotrexate and vitamin A therapy (retinoids).

Operative

Established keloid (*more than 6 months old*).

Management:

Can be treated by excision.

1. *Preoperative radiotherapy* (4 or 5 sittings are needed).
2. *Intralesional excision of keloid:* Incision is given in such a way as to leave a thin

peripheral rim of keloid. The defect is closed by:

(a) approximation of the margins of the wound by suture, or

(b) application of split skin graft.

Skin grafting should better be avoided, because there is a possibility of keloid formation at the donor site. If skin grafting is imperative, the donor site also should be irradiated as a prophylactic measure against formation of keloid.

3. *Postoperative superficial radiotherapy:* Both:

 (a) to the donor area, and

 (b) to the recipient area.

 Idea of giving radiotherapy – to reduce the chances of recurrence.

4. Laser excision with or without silicon gel cover.

5. Aldara (imiquimod 5%) cream may be used to prevent recurrence after excision of presternal keloid.

PILONIDAL SINUS AND FISTULA

The pilonidal sinus is a subcutaneous track containing hairs or their microscopic fragments. Pilonidal means a nest of hair (Latin *pilus,* hair; *nidus,* nest).

Sites

Pilonidal sinuses are found as small midline pits most often in the natal cleft overlying the coccyx or lower part of the sacrum behind the anal orifice. There may be lateral openings, particularly, if the disease is complicated by sepsis.

They may, however, occur in other regions, e.g. interdigital clefts of barber's finger, the umbilicus, the axilla, the face and amputation stump.

Aetiology

Not definitely known and two theories have been suggested.

(a) *Congenital theory:* When seen in children and young women. It has been suggested *that a developmental abnormality around the*

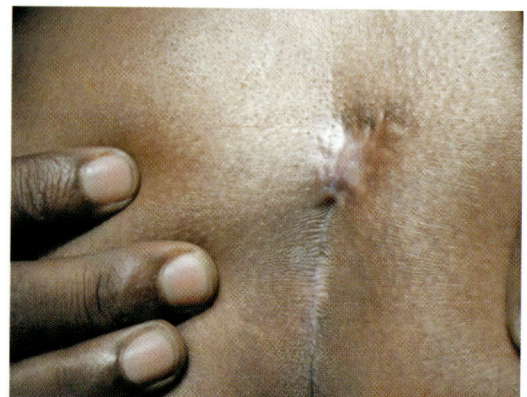

Fig. 2.75: Pilonidal sinus at the upper end of natal cleft with single opening.

sacrococcygeal region leads to the formation of an epithelial lined sinus which grows hairs at puberty. The lesion may be caused by any one of the following ways.

• The origin of the lesion is associated with the neuroenteric canal and is due to blockage of a congenital coccygeal sinus which is a remnant of this canal. *But the squamous lining of the tract contradicts this view and suggests rather an ecto-dermal origin.*

• The lesion may occur as a result of seques-tration or subcutaneous inclusion of epidermal structures due to the faulty fusion of the ectodermal lining at the cleft between the buttocks.

• It may result from excessive traction on the skin caused by the retrogression of the tail bud.

(b) *Acquired theory:* Recently this theory has won a major acceptance and claims that the sinus is nothing more than a foreign body granuloma, *the foreign body being hairs* which penetrate the skin through abrasions, sweat glands or hair follicles. *The reasons in favour of acquired origin of pilonidal sinus* can be summarised as follows:

• The occurrence of pilonidal sinuses else-where – *interdigital pilonidal sinus is an occupational disease of 'barbers'* but the hair within the interdigital cleft or clefts is that of the customers.

- Also the pilonidal sinus may occur in the umbilicus, the axilla, scalp or the face, following sutured lacerations. Rarely noted in the clitoris.
- The lesion occurs most often in the late teens or early adult life and this age incidence is in dissonance with the age of onset of congenital lesions.
- The presence of a granulation tissue inside the sinus track.
- *The sinus is lined by skin.*
- *The absence of hair follicles and sebaceous glands in the walls of the sinus.*
- The hair projecting from the sinus are *dead hairs* and their pointed ends are directed towards the blind end of the sinus. *The hair is the content of the sinus.*
- *The lesion is mostly common in men: Hairy obese men with deep cleft between the buttocks being most frequently affected.*
- Recurrence is common in spite of adequate excision of the sinus track.
- The condition rarely occurs in blondes.

Mode of origin of acquired pilonidal sinus

It is due to entrapment in the natal cleft of shed hairs of local origin or from the nape of the neck and subsequent penetration of the same in this region either through the intact skin via the openings of sudoriferous glands of the natal cleft or the raw skin due to fissure, abrasion, dermatitis or pustules. The embedded hair within the skin of natal cleft sets up chronic infection resulting in an abscess or a sinus. *Shedding of hairs is much augmented by the shearing strain in the buttock when one sits on a hard seat particularly in a moving vehicle for a prolonged period and shearing of hairs, subsequent entrapment and penetration are much more frequent in those who use toilet paper after evacuation.* Once a sinus has formed, there is possibility of other loose hairs being sucked into the pit by the intermittent negative pressure of the area.

The pilonidal sinus was *common among the jeep drivers in army* and has been referred to as 'jeep-driver's disease' by army surgeons: *Occupational hazard.*

Pathology

The sinus extends into the subcutaneous planes as a bulbous diverticulum with or without branching side channels.

Lining of the tract

Usually stratified squamous epithelium.

Contents

1. Granulation tissue.
2. Epithelial scales and debris.
3. Hairs: *These are dead hairs* and are found either:
   (a) lying loose in the sinus;
   (b) embedded in the granulation tissue; or
   (c) deep in the mature scar tissue.

Microscopically

Foreign body giant cells are commonly present.

Diagnostic criteria

1. *Age:* Common in late teens or early adult life.
2. *Sex:* Males are more commonly affected. Many of the patients are exceptionally hairy and are usually obese and overweight.
3. *Ethnic group:* More common in dark-haired hirsute men. The condition rarely occurs in blondes. Common in obese men.
4. *Occupation:* Common in 'jeep drivers' in army. *The hair here is from his own natal cleft.*

   Barbers may present with pilonidal sinus in the webs between their fingers. *The hair here is from the client.*
5. Presence of an infected cyst, sinus or sinuses in the midline in relation to the skin dimple at the tip of the coccyx, i.e. at the upper end of the cleft between the buttocks.
6. The sinus may have one or multiple openings and on gentle probing, the sinus passed upward and forward towards the sacrum.
7. Presence of a tuft of hairs projecting from its mouth.
8. The sinus may be discharging and the discharge from the sinus is either serosanguineous or purulent, and may be bloodstained. The discharge may be foul smelling due to sebum and may contain hairs.

9. Pain and/or tenderness at the bottom of the spine.
10. Occasionally the patient may present with an abscess when the mouth of the sinus is blocked.

Investigations

1. A sinogram may be done to identify the ramifications and their relationship to the underlying bony structure.
2. MRI may help to identify the topography of the lesion.
3. C&S of the discharge.
4. Investigation to exclude tuberculosis.
5. Biopsy of the excised tissue.

Complications

1. Recurrent inflammation.
2. Recurrent abscess formation.
3. Recurrence of sinus: Recurrence is probably due to the following reasons:
   (a) Inadequate excision: A diverticulum of the main tract has been overlooked at the primary operation.
   (b) Entry of new hair through the scar or skin.
   (c) If the natal fold is deformed by scarring after operation, the least trauma may cause tearing of the scar, and the resulting cervices may be contaminated with coliform and cutaneous bacteria, which lead to the formation of a dermal abscess and later a sinus.
4. Osteomyelitis of sacrum/coccyx.
5. Rarely squamous cell carcinoma.

Differential diagnosis

1. *Fistula-in-ano: In pilonidal sinus there is absence of an internal opening in the anal canal. The sinus tract also passes upward and forward towards the sacrum and not towards the anal canal.*

   In fistula-in-ano the opening is in between the tip of the coccyx and anus. *On probing, the tip of the probe enters the anal canal.*
2. *Sinuses secondary to suppuration of post-anal dermoid:* Here the opening of the sinus is in front of the sacrum and coccyx *and not*

behind. Rectal examination may reveal a cystic swelling in front of the sacrum deep to rectal mucosa.
3. Perianal suppurative condition.
4. Infected sebaceous or dermoid cyst.
5. Hidradenitis suppurativa.
6. Osteomyelitis of coccyx or sacrum.

Treatment

No single method of treatment is entirely satisfactory. The most effective treatment is complete excision of all the sinus tracks together with all their ramifications.

Operative treatment should be carried out at a time when the acute infection is quiescent.

To facilitate the excision, methyl blue may be injected as a guide to determine the extent of arborization of the sinus tract.

Following excision of the sinus, closure of the wound may be accomplished either primarily or by secondary intention. *So methods of treatment include:*

(a) *Excision of the sinus and primary closure:* An elliptical incision is used and the sinus and its ramifications are excised along with all the debris and hair. *The defect is then closed* either by suture, split-skin graft or Z-plasty or Rhomboid Limberg flap. The disadvantage of the primary closure is that there is a chance of haematoma formation and subsequent infection.

(b) *Excision of the fistula and closure by second intention:* Following excision, proper haemostasis is secured by diathermy and catgut ligature. The wound is then not sutured but kept open followed by regular packing with iodine or EUSOL gauze pieces and thus allowed to granulate and heal by second intention. This method is preferable in the presence of any infection.

(c) *Fistulotomy:* Laying open of the track and its ramifications and removal of all debris and hair followed by suturing of the edges to the skin (*thus marsupialization of the sinus*). Free drainage is thus established. *This procedure yields a good hairless scar.*

Prognosis after surgery is excellent. Recurrence or persistent disease is likely to be due to inadequate excision or missing of occult tracks.

Conservative approach of Maurice

The sinus tracks can be destroyed by careful installation of *full strength pure phenol by means of a syringe and needle* until the tracks are full and overflowing. The area is then squeezed until all phenol and debris are extruded and a second injection of phenol is repeated, which is also squeezed out. This approach may be repeated.

Treatment of pilonidal abscess

Incision and drainage is advised as a preliminary step to control overt sepsis before definitive surgery is planned.

Postoperative measures

1. Avoid prolonged sitting, e.g. driving a car for a long distance.
2. The site must be kept free of hairs by shaving or by using a depilatory cream to prevent further incursions of hair in future.
3. Reduce body weight and obesity.
4. Use of epilatory creams or lotions.
5. Avoid long distance drive at a stretch.

Note

Other sites of pilonidal sinuses are:

Umbilicus → Axilla → Clitoris → Scalp following sutured lacerations → Interdigital clefts of barber.

▌BASAL CELL CARCINOMA (BCC)

Syn. Rodent ulcer.

• It is a *slowly growing but locally invasive skin tumour* arising from the *pluripotential basal cells* of the epidermis of the skin. *Basal cells are present in the deepest layer of the epidermis.*
• It may also arise from the outer root sheath of hair follicles, sweat glands and sebaceous glands (pilosebaceous adnexa).
• It may be single or multiple.
• It is locally invasive.

• It is called **'rodent ulcer'** because the ulcer grows by burrowing the deeper tissues like a rat (rodent – a rat).
• The tumour spreads radially for an extended period of time before developing a vertical growth phase.
• It is also called **'field-fire type of cancer'** because it is found in some cases that the ulcer tends to heal at one place while breaking out in the adjacent area, i.e. *like field-fire, ulcers spread centrifugally.*
• Common in fair-skinned people.

Sites

1. It is one of the commonest tumours of the head and neck. *Face is the common site because it is mostly exposed to ultraviolet rays of the sun. Majority of the lesions occur on the face above an imaginary line joining the angle of the mouth and the lobule of the ear.* 90% of basal cell carcinomas are seen on the face.

   So, the commonest sites are:

   • on the nose;
   • near the inner and outer canthi of the eye;
   • on the cheek near the nasolabial fold;
   • on the forehead, particularly in females.

   It is also called **'tear cancer'** because it is commonly found along the region on the face where tears roll down.

2. Rarely it may occur on the other parts of the skin surface, i.e. on the other parts of the face, neck, scalp (specially the forehead and temple), pinna, very rarely on the trunk and limbs.

3. BCC at the centre of face, postauricular region, pinna and forehead are more prone to recur.

4. Very rarely it may occur on the squamous cell mucous membrane, e.g. tongue, oesophagus and anal canal.

Predisposing factors for basal cell carcinoma

• *UV light (most important):* Exposure to ultraviolet radiation (actinic rays) is the main cause of BCC. DNA present in the skin cells is damaged when UV rays hit the skin.

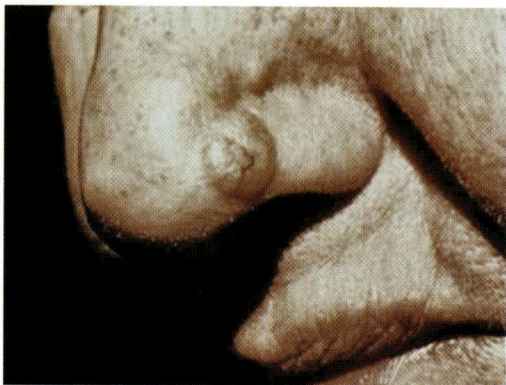

Fig. 2.76: Nodular type of BCC on the left alae of the nose.

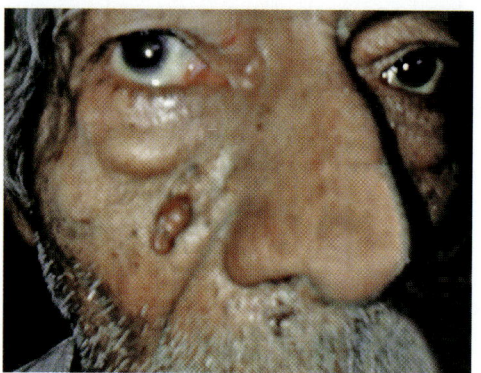

Fig. 2.77: Plaque type of BCC beside the right naso-labial fold.

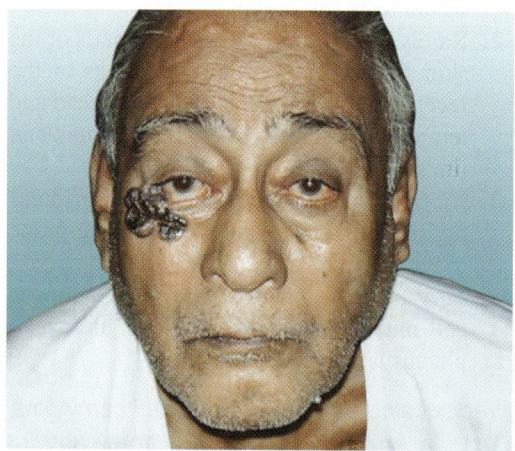

Fig. 2.78: Pigmented plaque type of BCC just below the right lower eyelid near the outer canthus. Note that all pigmented lesions are not melanoma.

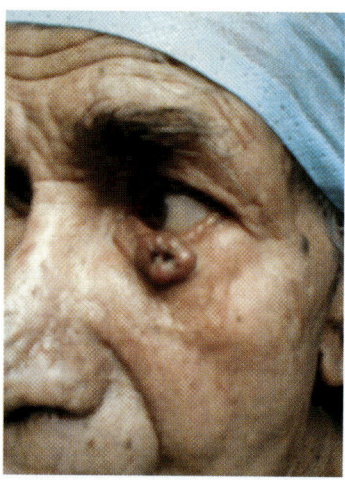

Fig. 2.79: Ulcerative type of BCC on the left lower eyelid near inner canthus. *Note the beaded appearances on the upper raised margin of the ulcer.*

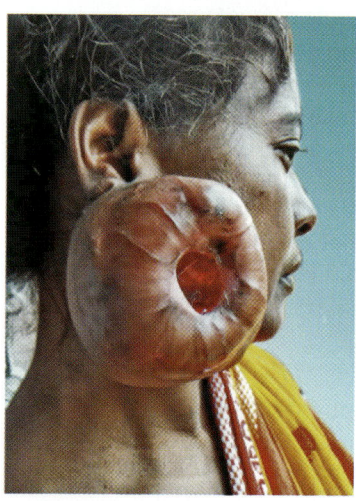

Fig. 2.80: BCC over the right parotid region of face. Note the fine blood vessels over the raised nodular margin of the ulcer.

- Arsenical compounds
- Coal tar
- Aromatic hydrocarbons
- Infrared rays
- Genetic skin cancer syndrome

Aetiopathology

1. It is a *low grade malignancy*. It arises mainly in late middle life, i.e. at or above 40 years of age.

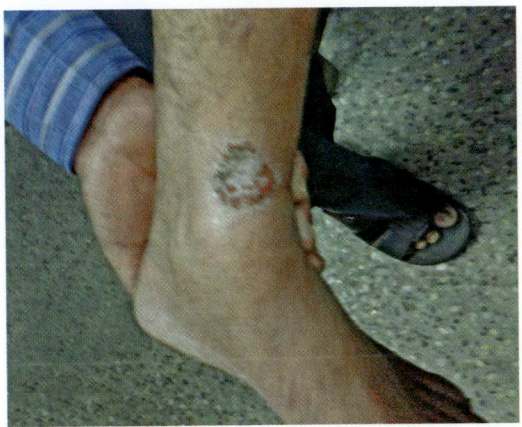

Fig. 2.81: BCC: Medial surface of the left leg—nodules at the margin.

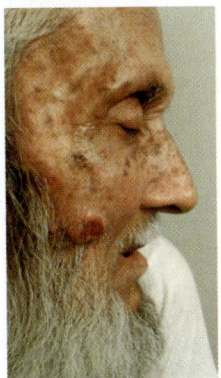

Fig. 2.82: BCC with nodules at the raised margins of the ulcer—over right cheek.

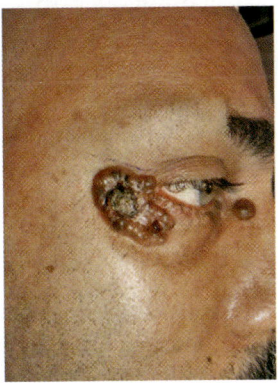

Fig. 2.83: BCC with pigmented nodular margin lateral to the outer canthus of the eye. Note also another pigmented nodule near inner canthus of the eye.

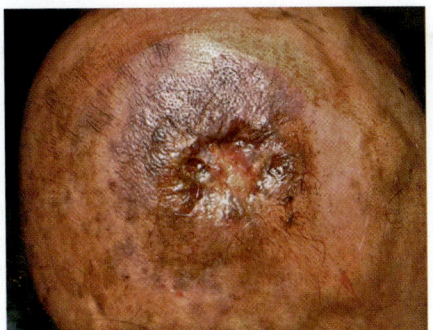

Fig. 2.84: BCC over the scalp.

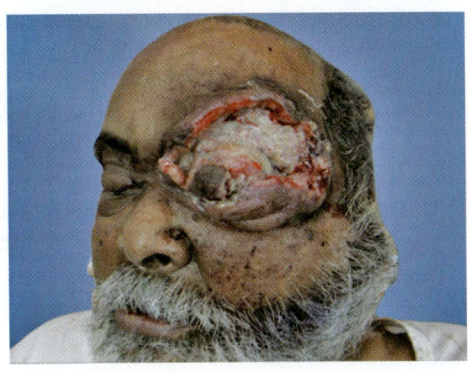

Fig. 2.85: Ulcerative type of BCC (rodent ulcer) extensively involving the left eye. *Both the burrowing (rodent)* and *spreading (field-fire)* characters were evident in this lesion. D/D: Seborrheic keratosis, keratoacanthoma, amelanotic melanoma and infected haemangioma. (*Courtesy:* Dr S Tibrewal, MS, MRCS, DNB, MNAMS)

2. *It affects males more than females.*
3. It is *prevalent in white-skinned people* in tropical regions due to extensive exposure to sunlight or actinic exposure (UV rays). *So particularly prevalent in Australia and New Zealand.*

    It is also *common in people suffering from xeroderma pigmentosa* due to inadequate repair of DNA after sunlight-induced injury.
4. It is *a very slowly-growing tumour* and often the lesion has been present for two or even three years before any treatment is sought.
5. It occurs in those parts of the skin which are unprotected from bright sunlight of high actinic value, *that is why face is common site.* There is often an *occupational factor –*

agricultural workers, fishermen and dedicated sunbathers being more prone to this lesion.

6. The tumour is frequently multiple. The multiple growths may be confined to one area, or they may occur in different areas.

7. The multiple basal cell carcinomas particularly develop in persons *who have an arsenical dermatitis* following the prolonged administration of arsenic. *Arsenic was once commonly used in skin ointments.*

Types

1. *Nodule:* Solid, non-fluctuant pearly swelling but may look cystic. Nodular and nodulo-cystic variants account for 90% BCC.
2. *Plaque:* Firm, raised and red or pink plaque.
3. *Ulcerative*
4. *Field-fire type*
5. *Morphic type* (rarest) appearing as red raised plaques or streaks surrounded by scar. Most aggressive type.
6. *Pigmented BCC:* Dark brown colour mimicking a melanoma; very rare.

Description of a typical lesion

At its inception it lies deep to the epidermis and *at this stage it appears* as a firm pearly papule or a flat or slightly raised plaque *with telangiectasia,* or a dark cystic swelling *with or without tiny venules coursing across the surface.*

Sooner or later the covering epidermis over the centre gives way and *the growth takes the form of an ulcer* with the following characteristic features:

1. *Edge of the ulcer* is raised and rounded but not everted. *The rolled edge may be beaded with pearly opalescent nodules.* Sometimes one edge of the ulcer undergoes partial healing while it is extending at another edge for a time, but later breaks out again. Initially the shape is circular but as the growth spreads the shape of the ulcer becomes irregular (*field-fire type*).
2. *Floor of the ulcer* first superficial, then becomes deep and even proceeds up to bone. Central part of the ulcer may show temporary evidence of healing by formation of a scab, but this scab goes on forming and breaking down. The scab is formed of dried serum and epithelial cells. If it is picked off, the floor will bleed slightly.

If the ulcer erodes deeper structures, the floor is covered with poor quality granulation tissue.

3. *Base of the ulcer* is indurated but less pronounced or barely perceptible, and may be fixed or freely movable over the deeper structures.

Histopathology

- It is composed of closely packed islands or nests of uniform basophilic epithelial cells (basiloid cells) disposed in rounded masses or columns set in a stroma of cellular connective tissue.
- Central cells are polyhedral containing large basophilic nucleus.
- The peripheral cells are columnar, more deeply staining and have a palisade nuclear arrangement (i.e. perpendicular to the surrounding connective tissue). *The most characteristic histological feature of BCC is nuclear palisading.*
- Prickle cells and cell nests are absent (cf. SCC).
- Mitotic figures are usually absent. Stromal component is composed of chronic inflammatory cells and benign fibrovascular tissue.

Spread

- *Local spread:* By direct infiltration *superficially* very common, or *deeply* to involve the other adjacent structures (e.g. cartilage, bone) is *very common.*
- *Lymph spread:* Lymph node metastasis, either regional or distant, is *very rare* even in a growth of long standing.
- *Blood spread: Extremely rare.*

Differential diagnosis

Seborrheic keratosis, keratoacanthoma, amelanotic melanoma, infected haemangioma.

Investigations

- In a small tumour less than 1 cm in diameter – *excision biopsy* is preferred which provides both tissue diagnosis and cure at the same time.

- In a larger lesion – *wedge biopsy* from the edge of the tumour or ulcer to confirm the diagnosis.
- X-ray of the lesion to look for bony erosion.

Treatment

1. Radiotherapy
2. Surgery – the treatment of choice
3. Other methods

Radiotherapy:

- *BCC is highly radiosensitive with 90% cure rate.*
- Superficial radiotherapy using 40–60 Gy (4000–6000 rads) after preliminary biopsy and histological proof will cure over 90% of the lesions. *Fractional doses over a few weeks* decrease scarring and necrosis. In elderly patient with a low risk of second malignancy, radiotherapy is ideally indicated.
- The tumour may be so small that biopsy and cure are identical – *the operation is called excision-biopsy. So, radiotherapy is avoided.*

Contraindication of radiotherapy:

1. Adherence to bone or cartilage, e.g. over the nose or ear because of the high chance of subsequent necrosis of cartilage or bone.
2. Lesions very close to the eye to prevent radiation damage to eye.
3. Lesions on the back of the hand are also best avoided by the radiotherapist.
4. Exposure to extreme cold (as in Arctic regions) – as the exposed irradiation scars are very much prone to frostbite.

Surgery – the treatment of choice:

Indications:

1. The causes where radiotherapy is contra-indicated – as mentioned above.
2. Recurrence after radiotherapy.
3. Appearance of a new lesion closely adjacent to previously treated areas, either by radiotherapy or by surgery.

Principle:

Adequate excision of the lesion *with a clear margin of at least 3 to 5 mm and more* where possible *as a fusiform eclipse.* Adequate excision should also take account of the depth.

Reconstruction may be by simple direct suture or may need the use of split or full thickness skin grafts, to cover the defects.

In larger, neglected and deeply invasive lesions – plastic reconstruction by rotation or advancement flaps or pedicle grafts may be required, for better cosmetic results.

Other methods of treatment:

Recently, in some centres, the following methods are practised particularly in places where multiple tumours are common. *The available methods are:*

1. Curettage followed by diathermy for lesion <1 cm in diameter.
2. Cryosurgery with liquid nitrogen at –196°C. Specially useful in elderly patient for small lesion.
3. *Laser beam destruction:* Nd:YAG or carbon dioxide laser. Useful for superficial BCC confined to the epidermis and papillary dermis.

   Disadvantages of these three methods are:

   (a) They destroy more tissues than are needed and thus result in retardation of healing.
   (b) They do not provide a tissue diagnosis.
   (c) They are not suitable for lesions situated over a bone or cartilage.

4. *Mohs micrographic surgery:* Recently tried for *BCC of less than 2 cm in diameter in the areas of eyelids or nose* – microscopically controlled tissue sparing surgery done in stages for better cosmesis. Cure rates of BCC treated by this technique are 99%. Indication for use of this technique – scar morpheaform of sclerosis of basal cell carcinoma. *Clinically suspected bone invasion is a contraindication to this technique.*

5. *Local chemotherapy* has been practised for some years in many centres – (i) *5-fluoro-uracil cream* is applied locally, and it is a simple and safe procedure particularly in flatter lesions, but recurrence is frequent, probably due to residual disease in the depth. (ii) *Immiquamod 5% (Aldara)* – local application 3 times per day for 6 weeks – histologically proven clearance rate is 75–80%.

Treatment of recurrence
Immediate excision of the lesion.

BASISQUAMOUS CARCINOMA

It is a condition where histological features of squamous carcinomatous changes are seen often at the edge of a basal cell carcinoma.

This type of lesion occurs more often in recurrent lesion or in the skin damaged by previous radiotherapy. It has higher growth rate as well as higher metastatic potential.

The lesion is more necrotic, friable and edge of the lesion is moist.

Lymphatic metastasis is a common possibility.

Diagnosis is confirmed only after biopsy.

Treatment should be done along the lines of squamous cell carcinoma.

CYLINDROMA (*Syn.* Turban tumour)

- *A peculiar benign variant of BCC. Also known as trichoepithelioma.*
- Generally seen over the scalp.
- Appears as multiple translucent cylinders, *forming an extensive turban-like swelling over the scalp* with little tendency to ulcerate.
- Less aggressive and carries better prognosis.
- Occasionally malignant transformation may occur.

Treatment
Adequate excision. The resultant defect is covered by a free skin graft or a flap.

Note
Other causes of turban tumour are multiple sebaceous cysts, multiple neurofibroma.

Note
BCC does not occur in mucosal areas which do not have pilosebaceous adnexa, i.e. in lip, tongue, cervix uteri, glans penis (cf. SCC).

Note
It may be associated with hereditary Gorlin's syndrome. This syndrome presents with numerous BCC tumours.

Note
BCC and SCC have been linked to chronic sun exposure typically in fair-skinned people.

Note
Recently Mohs micrographic surgery is also being tried in SCC and melanoma.

Note
Therapies currently used for BCC offer 85–95% cure rate.

Cause of death in BCC
- Direct intracranial extension by infiltration (Fig. 2.85).
- Erosion of major blood vessels.

KERATOACANTHOMA

- This is a *self-limiting* benign superficial cutaneous growth arising from the follicle-bearing area of the skin.
- It is a *self-healing nodular lesion with central ulceration.*
- *Etiology* – not clear; may be caused by papilloma virus infection of the hair follicle and is associated with smoking and/or exposure to chemical carcinogens or sun rays.
- It presents as a *cup-shaped growth that exhibits symmetry at the margin with a central crater filled with a plug of keratin.*
- *Margin of the swelling is not beaded (cf. BCC).*
- Common in white-skinned elderly men and *usually form on the face.* Size is between 1 cm and 3 cm.
- *It usually resolves spontaneously over 6 months after a rapid growth phase. Removal of the central keratin plug hastens the speed of resolution.*
- *Differential diagnosis:* Basal cell carcinoma, squamous cell carcinoma. So, some surgeons prefer *elliptical excision biopsy* which also results in better scar formation.

LEUKOPLAKIA

- Presents as elevated white papular lesion on the lip, cheek, gum, palate and tongue.

- *Predisposing factors* – smoking, tobacco chewing, gutka, Pan Bahar which are kept inside the oral cavity for longer time; sharp/septic tooth.
- Premalignant condition for SCC.
- An edge biopsy of the lesion may be done to exclude development of malignancy.
- Early symptoms are minimal. So, these are frequently ignored until pain and/or fibrosis develop leading to difficulty in speaking or eating.
- *Treatment:*
  - Immediate stoppage of smoking, chewing of tobacco, pan masala, betel quid, gutka.
  - Plenty of cabbage, spinach and carrots provide β-carotene and vit. A which reduce the oral leukoplakia and mucosal dysplasia.
  - Immune stimulants such as levamisole, Immumod found to be useful in the long run.
  - Close follow-up is necessary and repeat biopsy may be useful in the long run.
  - Excisional surgery is rarely needed if edge biopsy is negative for SCC.

SQUAMOUS CELL CARCINOMA

Syn. Epithelioma, epidermoid carcinoma. It is a malignant tumour arising from the squamous cells. *Second most common type of skin carcinoma.* Squamous cells are the uppermost lining of the epidermis.

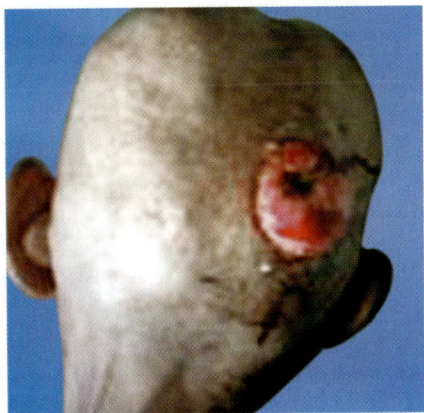

Fig. 2.86: Squamous cell carcinoma over the occipital region of the scalp—proliferative type with surface ulceration.

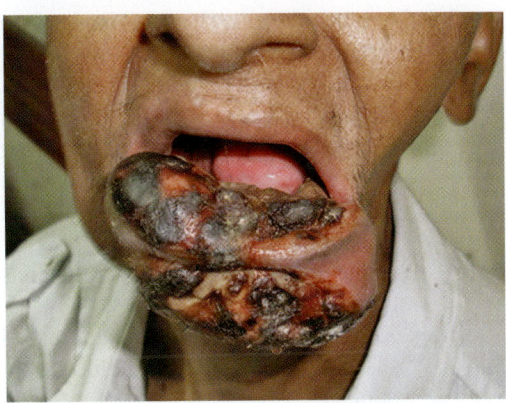

Fig. 2.87: SCC: Involving the lower lip and infiltrating the chin also.

In the case of skin, it is the prickle cell layer (keratinizing cells of epidermis and its appendages) from where squamous cell carcinoma arises.

Sites

1. *Any part of the skin or its appendages covered by stratified squamous epithelium,* e.g. in face, pinna, dorsum of the hands, palm, sole, etc.
2. *Junctional region of the skin and mucous membrane-mucocutaneous junction,* e.g. lip, penis (corona glandis), anal region, vulva, etc.

Aetiopathology

1. It usually occurs in elderly subjects.
2. It affects males more than females.
3. It is relatively common in white-skinned people in tropical regions due to excessive exposure to ultraviolet rays (of sunlight) especially during childhood. *In sunlight-induced cancers, ultraviolet-B rays are more carcinogenic.* So, common in fair-skinned people in Australia where people like to take prolonged sunbath on the seabeach for tanning of the skin.
4. It is more malignant and more rapidly growing than basal cell carcinoma.
5. *Origin:*
   (a) *De novo*, i.e. it may arise in a previously normal area exposed to prolonged sunlight (UV light).

(b) *On some preexisting skin lesion:* Premalignant lesions of the skin, e.g.
- Senile (or solar) keratosis.
- Bowen's disease – erythroplasia of Queyrat – carcinoma *in situ* occurring over glans penis: Lesion appears as reddened, scaly, slightly raised plaque.
- Leukoplakia.
- Lupus vulgaris (a type of cutaneous tuberculosis).
- Xeroderma pigmentosum: increased susceptibility to sunlight-induced skin damage.
- Chronic ulcer of long-standing, e.g. venous ulcer, burns, old scar or keloid, chronic discharging osteomyelitic sinus causing chronic irritation (Marjolin's ulcer).
- Radiodermatitis following irradiation.
- HPV5 and HPV16 virus infection. Commonly spread by sexual contact. May lead to genital warts or cancers of cervix, vagina, vulva or anus following anal sex, throat following oral sex.
- Chronic irritation of the skin such as following.
  - *Prolonged industrial exposure to certain chemicals (carcinogens),* e.g. pitch, tar, soot, dyes, arsenic and psoralen.
    Scrotal cancer was once common in workers of chimney sweeps (*chimney sweep cancer*) due to prolonged contact *with carcinogenic soot*. It still occurs in workers whose clothes become soaked in shell oil or creosote oil, pitch or paraffin tar, cotton oil (in cotton spinning mills).
  - Continuous application of heat by a charcoal burner (Kangri) to the abdomen, lower back of the body or back of the thighs may cause typical *Kangri cancer of Kashmir.* Kangri is an earthenware filled with burning charcoal. Kashmiris keep the Kangri on their abdomen to keep themselves warm. The warming appliance is also known as Kairo in Japan and Kung in China.
  - Sleeping on oven bed, which is often a habit of Tibetans, may cause *Kang cancer of back and buttocks, heels and elbows.*
  - Intensive use of arsenical preparations such as Fowler's solution for psoriasis of skin.
- Heavy alcohol and tobacco abusers.
- **Khainy** (mixture of tobacco and lime), *gutka* may develop SCC of mucocutaneous junctions especially lip and buccal areas.
- Mixture of betel nut and lime with *Pan; Pan Bahar/Pan masala.*
- Chutta cancer inside the mouth – common in persons who smoke with the lightened end of the *cigarette* or *biri* inside the mouth particularly after taking country liquor or Tari.
- Balanoposthitis – chronic irritation by the smegma collected in the preputial sac may cause carcinoma of penis.
- Mechanical – chronic irritation of gums and margins of tongue from ill-fitting dentures.
- Infections – secondary to chronic HPV viral infection. HPV16 and HPV18 most common subtypes *implicated following sex.* Most commonly a verrucous growth on the penile shaft, external labia, cervix or in the periungual region, anus (after anal sex), mouth and throat (after oral sex).

Progress

A squamous cell carcinoma may be invasive *ab initio*.

Occasionally, however, dysplastic changes occur in skin epidermal cells, which later progress and present with all the features of malignancy *with the exception of invasion. This later condition may involve any squamous epithelium, but is particularly common in the larynx or cervix and is called carcinoma-in-situ or intraepidermal carcinoma.* The latent period to the development of invasive cancer in such patients appears to be of the order of 10–20 years.

Types

1. Ulcerative type – common.
2. Proliferative type – exophytic or cauliflower type arising as a mass.
3. Ulceroproliferative.

Description of a typical ulcerative lesion such as occurs on the lip (see also chapter on carcinoma tongue and lip)

To start with, there is a slight thickening or a small nodule which breaks down to form an ulcer. *This ulcer refuses to heal and is covered with a crust.* Then, as the disease progresses, the ulcer becomes irregular and has the following characteristics:

- *Edge of the ulcer* is rolled out and everted.
- *Floor of the ulcer* is covered by greyish white necrotic slough, dried serum and blood. There may be pale unhealthy granulation tissue.
- *Base of the ulcer* is indurated and may be fixed to the deeper structures. In early stage, the ulcer can be moved freely with the skin over the underlying muscles and bone.
- The ulcer may bleed to touch (bleeding ulcerating nodule is seen more commonly in SCC than in BCC).
- Painless initially but later becomes painful as it invades the deeper structures.
- Enlarged lymph nodes may sometimes be the presenting feature before the primary tumour is noticed.
- Surrounding tissues look normal apart from adjacent inflammation.

Histopathology

It is composed of solid, irregular strands and columns of invading epithelium which infiltrate the subjacent connective tissue. In a well-differentiated case there is the presence of '*cell nests*' or *epithelial pearls of central keratin* surrounded by *large peripheral eosinophilic or prickle cells in a concentric manner like onion peel*. These cells may show signs of malignancy (hyperchromatic nuclei, loss of polarity, mitotic figures).

What are 'cell-nests'?

Epithelial cells of epidermis proliferate into the dermis in columns separated from one another by the connective tissue. In course of time the central cells, being the oldest, undergo some degenerative changes as found in normal surface epithelium and are finally converted into a hyaline structureless mass of keratin – *epithelial pearls (cell nests)* look red after eosin stain. This process is called keratinization or cornification. This is surrounded by large peripheral prickle cells in a concentric manner giving an *onion-peel appearance. These peripheral cells may show signs of malignancy.*

Peculiarities of cell-nests

1. *Well formed cell-nests in a squamous cell carcinoma indicate:*
   - a relatively slowly growing tumour;
   - high degree of cell differentiation;
   - poor sensitivity to radiotherapy.
2. Squamous cell carcinoma without cell-nests, but consisting of ill-differentiated or undifferentiated prickle cells with high mitotic figure, indicates:
   - a rapidly growing tumour;
   - sensitive to radiotherapy.
3. *Cell nests may be absent in a squamous cell carcinoma,* e.g.
   - in a rapidly growing or well-advanced tumour;
   - in the oesophagus and bladder, where cornification does not normally occur.
4. *Cell-nests may be found rarely in some lesions other than squamous cell carcinoma,* e.g.
   - pleomorphic adenoma of the parotid gland;
   - teratoma of the testis.

Microscopically

- *Carcinoma-in-situ:* Intraepithelial or pre-invasive.
- *Invasive carcinoma: Malignant cells invade the basement membrane* to involve the deeper connective tissue and muscles.

Spread
- *Local spread* – by continuity and contiguity into the surrounding tissues is generally slow.
- *Lymph spread* – by permeation and embolism reaching the lymph nodes, usually in the late stage. *Lymph node involvement varies with the site of the primary lesion.*
  1. It is common in cancer of the foot.
  2. It is frequent in cancer of the face or neck.
  3. It is late or absent in case of the hand of an old person, in case of a scar, or chronic ulcer.
  4. *It is absent in Marjolin's ulcer.*
     Less than 5% cutaneous SCC metastasize to lymph nodes.
- *Blood spread* – occurs only in very advanced stages to the lungs.

Differential diagnosis
1. Keratoacanthoma
2. Pyogenic granuloma
3. Amelanotic melanoma
4. Seborrhoeic keratosis

Note

Involvement of lymph node reduces survival considerably.

Note

Lymph node spread may be absent in following situations.
- When the lesion is developing in scar and chronic ulcer (Marjolin's ulcer).
- SCC in old age.

Note

Distant metastasis is likely to occur from SCC in scars and ulcers *even though lymph nodes are not involved.*

Note

SCCs on vulva and penis behave in a more aggressive fashion and thus have worse prognosis.

Investigation

To confirm diagnosis, *an incisional or wedge biopsy is taken from the edge of the ulcer or tumour,* i.e. from the junction of the tumour and normal skin. *The reasons for taking biopsy from the edge are:*

1. The edge is the growing part, so malignant cells are plenty.
2. Biopsy from the centre of the lesion may show only necrotic tissue.
3. Comparison with the normal skin is possible.

   For lesions ≤1 cm in diameter: Excisional biopsy is preferred which provides both tissue diagnosis and cure at the same time.

Other preoperative investigations
1. X-ray of the affected part to rule out bony involvement.
2. X-ray of the chest to rule out metastasis (though rare).
3. Routine preoperative investigation.
4. Role of FNAC for lymph nodes is limited since negative report has no value.

Treatment

I. Treatment of the primary lesion.
II. Treatment of the secondary lymph nodes.

Treatment of the primary lesion

Radiotherapy
- *Superficial radiotherapy after adequate biopsy and histological proof will cure over 80% of early lesions.*
- Radiotherapy is applied in the form of deep X-ray therapy, electron beams or local methods such as radium implants and moulds.
- *Radiotherapy is indicated in early lesion,* i.e. well-differentiated tumour with margins free of tumour.
- RT is also considered *when genital mutilation is undesirable in a young man with carcinoma penis.*
- *Radiotherapy is contraindicated* in certain areas such as:
  - Pinna, where radiation necrosis is a frequent and painful sequel.
  - Scalp, where radiation causes wide depilation, so this area is a cosmetic indication for surgery.
  - Lesion close to the eye.
  - Lesion involving underlying cartilage and bone.
  - Verrucous carcinoma.

Surgery

Indication

1. Lesions are large in size.
2. Involvement of the muscle, cartilage or bone.
3. Lesion close to the eye.
4. Lesion in the scalp, pinna.
5. Recurrence after radiotherapy.
6. Meagre facilities of radiotherapy, particularly in our country.

Principle

1. *Wide excision of the growth* with a margin of 1 to 2 cm of normal healthy tissue all around from the probable indurated edges of the tumour up to the deep fascia.
   Reconstruction: The resulting defect may be closed by simple direct suture of the apposed skin margins. *If the defect after excision is large*, split or full thickness graft may be required to cover the defect. Rotational flaps or pedicle grafts may be tried for better cosmetic result.
2. Amputations may be necessary in carcinoma of finger, toe or foot involving bones and tendons with one joint above.
3. Amputation of penis in carcinoma of penis.
4. Lesions of the ear are treated with wedge excision when possible.
5. Mohs microscopic surgery provides a cure rate for SCCs of 94–100% and has been of particular value in SCC with perineural invasion.
6. Circumcision for tumours confined to the foreskin.

Note

Genital mutilation is undesirable in a young man with carcinoma penis.

Treatment of the secondary lymph nodes

1. *Clinically no palpable nodes:* Regular observation is needed. *If nodes appear*, radical block dissection is to be performed after FNAC/FNAB of lymph nodes.

   In some centres, in absence of clinically palpable enlarged lymph nodes particularly in penile (or vulval carcinoma) without waiting for observation, SLNB is performed to note the presence of lymph node metastasis, if positive lymphadenectomy is performed.

2. *Lymph nodes are palpable but discrete and mobile:* It may be reactive due to infection rather than involved by metastasis.
   So, a course of antibiotics is given preoperatively for 3 weeks, and observe:
   • *If the nodes disappear or diminish in size* – suggestive of infective origin. So, no further treatment, but regular observation is required.
   • *If the nodes remain unaltered* – suggestive of malignant involvement. So radical block dissection is to be performed after FNAC/FNAB.
3. *Lymph nodes are palpable, hard, mobile* and are suspected of being involved due to metastasis – *radical block dissection is to be performed after nodal biopsy.*
4. *Regional LN dissection is only indicated for clinically positive nodal disease* or *lymphatic basin that is positive after SNL biopsy.*
5. *Lymph nodes are palpable, hard and fixed* – palliative external radiotherapy is given to palliate pain, fungation and bleeding.

   Chemotherapy has not been useful for the treatment of SCC.

Prognosis of SCC

1. *Size of the lesion* is the most important determinant of outcome of patients with SCC. *Lesions >2 cm* have a higher rate of regional recurrence and greater incidence of regional metastasis.
2. *Depth of invasion:* Tumours >4 mm depth of invasion have 5% risk of metastatic spread.
3. *Regional LN metastasis* occurs in 2–18% of patients with SCC and correlates with tumour size and differentiation. *Lymph node involvement reduces the survival rate considerably.*
4. *Perineural invasion* is associated with increased incidence of local recurrence.

Note

Variants of squamous cell carcinoma

1. Occult primary SCC may arise on sites other than skin.

- *On the mucous surface covered by stratified squamous epithelium*, e.g. glans penis particularly with phimosis and recurrent balanoposthitis – chronic irritation by smegma collected in the preputial sac may cause SCC.
- *On the columnar cells* undergoing metaplasia, e.g. (i) gallbladder with chronic cholelithiasis; (ii) bronchus with chronic and recurrent bronchitis.
- *On the mucous surface covered by non-stratified squamous epithelium*, upper air or nasopharyngeal passage, buccal cavity, oesophagus and uterine cervix.
- *On the papillary transitional cells* undergoing metaplasia, e.g. urinary bladder, pelvis of the kidney due to chronic irritation by a calculus.

2. *Verrucous carcinoma:* A slowly growing papillomatous mass seen on the sole of the foot or cheek – well-differentiated masquerading as a simple wart but burrowing into the deeper tissue. *The lesion is well-differentiated and metastasizes late.* Also known as *epithelioma cuniculatum*.
3. Marjolin's ulcer – common on scar, keloid or chronic venous ulcer.
4. Spindle or sarcomatoid epithelial cell carcinoma.

Note

BCCs and SCCs *have been linked to chronic sun exposure typically in fair-skinned people.*

MARJOLIN'S ULCER

It is actually a low-grade epidermoid or squamous cell carcinoma *arising from the epithelium covering the scar tissue, keloid or chronic ulcer.*

It may also develop on *long-standing venous ulcer, long-standing radiation ulcer, long-standing ulcer following thermal injury, or on chronically discharging osteomyelitic sinus.*

As the epithelium covering the scar tissues *contains no hair follicle, no nerves, no lymphatics*, the lesion has the following characteristic features.

Characteristic features

1. It may occur many years after the formation of scar.
2. Very slowly growing, due to relative avascularity of the scar tissue. It is also less malignant than a typical squamous cell carcinoma.
3. Painless, as the scar tissue contains no nerve.
4. Edge of such ulcer is not always raised and everted.

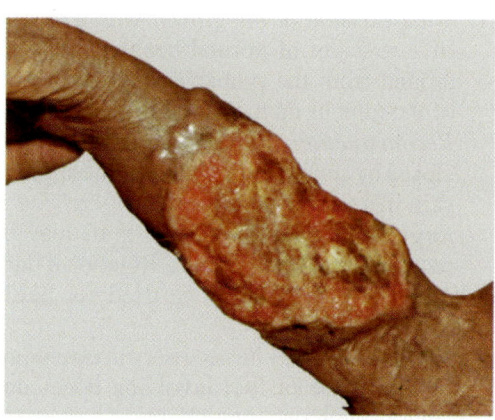

Fig. 2.88: Marjolin's ulcer—squamous cell carcinoma of right forearm. Ulcer developed over the post-burn wound. Note the surrounding scar following burn.

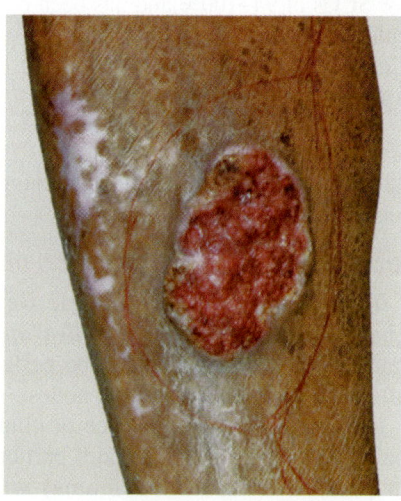

Fig. 2.89: Marjolin's ulcer (SCC) on the medial side of the right leg. Note the hypopigmented surrounding scar. Required wide excision and skin grafting. (*Courtesy:* Dr Sudeb Saha, MS, FAMS)

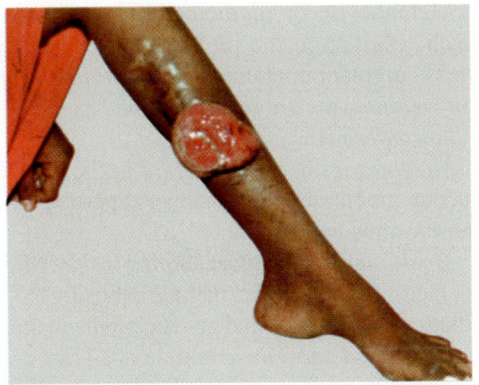

Fig. 2.90: Clinically Marjolin's ulcer of the left leg. Note the hypertrophied scar above the ulcer. But after excision, histopathology of the lesion revealed schwannoma. Patient was treated with wide excision of the lesion followed by delayed skin grafting. Patient also had a course of postoperative radiotherapy.

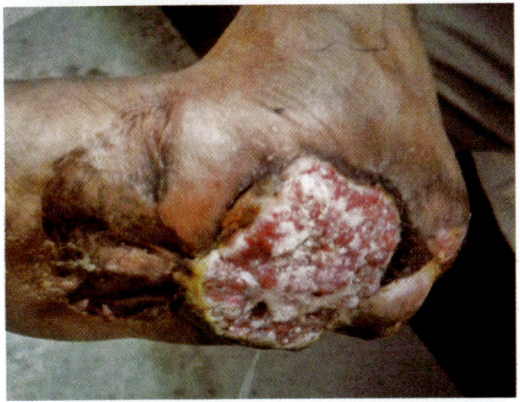

Fig. 2.91: Marjolin's ulcer over the scar on the sole of the right foot. Note the growth over the scar (SCC).

5. *No lymphatic metastasis:* As the lymphatics have been destroyed and occluded, unless the normal healthy skin adjacent to the lesion is involved when it presents the features of ordinary squamous cell carcinoma.
6. Radioresistant – due to avascularity. Usual squamous cell carcinoma is radiosensitive.

Treatment

After confirmation by biopsy:

1. If the site permits, wide tridimensional excision with a margin of at least 1 cm is

performed followed by skin grafting, either by split skin or full-thickness skin.
2. If the ulcer is very big one involving the distal part of the limb and excision is not possible, the treatment is amputation.
3. *Radiotherapy has no role.*

MELANOCYTIC TUMOURS AND MALIGNANT MELANOMA

Melanocytic tumours are melanin-containing tumours arising from the melanocytes or melanoblasts – *naevus cells*. These are cells of neural origin and originate from the neural crest and *are found in the basal layers of the epidermis*. Each melanocyte synthesizes the pigment melanin which protects the cell nuclei from ultraviolet radiation. Naevus cells in the dermis often produce less melanin.

Melanin is a sulphur-containing, iron-free black pigment. *It is an endogenous pigment* manufactured by these specialised cells (melanocytes and/or melanoblasts).

The melanocytes are also present in the following sites.

1. Leptomeninges
2. Adrenal medulla
3. Certain nerve cells, e.g. substantia nigra and locus ceruleus
4. Tela choroidea

Normally limited pigmentation may occur in *mucocutaneous junction*, e.g. mouth, anorectal junction, vagina, nail bed, and iris, ciliary body in eye.

The function of melanin is protective, and in human the melanin of the skin *appears to protect it against sunlight*.

Site of melanin formation

In the skin, melanin is formed in melanocytes or their precursors, the melanoblasts. Regarding the origin of these cells there are two views:

1. *Epithelial theory:* The melanocytes are specialised epithelial cells derived from the surface epithelium.
2. *Neurogenic theory:* The melanocytes are believed to originate from the neuroectoderm

of the embryonic neural crest and to migrate with the peripheral nerves to the basal layers of the epidermis (stratum basale): Masson's hypothesis.

Formation of melanin

The melanin is formed from the amino acid 'tyrosine'.

$$Tyrosine \xrightarrow{Tyrosinase} Dopa \xrightarrow{Dopa\ oxidase} Melanin$$

Melanin is intracellular and found near one of the poles of the cells as brown or black granules of uniform size. There are two varieties of cells – melanocytes and melanophores.

The melanocytes are the mature cells. They contain the pigment melanin and also the enzyme 'dopa oxidase'. The functions of melanocytes are both synthesis and carriage of melanin. Melanocytes are dopa-positive. *Normally, the melanocytes appear as clear cells in the basal layer of the epidermis*, but in melanotic condition they are increased in number with pigmentation.

The melanophores are phagocytes. They only carry the melanin pigment but cannot produce it as they do not possess the enzyme dopa oxidase. So, the *melanophores are dopa-negative*.

Role of hormone

Synthesis of melanin and its progress are hormone dependent. Hormones responsible are:

1. MSH (melanocyte-stimulating hormone), which is formed in the anterior lobe of the pituitary.
2. ACTH, to a slight extent.
3. Sex hormones:
   * Oestrogen
   * Androgen.

Surgical pathology

Melanocytic tumour may be benign or malignant.

BENIGN MELANOMA (Figs 2.92 to 2.96)

(*Syn.* Melanocytic naevus, pigmented naevus, mole)

Naevus is a general term referring to localised cutaneous malformations including moles and birth marks. *Naevus means a birth mark.*

Melanocytic or pigmented naevi are those which result from the proliferation of melanocytes – pigment containing cells. *In the normal skin melanocytes are present in the basal layers of the epidermis.*

Melanocytes are also present in the eye, the mucous membrane of the upper digestive tract, sinuses, anus and vagina.

Most common site of melanoma is skin. Major risk factors of melanoma include exposure to UV radiation (UVB rays) and genetic predisposition.

Pigmented naevi are common in all races and may be several in numbers. They may arise on any part of the skin surface and mucocutaneous junction of the body. They occur on the soles in about 10–15% of individuals.

Pigmented naevi may be present at birth, but more commonly they develop in childhood and at puberty or even later.

The following clinicopathological varieties of pigmented naevi are encountered.

* Congenital melanocytic naevi
* Acquired melanocytic naevi
  (i) Junctional naevus
  (ii) Compound naevus
  (iii) Intradermal naevus

Congenital melanocytic naevus

* Appears at birth
* Carries a risk of malignant change.

Acquired melanocytic naevus

* Appear after first 6–12 months of age.
* Enlarges with body growths and may regresses in later life.
* *In the normal skin, the melanocytes are present at the basal layers of the epidermis.*
* Initially, the naevus is junctional where *proliferating melanocytes (naevus cells) are present in clumps at the epidermodermal (ED) junction – junctional naevus.*
  Over a period of time, some of the melanocytes enter the dermis resulting in a *compound naevus* – the naevus cells being then present both at the epidermodermal junction and in the dermis.
* Later an *intradermal naevus* is developed, where the naevus cells are present only in the dermis.

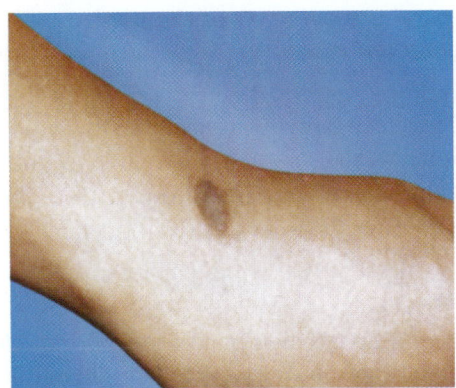

Fig. 2.92: Hairy pigmented mole over the dorsum of the right hand. This lesion *developed itching at adulthood* and so excised.

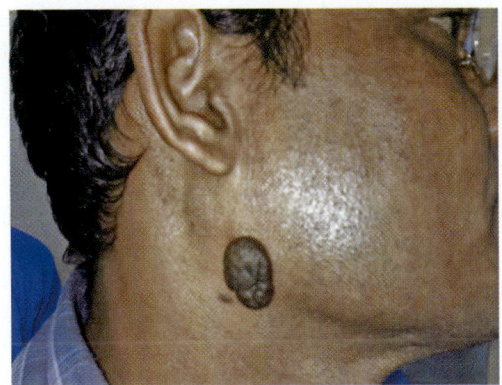

Fig. 2.95: Pigmented plaque type of lesion on right side of the face over the angle of the mandible since birth. Recently increasing in size during last 6 months with the development of satellitosis at the lower pole. Note that the lesion is also situated in an area subjected to repeated trauma from shaving. Total excision biopsy of the lesion including satellitosis and a margin of 2 mm of normal surrounding skin beyond the lesion and including satellitosis was performed. Fortunately, histopathology did not show any malignant change.

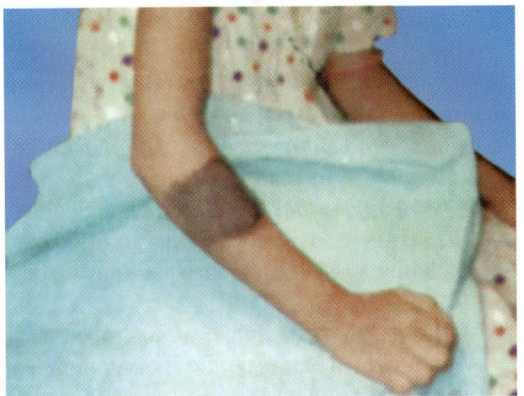

Fig. 2.93: Giant hairy mole over right forearm.

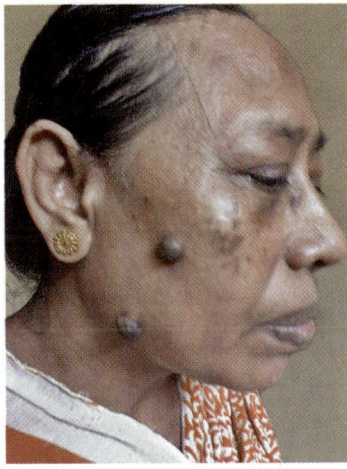

Fig. 2.96: Common pigmented moles: Intradermal naevus—right side of face. Recently increasing in size with itching—advised excision biopsy to exclude melanoma.

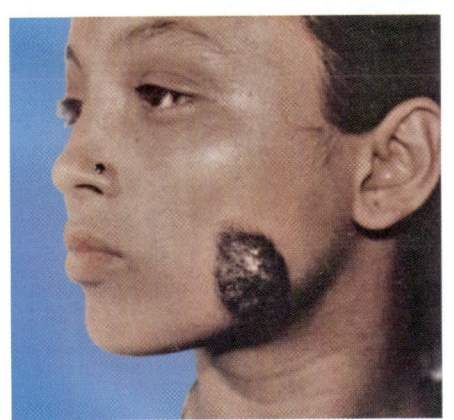

Fig. 2.94: Darkly pigmented hairy mole over the left side of face; recently being enlarged, thickened and darker. Suspect malignant change.

It is the junctional component of a naevus which is potentially dangerous, *because these are those cells which are liable to undergo proliferation from time-to-time. This is called junctional activity. If this activity occurs in a* naevus of an adult over the age of 30 years, the matter is serious, it may be the first indication of malignancy.

Characteristic features of each variety

Junctional naevus

- Most acquired melanocytic naevi in children *appearing before puberty* are of junctional type. This lesion *occurs at the basal or junctional layer of the epidermis and dermis* and *is essentially made of immature cells with a high degree of malignancy.*
- Can occur anywhere on the body and at any time after birth to puberty.
- *Commonly occur in the palms, soles, digits and nail beds*, i.e. *acral naevus*, and *genitals.*
- *Usually hairless.*
- *It is presumed that majority of malignant melanomas (90%) begin in junctional naevi*, but all junctional naevi do not change into malignancy.

Compound naevus

- Combination of both junctional and intra-dermal components.
- The intradermal components are inactive. *But the junctional components are very much prone to malignant change.*
- More common in older children and adults.
- *Appear as dome-shaped pigmented nodules.*
- *Many lesions may bear hair.*

Note

Junctional naevus and compound naevus are definitely premalignant.

Intradermal naevus (Common mole)

- Found in adult and elderly subjects.
- Appear as an elevated, dome-shaped, soft, smooth or warty lesion.
- Skin colour is light brown with or without telangiectasia.
- *Mostly hairy*, hence popularly known as *hairy mole.*
- Lesion can occur at any part of body except the soles, palms or genitalia. *Mostly common on the face.*

Clinical presentation of the benign pigmented mole

- Multiple pigmented naevi
- Congenital hairy pigmented naevus
- Spitz naevus
- Blue naevus
- Dysplastic naevi
- Freckle

Note

Except multiple pigmented naevi all the other lesions may undergo malignant change and should be followed up carefully.

Clinical evidence of malignant change in a naevus

1. *Increase in size peripherally.*
2. *Change in thickness:* Thicker, more palpable and nodular.
3. *Change in outline:* The edges become irregular.
4. *Change in colour:* Increasing pigmentation, irregular pigmentation, depigmentation.
5. *Change in surface characteristics:* Scaling, crusting, erosion, ulceration, oozing, bleeding, loss of hair from a previously hairy lesion.
6. *Change in surrounding tissues:* Appearance of pigmented halo, satellite spots or nodules, spread of pigment from the edge of naevus to the normal skin, inflammation around the skin.
7. *Development of symptoms:* Itching, aware-ness of the lesion, serous discharge, bleeding, pain from inflammation.
8. *Doppler positive pigmented lesion using hand-held doppler* – more than 1 mm thick lesion.
9. *Regional lymphadenopathy.*

Any change in a naevus as mentioned above deserves immediate attention to exclude malig-nant change. *Always do excisional biopsy a suspect pigmented lesion.*

Note

Infiltration into deep fascia by melanoma is rare in initial stage as deep fascia acts as a strong barrier.

Treatment of naevus

Most naevi pursue an uneventful course. They usually grow very slowly, remain quiescent for long time and gradually atrophy. Hence, rarely require active treatment/interference.

Surgical excision is indicated under the following circumstances.

1. *For cosmetic reasons:*
   (a) Naevi appearing at birth – usually innocent.
   (b) Naevi appearing before puberty – usually junctional naevi.
2. *Any naevi situated in the potentially dangerous areas* like soles, palms, digits, genitalia, and mucous membrane.
3. *Any naevi situated in the area subjected to repeated trauma,* e.g. rubbing by clothes, brassiere strap, belts, or cuts while shaving.
4. *Giant hairy mole.*
5. *Suspicion of, or clinical evidence of, malignant change in a mole.*

A *total body examination is to be done* for number of pigmented lesions and number of atypical (dysplastic) lesions.

Principles of excision

The operation is called **total excision biopsy**.

1. Naevi appearing at birth or before puberty, *can be excised close to their margins with at least 2 mm beyond the margin of lesion.*
2. All other naevi, particularly the suspicious lesion, *the excision should be complete and should include a margin of normal skin **at least 5 mm** beyond the margin of the lesion.*

Any excised naevus should be sent for histopathological study. If histopathology confirms the diagnosis of malignant changes with positive margin, then *a wider excision is performed depending on the thickness of the tumour.*

Histological features of malignancy in naevus

1. Increase in junctional activity.
2. Increase in nuclear cytoplasmic ratio.
3. Increase in cell size.
4. Cytoplasm is filled with fine melanin granules.
5. Vacuolated cells in the epidermal layer.

6. Tumour cells clump in the subepidermal lymphatics.
7. Lymphocytic invasion.

MALIGNANT MELANOMA

This is a malignant tumour arising *from the epidermal melanocytes* which are normally located in the basal layer of epidermis. *Melanocytes are cells of neural origin. They are pigment-producing cells.*

Malignant melanoma may develop in any area of the skin – **cutaneous melanoma**.

Malignant melanoma may also arise in the:

- Pigmented area of the eye:
  (a) Uveal tract
     · Iris
     · Ciliary body   } **Ocular melanoma**
     · Choroids
  (b) Retina
  (c) Conjunctiva
- Mucocutaneous junction – anus, vagina – mucosal melanoma.
- Meninges

CUTANEOUS MELANOMA

This is one of the most malignant and dangerous forms of cancer of the skin. This is also a most rapidly infiltrating tumour. Fortunately this is a rare tumour accounting for only 3% of all malignant tumours of the skin.

Origin

1. *In some preexisting mole* such as junctional naevus, compound naevus, freckles – 90% of cases.
2. *De novo* – 10% of cases.

Aetiology

1. *Age:* Common after puberty, usually third decade, i.e. usually in the 20 and 40 years of age. This tumour is unknown before puberty.
2. *Sex:* Occurs most commonly in the female. But mortality is slightly higher in male.
3. *Race: More common in fair-skinned people who have been exposed to sunlight for a longer period,* that is why it is more frequent in Queensland, Australia.
   Rare in Blacks, but survival is poor in Blacks.

4. *About 50% melanomas arise from a preexisting lesion* – junctional/compound naevus.

5. *Factors associated with increased risk*
   (a) Genetic predisposition
       • Fair-skinned persons with red hair, blue eyes and freckles, specially Caucasians (more in Australians). Blacks are rarely affected.
       • Albinism
       • Multiple atypical or dysplastic naevi
       • Xeroderma pigmentosa
       • Persons born with congenital giant melanocytic naevi
       • Family history of melanoma.
         (i) About one in every ten patients diagnosed with this disease has a family member with a history of melanoma.
         (ii) Each person with a first degree relations diagnosed with melanoma has a 50% greater chance of developing this disease (cf. breast carcinoma).
         (iii) FMMM (familial atypical multiple mole melanoma) syndrome: People with this syndrome are at greater risk of developing melanoma. Gene mutations to p53 and BRAT have been associated with familial melanoma.
         (iv) Children of melanoma prone families may develop melanoma before adolescence.
   (b) Environmental factors:
       • *Sun exposure is the only avoidable factor.*
       • Ultraviolet radiation (UVA and UVB) are demonstrated to be carcinogenic. Specially UVB rays.
       • Increased incidence at the sites exposed to sunlight. Rarely occurs on double covered areas.
       • Solar irradiation is becoming much more dangerous due to the decreasing ozone layer in the atmosphere.

   (c) Increased incidence of melanoma has been noted in immunosuppressive patients as in patients with renal transplantation and leukemia.

6. *Role of trauma:* Not well-defined *but high incidence of melanoma in the sole has been observed in Bantu-blacks who walk barefoot.*

7. *Role of pregnancy:* Pregnancy is wrongly alleged to provoke malignant change in a naevus. Though pigmentation is increased during pregnancy, it has no effect on melanocytic neoplasm.
   • The treatment policy should not be altered in pregnant women.
   • Women who have had treatment of melanoma are advised to avoid pregnancy for 3 years.
   • Often there is a tendency for malignant melanoma to regress during pregnancy.

8. *Site of predilections*
   • Cutaneous melanomas can occur in any part of the body including genitals.
   • Distribution:
     • 25% in head and neck
     • 25% over trunk
     • 25% in lower limb
     • 11% in upper limb
     • 14% on genital
   • Melanomas located in the thick areas of skin have a worse prognosis. These areas are collectively grouped as '**BANS**': Upper **B**ack, upper **A**rm, posterior **N**eck and posterior **S**calp.
   • *In females:* Lesions are more common on the lower extremities.
   • *In males:* Lesions are more common on the trunk and head and neck.
   • *In Whites* – more than 90% of melanomas occur on the sun exposed skins.
   • *In Blacks* – more than 60% of melanomas arise on non-sun exposed skin, involving in particular planter, subungual and mucosal surfaces. *In Bantu tribe, sole is the commonest site.*
   • 70% of melanomas in Blacks are found on the lower limb and 90% of the lesions of the leg occur below the ankle.

- Other sites of melanoma:
  - Mucocutaneous junction (anorectal region, genitals)
  - *Those located over genitals, palms and soles have the highest malignant potential.*
  - Eyes (iris, ciliary body, choroids)
  - Head and neck (meninges, nasopharynx, paranasal sites).
9. *Progress*
   - The course of the disease is unpredictable. As a rule there is early and widespread dissemination which leads to high mortality.
   - *It has been reported that spontaneous regression may occur in exceptional cases.*

Surgical pathology

Pathologically malignant melanoma is regarded as *melanocarcinoma*. Rarely it may appear like a sarcoma.

Clinicopathological classification of malignant melanoma

Lentigo maligna melanoma (LMM)

- *Least common and least malignant.*
- Linear pattern of melanocyte proliferation in the epidermal basal cell layers – may be reactive or neoplastic *in situ type.*
- Slowly growing and remains non-invasive for many months.
- Often arises in Hutchinson's melanotic freckle (HMP) consequent often on prolonged solar irradiation.
- *Most frequently seen in elderly.*
- *Developed on the skin areas with high levels of sun exposure, e.g. in the face or arms.*
- Often present as a slowly growing brown or black stain on the skin (macular lesion).
- Lymph node metastases are rare and occur later in clinical history.

Superficial spreading melanoma (SSM)
(Fig. 2.90)

- *Most common variety but less aggressive lesion.*
- Occurs on any part of the body but commonly on lower limbs in women and trunk in man.
- Commonly arises on a preexisting naevus.

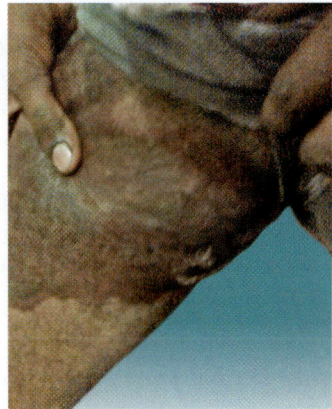

Fig. 2.97: Large pigmented lesion involving the anterior upper third of right thigh extending to adjacent lower abdomen—spreading melanoma.

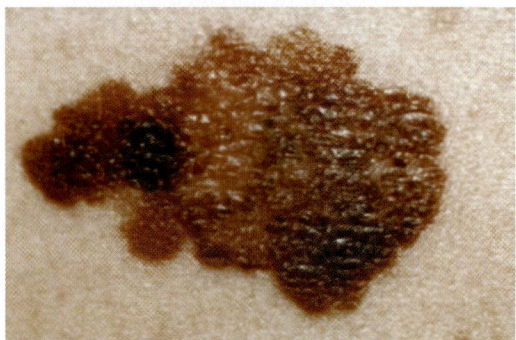

Fig. 2.98: Superficial spreading melanoma over the trunk. Note the irregular margin of the lesion with spreading orientation, colour variation from brown to black, and irregularity of the surface (cf. Cafe au lait spot).

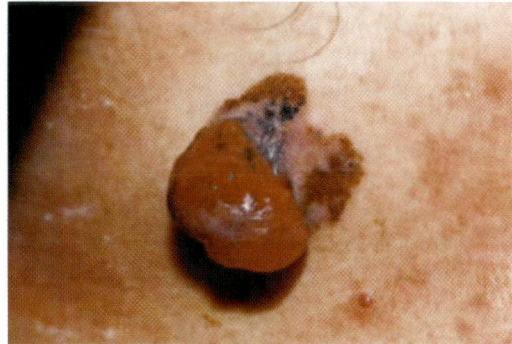

Fig. 2.99: Nodular melanoma. Note the well demarcated smooth reddish lump arising on a pigmented mole.

- Age group is younger than in LMM.
- The lesion is usually present as *a flat or elevated plaque* (**papular**) *with irregular border and surface and spreading orientation on the skin with colour variation* – brown, black, blue or pink. May be palpable.
- *Intermittent itch is a common symptom.*
- Lateral or radial growth predominates.
- Lymph node metastasis is rare until a nodular component develops.

Nodular melanoma (NM) (Fig. 2.99)
- *Least common but most aggressive; worst prognosis.*
- It can occur on any part of the body.
- *Nearly all mucosal, genital and anal melanomas are nodular ab-initio.*
- *Presents as a well-demarcated smooth nodule or lump* (**nodular**) *and well-pigmented.* It appears in a mole or on normal skin.
- It rapidly grows larger over weeks or months. *Vertical growth is the prominent features in contrast to the SSM where lateral growth predominates.*
- Frequently exophytic, i.e. it demonstrates outward growth beyond the surface.
- *Itch is common* and *ulceration occurs more frequently* leading to weeping or bleeding.

Acral lentiginous melanoma (ALM)
(Figs 2.100 to 2.102)
- Most aggressive lesion with early metastasis.
- Such lesions are more common in oriental and black persons (dark-skinned persons).
- *Occurs mainly in the **skin of palm and sole, and under nail plate** (**subungual melanoma**)*
- A variety of SSM but occurs on sites that are protected from sun burn by a thick layer of keratin.
- **Special varieties of ALM**
  (a) *Plantar melanoma:* Common in blacks. Usually heavily pigmented (Fig. 2.103). Ulceration and fungation occur in advanced lesions.
  (b) *Subungual melanoma:*
   · Usually begins as a pigmented linear streak in the nail bed – *involving nail-fold matrix.*
   · Symptomless in early stage. Often attention is drawn to the lesion only after injury.

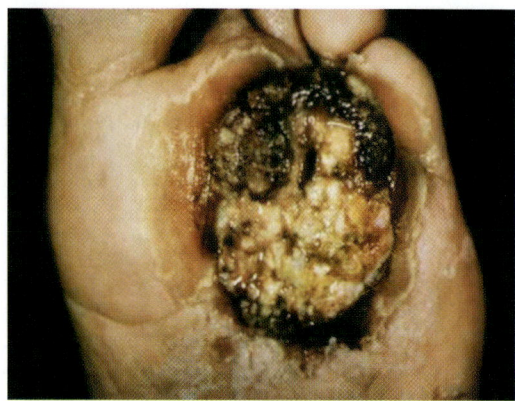

Fig. 2.100: Acral lentiginous melanoma. Note the pigmented proliferative lesion on the sole of the left forefoot. Wedge biopsy suggested malignant melanoma. Conservative below knee amputation was performed. Patient was sent to oncologist for further therapy.

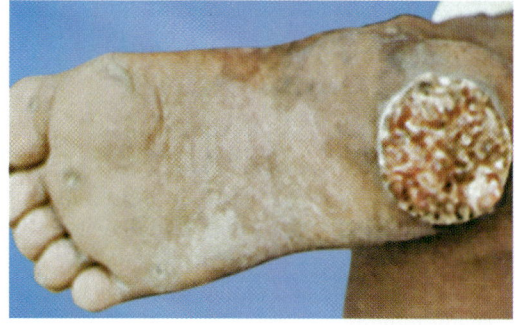

Fig. 2.101: Acral lentiginous melanoma over right heel. Requires conservative below knee amputation.

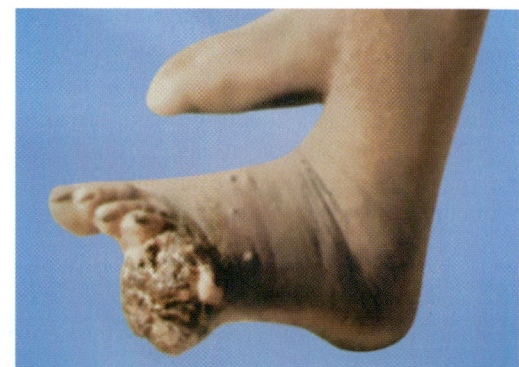

Fig. 2.102: Acral lentiginous malignant melanoma involving the little toe. Note also the subcutaneous nodules (satellite nodules) on the dorsum of the foot. Requires conservative below knee amputation.

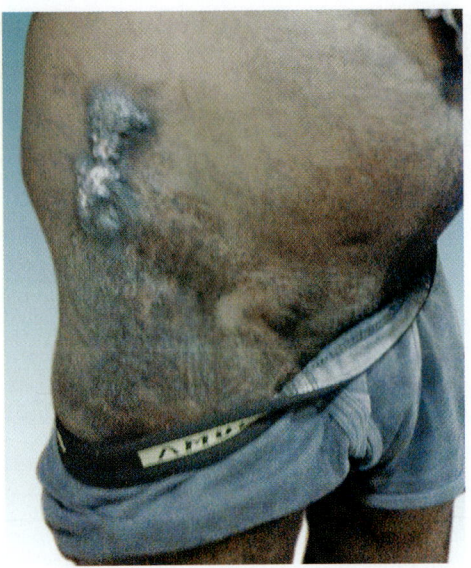

Fig. 2.103: Pigmented hairy mole of the anterolateral aspect of right thigh extending to abdomen. Note also the raised nodules over the abdominal wall—malignant melanoma.

· Distal migration of pigment away from the nail bed, pigmentation of lateral nail fold (Hutchinson's sign) and progressive elevation of the nail from the nail bed will lead to suspicion of subungual melanoma. In late stage, the tumour may extrude through the nail plate when ulceration, secondary infection and bleeding are common.

D/D of subungual melanoma: Subungual melanoma should be differentiated from the following lesions.

· Subungual haematoma
· Pyogenic granuloma
· Chronic paronychia
· Bacterial and fungal infections
· Rare vascular tumour

Growth pattern of melanoma

Most malignant melanoma grow in two phases:
* *Phase of radial growth (superficial growth):* Lesion extends superficially and laterally. The neoplastic cells are confined to the epidermis.
* *Phase of vertical growth:* Malignant cells invade the dermis and deeper tissues.

Vertical growth has a worser prognostic variable than radial growth.

Vertical growth can be evaluated by two ways:

(i) Clark's anatomic level of invasion.
(ii) Breslow's tumour depth measurements.

Both the 'Clark level' and 'Breslow's tumour depth' *refer to the microscopic depth of tumour invasion.*

Clark's anatomic level of invasion

Based on depth of invasion in the dermis on histopathology

Level I • *Tumour cells confined to the epidermis* above basement membrane – **melanoma-*in-situ*.**
 • *Do not develop metastasis,* i.e. non-invasive

Level II • *Tumour cells invade the papillary dermis after having broken through the basement membrane.*
 • *Rarely produce metastasis.*

Level III • *Tumour cells extend to the interface between papillary and reticular dermis.* A portion may protrude, but does not invade the reticular dermis.
 • *A small but significant proportion will develop metastasis.*

Level IV • *Tumour cells extend into the reticular dermis; develop metastasis.*

Level V • *Tumour cells extend into the subcutaneous tissue – subdermal fat involvement; develop metastasis*

• *A lesion when reaches level III – poor prognosis because of risk of metastasis.*
• Nodular melanomas are regarded as being at least level III in depth of invasion.

Breslow's tumour depth (thickness) measurement

• *Measured the vertical thickness of tumour in millimetres to assess the depth of involvement:* Breslow introduced staging by measuring the maximal vertical thickness of the melanoma from the top of the granular layer of the epidermis to the deepest melanoma cells in the dermis.

- Breslow's method of measurement requires an optical micro-callipers fitted to the ocular position of a standard microscope.
- *Breslow's tumour depth measurement is reliable and more accurate as a prognostic index and thus is important determinant of therapy.*

Stages and thickness of Breslow's tumour

Stage I   Thickness 0.75 mm or less

Stage II   Thickness 0.76 to 1.50 mm, i.e. <1.51 mm

Stage III Thickness 1.51 to 3.00 mm, i.e. ≤3.00 mm

Stage IV   Thickness more than 3.00 mm

A comparison of Clark's level of invasion and Breslow's tumour depth can be assessed to predict the virulence of the lesion (Fig. 2.104 and Table 2.1).

All subtypes except nodular melanoma are characterised by radial growth which may last for many months to years before a dermal expansile nodule (vertical growth) develops.

Spread

Malignant melanoma may spread by local extension, by lymphatics or by blood stream.

Table 2.1: Comparison of Clark's level and Breslow's tumour depth before spread

Clark's level of invasion	Breslow's tumour depth	Virulence
Level I	0.75 mm from the surface of the skin (epidermal lesion)	Low risk primary tumour. Do not metastasize at any site
Level II ⎫ Level III ⎬	0.76 to 1.50 mm	Intermediate risk. 25% incidence of metastasis.
Level IV ⎫ Level V ⎬	1.51 mm deeper below the skin surface, i.e. sub-dermal fat involve-ment	High risk. 60% incidence of metastasis.

Local spread

- Initially, the growth spreads *laterally* by continuity and contiguity within the epidermis, i.e. intraepidermal growth – *radial growth phase.* Metastasis is unusual.
- Later the growth spreads vertically within the dermis – *vertical growth phase.*
- Normally the radial growth phase precedes the vertical growth phase except the nodular melanoma in which vertical growth phase occurs early.

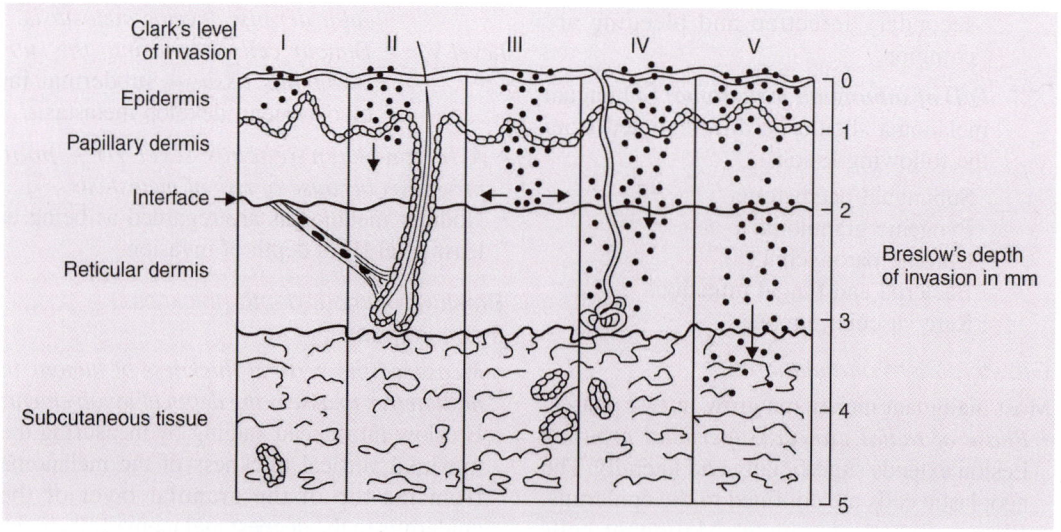

Fig. 2.104: Comparison of Clark's level of invasion and Breslow's tumour thickness.

- *Vertical growth has a worse prognostic variable* than the radial growth because of increased metastatic potential.
- *The deep fascia acts as a strong barrier to the spread of melanoma to the deeper tissues.*

Lymph spread

- *Regional lymph nodes are most common site of metastasis: poor prognostic sign.*
- The tumour spreads mainly and at first exclusively by lymphatics before spreading elsewhere. The lymphatic spread usually precedes blood spread.
- The lymphatic spread is usually circumferential and wide.
- The spread is either *by emboli* to regional lymph nodes, or *by permeation* of the dermal lymph channels when giving rise to secondary deposits, e.g. local *satellite nodules* near the site of within 5 cm of the primary tumour (*satellitosis*) *and/or in-transit deposits* between the primary tumour and the regional lymph nodes. *Satellite lesion represents an aggressive tumour and microinvasion.*
- Secondary lymphoedema may occur.
- *Lymphatic spread is seen very early in mucosal melanoma,* such as anal canal, due not only to the fact that it is rich in lymphatics, but also to frequent movements, propelling the lymph.
- *Single most important prognostic index. It signifies stage III disease.* When regional lymph nodes are involved 5 years survival decreases to about 30%.
- *Lymphatic spread is not seen in melanoma of the choroid plexus since CNS has no lymphatics.*

Blood spread

- *Dissemination by blood is usually late development.*
- In most cases metastases appear at multiple sites.
- Most commonly to brain, lungs and liver; less commonly in the skin, bone and gastrointestinal tract.
- *Secondary deposits are usually black,* but sometimes contain little or no melanin, even when the primary lesion is heavily pigmented.

- *Extensive visceral involvement may cause melanuria.*
- Overall prognosis is poor in presence of distant metastases.
- *One peculiar characteristic of malignant melanoma* is the occasional tendency for highly invasive metastases to appear many years after the apparently adequate excision of the primary lesion.
- *Eye lesions can metastasize to the liver many years after enucleation.*
- *A history of loss of an eye by enucleation from the disease (not known) long ago and appearance of an enlarged liver recently should suggest an ocular melanoma.* Beware of enlarged liver in a patient with glass eye.

Progress

Prognosis depends on:

1. Clark's anatomical level
2. Breslow's tumour depth (thickness) of invasion
3. Spread – local, lymphatic, blood spread

The course of the disease is unpredictable. As a rule, there is early and widespread dissemination which leads to high mortality.

It has been reported that spontaneous regression may occur in exceptional cases.

Spontaneous regression

Spontaneous regression may occur in melanoma usually in superficial spreading melanoma (SSM) and lentigo maligna melanoma (LMM). Regression may be partial or complete.

It is presumed that this regression phenomenon represents *tumour cells which have invaded into the dermal collagen and have been destroyed by the body's natural defence mechanism.* Histologically, the regression is considered as an area with a normal appearing epidermis overlying a thickened fibrotic stroma, devoid of tumour cells, but containing a variable number of melanophages, lymphocytes, plasma cells and new blood vessels.

Thin tumours with regression should be treated as they were 1 mm or more in tumour thickness and so wide excision is necessary.

Note

There is a tendency for malignant melanoma to regress during pregnancy.

Note

Spontaneous regression is also seen in:

1. Retinoblastoma
2. Choriocarcinoma
3. Salmon pink patch
4. Strawberry angioma

Amelanotic melanoma

Generally, the malignant melanoma and its metastatic deposits are well-pigmented, *but sometimes they contain no or very little pigment. This is called amelanotic melanoma.* The cells lose their capacity to produce melanin, though they contain the precursor of melanin pigment. *Most commonly occurs in the setting of melanoma metastases to the skin* when appears as pink or flesh-coloured lesion after mimicking BCC or SCC or soft tissue sarcoma.

Such tumour is difficult to distinguish from an anaplastic carcinoma or sarcoma, *but the Dopa reaction is helpful in the diagnosis, which will be positive in melanoma.*

Diagnostic criteria of malignant melanoma

1. *Age:* Malignant melanomas are *rare before puberty* but can occur in children.
2. *Sex: Females* are more frequently affected.
3. *Race: Common in Caucasians* and rare in Blacks.
4. *Occupation:* It is prevalent in white-skinned people living in those parts of the world which enjoy excess sunlight, such as Australia and the west coast of America. Outdoor workers, e.g. agricultural workers, fishermen, and dedicated sunbathers are more prone to this lesion.
5. The patient presents with a pigmented lesion on the body. *A malignant melanoma usually does not occur before puberty.* After puberty, the lesion may present in one of the following ways.

   (a) *Preexisting benign mole undergoing malignant change* (the features are already described).
   (b) *Arising de novo:* A pigmented lesion appears after puberty and grows progressively, sometimes rapidly over a period of months. It may ulcerate and bleed shortly after its appearance.
6. Melanoma often itches but is not painful.
7. Sometimes the patient may present with lymph node enlargement being unaware of the existence of the primary lesion (*occult melanoma*).
8. In late cases, the patient may present with the symptoms of distant metastases such as weight loss, dyspnoea, jaundice or neurological abnormalities.
9. *The patient may present because of cosmetic disfigurement, ulceration with or without bleeding.*

Local examination (see clinicopathological classification)

10. *Site:* Melanoma can arise on any part of the body – palms, soles, extremities, arms, chest and mucocutaneous junction. *In case of females,* more frequently on the lower extremities, and *in case of males,* more commonly on the arms and chest.

    A particularly common site is on the sole of the foot. It is interesting to note that it is the only site in which a melanoma is at all common in the coloured people.

    It may also occur beneath the nail (subungual melanoma), especially of the thumb and great toe.

    It is also seen at the mucocutaneous junction, e.g. the mouth, anus, vulva, or in the genitalia.

    Melanomas also occur in the eye, in the choroid, conjunctiva or retina. *Retinal melanomas have a poor prognosis and a remarkable predilection for early metastasis to the liver.*

    The other parts of the body must be searched for multiple pigmented lesions.
11. *Colour: Usually black in colour,* but a wide variety of colour changes including red, grey,

violaceous blue are noted in melanoma. By contrast, *the benign mole is usually brown or various shades of brown.*

Virulent amelanotic melanoma may appear as pink and fleshy lesion like in SCC.

The presence of an *inflammatory (or depigmented) halo,* in the surrounding skin is sometimes noted.

A depigmented halo is rare in melanoma but common around benign naevi.

12. *Surface:* Varies (*see* clinicopathological classification). It may be *macular, papular, nodular, or include all the varieties in one lesion.* The early lesion is smooth but later ulceration develops from ischaemic necrosis. The ulcer is covered with a crust of blood and serum. Bleeding is common on the surface. A big melanoma may look wet, soft and boggy from infection and bleeding.

13. *Size and shape:* Varies, the border is usually irregular. *A neglected nodular melanoma* will become a large florid tumour which protrudes from and overlaps the surrounding skin.

14. *Consistence:* The primary tumour feels firm and solid. The satellite nodules feel hard.

15. *Temperature and tenderness:* Temperature remains the same as that of the surrounding skin. *The tumour is also not tender.*

16. *Mobility:* The tumour is intimately fixed to the skin and moves with the skin. It can be easily lifted up from the deeper structures.

17. *Surrounding skin:* There may be *inflammatory halo* or a *halo of brown pigment* in the skin around the tumour.

   Satellite nodules, pigmented or depigmented, in-transit metastasis, may be seen or felt in the skin and subcutaneous tissues between the primary tumour and the nearest draining lymph nodes.

18. *Regional lymph nodes:* Should be examined. They may be enlarged.

General examination

19. One should examine for distant metastases, e.g. *liver* (hepatomegaly, jaundice), *lungs* (pleural effusion), *brain* (neurological abnormalities), *bones* (pathological swelling or fracture).

Five important features of melanoma suspicion in a pigmented lesion: ABCDE.

* **A**symmetry
* **B**order irregularity
* **C**olour variation
* **D**iameter >6 mm
* **D**evelopment of symptoms
* **E**levation – elevated or enlarging surface

Clinical staging

Clinical staging *depends on* the tumour thickness, ulceration, presence or absence of satellite nodules, in-transit metastasis, clinically involved lymph nodes and/or distant metastases.

Stage 0   *Melanoma-in-situ.* The melanoma cells are found only in the outer layer of the skin and have not invaded the deeper tissues, i.e. *intraepidermal growth.*

   No nodal involvement. Thus, localised to the site of origin (cf. Clark's Level I).

Stage I   Thin melanoma (≤1.50 mm)

   Rarely nodal involvement (cf. Clark's Levels II and III).

Stage IIA   Thick melanoma between 1.51 to 4 mm (cf. Clark's Level IV).

Stage I and Stage IIA: Localised cutaneous disease.

Stage IIB   Thick melanoma more than 4.00 mm or *penetration into the subcutaneous tissue* (cf. Clark's Level V) or 2 mm thick melanoma with surface ulceration.

Stage III   Any tumour size + *spread beyond the primary site of origin,* i.e. presence of satellitosis, in-transit metastasis, regional lymph node metastasis or all of them.

Stage IV   Any of the above + *distant metastasis* such as involvement of two or more groups of lymph nodes; visceral metastases, e.g. lung, liver, bone and brain are the more frequent sites; disseminated cutaneous metastasis.

Investigations

- Edge or wedge biopsy including junction of normal skin should be done at the earliest.
- Chest X-ray, ultrasound of liver and liver function tests are mandatory in all cases.
- CT brain and skeletal survey may be done only if indicated.
- Lymphangiography and lymphoscintigraphy are of limited value and so not routinely done.
- FNAC/FNAB of the lymph nodes for metastasis.
- Tomographic Gallium-67 citrate scans are *helpful for detecting metastatic melanoma in a number of distant sites:* Metastasis in lymph nodes, abdominal viscera and other soft tissues. But they are less helpful for detecting metastasis in the lung and brain.

Note

Melanuria is seen in disseminated tumours where the urine is dark-stained or turns dark on waiting for few minutes.

Treatment

1. Treatment of the primary lesion.
2. Treatment of the regional lymph nodes.

Treatment of the primary lesion

- *Surgical excision of the primary lesion after confirmation of diagnosis by adequate biopsy is the treatment of choice.*
- Radiotherapy and chemotherapy have no role in the management of primary melanoma.

Establishment of diagnosis

- *Excision biopsy of a suspected lesion is only recommended* to confirm diagnosis and provides histopathological information that guides further surgical strategy. **No incisional or core biopsy.**
- *A tridimensional excision biopsy should be performed with a margin of at least* **2 mm lateral clearance** *beyond the extent of the lesion.*
- *The orientation of incision should be elliptical in shape in the direction of Langer's line* to allow tension free closure.

- *The excision must include underlying cuff of subcutaneous tissue deep to the tumour up to the deep fascia so that complete histological data including* Clark's levels of invasion and Breslow's tumour depth can be assessed. *Prognosis depends upon the depth of the tumour.*

  All corners of the excised specimen are properly identified and labelled and should be examined histologically to ascertain the adequacy of clearance.
- *The deep fascia should not be interfered with or dissected* to avoid spread of melanoma to the tissues deep to the deep fascia.
- *Excision biopsy on the extremities* should be in the longitudinal direction of the limb to allow for a primary wound closure.
- *Use of wide local excision (WLE) as an initial biopsy may reduce the efficacy of subsequent lymphatic mapping required to know the lymphatic spread.*
- *Incision and needle biopsy should be avoided in melanoma* because of the risk of transferring melanoma cells to the subcutaneous fat and deeper tissues and thus conversion of a superficial melanoma to a deep melanoma.
- *A punch biopsy or excision of a segment of the lesion* may be appropriate if complete excision causes unreasonable deformity, e.g. in large lesions of the face for cosmetic reason.
- *Shave biopsy or curettage should not be used* when melanoma is suspected because the cancer cannot be staged accordingly.
- *For any suspicious or persisting lesions of the nail,* an adequate biopsy material is required for histological examination and *should include a portion of the proximal terminal of the nail matrix, the nail bed and the nail plate.*

Once the diagnosis of melanoma is confirmed, investigations to look for lymphatic spread and metastasis are carried out.

(a) *Investigations for lymphatic spread*
  (i) *In presence of enlarged regional lymph node(s):* FNAC/FNAB of the enlarged node(s) is helpful to detect the lymphatic spread and to stage the disease.

(ii) *In absence of enlarged lymph nodes:* Sentinel lymph node biopsy (SLNB) *following lymphatic mapping with the use of dyes and radioactive substances* is required to detect the lymphatic spread.

If positive, complete block dissection is to be performed. *Lymph node involvement indicates stage III disease.*

(iii) Lymphangiography and lymphoscintigraphy are of limited value and so not routinely done.

(b) *Investigations for metastasis*
   (i) Chest X-ray
   (ii) LFT
   (iii) LDH
   (iv) Preoperative liver, brain and bone scan – U/S, CT:
      • Not mandatory, for clinical stage I lesion.
      • Should be done if LFT, LDH is abnormal.
      • Extraordinarily high LDH often indicates metastatic spread to the liver.

(c) *Melanuria*
   • *Urine test for melanuria:* Melanuria is seen in disseminated tumours, where the urine is dark-stained or turns dark on waiting for a few minutes. *Melanuria signifies advanced disease.*

Note

Tumour markers for melanoma

1. LDH
2. S-100 – positive in 90% melanoma
3. Melan-A
4. HMB45 (hydroxy methyl bromide)
5. Dopa: Dopa reaction is *helpful in the diagnosis of amelanotic melanoma.*

Treatment of the primary melanoma

• *Surgical resection of primary melanoma is the treatment of choice.*
• After histological diagnosis, *the site of the original lesion is usually re-excised with adequate margins dictated by the tumour thickness.* Often this is done by a *wide local excision* (WLE) with 0.5 to 3 cm margins all around (Table 2.2). *This wide excision aims to reduce the rate of tumour recurrence at the site of the original lesion.*

Table 2.2: Recommended margins for surgical resection of primary melanoma

Primary melanoma thickness	Margin radius (cm)
(i) Melanoma-in-situ	0.5 cm
(ii) <1.0 mm	
(iii) = 1.0 mm	1.0 cm
(iv) >1–2 mm	2.0 cm
(v) >2 mm	3.0 cm

• *The 3 cm margin of excision* is also advocated for tumours with regression noted on histological examination.
• *For lesion in the face,* maximum safe margin of excision is *2.5 cm for cosmetic reason.*
• *The deep fascia is not included in the excision* because it is noted that *the deep fascia limits the local spread or 'in-transit' recurrence to the subcutaneous tissue.*
• The residual defect following WLE *is preferably closed directly by primary suture. Where direct closure is not technically possible a split-skin graft can be used.*

Closure developed by rotational or advancement flaps or pedicle flap is better avoided *because a thick flap may hide a local recurrence for longer period of time.*

SUBUNGUAL MELANOMA

Amputation at the metatarsophalangeal or metacarpophalangeal joint is the optimal treatment. Cade advised removal of the metatarsal or metacarpal also (i.e. *Ray amputation*).

MELANOMA OF THE SOLE OF THE FOOT OR PLANTAR MELANOMA

(i) *Amputation is seldom performed nowadays,* because of improvements in non-ablative therapy available in certain centres.
(ii) *Wide excision of the lesion with a large surface area is combined with isolated limb perfusion with Melphalan.* This

combined therapy is found to be *effective in patient with planter and subungual melanoma with minimal morbidity.*

The residual large defect may present a difficult problem during reconstruction. A split skin grafting generally provides effective cover and patients are able to walk on the grafted foot with little difficulty after using a special foot wear.

(iii) *Limited amputation of the limb* may be justified in advanced case *to remove a foul smelling fungating mass.*

Treatment of regional lymph nodes

- No role of prophylactic lymph node dissection (PLND) because of many postoperative complications but without any survival benefits.
- SNLB is performed both in clinically palpable or non-palpable sentinel lymph nodes (SLNs) to note the presence of LN metastasis to justify lymphadenopathy.
- SLNB is advocated in following conditions.
  (i) Primary tumour thickness ≤1 mm but with surface ulceration
  (ii) Primary tumour thickness >1 to 2 mm
  (iii) Primary tumour of the limb
- Alternatively in presence of clinically palpable node/nodes, FNAC is performed.
- *In presence of lymph node involvement* detected by SLNB or FNAC, therapeutic lymph node dissection (TLND) is performed.
- TLND is also advocated, if during follow up previously normal lymph nodes become enlarged and suspicious.
- *TLND should be avoided in patients with primary lesions greater than 4 mm in thickness* because of the high risk of blood borne metastasis at the time of initial diagnosis.
- *TLND is also avoided in patients with stage IV diseases with distant metastases*, or with advanced age and/or poor physical state as the long-term survival is poor.
- *Where inguinal nodes are involved, radical ilio-inguinal dissection (used to be performed before) is not justified* because long-term survival after removal of involved iliac nodes is extremely poor.
- After radical inguinal node dissection trans-

position of the sartorius is done to cover the femoral vessels.

Monoblock dissection

During TLND, where possible, i.e. on the trunk, on the limbs above the elbow or knee joints, on the face, *the primary tumour is excised along with block dissection of the regional nodes in continuity (monoblock dissection).* Monoblock dissection removes all the potentially contaminated tissues between the primary lesion and the draining lymph nodes, thus prevents in-transit recurrence.

For facial primary lesion – superficial parotidectomy is also advised.

Treatment of metastatic malignant melanoma

Metastatic malignant melanoma is refractory to most modalities of treatment. In general, *this tumour is highly radioresistant and relatively chemoresistant. Immunotherapy remains still in the experimental stage.* All these modalities are still considered palliative at the present time.

Prognosis

- The prognosis varies with the pathological type of the lesion, level of invasion, tumour thickness, clinical staging, site, sex and age, mucosal involvement.

5-year survival predictions

- *Low risk primary tumour, i.e. Clark's level I or Breslow's tumour depth ≤0.75 mm: 95–100%* chance of a 5-years cure with conservative surgical treatment.
- *Intermediate risk tumour: 85–95%* chance of a 5-years cure.
- *High risk tumour: 15–50%* chance of a 5-years cure.
- *If lymph node metastasis is present* the prognosis becomes worse.
- *Surface ulceration of the lesion* lowers the survival rates for tumours of comparable thickness.
- *Melanoma of the face* has a better prognosis.
- *Subungual melanoma* has a relatively good prognosis.
- *Women overall* have a 10% survival advantage.
- Worst prognosis is seen in amelanotic melanoma.

PYOGENIC GRANULOMA

It is an exuberant overgrowth of granulation tissue producing a red, soft or moderately firm, polypoid lesion typically 5 to 10 mm across. The lesion looks like a lobular capillary haemangioma but has a typical natural history. It develops due to abnormal inflammatory reaction in response to trauma or a foreign body, such as a splinter. It usually appears on the skin of the upper extremity and the glabrous surface of the digit, in the nail fold (periungual), within the web space and flexion creases.

Persistent ulceration with or without bleeding is common when differential diagnosis from malignant lesion is very difficult. Resolution is very slow. The history of trauma may not be remembered by the patient.

Treatment is complete excision. Skin coverage may be necessary for large resulting defect. Recently, laser therapy has become helpful.

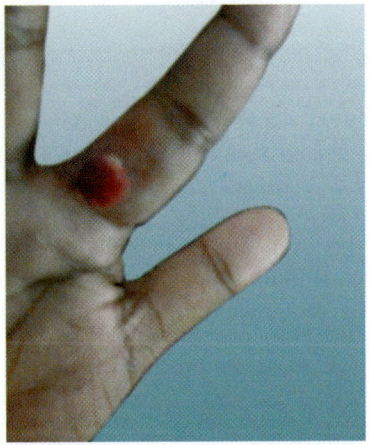

Fig. 2.107: Pyogenic granuloma at the base of the right index finger.

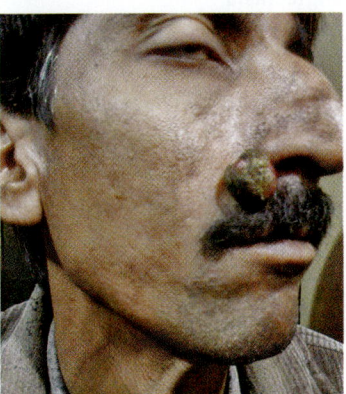

Fig. 2.108: Pyogenic granuloma at the angle of right alae nasi.

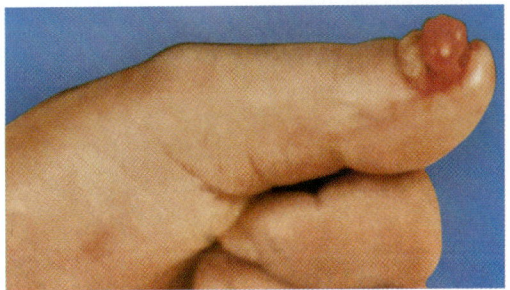

Fig. 2.105: Pyogenic granuloma at the nail bed of the left thumb. D/D: Haemangioma, malignant melanoma.

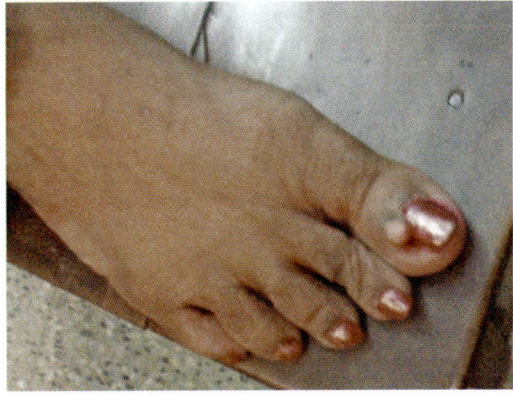

Fig. 2.109: Pyogenic granuloma with ingrowing toe nail—right great toe.

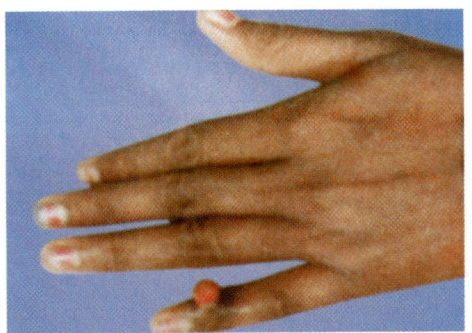

Fig. 2.106: Pyogenic granuloma of left little finger.

Note

Pigmented lesions of the skin other than melanoma

1. Seborrhoeic keratoses or warts
2. Pigmented basal cell carcinoma or squamous cell carcinoma
3. *Cutaneous angiomata:* The soft consistency of the lesion and blanching on pressure are often helpful in making the diagnosis.
4. Pyogenic granuloma
5. Subungual haematoma
6. Glomus tumour
7. Kaposi's sarcoma
8. Histiocytoma
9. Keratoacanthoma
10. Epidermal naevus
11. Telangiectasia

When doubt exists in the diagnosis, excision biopsy is indicated in the above mentioned lesions to exclude malignant melanoma.

12. *Cafe au lait patch:* This is an area of pale brown milk-coffee coloured pigmentation in the skin. This is often associated with neuro-fibromatosis and sometimes with pheo-chromocytoma. This is present at birth and never undergoes malignant change.
13. *Multiple circumoral melanosis* associated with the Peutz-Jeghers syndrome. The Peutz-Jeghers syndrome is a familial condition, an autosomal dominant syndrome and consists of:
    - Multiple intestinal polyposis, and
    - Multiple melanin spots around the mouth, on the lips and in the buccal mucous membrane. These moles and polyps never turn malignant.
    - Intestinal polyps may cause intussus-ception and bleeding which need urgent intervention.

Notes on melanoma:

- Most common type – superficial spreading
- Least common type – Lentigo maligna
- Most benign form – Lentigo maligna
- Most of the melanoma are pigmented. But pigmentation is not mandatory for diagnosis of melanoma – *amelanotic melanoma.*

- Most arise from preexisting lesion.
- Most malignant type – nodular type
- Most common site in males – *torso,* i.e. lower front and back
- Most common site in females – *lower leg*
- High risk factors for melanoma spread:
  - More than 50-fold increased risk with *persistently changing mole*
  - Atypical moles in patients with history of melanoma in two family members
  - >50 naevi with >5 mm diameter
- Poor prognosis:
  - Lesion in the scalp, hand, foot (acral lentiginous) and in mucous membrane
  - Presence of an ulcer on melanotic patch
  - Presence of satellite lesion
  - Thickness of the lesion – most important factor
    - (i) Stage IV (thickness <3 mm) – lesion extends to reticular dermis
    - (ii) Stage V (thickness >3 mm) – lesion extends to subcutaneous tissue
- Worst prognosis:
  - Amelanotic melanoma
  - Mucosal melanoma is more aggressive than cutaneous form and carries poor prognosis
- Occult melanomas
  - Primary unknown
  - Common in genitalia, anus, scalp, eye, external auditory canal, nail bed, adrenal medulla
- Lymphatic spread – *single most important prognostic factor.* It signifies stage III disease.
  - Number of nodes more important than size.
  - *Proceeds as an orderly process.* Thus evolved the concept of the first node to get involved which is known as *sentinel node.*
  - *In thick melanoma* – a sentinel node biopsy (SLNB) to be performed. *If positive,* lymph-adenectomy is to be performed.
  - *In-transit nodules or satellite nodules* are seen on the skin between the primary lesion and regional lymph nodes and is due to retrograde spread to dermal lymphatics.
- *Features of blood spread:*
  - Liver – massive hepatomegaly, ascites
  - Lung – cannon ball metastasis, pleural effusion

- Brain – convulsions, raised intracranial pressure
- Bone – bone pain, pathological fracture, vertebral metastasis, paraplegia
- Skin – cutaneous nodules, mostly pigmented
- Extensive visceral metastases – cause melanuria

Note

Points to be remembered:

- No incisional biopsy in melanoma.
- No induration occurs in melanoma.
- No role of radiotherapy.
- Usually rare before puberty.
- Amelanotic melanoma can be diagnosed by histochemical studies showing S-100 protein, MART-1 and HMB-45 reactivity.
- Spontaneous regression may occur in malignant melanoma.
- Malignant melanoma is highly radioresistant.

Note

Malignancies which can spread from mother to foetus

- Malignant melanoma
- Lymphosarcoma

Note

SLNB is practised in the following malignant lesions:

1. Malignant melanoma
2. Carcinoma penis
3. Carcinoma breast

Methods used for identifying SNLB:

- No special OT is required.
- SLN biopsy is usually done intraoperatively by using isosulphan blue dye (lymphazurin) and/or radioactive Tc-99 labelled sulphur colloid.
- Accuracy of detection of SLN is best when both the methods are combined.
- Gamma camera detects the SLN when radioactive colloid is used.

- Blue dye colours the SLND, hence aids in identification of lymph node at operation.
- *Contraindication of SLNB in palpable lymphadenopathy* prior to surgery, chemotherapy or radiotherapy, and multifocal lesions.

Note

Melanoma located in the thick area of the skin has worse prognosis. These areas are collectively grouped as BANS which stands for: B – upper **B**ack, A – upper **A**rm, N – posterior **N**eck, S – **S**calp.

Note

Non-cutaneous melanoma

- Mucosal melanoma
- Ocular melanoma
- Rarely, melanoma may be found in the intestines and in the meninges.

Note

Mucosal melanoma

- Common in Blacks.
- Involves the mucosa of the lips, nose, palate, genital tract and anorectal regions.
- Usually lightly pigmented.
- Irrespective of the site, associated with poor prognosis owing to early lymphatic spread and advanced stage of the disease.
- Resistant to radio- and/or chemotherapy.
- Anorectal melanoma is treated by abdominoperineal resection.
- Melanoma vulva is treated by vulvectomy with plastic reconstruction.

Note

Some superficial melanomas (lentigo maligna) have resolved with topical application of imiquimod (Aldara) cream, an immune enhancing agent.

Note

Antiestrogen-like tamoxifen have been tried in presence of systemic diseases from melanoma spread with a response rate of 15–20%.

Swellings in the Neck

Swellings in the neck are caused by innumerable pathological lesions arising from the anatomical structures lying therein.

Skin and superficial fascia
- Sebaceous cyst
- Lipoma
- Fibroma

Lymphatics
- Cystic hygroma
- Solitary lymphatic cyst

Lymph nodes
- Inflammatory lymph nodes and cold abscess
- Neoplastic
- Reticuloses

Blood vessels
- Aneurysm
- Haemangioma
- Carotid body tumour

Nerve tissue
- Neurofibroma

Thyroid gland
- Inflammatory
- Neoplastic
- Autoimmune disease
- Physiological goitre

Pharynx
- Pharyngeal pouch

Larynx
- Laryngocele

Branchial arch remnant
- Branchial cyst

Thyroglossal duct remnant
- Thyroglossal cyst

Salivary glands
- Inflammatory
- Neoplastic
- Autoimmune disease

Most of the neck swellings can often be diagnosed from the history and physical signs alone.

The most common swellings in the neck are of lymph node origin and the most likely causes of lymphadenopathy are infections and metastatic spread of cancer.

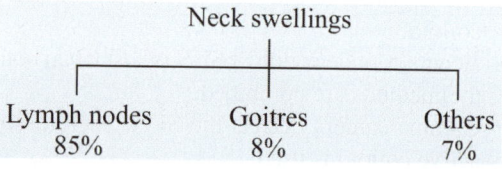

Neck swellings — Lymph nodes 85% — Goitres 8% — Others 7%

Lymph nodes are recognised by their physical signs more easily when multiple than when solitary. *Solitary lymph node swelling* presents the greatest diagnostic challenges.

Goitres are swelling of the thyroid gland. They are distinguished from other lump in the neck by the fact *that they move on swallowing.*

Others are solitary swellings arising from variable structures.

Any solitary swelling in the neck must be distinguished from an isolated enlarged lymph node.

SURGICAL ANATOMY

Triangles of the neck (Fig. 3.1)

The anterolateral part of the neck is conventionally divided into an anterior and a posterior triangles by the diagonally running sternomastoid muscle. *By pressing the jaw laterally against resistance of one's hand, the opposite sterno-mastoid becomes taut.* This muscle helps to define two triangles.

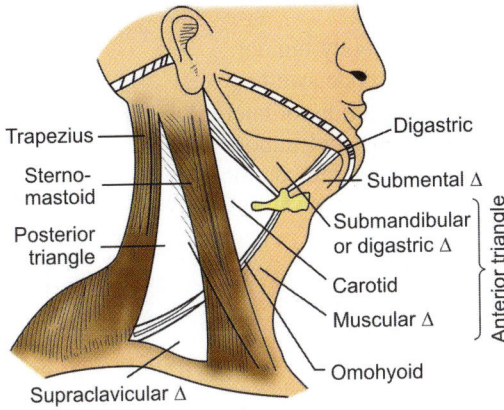

Fig. 3.1: Triangles of the neck. Some swelling is peculiar to a particular triangle, e.g. cystic hygroma in the posterior triangle.

The anterior triangle is bounded by the midline from chin to manubrium, posteriorly by the anterior border of the sternomastoid and above by the lower border of the mandible. It can be subdivided by the digastric muscle and the omohyoid muscle into the suprahyoid – *submental and submandibular triangles,* and the infrahyoid – *carotid and muscular triangles.*

The posterior triangle is bound anteriorly by the posterior border of the sternomastoid, posteriorly by the anterior border of the trapezius and below by the middle third of the clavicle.

For clinical evaluation, the swellings in the neck can be grouped in one of these easily definable triangles.

CLASSIFICATION

The swellings of the neck can be classified in two groups: Those situated in the midline and within approximately 2 cm on either side of the midline (*midline swellings*), and those situated lateral to this area (*lateral swellings*).

Midline swellings (Cystic and solid) (Fig. 3.2)

Cystic swellings

1. Ranula
2. Cervical dermoid
3. Subhyoid bursal cyst
4. Thyroglossal cyst
5. Cyst in relation to the isthmus of the thyroid gland
6. Cold abscess in the space of burns
7. Aneurysm of the innominate artery
8. Ludwig's angina.

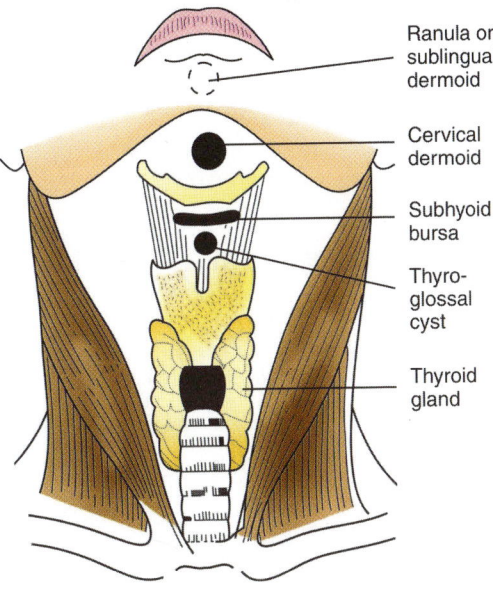

Fig. 3.2: Midline swellings of the neck.

Solid swellings

1. Lymph node swelling
   - Submental
   - Pre-laryngeal
   - Pretracheal
2. Thyroid gland swelling (*moves up with swallowing*)
   - Diffuse swelling
   - Solitary nodule
   - Multinodular
3. Bony growth arising from the manubrium sterni
4. Rarely persistent thymus
5. Rarely ectopic thyroid

   All the midline swellings are included within the anterior triangle.

Lateral swellings (Cystic and solid)
(Fig. 3.3)

For better clinical assessment lateral swellings can be grouped according to their locations within any of the three triangles of the neck:
   (a) submandibular triangle;
   (b) carotid triangle; and
   (c) posterior triangle.

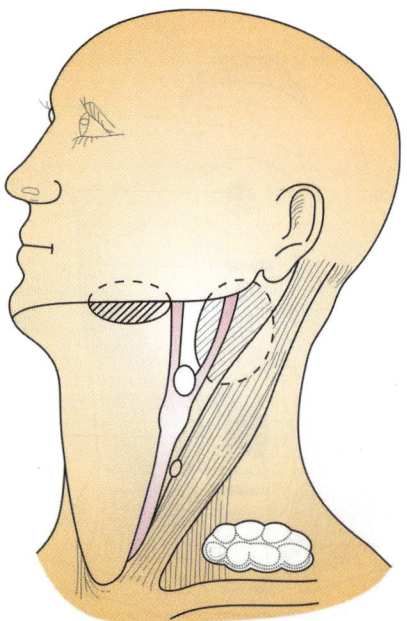

Fig. 3.3: Lateral swellings of the neck.

Submandibular triangle
Cystic swellings

1. Plunging ranula
2. Lateral variety of sublingual dermoid
3. Retention cyst of salivary gland

Solid swellings

1. Submandibular salivary gland
   - Tumours
   - Sialitis
   - Sialolithiasis
   - Sjogren's syndrome
2. Lymph node swelling

Carotid triangle
Cystic swellings

1. Branchial cyst
2. Abscess in the lymph glands, e.g. cold abscess
3. Carotid aneurysm
4. Cystadenoma of lateral lobe of thyroid
5. Laryngocele

Solid swellings

1. Carotid body tumour
2. Lymph node swelling
3. Solid swelling of lateral lobe of thyroid
4. Sternomastoid tumour
5. Branchiogenic carcinoma

Posterior triangle
Cystic swellings

1. Cystic hygroma
2. Solitary lymphatic cyst
3. Abscess in the lymph nodes, e.g. cold abscess
4. Pharyngeal pouch
5. Subclavian aneurysm

Solid swellings

1. Lymph node swelling
2. Cervical rib

Swellings anywhere in the neck

In addition to the above mentioned lesions the following lesions can occur anywhere in the neck. These are:

1. Sebaceous cyst

2. Lipoma
3. Fibroma
4. Neurofibroma
5. Haemangioma.

Pulsatile swellings in the neck

1. Aneurysm of carotid, subclavian, innominate arteries
2. Prominent subclavian pulse over a cervical rib
3. Carotid body tumour
4. Vascular toxic goitre
5. Tortuous vessel
6. AV malformation
7. Transmitted pulse by a solid swelling

RANULA

Ranula is a soft, cystic and bluish swelling simulating frog's belly. The term '*ranula*' is derived from the Latin word, *Rana*, which means a little frog.

Origin

It is a *mucus-retention cyst* arising from the mucous glands situated on the floor of the mouth and the undersurface of the tongue due to obstruction to the ducts secreting mucus. The names of the glands are *glands of Blandin and Nuhn*. The swelling is mostly, if not entirely, unilateral and presents as swelling in the floor of the mouth. If extending beyond the mylohyoid muscle, it presents as a swelling in the sub-mandibular region also.

According to some, it is a dilatation of the Wharton's duct of the submandibular gland though this theory is not universally accepted (W. Boyd).

Pathology

Lining of the cyst wall: The wall of the cyst is lined by either columnar or cuboidal epithelium or by fibrous tissue.

Contents: Viscid and glairy or jelly-like fluid.

Diagnostic criteria

Once seen, diagnosis is never to be in doubt. It is obvious from its site and appearance.

1. *Age:* Mostly seen in young children and adolescence.
2. *Sex:* Both the sexes are equally affected.
3. Patient presents with *swelling in the floor of the mouth* which may be painful.
4. Intrabuccal swelling situated in the floor of the mouth between the undersurface of the tongue and the symphysis menti (Fig. 3.4); *mostly unilateral, on one side of the frenulum linguae (patient should be asked to show the undersurface of the tongue).*

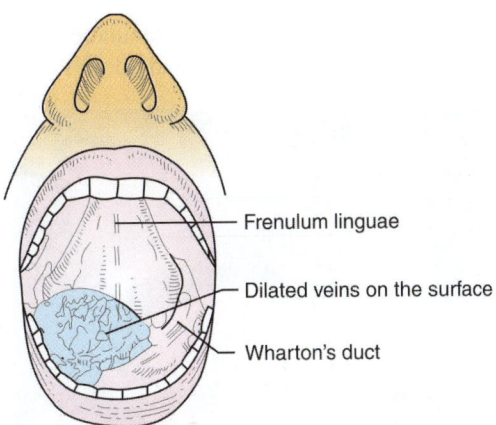

Frenulum linguae

Dilated veins on the surface

Wharton's duct

Fig. 3.4: Ranula. A typical ranula passing sub-mucosally across the floor of the mouth with dilated veins on the surface which gives the appearance resembling a frog's belly.

5. *Shape and size:* Spherical cyst varies from 1 to 5 cm in diameter but only the top half is visible.
6. *Colour is pale blue with characteristic semi-transparent appearance* and with the presence of ranine vein (deep lingual vein) found as a bluish line over the surface.
7. Surface is smooth and mucous membrane is mobile over the swelling. The edge of the swelling is difficult to feel. The swelling is not tender.
8. *Cystic swelling: Fluctuation is positive.* (Fluctuation is elicited with the tip of the index finger, and is called Paget's test, as a cystic swelling feels more cystic in the centre.)
9. *Transillumination: Positive.* During trans-illumination amidst the reddish glow there

is the presence of white opaque strands which indicate either the presence of deep lingual veins running along the wall of the cyst, or Wharton's duct.

10. Patient may give the history of bursting of the ranula with subsequent reformation.
11. May or may not have prolongation in the neck.
12. Cervical lymph glands are usually not enlarged.

Types of ranula

Oral type (Fig. 3.5): Simple ranula restricted to the oral cavity (features already described).

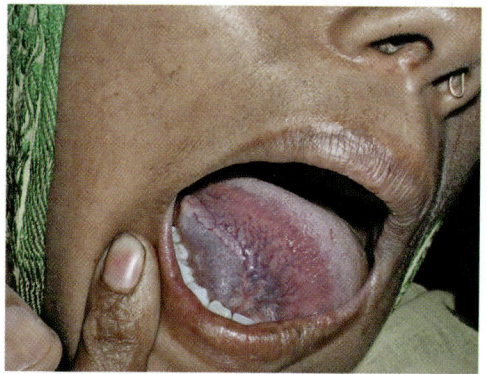

Fig. 3.5: Ranula on the floor of the mouth on the right side of frenulum linguae.

Plunging type: When the oral variety extends into the neck (particularly submandibular region) passing beyond the floor of the mouth along the posterior border of mylohyoid muscle and appears in the submandibular region.

Diagnosis of plunging ranula: By bidigital palpation of the swelling (cross fluctuation test). One finger is placed in the oral cavity and the other on the neck. If the pressure is given from the neck, finger in the oral cavity is pushed up, and vice versa.

Therefore, in all cases of ranula, one should examine the submandibular region for any cervical prolongation.

Complications

1. Repeated trauma
2. Bursting and reformation

3. Infection
4. A big ranula may cause difficulty in speech or eating or mastication due to restricted movements of the tongue.

Differential diagnosis

1. *Sublingual dermoid:* Midline swelling; transillumination is negative.
2. *Haemangioma:* Compressible; trans-illumination negative.
3. Mucous cyst.

Treatment

1. Complete excision which includes the removal of the affected glands.
2. Partial excision with 'marsupialization'.

Complete excision is ideal, but it is difficult and tedious, because it almost always bursts on attempted dissection, and there is a chance of incomplete removal and so, a chance of recurrence. *Moreover, there is every chance of injury to the lingual nerve and the submandibular duct (Wharton's duct).*

Partial excision with marsupialization: The top of the cyst is excised. The cut edge of the cyst wall is sutured with the adjacent mucous membrane covering the floor of the mouth. Thus the bottom of the ranula becomes part of the floor of the mouth.

Every care should be taken not to injure the Wharton's duct. *Marsupialisation avoids surgical dissection and chances of injury to the sub-mandibular duct and lingual nerve.*

Plunging type ranula is better approached through the neck along the Langer's line over the submandibular region.

Note

Plunging ranula may also be treated by one of the methods described above, ensuring good drainage of cervical extension. *It avoids a cosmetically undesirable scar from cervical incision.*

Note

The sublingual glands secrete saliva irrespective of stimulation to keep the mouth cavity moist and smooth.

CERVICAL AND SUBLINGUAL DERMOID

This is a form of congenital sequestration dermoid arising due to inclusion of the surface ectoderm at the fusion line of the 1st branchial arches or mandibular arches.

Common age of appearance

Though congenital, it does not appear before the age of ten. The usual time of appearance is between 10 and 25 years.

Pathology

Sublingual dermoid is a thin-walled cystic lesion.

- *Lining of the cyst wall:* As it is a *congenital ectodermal* swelling, it is lined by squamous epithelium.
- *Contents:* Cheesy material or sebaceous material. It never contains hair as in other dermoids.

Types

According to position:

1. Median variety
2. Lateral variety (uncommon)

Each variety is again either above the mylohyoid muscle or below the mylohyoid muscle. So, anatomically it is of two varieties:

1. Supramylohyoid or sublingual
2. Inframylohyoid or cervical.

Pathogenesis

During fusion of the two halves of the mandibular arches some ectodermal cells may be sequestrated into the underlying mesoderm. In future these ectodermal cells may proliferate and ultimately liquefy to form the cystic swelling. The swelling may be projected below the mylohyoid muscle (inframylohyoid variety), or above the mylohyoid muscle (supramylohyoid variety) in the floor of the mouth below the undersurface of the tongue and hence is called sublingual dermoid (Fig. 3.6).

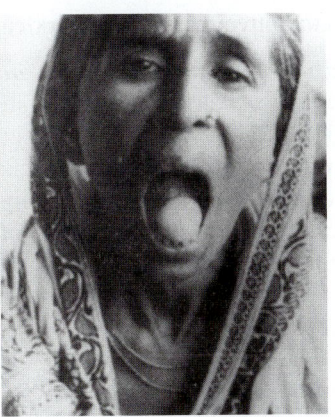

Fig. 3.6: Sublingual dermoid. Patient having this swelling in the floor of the mouth beneath the tongue. Duration—for the last 20 years. Fluctuant, non-opaque swelling. Patient did not have difficulty in eating but she had some difficulty in speech.

According to some, the cervical type of dermoid is derived from the 2nd branchial cleft, particularly the lateral variety.

Diagnostic criteria

The patient may present with the swelling in different manners according to the positions.

I. Median variety

(a) Supramylohyoid variety or sublingual variety

1. *Midline cystic swelling in the floor of the mouth between the tongue and the jaw.* A sequestration dermoid in the floor of the mouth beneath the tongue is due to entrapped ectoderm at the level of the 1st branchial arch fusion. It is typically a midline swelling, either supra- or inframylohyoid, rarely may be paramedian.
2. *Shape and size:* Spherical cyst varies from 2 to 5 cm in diameter.
3. Surface is smooth. The swelling is not tender.
4. Cystic swelling – *fluctuation is positive.*
5. Transillumination – *negative* (cf. ranula).

Differential diagnosis:

- Ranula – transillumination positive.
- Hamartoma and benign tumours of the tongue – usually they are attached to the tongue.

(b) Inframylohyoid variety or cervical variety

1. *Midline cystic swelling just below the symphysis menti* (i.e. in the submental region). The swelling is sometimes so prominent that the patient seeks advice because of 'double chin' appearance.
2. Does not move with deglutition (cf. thyroid swelling).
3. Does not move on protruding the tongue (cf. thyroglossal cyst).
4. Fluctuation – *positive*.
5. Transillumination – *negative*.
6. Bimanually palpable with one finger in the mouth and one beneath the chin.

Differential diagnosis:

1. Ectopic thyroid
2. Suprahyoid thyroglossal cyst
3. Submental lymph node swelling.

II. Lateral variety

(a) Supramylohyoid or sublingual

- Cystic swelling in the floor of the mouth placed laterally.
- Transillumination – negative (cf. ranula).

(b) Inframylohyoid or cervical

- Cystic swelling in the region of the sub-mandibular salivary gland.
- Transillumination – negative.

Differential diagnosis:

1. *Plunging ranula:* Bidigitally palpable; *trans-illumination is positive.*
2. *Submandibular salivary gland swelling: Solid swelling.*
3. *Submental lymph node swelling: Solid swelling,* usually other nodes are involved and usually not bimanually palpable.
4. *Thyroglossal cyst: Moves up with deglutition* whereas a sublingual dermoid cyst does not.

Investigation

CT scan may be useful to show the extension of sublingual dermoid.

Complications

1. Cosmetically looks ugly.

2. If too big, may cause difficulty in speech or eating, respiratory difficulty.
3. Infection.
4. Repeated trauma.

Treatment

Complete excision.

Sublingual dermoids are approached through the floor of the mouth.

Cervical dermoids are approached via a curved incision along the Langer's line over the submental or submandibular region. Sometimes the dissection is to be carried out from the neck into the oral cavity by retracting the posterior border of the mylohyoid muscle.

Note: See p. 30 for dermoid cyst (Chapter 2).

THYROGLOSSAL CYST

It is a cystic swelling arising from the remnant of the thyroglossal duct. It is regarded as tubulo-dermoid.

Surgical anatomy

The thyroglossal duct extends as a downgrowth of solid column of cells from the foramen caecum at the base of the tongue to the isthmus of the thyroid gland. Subsequently the solid column undergoes canalisation. This duct ultimately disappears when its function is over. The other name of the duct is *median thyroid diverticulum*.

Path of the duct

It starts from the foramen caecum of the tongue and descends through the genioglossi muscles up to the hyoid bone (Fig. 3.7). At the region of the hyoid bone it descends:

(a) either in front of the hyoid bone, or
(b) through the hyoid bone, or
(c) it hooks below and behind the hyoid bone (Fig. 3.8).

Then it descends up to the level of the upper border of the thyroid cartilage.

Fate of the duct

1. It completely atrophies except at the lower part where it forms *the isthmus of the thyroid gland*, and *the pyramidal lobe*, if present.

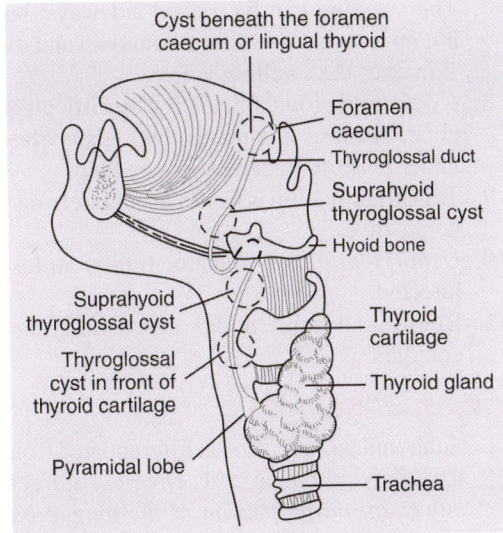

Fig. 3.7: The course of the thyroglossal duct and different sites of the thyroglossal cyst.

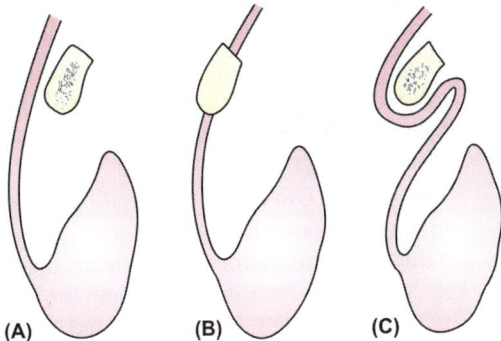

Figs 3.8 A to C: Relation of the thyroglossal duct with the hyoid bone: (A) In front of the hyoid bone; (B) Through the hyoid bone; (C) Hooks below and behind the hyoid bone.

2. Part from foramen caecum up to the hyoid bone disappears. The rest persists as *levator glandulae thyroidae*.
3. From the portion of the diverticulum ectopic thyroid tissues may develop which in adult life are situated along the course of the diverticulum. When present in the region of the tongue, it is called *lingual thyroid. A lingual thyroid looks like a flattened strawberry sitting on the base of the tongue. It may be the only thyroid tissue present in the body.*

4. A portion of the duct may remain un-obliterated and gives rise to a cystic swelling due to accumulation of secretions – *thyroglossal cyst.*

Sites where thyroglossal cyst may occur

Anywhere along the course of the duct (Fig. 3.7), e.g.

1. Subhyoid region (commonest: Over 80%).
2. Suprahyoid region – double chin appearance.
3. In front of the thyroid cartilage (second common site).
4. In front of the cricoid cartilage (rare).
5. In the floor of the mouth.
6. In the substance of the tongue beneath the foramen caecum (rarest).

Pathology

- *Lining of the cyst wall:* Cyst is lined by columnar, cuboidal or squamous epithelium and surrounded by a shell of lymphoid tissue (so, prone to infection). It may contain thyroid tissue.
- *Contents:* Transparent, thick, jelly-like fluid; cholesterol crystal may be present. Occasionally clotted blood may be present.

Diagnostic criteria

1. *Age:* Commonly found in children but may occur at any age.
2. *Sex:* More common in women.
3. *Midline cystic swelling* (Figs 3.9, 3.10 A and B): Thyroglossal cyst usually presents as an asymptomatic swelling in the upper part of the neck in the midline. It is usually present around the hyoid bone. Cyst in front of thyroid cartilage is situated slightly lateral to the midline, usually to the left.
4. *Usually elongated in shape having its long axis along the long axis of the neck* (cf. subhyoid bursal cyst). The size varies from 0.5 to 5 cm in diameter.
5. *Moves upward with deglutition* (because the swelling is attached to hyoid bone by fibrous tissue).
6. *Swelling also moves up on protrusion of the tongue* (because the swelling is attached to the tongue by the persistent obliterated thyroglossal duct) (Figs 3.10 A and B).

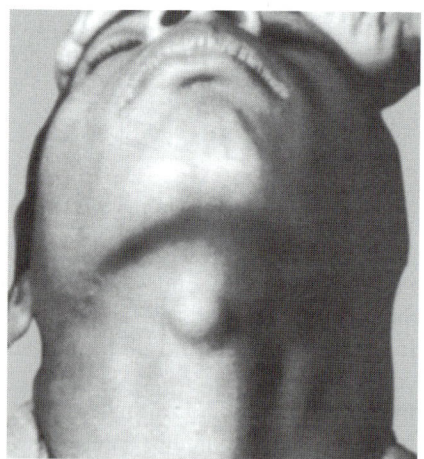

Fig. 3.9: Thyroglossal cyst. Midline cystic swelling in front of the hyoid bone.

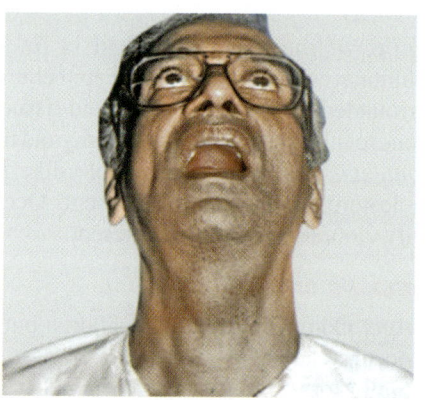

Fig. 3.10A: Thyroglossal cyst. Midline cystic swelling in front of upper border of thyroid cartilage.

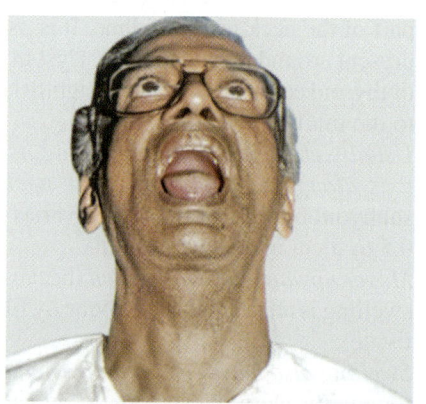

Fig. 3.10B: Same patient. On protrusion of the tongue the swelling moves up towards the chin.

7. The swelling can be moved sideways, but not up and down. Surface is smooth and the skin over the swelling is free.
8. *Cystic in feel* but fluctuation is difficult to elicit, because it contains thick glairy fluid under tension. Paget's test may help.
9. Transillumination is negative but rarely may be positive.
10. *Usually painless* and not tender unless infected.
11. Regional lymph nodes are usually not enlarged.

Differential diagnosis

1. Subhyoid variety is to be differentiated from the subhyoid bursal cyst. *Thyroglossal cyst moves up on protrusion of the tongue but not the subhyoid bursal cyst.*
2. Suprahyoid variety is to be differentiated from the cervical dermoid cyst situated below the mylohyoid (inframylohyoid) – same as above.
3. Thyroglossal cyst in front of thyroid or cricoid cartilage is to be differentiated from a cystic swelling in connection with the thyroid gland particularly related to the isthmus of thyroid.

   In both the conditions the swelling moves up with deglutition.

   But on protrusion of the tongue the thyroglossal cyst only moves up but not the cyst in connection with the thyroid gland.

Note

In doubtful case, U/S or radionuclide thyroid scan and thyroid function tests may be performed preoperatively to demonstrate that normally functioning thyroid tissue is present in its usual position.

Complications

1. Recurrent infection (because the cyst is surrounded by a shell of lymphoid tissue).
2. Fistula formation.
3. Malignancy – Papillary carcinoma can occur rarely in the thyroglossal duct remnants.

Treatment

Complete excision of the cyst with transverse incision.

Note

What are the swellings that move with deglutition?

1. Thyroid swellings
2. Cyst in relation to the isthmus of the thyroid gland
3. Ectopic thyroid
4. Thyroglossal cyst
5. Subhyoid bursal cyst
6. Enlarged pretracheal glands
7. Laryngocele

But only the thyroglossal cyst moves up also on protrusion of the tongue.

THYROGLOSSAL FISTULA

Aetiology

1. *Congenital:* Very rare, when the cellular median thyroid diverticulum communicates with the skin of the neck.
2. *Mostly acquired* because of:
   - bursting of the infected thyroglossal cyst;
   - inadvertent incision over the infected cyst mistaking it for an abscess;
   - incomplete removal of the thyroglossal cyst.

Though the fistula is mostly acquired, the persistence of the tract is always a congenital anomaly.

Pathology

- *Lining of the tract:* Usually by columnar cell epithelium.
- *Nature of the discharge:* Serous or mucoid; if infected, purulent.

Diagnostic criteria

1. Usually found in children or young adults. Rarely may be present at birth. (So, ask about duration – congenital or acquired.)
2. *Small fistula's opening in the midline of the neck* usually below the hyoid bone, hence also known as *median fistula of the neck* (cf. branchial fistula which is known as lateral fistula of the neck).
3. The fistula may be infected with purulent

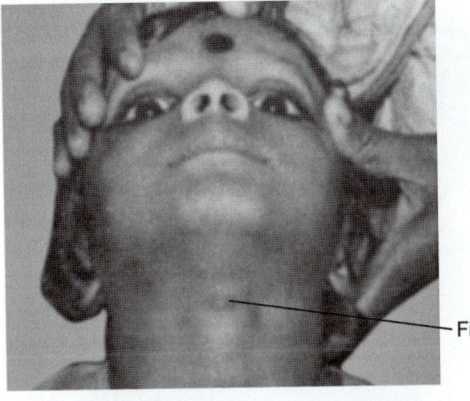

Fig. 3.11A: Thyroglossal fistula—midline fistula. So, known as the median fistula of the neck.

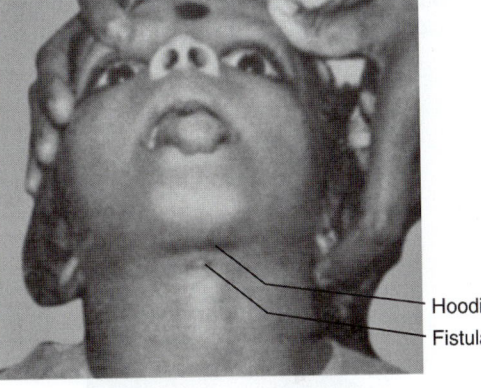

Fig. 3.11B: Same patient. Fistula moves up on protrusion of the tongue. Note the hooding of the skin above the fistula (*see* text).

discharge. In the quiescent stage there may be mucoid discharge.
4. *The fistula's opening moves up on protrusion of the tongue* (because of the persistence of the tract which is attached to the base of the tongue).
5. *Characteristic feature is the hooding of the skin above the opening,* i.e. a crescentic fold of skin with the concavity downwards, overlying the fistula's opening. This hooding of the skin becomes more prominent on protrusion of the tongue (Fig. 3.11B).
6. The fistula may close intermittently with recurrence of pain and inflammation.
7. Enquire about any previous swelling which might have burst or been incised.

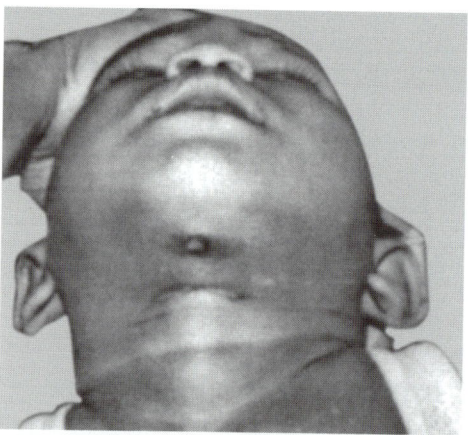

Fig. 3.12: Recurrent thyroglossal fistula. Most probably due to inadequate excision. Note the previous scar mark below the fistula. Sistrunk's operation is always advisable.

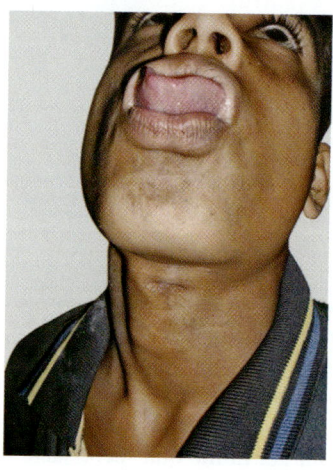

Fig. 3.13: Recurrent thyroglossal fistula—moved up on protrusion of the tongue. Note the scar mark from previous operation. Sistrunk's operation is always advisable. (*Courtesy:* Professor Sudeb Saha, MS, FAMS)

Treatment of thyroglossal fistula

Complete excision of the fistula tract with the removal of every vestige of the thyroglossal tract as close as possible to the base of the tongue up to the foramen caecum, may require multiple transverse incisions on the neck. Otherwise there may be recurrence of thyroglossal fistula. *Sistrunk's operation is for thyroglossal fistula, not for thyroglossal cyst.*

Sistrunk's operation

Where, in addition to the above measures, a portion (particularly the central) of the hyoid bone is excised along with intact tract within. Because the body of the hyoid bone may obstruct the dissection particularly when the tract is hooking below and behind the hyoid bone or passing through its substance during its descent.

Preoperative precautions and measures

1. *The suspected swelling may be due to ectopic thyroid tissue.* So, before excision, if it is doubtful, one should confirm that it is not the only thyroid tissue present in the body, otherwise its excision will be followed by hypothyroidism.
   So, in case of any doubt, it is to be confirmed by radioactive iodine uptake test.
2. For better visualisation of the tract, methylene blue may be injected into the cyst. *When the fistula is present*, the dye is pushed through the fistula's opening on the night before operation, and the opening of the fistula is closed with a purse-string suture. This procedure helps in better visualisation of the tract during operation.
3. If there are any features of infection, they should be controlled with antibiotics prior to surgery.

PUBERTY GOITRE

- Any enlargement of the thyroid gland is called the goitre.
- The goitre presents as a lump on the anterior aspect of the neck.
- Diffuse hyperplastic goitre may be noticed at puberty or pregnancy.

Aetiology

When the metabolic demands are high during puberty or pregnancy, TSH levels become high. TSH levels become high to stimulate the thyroid gland to provide the increased demands of T_3 and T_4 during puberty or pregnancy. HCG also has TSH receptor-stimulating property which may explain goitre developing during pregnancy. *This is also termed as physiological or stress-induced goitre.*

Diagnostic criteria

1. Commonly seen in female during puberty or pregnancy.
2. Goitre presents as a lump in front of the neck.
3. The lump in the neck *moves upwards on swallowing or deglutition* – both visible and palpable.

   Swallowing test: Give the patient a glass full of water. The patient is asked to take sips of water but will not swallow it till asked for. *Now, with the neck straight or slightly extended and looking straight ahead horizontally, the patient is asked to swallow the water. Note the movement of the swelling over the neck, whether the swelling moves up on swallowing of water.*

   Note: Do not hesitate to ask for a glass of water which is usually kept on the examiner's table.
4. But the lump does not move up on protrusion of the tongue (cf. thyroglossal cyst).
5. *Pizzillo's method of inspection:* To render the swelling prominent for inspection easier, one can perform Pizzillo's method – by asking the patient to put her head backwards and press against her hands placed over the occiput, *to make a minimally enlarged gland more prominent.*
6. Surface is smooth, soft to firm, not irregular or nodular.
7. Not tender. No local rise of temperature (cf. local rise of temperature is a feature of thyroid toxicity).
8. *No protrusion of eyeball (proptosis or exophthalmos) or (visible sclera between the cornea and upper eyelid)* while patient looks straight ahead horizontally.
9. Mobility of the swelling is not restricted when examined from front and behind (cf. malignancy of thyroid) – on inspection or palpation.
10. *There will be no features of thyroid toxicity* like increased sweating, tremor of the outstretched fingers, increased pulse rate or heart rate or proptosis.

Examine these features to exclude thyroid toxicity.

Differential diagnosis

Thyroglossal cyst where the swelling moves upwards on protrusion of the tongue.

Investigation

- T_3/T_4/TSH: T_3 and T_4 remain normal. *TSH levels may be high during puberty or pregnancy* which stimulate the thyroid gland. HCG may be marginally raised which has TSH receptor-stimulating property, which may explain goitre developing during pregnancy.
- Ultrasound of the neck – to assess the size of the gland and to assure the parents and patient and her husband that there is nothing abnormal.

Treatment

- Wait and watch – assurance to the patient and parents or husband.
- Continue with the normal diet. *Avoid cabbage in the diet.*
- Tab thyroxine – 0.2 mg/day to suppress the high level of TSH for over a year to make the gland regress. Rarely, it may fail to do so, transforming itself into a colloid goitre.
- Repeat examination every 6 months till puberty and pregnancy are over.

Note

Size of goitre

- Large goitre – protrusion of the goitre beyond the chin or jaw.
- Largest neck circumference crossing the goitre is 40 cm or more.

Grading of goitre (WHO classification)

Grade Ia Not visible but palpable lump in the neck consistent with thyroid swelling.

Grade Ib Visible with neck in the extended position.

Grade II Visible and palpable with the neck in the normal position.

Grade III Visible large gland evident from a distance and palpable.

Note

Different types of goitre

'Goitre' denotes enlargement of thyroid gland irrespective of its causes. It is classified as:

1. *Simple goitre*
   (a) Diffuse hyperplastic goitre
   (b) Nodular goitre
   (c) Colloid goitre
2. *Toxic goitre*
   (a) Diffuse toxic goitre (Graves' disease)
   (b) Toxic nodular goitre
   (c) Toxic nodule
3. *Neoplastic goitre*
   (a) Benign
   (b) Malignant
4. *Thyroiditis*
   (a) Autoimmune thyroiditis
   (b) Subacute or granulomatous thyroiditis (de Quervain's)
   (c) Riedel's thyroiditis
5. *Stress-induced goitre:* Physiological goitre
   • During puberty
   • During pregnancy

Note

Puberty goitre may be given as a short case also during postgraduate examination.

SUBHYOID BURSAL CYST

It is the accumulation of inflammatory fluid giving rise to *a cystic swelling of the subhyoid bursa.*

The subhyoid bursa is situated over the thyro-hyoid membrane below the hyoid bone slightly posterior to its lower border.

Pathology

Lining of the cyst – epithelium.
Contents – turbid or clear fluid.

Diagnostic criteria

1. History of painful onset with features of mild inflammation.
2. Midline swelling but transversely elongated – discoid-shaped cystic swelling (cf. thyroglossal cyst).
3. Situated below the hyoid bone.
4. Moves with deglutition (as attached to hyoid bone).
5. But no movement on protrusion of the tongue (cf. thyroglossal cyst).

6. Cystic in feel – fluctuation is positive.
7. Transillumination – usually negative; may be positive if fluid is clear.

Treatment

Complete excision by skin crease incision.

BRANCHIAL CYST AND FISTULA

Before considering the cysts and fistula, a short account of branchial arches and their derivatives is presented here.

The matured structure of head and neck are embryologically derived from the six pairs of branchial arches.

DEVELOPMENT OF BRANCHIAL ARCHES

In the developing embryo surrounding the primitive pharynx (or cephalic part of the foregut) six pairs of mesodermal condensation appear in the form of branchial or visceral arches, derived from the lateral sheet mesoderm (Fig. 3.14).

In between the arches, there are depressions or spaces both inside and outside the pharynx. *Internally*, these spaces are lined by endoderm and are called branchial or pharyngeal pouches. *Externally*, these spaces are lined by ectoderm and are called branchial or pharyngeal clefts. So, between the two is the cleft membrane, which is lined internally with columnar and externally with squamous epithelium. The cleft membrane never disappears in human body (in contrast to fishes), because a little mesodermal element always persists between the entoderm and ectoderm.

Each branchial arch has a central plate of cartilage (which later gives rise to bone), a muscle mass, a nerve (to supply the derivatives of the arch) and an artery.

Mesodermal derivatives of the branchial arches

First arch or mandibular arch

A. *From the cartilage:*
   1. Malleus

2. Incus
3. Lingula of the mandible
4. Mental ossicles, if present.

B. *From the sheath around the cartilage:*
   1. Anterior ligament of malleus
   2. Sphenomandibular ligament
   3. Body and ramus of the mandible.

C. *From the muscle mass or myotomep:* All the muscles supplied by mandibular nerve:
   1. Muscles of mastication – masseter, temporal, lateral and medial pterygoids
   2. Tensor palati
   3. Tensor tympani
   4. Mylohyoid
   5. Anterior belly of digastric.

D. *Nerve of the first arch:* Mandibular nerve (a branch of trigeminal nerve or 5th cranial nerve).

E. *Artery of the first arch:* Maxillary artery (remnant of the 1st aortic arch).

Second arch or hyoid arch

A. *From the cartilage (Reichert's cartilage)*
   1. Stapes
   2. Styloid process of the temporal bone
   3. Lesser cornu and upper half of the body of the hyoid bone.

B. *From the sheath around the cartilage:* Stylo-hyoid ligament

C. *From the muscle mass or myotome:* All the muscles supplied by the facial nerve:
   1. Muscles of facial expression including occipitofrontalis and buccinator
   2. Platysma
   3. Posterior belly of digastric
   4. Stylohyoid
   5. Stapedius.

D. *Nerve of the 2nd arch:* Facial nerve (7th cranial nerve).

E. *Artery of the 2nd arch:* Stapedial artery (remnant of the dorsal part of 2nd aortic arch).

Note

Second branchial arch remnants cause cyst or sinus/fistula with the external opening along the anterior border of sternomastoid muscle.

Third arch

A. *From the cartilage:* Greater cornu and lower half of the body of the hyoid bone.

B. *From the muscle mass or myotome:* A muscle supplied by the glossopharyngeal nerve – stylopharyngeus muscle.

C. *Nerve of the 3rd arch:* Glossopharyngeal nerve (9th cranial nerve).

D. *Artery of the 3rd arch:* Internal carotid artery (remnant of the dorsal part of 3rd aortic arch); common carotid artery (remnant of the ventral part of the 3rd aortic arch).

Fourth arch

A. *From the cartilage:*
   1. Thyroid cartilage
   2. Epiglottis.

B. *From the muscle mass or myotome:* All the muscles supplied by the external laryngeal nerve which is a branch of superior laryngeal nerve:
   1. Cricothyroid
   2. Inferior constrictor of pharynx.

C. *Nerve of the 4th arch:* Superior laryngeal nerve, a branch of vagus nerve.

D. *Artery of the 4th arch:*
   1. Right side, first part of the subclavian artery.
   2. Left side, main part of the arch of the aorta (both are remnants of the 4th aortic arch).

Fifth arch

Disappears.

Sixth arch

A. *From the cartilage:*
   1. Cricoid cartilage, arytenoid cartilage (probably corniculate and cuneiform cartilages).
   2. Rings of trachea and bronchi.

B. *From the muscle mass or myotome:* All the muscles supplied by the cranial accessory nerve carried via the recurrent laryngeal nerve:
   1. All the intrinsic muscles of the larynx except the cricothyroid.
   2. All the muscles of the pharynx except the stylopharyngeus.

3. All the muscles of the palate except the tensor palati.

C. *Nerve of the 6th arch:* Recurrent laryngeal nerve – a branch of the vagus nerve (10th cranial nerve) but carrying the fibres of cranial accessory nerve.

D. *Artery of the 6th arch:*
1. Ventrally – main part of the pulmonary artery.
2. Dorsally – on the right side the artery disappears; on the left side the artery persists as the ductus arteriosus (both are the remnants of the 6th aortic arch).

BRANCHIAL CYST

It is a cystic swelling arising in connection with the persistent cervical sinus which is formed due to the fusion of overgrowing 2nd branchial arch with the 6th branchial arch. (For branchial cyst, *see* Figs 3.14 and 3.15.)

Pathogenesis

Conventional theory

The 2nd branchial arch migrates towards the surface and overgrows the 3rd and 4th arches (Fig. 3.14A) and ultimately fuses with the 6th arch forming a cavity called cervical sinus (5th arch disappears completely). Normally this sinus disappears. But if it persists, accumulation of fluid occurs inside the sinus and gives rise to a cystic swelling called branchial cyst. The secretion usually comes from the appendages of the ectodermal lining of the enclosed space, sweat and sebaceous glands.

The branchial cyst usually lies superficial to the structures derived from the 2nd and 3rd branchial arches, i.e. the lesser cornu of hyoid bone, posterior belly of digastric muscles, facial nerve, external carotid artery.

Sometimes the 2nd arch fails to fuse with the 6th arch and thus gives rise to branchial sinus or fistula (Fig. 3.14B).

Other theories of origin of branchial cyst

1. One theory suggests that the cervical sinus is closed from the bottom to the surface and during this process ectodermal epibranchial

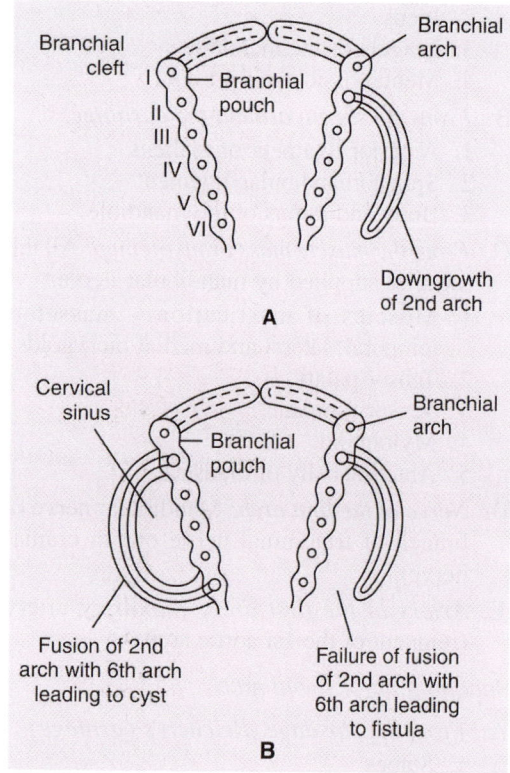

Figs 3.14 A and B: The method of formation of branchial cyst and branchial fistula.

placodes grow inwards. The placodal vesicles usually disappear after organising the development of the ganglion connected with some cranial nerves. If the placodal vesicles persist, they are expressed as branchial cyst.

2. It has been suggested that the branchial cyst may develop from the inclusion of the parotid epithelium in the upper deep cervical lymph nodes (*Illingworth*) (cf. Warthin's tumour).

3. Another theory: Entrapment of the 1st and 2nd branchial cleft ectoderm in the depth within a lymph node forming a cyst lined by squamous epithelium containing cholesterol crystals.

Pathology

• *Lining of the cyst wall:* Squamous epithelium (rarely columnar) surrounded by a large

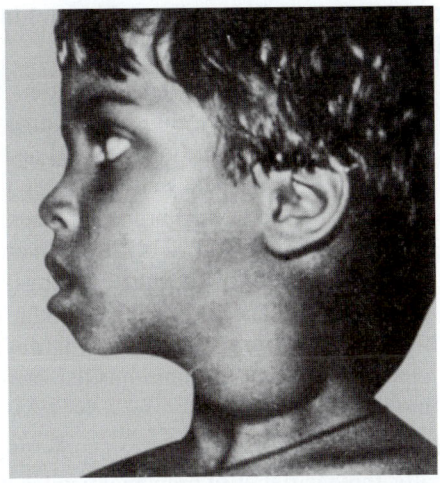

Fig. 3.15: Branchial cyst. A cystic swelling at left carotid Δ below the angle of the mandible. Posterior margin of the swelling overlapped left sternomastoid. Transillumination negative. Here the age of presentation is 10 years.

amount of lymphoid tissue, so prone to infection.

• *Contents:* Cheesy material derived from desquamated epithelial cells. It may resemble the appearance of cold abscess. But its characteristic feature is *the presence of cholesterol crystals* in large numbers.

Diagnostic criteria

1. *Age:* Although congenital, it first appears in late childhood around 10 and 15 years, but its advent may be postponed till the 30th year. (Why? Because the fluid which it contains accumulates very slowly.)
2. *Sex:* Equally common in both sexes.
3. The patient presents with *a slow growing painless lump in the upper lateral part of the neck inferior to the angle of the mandible.*

Examination:

4. *Site:* The lump lies below the angle of the jaw, beneath the upper third of the sterno-mastoid muscle and *bulges forward around the anterior border of the muscle into the carotid triangle.* Very rarely the cyst can bulge backwards behind the muscle.
5. *Shape and size:* Usually ovoid and varies from 5 to 10 cm in width.

6. *Surface:* Smooth and the edge is distinct. Overlying skin is free and looks normal unless infected.
7. The lump is a firm, *cystic swelling. Fluctuation is positive.* The fluctuation is not always easy to elicit, specially when the cyst is deep to the upper part of the sternomastoid muscle. *The lump is usually non-tender unless infected.*
8. The lump is not very mobile as it is closely tethered to the surrounding structures.
9. *Transillumination: Negative* because of its thick contents. The cyst contains yellow thick fluid with cholesterol crystals and epithelial debris: Mucoid or rarely purulent.
10. *Lymph nodes:* The local deep cervical lymph nodes should not be enlarged. If they are, one should reconsider the diagnosis in favour of cold abscess rather than a branchial cyst.
11. *On aspiration:* The aspirated materials resemble the appearance of cold abscess. But the aspirate may demonstrate fat globules, and *cholesterol crystals* secreted by the sebaceous glands in the epithelial lining.

Differential diagnosis

1. *Cold abscess in the neck:* A caseating tuberculous lymph node may simulate a branchial cyst. But the presence of enlarged matted lymph nodes in the neck along with other features of tuberculosis, such as evening rise of temperature, loss of weight, anorexia, excessive sweating etc., are helpful in the diagnosis of tuberculous lymphadenitis with abscess. *Aspiration from the cold abscess does not show any cholesterol crystals.*
2. *Cervical dermoid (inframylohyoid variety):* Aspiration from dermoid does not show cholesterol crystals.
3. *Plunging ranula:* Transillumination is positive.
4. *Cystic hygroma:* Transillumination is brilliantly positive and commonly situated in the posterior triangle.
5. *Carotid body tumour:* Solid swelling.
6. *Solitary enlarged cervical lymph node:* Solid swelling.
7. *Submandibular salivary gland swelling:* Solid swelling.

Complications

1. Recurrent infection (because of the presence of lymphoid tissue in the wall) producing cellulitis and abscess formation.
2. Followed by bursting, resulting in fistula formation.
   When there is infection of the branchial cyst, it may look like a hot abscess and when it is inadvertently incised branchial fistula is formed.
3. Branchiogenic carcinoma, usually a squamous cell carcinoma.

Treatment

Excision of the cyst through incision along the Langer's line – early in life to prevent recurrent infection.

Precautions during operation

1. The cyst wall is thin and delicate, so not to be held by any tissue forceps.
2. Avoid injury to the following structures deep to cyst.
   • Hypoglossal nerve, glossopharyngeal nerve and spinal accessory nerves.
   • Carotid arteries.
   • Wall of the pharynx close to the posterior pillar of tonsils.

BRANCHIAL SINUS OR FISTULA

This may be either congenital or acquired.

1. *Congenital: Commonest.* It is due to either:
   • failure of fusion of the 2nd branchial arch with the 6th branchial arch (Fig. 3.14); or
   • disappearance of the membrane (cleft membrane) connecting these two arches.
2. *Acquired:* It is due to either:
   • bursting of the infected branchial cyst; or
   • inadvertent incision over the infected branchial cyst when mistaken for an abscess;
   • recurrence or fistula formation due to incomplete removal of the cyst.

Note

Some others suggest thymopharyngeal duct as the origin of branchial fistula.

Types of congenital variety of branchial fistula

1. *Incomplete: Commonest.* It does not communicate with the cavity of the pharynx and remains blind at the inner end against the lateral pharyngeal wall. So, this type should better be termed branchial sinus.
2. *Complete variety* (Fig. 3.14): In this variety both external and internal openings are present, and hence the branchial fistula. The internal opening may open inside the pharynx either at the intratonsillar cleft or in the pyriform fossa.

Considering the above discussion, theoretically, three varieties of branchial fistulae may be recognised.

(i) *A complete fistula* with an external opening on the skin, and an internal opening in the pharynx (Fig. 3.16). This is usually the result of inadvertent trauma during exploration of the tract by a probe which ruptures the tridermal-cleft membrane, separating the tract from the pharynx (McGregor).

(ii) *Only an internal opening* in the pharynx (only theoretically possible).

(iii) *Only an external opening* on the skin (*commonest*).

Path of the fistula tract

The superficial and deep relations of a branchial fistula are the same as in the case of a branchial cyst.

Traced from below, the tract pierces the deep fascia at the upper border of thyroid cartilage – then passes between the fork of the common carotid artery lying superficial to internal carotid artery (3rd arch derivative) but deep to external carotid artery and its branches (Fig. 3.16). When traced further towards the pharynx, the tract lies superficial to stylopharyngeus muscle, glosso-pharyngeal nerve (3rd arch derivative) but deep to the hypoglossal nerve and the stylomandibular ligament. The internal opening lies at the tonsillar fossa found between the palatoglossal and palatopharyngeal arches.

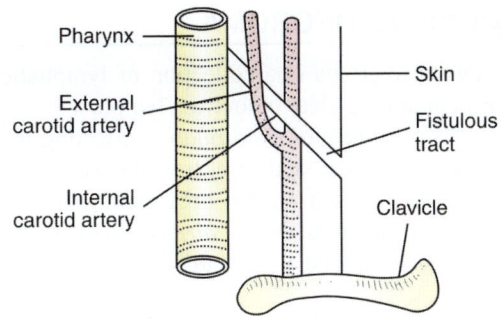

Fig. 3.16: The course of a branchial fistula—a complete variety.

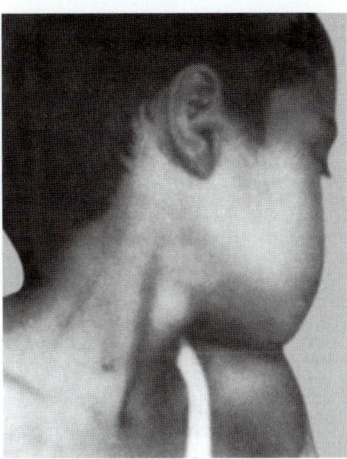

Fig. 3.17: Branchial fistula. Note the external opening at the junction of lower one-third and upper two-thirds of the sternomastoid muscle (cf. branchial cyst).

Pathology

- *Lining wall of the sinus:* Squamous epithelium or pseudostratified ciliated columnar epithelium deep to which is a layer of lymphoid tissue.
- *Nature of discharge:* Mucoid or mucopurulent with or without excoriation of the surrounding skin.

Diagnostic criteria

1. May be found at any age but usually seen in growing adults.
2. Equally common in male and female.
3. May be unilateral or bilateral.
4. *Site of external opening:* In congenital variety a small dimple or an external opening is situated at the typical site, i.e. at the anterior border of sternomastoid at the junction of the lower one-third and upper two-thirds (Fig. 3.17) (cf. branchial cyst).

   But in the acquired variety, the dimple will be at a higher level, i.e. at the level of branchial cyst.

   Branchial fistula is also called *lateral fistula of the neck* (cf. thyroglossal fistula, which is called *median fistula of the neck*).
5. Swallowing may accentuate the dimple on the skin.
6. Mucoid or mucopurulent discharge.
7. Excoriation of surrounding skin may be present.
8. Branchial cartilage may be present on palpation.

Note

Clinically, sinuses and fistulas are present at birth whereas cysts usually appear in childhood and adult life.

Treatment

Complete excision of the tract after thorough dissection starting from the cutaneous opening up to the wall of the pharynx to prevent recurrent infection.

Preoperative measures

Sinogram: Injection of radio-opaque dye into the fistulous tract followed by straight X-ray in order to assess the upper limit and extent of the fistula. This may be of some help during excision of the tract.

Steps of operation

1. Under general anaesthesia, methylene blue is injected into the track. A probe may be passed into the fistulous track.
2. *Incision:* An elliptical incision along the Langer's line encircling cutaneous opening of the fistula.
3. After cutting superficial fascia, platysma, the tract is dissected from below up as high as possible.

Gentle traction on the tract, by pulling the excised cutaneous opening, facilitates identification and proximal dissection of the tract.

4. Sometimes a second incision is needed above the upper border of thyroid cartilage. *This second incision* is made parallel to the first incision and the dissected tract is taken out through the second incision. This is known as '*stepladder pattern*' of dissecting a branchial fistula.

It is generally possible to trace the fistula up to the lateral wall of the pharynx, where it is ligated and excised.

5. After removal of the tract, the skin is closed with or without a drain.

Precautions during operation

1. As the tract passes through the bifurcation of the common carotid artery, the vessels should be protected.
2. Care should be taken not to injure the hypoglossal nerve which lies superficial to the tract.
3. Complete removal is necessary, otherwise persistence of the tract will cause recurrence.

Note

In addition to branchial cyst or fistula, two other abnormalities in relation to branchial apparatus may be occasionally found.

    (a) Branchial cartilage
    (b) Cervical auricle.

Branchial cartilage

It is an elongated piece of cartilage embedded in the skin, situated deep to the cutaneous dimple in relation to the external opening of the branchial fistula.

Cervical auricle

A hood of skin looking like an ear, containing yellow or elastic fibrocartilage, is found in relation to the external opening of the branchial fistula.

What is branchiogenic carcinoma?

It is a rare neoplasm arising from the remnants of the branchial clefts. The condition is very rare. Existence of a proved case is extremely doubtful.

CYSTIC HYGROMA

A cystic hygroma is a collection of lymphatic sacs containing clear colourless lymph.

It is a *congenital malformation* affecting the lymphatic channels and arises from the congenital lymph sacs which are the precursors of adult lymphatic channels. *It is a variety of cavernous lymphangioma*, and also regarded as hamartoma.

Pathogenesis

At the 6th week of intrauterine life three pairs of lymph sacs appear in the embryo from which the adult lymphatic channels are derived.

- One pair in the neck – jugular lymph sacs.
- One pair in the retroperitoneum.
- One pair near the inguinal region below the bifurcation of the common iliac vein – posterior lymph sacs.

By and large, cystic hygromas develop from these primitive sacs. *In the neck, cystic hygroma develops from the remnants of the jugular lymph sacs.*

The jugular lymph sacs in the neck appear one on either side, at the junction of the internal jugular vein and subclavian vein (Fig. 3.18). In the lower animals these lymph sacs are called primitive lymph heart.

During development, a portion of this lymph sac along with its lymphatic channels may be sequestrated into the surrounding mesoderm (Fig. 3.18). This sequestrated portion of the lymph sac ultimately loses its communication with the primitive lymph sac.

Later, this isolated portion of the lymph sac lined by columnar epithelium secretes lymph and gets distended to give rise to a lymphatic swelling known as cystic hygroma.

Pathology

1. It appears very early and may be found at birth or within the first few years of life. *Of all the congenital swellings, it is the earliest tumour to develop after birth, even before sternomastoid tumour.*
2. It is a type of cavernous lymphangioma.
3. *It consists of multiple cysts,* so, multilocular and multilobular.

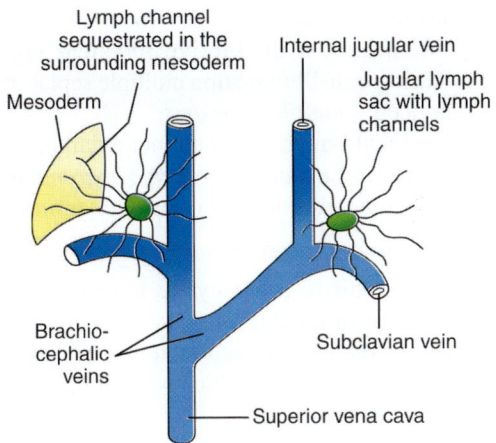

Fig. 3.18: The method of formation of cystic hygroma.

4. The cysts are filled up with clear lymph.
5. The larger cysts are situated at the periphery and the smaller cysts at the centre.
6. Many of the cysts may intercommunicate with one another.
7. *Lining of the cyst:* Each cyst is lined by a single layer of columnar epithelium and covered externally with a shell of lymphoid tissue.
8. *Contents:* Clear and watery or straw-coloured fluid consisting of cholesterol crystals, lymphocytes. The fluid does not coagulate.
9. Though cystic hygromas infiltrate into the surrounding tissues, *they never turn malignant.*

Usual sites of cystic hygroma

1. *Root of the neck in the posterior triangle:* Jugular lymph sac – 75%. Commonest site. It may extend upwards towards the ear or downwards towards the axilla and/or mediastinum.
2. Axilla – 20%
3. Groin or inguinal region
4. Mediastinum
5. Retroperitoneum
6. Tongue, buccal mucosa of the cheek and floor of the mouth. Usually lymphangiogenetic macroglossia occurs in connection with the cystic hygroma.

So, these sites are also to be examined during examination of a cystic hygroma in the neck.

Diagnostic criteria

1. *Age:* Infants or young children.
2. *Site:* Commonly at the root of the neck in the left posterior triangle, deep to the sterno-mastoid (Figs 3.19 and 3.20). Eventually, it may extend upwards in the neck, into the anterior triangle or downwards into superior mediastinum. Benign lesion but can be disfiguring.

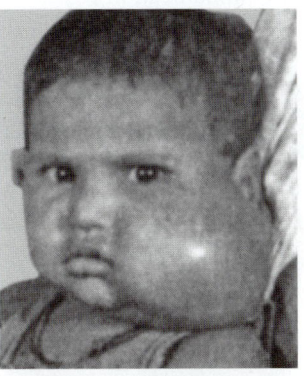

Fig. 3.19: Cystic hygroma of the left neck extending to the face raising the lobule of the ear. Trans-illumination was highly positive.

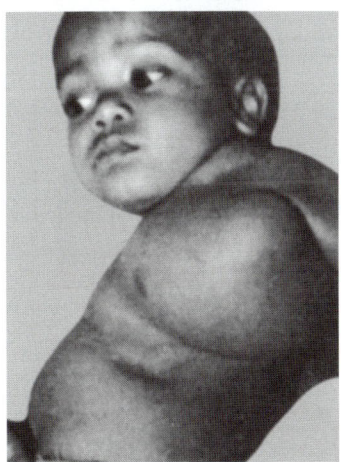

Fig. 3.20: Cystic hygroma involving neck and axilla (armpit). Axillary swelling was very big in this case. So, always examine the axillae, groins in addition for a second swelling in a patient with cystic hygroma. Transillumination is brilliantly positive.

3. The swelling increases in size and becomes prominent when the child cries or strains (due to rise of intrathoracic pressure which is transmitted through the root of the neck). This feature may be informed by the parents or can be observed (Figs 3.21 A and B).
4. *Soft cystic swelling – fluctuation positive.*
5. Surface is *smooth or lobulated.* The overlying skin is free and normal unless infected.
6. Margins are not well-defined on all sides, as it burrows into the tissue space.
7. Sometimes, partially compressible (because of intercommunication).

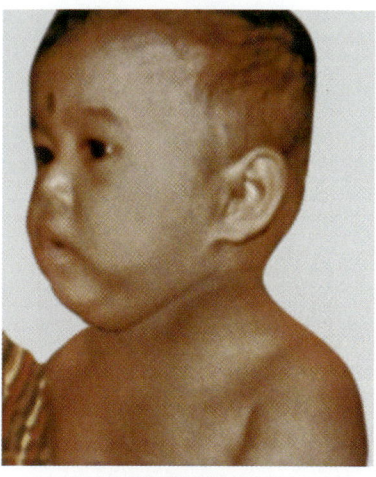

Fig. 3.21A: Cystic swelling at the root of the neck. Transillumination is highly positive.

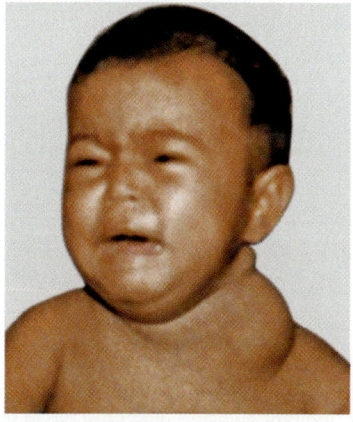

Fig. 3.21B: Same patient. The swelling becomes more prominent when the baby cries—cystic hygroma with possible extension into the thorax.

8. *Transillumination: Brilliantly transilluminant*, a distinctive physical sign. During transillumination multiple septae are noticed – *multilocular cyst.*
9. Regional lymph nodes are not enlarged.
10. *Other sites usual for the cystic hygroma are also to be examined (e.g. axillae, groin).*

Atypical presentation of cystic hygroma

1. During birth, a big cystic hygroma may cause obstructed labour.
2. Due to recurrent infection, it may present as a pyogenic abscess which is painful, tender, warm, soft swelling.
3. Cystic hygroma in the mediastinum may present as a growth in the mediastinum with mediastinal syndrome characterised by dyspnoea, dysphagia, etc. Clinically, it is very difficult to differentiate mediastinal cystic hygroma from a mediastinal tumour. Many a time the dispute is settled at the operation table. CT/MRI may be helpful.

Differential diagnosis

1. Branchial cyst.
2. Cold abscess in the neck.
3. Sometimes a collar-stud abscess.

In all the above mentioned cases transillumination is negative, but *in cystic hygroma transillumination is brilliantly positive.*

4. *Solitary lymph cyst:* This is a *single cyst* containing lymph and develops in the same process as cystic hygroma. Though congenital, it usually *appears in adult life* and is commonly found in the supraclavicular region (Fig. 3.22, *a solitary cyst*, in this case in a child). *Transillumination is positive.*

Complications

1. Recurrent infection – because the cyst is surrounded by a shell of lymphoid tissue. Infection → Abscess → Septicaemia may develop.
2. Haemorrhage within the mass.
3. Sudden increase in the size of the cyst may cause respiratory distress when the treatment is aspiration of the cyst with or without tracheostomy.

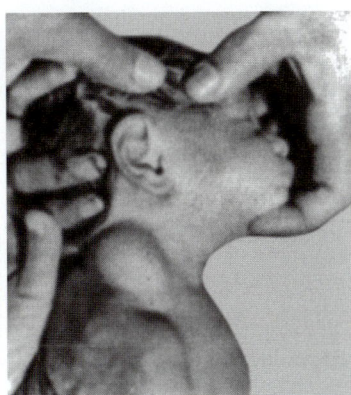

Fig. 3.22: A cystic swelling in the supraclavicular region. Brilliantly translucent cyst without any septae within (i.e. not multiloculated)—solitary lymphatic cyst (cf. cystic hygroma—multilobular cyst).

4. Never turns into a malignancy.
5. Surgery itself may cause torrential haemorrhage.

Can spontaneous recovery take place?

Yes, and when it occurs it will take about 2 years to recover.

Treatment

1. If there is no urgent indication, the operation can be delayed, and the child is observed for 3 years, because there is a chance of spontaneous recovery.
2. Before commencing any treatment, *X-ray of the chest is to be done to see any evidence of mediastinal cystic hygroma.* X-ray may reveal shadow at the hilar region or in any part of the mediastinum. An USG/CT scan or MRI may be helpful in delineating the topography of the lesion.
3. **Conservative:**
   (a) *Aspiration alone,* particularly when the cyst is big enough to cause pressure symptoms.
   Fallacy:
   • There are multiple cysts with intercommunication between them. Therefore, *single aspiration cannot bring about permanent cure.*
   • *Repeated aspiration leads to infection.*

   (b) *Aspiration followed by injection of hot water or sclerosant* such as hypertonic saline, STD, ethoxysclerol into the cysts. *Advantage:* Injection of sclerosing agents causes fibrosis of the capsule with the following advantages.
   • The size diminishes;
   • The cyst becomes more localised;
   • Dissection is easier because the cyst wall becomes thick.
4. **Operative:** Complete excision of the cyst is the treatment of choice undertaken at an optimal age of 3 years.
   Precautions during excision:
   (a) Cyst wall should never be held with tissue forceps because the wall is very thin, delicate and it will give way, so chances of incomplete removal.
   (b) There are finger-like projections from the cyst wall invading the surrounding structures. So, every care should be taken for complete excision.
   Dangers of incomplete removal:
   • Fluid and electrolyte loss leading to dehydration may rarely develop, which is very difficult to correct in a child.
   • Wound infection.
   • *Recurrence:* Residual or recurrent disease is best treated by sclerotherapy.
   Sometimes, thoracotomy may have to be done for mediastinal extension of cystic hygroma. Occasionally, tracheostomy may have to be done if there is prolonged tracheal compression.
5. *Radiotherapy:* Cystic hygroma is relatively radioresistant. But it may be used in case of recurrence, or when the surgical treatment is not feasible.

Complications of surgery of cystic hygroma

1. Injury to spinal accessory, vagus, cutaneous nerves and jugular veins.
2. Surgery itself may cause severe haemorrhage.
3. Collection of blood and lymph under the flaps may be treated by aspiration under aseptic conditions.
4. Flap necrosis, chylous fistula, lymphorrhoea.
5. Secondary haemorrhage.

Note

Name the cysts containing cholesterol crystals:

1. Branchial cyst
2. Cystic hygroma
3. Thyroglossal cyst
4. Dental cyst
5. Dentigerous cyst
6. Old hydrocele, occasionally.

Note

Sclerosing agents: Hypertonic saline, STD (sodium tetradecyl), ethoxysclerol, bleomycin, doxycycline, ethanol, picibanil (OK-432) (derivative of *Streptococcus pyogenes*).

Note

Advance prenatal imaging modalities, e.g. *ultrasound* of the mother's belly during checkups helps in early diagnosis and useful coordination for surgical intervention of cystic hygroma at the time of delivery.

▌ PHARYNGEAL POUCH

It is a protrusion or herniation of the mucosa of the pharyngeal wall through the *Killian's dehiscence*, the weak area in the posterior pharyngeal wall between the oblique (thyropharyngeus) and the sphincter-like transverse fibres (cryco-pharyngeus) of the inferior constrictor muscle of the pharynx. Truly, it is a pressure diverticulum or *Pulson diverticulum of the pharynx*. Also known as Zenker's diverticulum.

Surgical anatomy

Killian's dehiscence (Fig. 3.23)

The inferior constrictor muscle has got two parts:

(i) upper oblique fibres (thyropharyngeus), and
(ii) lower horizontal fibres (cricopharyngeus).

In between these fibres on the posterior aspect of pharyngeal wall there is a potential area of weakness which is known as 'Killian's dehiscence'. At this site often there is a depression called pharyngeal dimple.

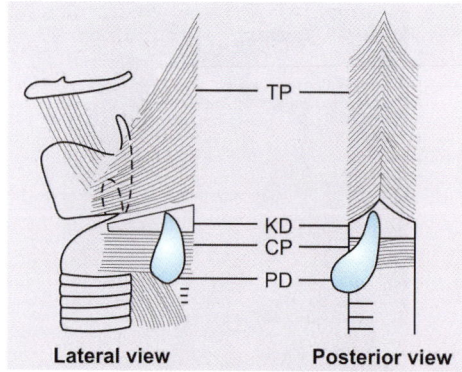

Fig. 3.23: The pharyngeal diverticulum. TP, thyropharyngeus part of inferior constrictor; KD, Killian's dehiscence; CP, cricopharyngeus part of the inferior constrictor; PD, pharyngeal diverticulum.

Both these fibres of inferior constrictor are different in their arrangements of fibres, nerve supply and functions.

Arrangement of fibres

- *Thyropharyngeus:* The fibres are oblique in direction and are inserted into the median raphe. This median raphe does not extend below the level of vocal cord.
- *Cricopharyngeus:* The fibres are horizontal in direction, around the upper end of the oesophagus and are continuous with the similar fibres of the opposite muscle. No median raphe exists here.

Nerve supply

- *Thyropharyngeus:* Supplied by the pharyngeal plexus carrying the fibres from the cranial part of the accessory nerve.
- *Cricopharyngeus:* Supplied by the recurrent laryngeal and external laryngeal nerves.

Functions

- *Thyropharyngeus is propulsive in function*, i.e. it propels the food downward during deglutition.
- *Cricopharyngeus is sphincteric in action* and is normally kept closed except during the act of deglutition when it relaxes to allow the food in the oesophagus.
- *When thyropharyngeus contracts, crico-pharyngeus relaxes and vice versa.*

Clinical basis of development of pharyngeal pouch

Due to neuromuscular imbalance when both the parts contract simultaneously, intrapharyngeal pressure rises and the mucous membrane bulges through the Killian's dehiscence forming a pharyngeal diverticulum. This is called Pulson diverticulum which is the beginning of pharyngeal pouch to appear beneath sternomastoid muscle. This may be due to different nerve supply of the two parts of the inferior constrictor muscles.

Course of the diverticulum

Initially it starts in the midline posteriorly. But posteriorly lies the rigid vertebral column. So, it deviates on either side, mostly to the left. Mouth of the sac becomes wider than the oesophagus lumen, so food from oesophagus enters the pouch as the pouch communicates with the pharynx.

Diagnostic criteria

1. Common in middle and old age. More common in men.
2. Symptoms vary according to the pathological stages.
   • *Stage I or stage of initial bulging:* There is formation of a small diverticulum directed posteriorly and it is usually symptomless. There may be symptoms of foreign body sensation in the throat.
   • *Stage II or stage of well-formed diverticulum:* The diverticulum becomes larger and globular in shape and still remains in the midline posteriorly with a tilt to one side; the mouth of the diverticulum is vertical giving rise to following symptoms.
   · Sense of suffocation, cough, mild dysphagia.
   · Regurgitation of food, during the next meal or when the patient turns from side-to-side. This may rarely cause aspiration pneumonia.
   • *Stage III or stage of big diverticulum:* The diverticulum becomes larger and pushed commonly to the left; the mouth being horizontal. The fundus of the sac becomes dependent and may cause extraneous pressure over the oesophagus.

Patient complains of:
· Gurgling sounds in the neck especially when the patient swallows (the diverticulum being filled up with food materials, liquid and air).
· Dysphagia.
· Vague soft swelling in the neck mainly on the left side.
· Aspiration of the contents of the pouch leading to features of aspiration pneumonia, lung abscess, mediastinitis.
· Features of cachexia due to starvation.
· Some patients can reduce the pouch after meal.

3. *Site:* When presented with swelling, the pharyngeal pouch appears as *a bulge beneath the sternomastoid muscle below the level of thyroid cartilage on the left side*. The bulge lies deep to the deep fascia and is fixed deeply.
4. *Shape and size:* Variable.
5. Surface smooth and *the edge is not palpable*.
6. *Soft swelling and indentable. It can be compressed and sometimes emptied.*
7. Fluctuation may be positive but trans-illumination is negative.

Investigations

1. *X-ray:* A barium swallow study using a thin barium reveals compression of the postero-lateral oesophageal wall and filling of the pouch. The contents of the pouch will spill into the oesophagus on compression of the swelling in the neck.
2. *Oesophagoscopy:* Dangerous.
3. CT/MRI scan of neck may define the topography as well as any local complication.

Treatment

• *Stage I:* Wait and watch.
• *Stage II and stage III:* Excision of the diverticulum either after a feeding gastrostomy or without it. *Approach to the diverticulum from the left side* with a longitudinal incision along the anterior border of sternomastoid muscle which was retracted posteriorly. Omohyoid muscle is severed for better exposure of the sac. *Excision of the diverticulum is performed*

after horizontal clamping of the mouth of the sac. The sac is removed and the mouth of the sac is sutured transversely in two layers. If required, myotomy of the hypertrophied crico-pharyngeal muscle is also performed. The wound is closed with a suction vacuum drain.

Dahlman's procedure may be done in poor-risk debilitated patient. The partition between the oesophagus and the pouch is divided by diathermy – *myotomy only.*

LARYNGOCELE

It is a diverticulum containing air, formed due to herniation of laryngeal mucosa through the thyro-hyoid membrane. *It is mostly unilateral and communicating with the cavity of the larynx.* It simulates cervical air pouches found in many mammals (e.g. monkeys) who inflate them voluntarily.

Diagnostic criteria

1. *Mostly acquired.* Commonly found amongst the professional trumpet players. May be found in glass blowers and in persons suffering from the chronic cough. May present with dysphonia or a swelling in the neck.
2. When the sac enlarges, it gives rise to a visible lateral swelling in the neck *over the thyroid cartilage.*
3. *The swelling becomes visible or prominent when the patient is asked to blow or breathe out against closed mouth and nose (Valsalva manoeuvre).*
4. Boggy in feel and non-tender.
5. May be resonant on percussion.
6. History of appearance and disappearance of the swelling.
7. *This swelling moves up with the larynx on swallowing. This is quite diagnostic.*
8. History of hoarseness of voice may be present.

Complications

1. Sudden death due to asphyxia from rapid distension of laryngocele—a rare pheno-menon.
2. Infection leading to laryngopyocele.

Investigations

Plain X-ray, especially after Valsalva manoeuvre, U/S, contrast CT, MRI may be helpful.

Treatment

Complete excision of the sac through neck incision after thorough dissection followed by invagination of the stump.

CAROTID BODY TUMOUR

It is a tumour arising from chemoreceptor cells of the carotid body. The carotid body is situated at the bifurcation of common carotid artery. The other name of the tumour is *chemodectoma* or *potato tumour.*

Carotid body

1. The carotid body is a flattened brownish nodule, a few millimetres in diameter.
2. It is situated within the adventitious coat on the posterior aspect of the common carotid artery at or just below the bifurcation.
3. It consists of parenchyma cells embedded in a fibrous stroma richly supplied with vessels and nerves.
   The parenchyma cells are of two types:
   (i) Chief cells containing granules of cate-cholamine.
   (ii) Sustentacular cells having long pro-cesses embracing adjacent capillaries.
4. It belongs to the chemoreceptor system.
5. *The role of carotid body is to monitor oxygen content of blood before it reaches the brain.*

Sites where other chemoreceptor apparatus present in the body (Fig. 3.24)

1. *Aortic bodies:* These lie near the points of origin of the left coronary artery, the innominate artery, bifurcation of the pulmonary trunk in relation to ligamentum arteriosum, arch of aorta.
2. *Glomus jugulare:* It lies in the adventitia of the bulb of the jugular vein.
3. *Glomus intravagale:* It is associated with the ganglion nodosum of the vagus nerve.
4. *Paraganglion tympanicum:* It lies along the tympanic ramus of the glossopharyngeal nerve.

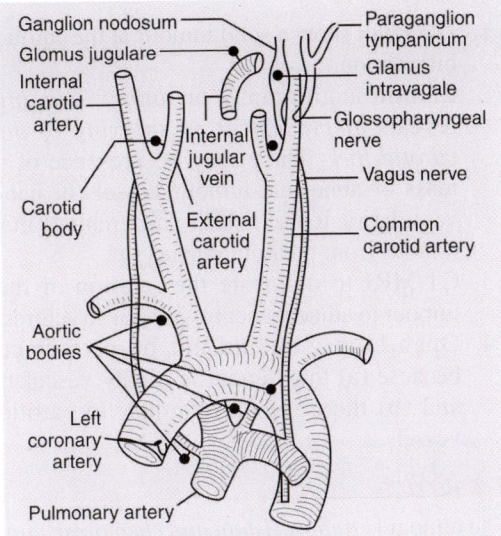

Ganglion nodosum
Glomus jugulare
Internal carotid artery
Internal jugular vein
Carotid body
External carotid artery
Aortic bodies
Left coronary artery
Pulmonary artery
Paraganglion tympanicum
Glamus intravagale
Glossopharyngeal nerve
Vagus nerve
Common carotid artery

Fig. 3.24: Different sites of chemoreceptor.

5. In addition, chemoreceptor apparatus may be found:
   • in relation to inferior alveolar artery in the orbit;
   • in relation to femoral artery in the femoral canal;
   • in the small bowel mesentery;
   • in the retroperitoneum;
   • in the nail beds.

Functions of chemoreceptors

The functions of the chemoreceptor cells are not clear. They are sensitive to the change of pH and carbon dioxide and oxygen tensions in the circulating blood and help in physiological feedback to medulla oblongata about arterial pO_2, pCO_2 and pH to modulate respiratory and cardiovascular functions. *Lack of oxygen produces hyperplasia of these cells.*

Pathology of carotid body tumour

1. It is regarded as non-chromaffin paraganglioma and is akin to glomus tumours of the skin and neuroblastoma of the sympathetic nervous system.
2. The tumour is hard and white-yellow, or spongy and vascular.
3. The tumour is well-encapsulated with a yellow or orange cut surface and with dense

fibrous septae. The tumour blends with bifurcation of the carotid artery.

4. Histology reveals solid masses resembling the chief cells set in a fibrous stroma. The cells may show nuclear pleomorphism.
5. The cells of the tumours stain black to brownish black with chromic acid, like some of the adrenal medullary tumours, *but do not produce catecholamines.* (Recently it has been shown that normal carotid body and its tumour sometimes contain considerable amounts of noradrenaline – W. Boyd.)
6. Previously the tumour was thought to be benign. But cases have been reported with metastases. Regional metastases occur in about 20% cases but distant metastasis is negligible.
7. *The tumour is radioresistant.*

Diagnostic criteria

1. *Age:* Common in middle-aged individual (between 40 and 60 years).
2. *Sex:* Equally common in both sexes.
3. *The patient presents with a painless slowly growing lump in the upper anterolateral part of the neck, i.e. carotid triangle, beneath the anterior border of sternomastoid deep to the deep cervical fascia.* The patient may notice that the lump pulsates. The lump increases very slowly and usually there is a long history.
4. Most commonly seen *in people who live at high altitude* because of chronic hypoxia leading to carotid body hyperplasia.
5. He may also suffer from occasional fainting attack or blackout (transient cerebral ischaemia). This symptom is due to impaired cerebral circulation following compression of the internal carotid artery by the tumour at a certain posture. On application of pressure on the lump this syncopal attack may be produced.

Examination:

6. The lump is mostly unilateral.
7. *Site:* The lump is situated in the upper and lateral parts of the anterior triangle of the neck deep to the deep cervical fascia, *beneath the anterior edge of sternomastoid*

muscle at the level of the upper border of thyroid cartilage (level of bifurcation of the common carotid artery).

8. *Size:* It varies but rarely exceeds the size of potato.
9. *Shape:* Initially spherical but becomes irregular as it grows.
10. *Surface:* Usually smooth but may be bosselated. The edge is well defined.
11. *Consistence: Solid swelling*, firm to hard in feel. The tumour is often called as *'potato tumour'* because of its consistence, shape and size.
12. The tumour is not tender or hot. The overlying skin looks normal.
13. *Sometimes the tumour may pulsate*. This is either a transmitted pulsation from the adjacent carotid arteries, or a palpable external carotid artery which is pushed forward. Rarely, the tumour is itself a vascular one causing pulsation.
14. *The lump is mobile from side-to-side, but not up and down.*

Differential diagnosis

1. Solitary metastatic neck lymph gland – solid.
2. Koch's lymphadenitis – solid.
3. Sternomastoid tumour – solid.
4. Solid swelling in relation to the apex of the thyroid lobe – solid.
5. Paraganglioma from the cervical sympathetic chain – solid.
6. Other soft tissue tumours such as lipoma, neurofibroma arising from vagus, fibromyxoma – solid.
7. Branchial cyst – cystic.
8. Aneurysm of carotid artery – pulsatile soft swelling – both transmitted and expansile.

Complications

1. *Transient cerebral ischaemia leading to fainting attack,* due to impaired cerebral circulation following compression of the internal carotid artery by the tumour at a certain posture.
2. Dysphagia due to direct compression – rare.
3. Change of voice following interference with the function of vocal cords due to pressure on the vagus nerve – rare.

Investigations

1. USG will show a solid tumour at the carotid bifurcation.
2. Carotid angiography or *duplex imaging* reveals *displacement or splaying of the carotid fork*. There may be presence of a mass of abnormal tumour vessels or neovascularity. It also helps to differentiate this tumour from a carotid aneurysm.
3. CT/MRI to delineate the relation of the tumour to adjacent neurovascular structures.
4. Open biopsy should not be performed because (a) this tumour is highly vascular; and (b) there is risk of injury to carotid vessels.

Treatment

The tumour is *radioresistant and chemoresistant.* So, *surgical removal is the treatment of choice.* Total excision is the most successful form of treatment, if failed, partial excision and postoperative radiotherapy may be considered.

In some cases, the tumour can be separated from the fork of the carotid artery without injuring it by blunt and sharp dissection, and so removed.

In other cases, the tumour is large enough and inseparable from the fork of the carotid artery. So, the tumour is removed along with resection of arteries followed by a graft, e.g. autogenous vein or synthetic Dacron/PTFE graft between common and internal carotid arteries *to maintain the blood supply to the brain.* This requires the use of hypothermia or some form of temporary bypass to perfuse the brain.

Danger during operation

Injury to the internal carotid artery – impairment of blood supply to the brain leads to contralateral hemiplagia.

Adjuvant RT is advisable following resection, either total or subtotal excision. Palliative RT may be tried when resection is difficult or when the patient is unfit for surgery.

Cautions

1. A general surgeon meeting unexpectedly with a carotid body tumour is best advised to confine himself to biopsy of the tumour:

FNAC/FNAB. Most tumours may bleed profusely during dissection and on open biopsy.

2. Palliative radiotherapy may be considered for those with difficult non-resectable malignant tumours and those who are unfit for surgery.

3. *In case of the old and enfeebled individuals with a long history of the lump the tumour may be left as it is without any interference. The lump may be covered with a scarf or muffler to divert attention of the relatives, friends or passersby.*

STERNOMASTOID TUMOUR AND CONGENITAL WRY NECK (TORTICOLLIS)

This is a twisted deformity of the neck *charac-terised by tilting of the head towards the shoulder along with torsion of the neck (a twisted neck) and deviation of the head to the opposite side.* In about 20% of cases, to start with, there is a hard lump over the central part of the sternomastoid muscle noticed between 1 and 4 weeks; it disappears within a few months.

Causes

There are many theories to explain the develop-ment of this lesion.

1. *Ischaemia:* Probably there is an interference with the blood supply of the sternomastoid muscle, *caused by injury during birth.* It is held that the middle part of the sternomastoid muscle is supplied by an 'end artery', sternomastoid branch of the superior thyroid artery, and in wry neck the lumen of the sternomastoid artery has been found obliterated at the anterior border of the muscle. It is suspected that the sternomastoid arteries might be obstructed during difficult labour, with subsequent fibrosis.

2. *Trauma:* The sternomastoid muscle might conceivably be torn *during birth* with the formation of haematoma. In the early months of life this haematoma appears as a lump (*the sternomastoid tumour of infancy*); but the lump is too discrete to be a haematoma, and microscopically contains no haemosiderin. *The haematoma subsequently undergoes fibrosis followed by contracture.* Muscular injury is most common in breech delivery.

3. *Congenital:* Hereditary theory is suspected by some authors, because such deformity may appear alone or also be associated with other congenital deformities such as clubfoot, congenital dislocation of hip, etc.

4. Other local congenital deformities are also responsible like hemivertebrae of cervical spine, unilateral atlanto-occipital fusion, Klippel-Feil syndrome, unilateral absence of sternomastoid, pterygium coli (a congenital band of fascia extending from the mastoid process of the temporal bone to the clavicle).

5. *Other theories:* Venous thrombosis or infective myositis has been suspected, but there is little convincing evidence.

Note

Sternomastoid muscle is supplied by the following arteries: (i) occipital artery, (ii) thyro-cervical trunk, and (iii) superior thyroid artery.

Diagnostic criteria

1. During the first few weeks of life, the mother notices an *elongated swelling in the middle of the sternomastoid muscle of the baby.* Right side is more often involved.

2. The swelling is hard in feel and tender, and the baby cries bitterly when it is palpated, or if the muscle is stretched in any way.

3. *Shape and size:* The lump is fusiform with its long axis along the line of sternomastoid muscle. It varies in size from 1 to 2 cm across.

4. *Surface and edge:* The anterior and posterior edges of the lump are well defined but the inferior and superior edges are ill-defined.

5. Gradually the swelling and tenderness subside within a few months and the muscle becomes tense and contracted with the *development of characteristic attitude of sustained turning, tilting towards the opposite side with flexion of the neck.* On examination at this stage the contracted muscle is felt as a tight cord.

6. *Examine the spine gently.* Neck movements are usually normal. There may be restriction of movements due to spasm of the sterno-mastoid muscle.

7. *Examine the eyes to exclude squint.* The torticollis may be secondary to squint.

Secondary changes

1. If the deformity is not corrected early, asymmetry of face (*plagiocephaly*) develops due to adaptive shortening of the other soft tissue parts on the affected side. There are thickening and contraction of the deep cervical fascia, scalenus anterior muscle etc. The vessels also become shortened.

2. *If uncorrected, facial asymmetry may develop with flattening of the face on the affected side. So, the torticollis should be corrected before the age of 1 year.*
   Facial asymmetry is rare with acquired type torticollis.

3. There may be secondary scoliotic deformity of the cervical and upper thoracic spines.

X-ray: Every case should be X-rayed to exclude any vertebral anomaly (e.g. hemi-vertebrae) which may be the primary error.

Treatment

1. *Prophylaxis: If the sternomastoid tumour is detected immediately after birth,* every effort should be made to prevent torticollis from developing. The neck should be manipulated daily into a position which elongates the affected sternomastoid to the full. The baby is laid on the bed in lateral position to sleep on alternate sides. *Spontaneous correction* may occur at this stage.

2. *When the condition is detected only after the torticollis has been developed:*
   (a) Daily physiotherapy to stretch the muscle and use of corrective brace – *torticollis harness* may be tried, but usually there is recurrence.
   (b) **Operation around the age of 12 months:**
      • *Subcutaneous tenotomy at the lower end* – in an early and mild case, *and*

where only the sternal head appears to be contracted. The danger is injury to blood vessels particularly internal jugular vein deep to the sternomastoid. The advantage is only for cosmetic reasons as the operation leaves no visible scar.

• *Open division of both the heads of sternomastoid at the lower end.* Along with it, the deep cervical fascia, and if necessary the carotid sheath and scalenus anterior muscle, are also divided. The phrenic nerve and the internal jugular vein should be identified and safeguarded.

• *Open division of the upper end of the sternomastoid* may be performed alone, or may be combined with the above procedure. The spinal accessory nerve should be safeguarded. *The advantage is that the scar is hidden by the hair.*

After-treatment

After operation, the correction must be maintained by torticollis harness which should be worn for about 6 months. Physiotherapy, both active and passive movements of the neck should be continued for 6 months.

Note

Congenital torticollis may be associated with hip dysplasia. So, the hips should also be examined carefully in children with torticollis.

SPASMODIC TORTICOLLIS

It is due to dystonia of cervical muscles. It usually begins in adult life. It involves SCM with or without trapezius.

Characteristics of the disease

• Sustained turning, tilting with flexion or extension of the neck.
• The head shifted laterally or anteriorly – involuntarily.
• The shoulder is usually displaced anteriorly on the side to which chin turns.

- Neck movements, both active and passive, are usually very painful.
- Local tenderness over SCM muscles.
- There will be no hard lump felt at the sternomastoid muscle.
- Agony – from pain.

Treatment

- Conservative by local heat application, ultraviolet light or SWD, oral analgesics and calmpose. Local application of ointment *but no massage.* Cervical collar may be helpful during waking hours.
- Gradual manipulation of the neck daily within the limits of pain tolerance is also helpful.

▎COLD ABSCESS IN THE NECK

On many occasions, a soft swelling, cold abscess due to accumulation of pus of tuberculous origin, may be encountered in the region of the neck, commonly in the posterior triangle.

Why is it called cold abscess?

Because:

- There is no sign of inflammation and so the abscess is not hot and red as in pyogenic abscess;
- The abscess is a low tension abscess, so it is much less painful than pyogenic abscess.

Source of cold abscess in the neck

It may be:

1. *Due to caseation of tuberculous lymph adenitis in the cervical region (Koch's lymphadenitis):* Commonly found in the upper half of the anterior triangle of the neck.
2. *Secondary to tuberculosis of the cervical spine (caries spine):* Commonly found in the posterior triangle of the neck.

1. From Koch's lymphadenitis

Usually one group of cervical lymph nodes is infected, most frequently the upper jugular group of nodes is affected. The organism is tubercle bacilli, mostly 'human type'. Tubercle bacilli most commonly reach a lymph node *by lymphatics,* when the tubercles first form in the cortex. *Blood-borne infection* sometimes occurs,

in which case the medulla of the lymph node is the first to be affected. The tubercle bacilli usually gain entrance through the tonsil of the corresponding side. The infective process passes through three stages.

- *1st stage: It is the stage of lymphadenitis. In this stage the lymph nodes become enlarged and slightly tender but remain discrete.* If the resistance of the patient is good, the nodes may resolve with fibrosis and calcification.
- *2nd stage: In this stage, the lymph nodes become matted with perilymphadenitis.*
- *3rd stage: In this stage, the caseating materials liquefy and break through the capsules of the lymph nodes to form a 'cold abscess'.* In the beginning the abscess remains deep to the deep cervical fascia. Ultimately the fascia is eroded at one point and the pus tracks into the superficial space. Now it is called *'collar-stud abscess'.* The superficial abscess gradually enlarges and becomes obvious on inspection. In untreated cases, the overlying skin becomes ischaemic and reddish blue at the centre of the abscess. Ultimately the skin at the centre necroses and gives way leading to a chronic discharging sinus.

2. From caries spine of the cervical region

The tuberculous process of the cervical spine may break through the bone and give rise to formation of cold abscess.

It may rupture anteriorly or posteriorly:

(a) *When it ruptures anteriorly,* the pus will appear anteriorly first deep to the prevertebral layer of the deep cervical fascia from where the pus may travel in one of the following ways.
  - In the upper cervical region, the pus may pass forward and bulge anteriorly into the posterior wall of the pharynx when it will cause a chronic midline deep-seated swelling (cf. *retropharyngeal abscess* which will cause an acute superficial swelling situated on one side of the midline).
  - In the lower cervical region, the pus may press the oesophagus and trachea forward.

- The pus may track downward behind the prevertebral fascia and enter the superior mediastinum.
- The pus may track laterally deep to the prevertebral fascia and behind the carotid sheath to reach ultimately the posterior triangle beyond the posterior border of sternomastoid and *thus form the cold abscess in the posterior triangle of the neck* (Fig. 3.25).

(b) *When it ruptures posteriorly*, the pus enters the spinal canal. From here the pus may follow the anterior primary division of the cervical spinal nerves and thus appear in the posterior triangle of the neck (Fig. 3.25).

From the posterior triangle the pus can travel into the axilla along the axillary sheath which is the prolongation of prevertebral fascia through the apex of the axilla dragged down by the cords of the brachial plexus and the subclavian artery. From the axilla it may travel further down along the course of the brachial artery.

Diagnostic criteria

1. *Age:* Common in children, young adults, and in the elderly.
2. *Sex:* Equally common in both sexes.
3. The patient presents with *a swelling in the neck which gradually increases in size*. It is usually *painless*.

4. The patient may give history of previous solid neck swelling (i.e. enlarged neck lymph nodes) on which the area of softening has occurred.
5. Features of tuberculous toxaemia almost always present, i.e. evening rise of temperature, sweating, anorexia, loss of weight.
6. Family history of tuberculosis may be present.
7. *Examination:*
   - *Site:* The lump is commonly found in the upper half of the anterior triangle of the neck. It may be found in the posterior triangle.
   - *Size and shape:* Varies.
   - *Surface:* Irregular and indistinct. The overlying skin may be discoloured, *but there is no sign of inflammation* (particularly brawny induration of pyogenic abscess) unless secondarily infected.
   - *Edge:* Usually indistinct unless the abscess is tense.
   - *Consistence: A soft cystic swelling. Fluctuation is positive.*
   - *Usually not tender.*
   - A peculiar rim of thickening surrounding the central soft area may be present.
   - *Matted lymph nodes* may be palpable on the deeper aspect when the abscess is secondary to tuberculous lymphadenitis.

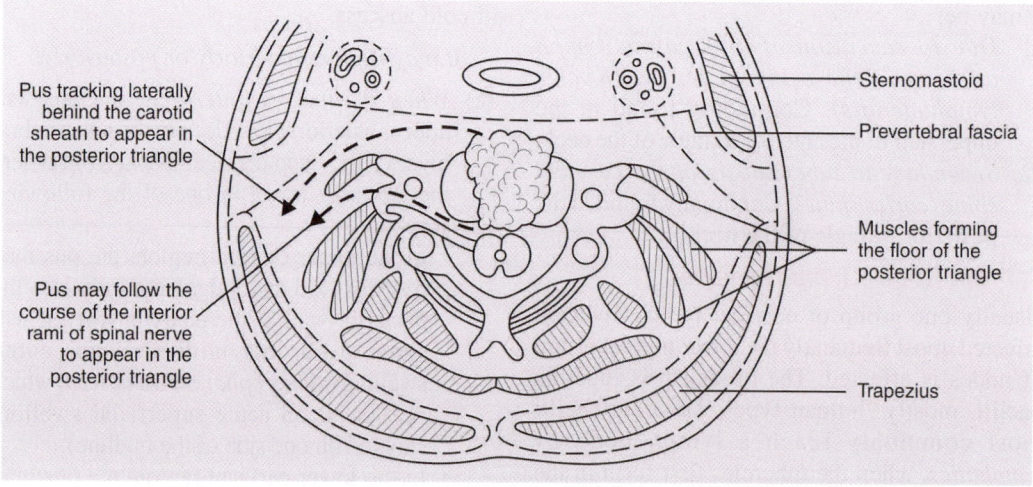

Fig. 3.25: The spreading of pus from the vertebral body to the posterior triangle.

- *Transillumination – negative* (cf. cystic hygroma).
- *The cervical spine should always be examined* to find:
  - tenderness in the cervical spine;
  - limited movements of the neck;
  - rigidity of the spinal muscles.
- General examination should be performed to see evidence of tuberculosis elsewhere, e.g. other lymph nodes, the lungs and the urinary tract.
- *Aspiration of the abscess will show caseous material* with no demonstrable cholesterol crystals (cf. branchial cyst).

Investigations

1. *Blood examination:*
   - Hb% – anaemia.
   - WBC – leucocytosis with lymphocytosis.
   - ESR – raised.
2. *Mantoux test* – positive.
3. *X-ray of the chest* may show evidence of primary complex with enlarged mediastinal lymph nodes.
4. *X-ray of the neck:* AP and lateral views may show:
   - calcified lymph nodes;
   - osteoporosis, joint space diminution, areas of destruction in the cervical vertebrae;
   - soft tissue shadow, i.e. paravertebral shadow.
5. *Sputum* may or may not show acid-fast bacilli.
6. *Aspiration of the abscess material* and examination for *Mycobacterium tuberculosis:*
   - *Staining: Ziehl-Nielsen stain for acid-fast bacilli.* Gram stain to exclude secondary infection.
   - Culture in Lowenstein-Jensen media.
   - Guinea pig inoculation test.

   All the examinations will show positive results.
7. *Lymph node biopsy,* when the surrounding lymph nodes are palpable, confirms the diagnosis showing central area of caseation, surrounded by lymphocytes and giant cells.

Differential diagnosis

1. *Branchial cyst:* Here, the aspiration shows the cheesy material which contains cholesterol crystals.
2. *Cystic hygroma:* Here transillumination is brilliantly positive.

Treatment

1. General treatment, and
2. Treatment of the local condition.

General treatment

1. *Anti-Koch's therapy:* Antituberculous drugs are to be used routinely and should be continued for a period of 18 months.
   - Inj. streptomycin—0.75–1 gm daily for a total of 90–120 injections.
   - INH (isonicotinic acid hydrazide) – 300 to 400 mg daily.
   - PAS (para-aminosalicylic acid) – 10 gm daily.

   The usual plan is to start with three drugs at the same time.

   (Presently newer antituberculous drugs are available which are most sensitive and thus shorten the duration of treatment from 18 months to 9 months. These are:
   - Rifampicin   15 mg/kg body weight
   - Ethambutol   25 mg/kg body weight
   - Pyrazinamide   20–30 mg/kg body weight
2. Vitamins particularly B-complex and C. Minerals – iron preparation. Good food and healthy surroundings.

Local treatment

Includes treatment of the abscess and treatment of the primary source, if any.

A. *Treatment of the abscess:* Usually the small abscess subsides with the general conservative treatment. If the abscess is a bigger one then aspiration, in addition, is helpful. *Techniques of aspiration:* The needle of aspiration should be insinuated through the healthy skin; otherwise, there is a chance of sinus formation if the damaged skin is punctured. The aspiration should be done from a higher level and never at dependent part. Otherwise, there is a chance of sinus formation along the track of the needle.

B. If there is associated glandular enlargement not responding to conservative treatment – excision biopsy of the tubercular lymph glands as a whole may be done.

C. *When the lesion is secondary to Koch's vertebrae:*

1. Immobilisation of the cervical spine with the help of plaster jacket (Minerva jacket).

   Extent of Minerva jacket:
   • Below: Middle of the chest or nipple line.
   • Above: The plaster extends above to cover the neck and scalp exposing the ear and face.

   The plaster immobilisation is continued for 3 to 6 months.

2. *Operation:* Cervical spine fusion. It may be done when the plaster immobilisation fails, or in the beginning.

COLLAR-STUD ABSCESS

It is a bilocular abscess with an intervening narrow communication (Fig. 3.26).

Causes

1. *Pyogenic:* Commonly found in the palm. The superficial loculus lies superficial to the palmar fascia and the deep loculus is situated deep to the palmar fascia with a narrow communication connecting the two. The communication occurs either due to erosion of the fascia or due to rupture of the fascia by increased tension.

2. *Tuberculous:* Commonly found in the neck,

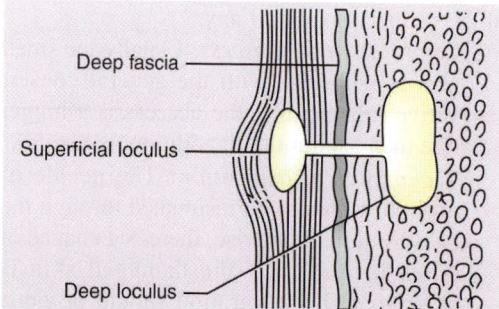

Fig. 3.26: The superficial and deep loculi of a collar-stud abscess.

Deep fascia

Superficial loculus

Deep loculus

due to caseation of tubercular lymph node followed by formation of cold abscess. For some time the abscess remains limited by the resistance of the deep cervical fascia. Ultimately the deep fascia is eroded at one point and the pus tracks into the superficial space.

Causes of non-tuberculous cold abscess

1. *Leprosy:* Nodular leprosy with degeneration.
2. *Actinomycosis:* Abscess following actinomycotic infection.
3. Gumma degeneration.

Differential diagnosis of neck swellings
(Flowchart 3.1)

While examining a neck swelling one should first observe *where the lump is situated – anterior triangle or posterior triangle.*

All midline swellings are included within the anterior triangle. If the lump is situated in the anterior triangle observe *whether the lump moves on swallowing* (thyroid swelling).

If it moves on swallowing observe *whether the lump moves up on protrusion of the tongue* (thyroglossal cyst).

Then one should examine the lump for other clinical characteristics such as single or multiple, solid or cystic, pulsatile or non-pulsatile, transilluminable or not. This protocol helps to define a lump clinically in most of the cases. *Multiple lumps are invariably lymph nodes. One should note that the commonest lump in the neck is of lymph node origin.*

Any swelling behind the posterior border of sternomastoid is in the posterior triangle.

One should remember also that any lump arising from skin and subcutaneous tissue such as, lipoma, fibroma, neurofibroma, sebaceous cyst, and haemangioma can occur anywhere in the neck.

Note

Solid swelling in the neck
• Enlarged lymph nodes
• Carotid body tumour
• Thyroid swellings
• Cervical rib

Note

Cysts presenting with midline neck mass

- Thyroglossal cyst
- Sublingual dermoid or cervical dermoid
- Subhyoid bursal cyst
- Deep plunging ranula
- Thymic cyst

Note

Cysts presenting as lateral neck mass

- Branchial cyst
- Laryngocele
- Lymphangiomas or cystic hygroma

Note

Cysts that contain cholesterol crystals

- Branchial cyst
- Dental cyst
- Dentigerous cyst (rare)
- Thyroglossal cyst (rare)
- Old hydrocele

Note

Cystic hygroma can be associated with:

- A nuchal lymphangioma or a foetal hydrops.
- A soft lump in the mouth, cheek or tongue (lymphangioma).
- Turner syndrome.
- Noonan syndrome.
- Cowchock Wapner Kurtz syndrome, where in addition to cystic hygroma includes cleft palate, lymphoedema, a soft lump in the mouth, cheek or tongue – examine the oral cavity.
- Can be diagnosed with prenatal U/S.

Note

Pulsatile swellings in the neck

1. Aneurysm of the carotid artery.
2. Aneurysm of the subclavian artery.
3. Carotid body tumour – transmitted pulsation.
4. Lymph node swelling in relation to the carotid artery – transmitted pulsation.
5. Primary toxic goitre – occasionally.

Note

Varieties of oesophageal diverticulum

1. *Pulsion diverticulum:* Pharyngeal pouch – through Zenker's or Killian's dehiscence.
2. *Traction diverticulum:* Occurs in the mid-oesophagus or in the parabronchial region due to mediastinal granulomatous disease like tuberculosis causing fibrosis and traction.
3. *Epinephric diverticulum:* Occurs in lower oesophagus, usually towards right side, due to obstruction in distal oesophagus or due to incoordinated lower oesophagus relaxation.

Note

Sclerosing agents for injections

- Absolute alcohol
- Picibanil (OK-432), contains penicillin and streptococci, may be used with or without steroids.

Note

Causes of thyroid swellings

1. *Simple goitre*
   - *Physiological:* Puberty, pregnancy, lactation
   - *Pathological:* Iodine deficiency, goitrogens
2. *Multinodular goitre*
3. *Inflammatory goitre:* Thyroiditis (Hashimoto's, De Quervain's, Riedel's)
4. *Neoplastic*
   - Papillary
   - Follicular (Hurthle)
   - Anaplastic
   - Medullary
   - Lymphoma
5. *Toxic*
   - Graves' disease
   - Solitary toxic nodules/adenoma
   - Multinodular goitre (Plummer's disease)
6. *Rare* – TB, sarcoid, amyloid, HIV

Flowchart 3.1: Algorithm for examination of neck swelling

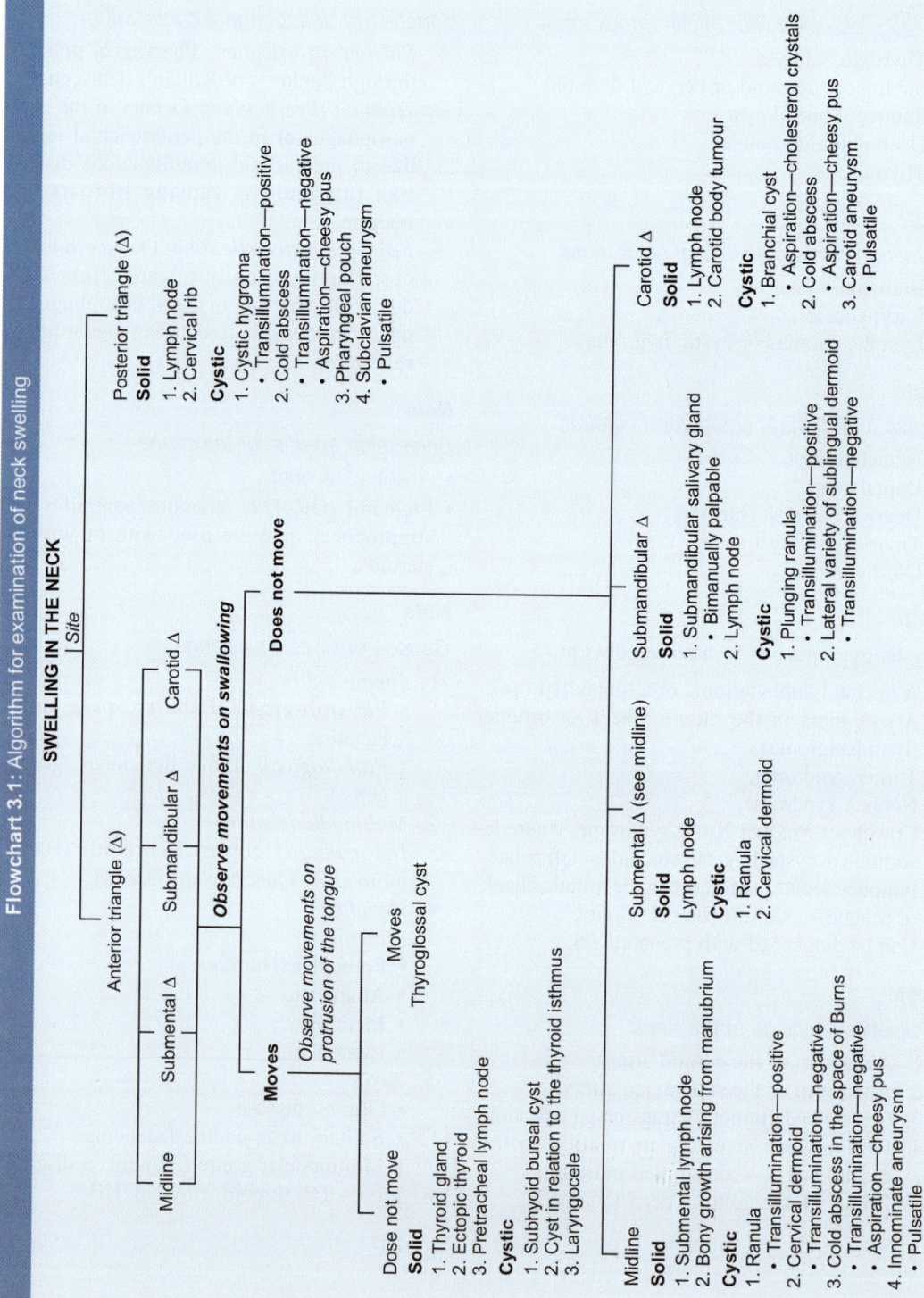

SWELLING IN THE NECK
| Site

Anterior triangle (Δ)

Midline
Submental Δ
Submandibular Δ
Carotid Δ

Observe movements on swallowing

Moves

Does not move

Moves → Thyroglossal cyst

Observe movements on protrusion of the tongue

Dose not move

Solid
1. Thyroid gland
2. Ectopic thyroid
3. Pretracheal lymph node

Cystic
1. Subhyoid bursal cyst
2. Cyst in relation to the thyroid isthmus
3. Laryngocele

Submental Δ (see midline)
Solid
Lymph node

Cystic
1. Ranula
2. Cervical dermoid

Midline
Solid
1. Submental lymph node
2. Bony growth arising from manubrium

Cystic
1. Ranula
 • Transillumination—positive
2. Cervical dermoid
 • Transillumination—negative
3. Cold abscess in the space of Burns
 • Transillumination—negative
 • Aspiration—cheesy pus
4. Innominate aneurysm
 • Pulsatile

Submandibular Δ
Solid
1. Submandibular salivary gland
 • Bimanually palpable
2. Lymph node

Cystic
1. Plunging ranula
 • Transillumination—positive
2. Lateral variety of sublingual dermoid
 • Transillumination—negative

Carotid Δ
Solid
1. Lymph node
2. Carotid body tumour

Cystic
1. Branchial cyst
 • Aspiration—cholesterol crystals
2. Cold abscess
 • Aspiration—cheesy pus
3. Carotid aneurysm
 • Pulsatile

Posterior triangle (Δ)
Solid
1. Lymph node
2. Cervical rib

Cystic
1. Cystic hygroma
 • Transillumination—positive
2. Cold abscess
 • Transillumination—negative
 • Aspiration—cheesy pus
3. Pharyngeal pouch
4. Subclavian aneurysm
 • Pulsatile

Cervical Lymphadenopathy

DISTRIBUTION OF CERVICAL (NECK) LYMPH NODES

Lymph nodes in the neck are arranged in two groups:

 I. *Superficial group:* These are a few and are scattered superficial to the investing layer of deep cervical fascia.

 II. *Deep group:* These are situated deep to the investing layer of deep cervical fascia and are distributed in two groups:
   1. Vertical group
   2. Circular group

Vertical group

Lying in relation to the internal jugular vein and deep to the sternomastoid muscle.

 1. *Jugulodigastric nodes:* Lying below the posterior belly of digastric muscle as it crosses the internal jugular vein. It also includes the tonsillar lymph node.

 2. *Juguloomohyoid nodes:* Lying behind the internal jugular vein where it is crossed by the anterior belly of the omohyoid muscle. All the lymph from the tongue ultimately reaches this group.

 3. *Supraclavicular nodes:* Lying around the inferior part of the internal jugular vein behind the sternomastoid muscle extending into supraclavicular region.

Virchow's glands

These are medial groups of left supraclavicular group of lymph glands lying *between the two heads of sternomastoid*. These are the common sites of metastases from the gastric carcinoma, testicular tumour, oesophageal carcinoma, and when involved, the prognosis is grave.

Enlargement of these nodes with abdominal malignant growths is known as *Troisier's sign*.

Circular or horizontal group

From anterior to posterior:
 1. Submental
 2. Submandibular
 3. Preauricular
 4. Postauricular
 5. Occipital.

The cervical groups of lymph nodes can also be described as six levels of lymph nodes from level I to level VI to facilitate lymph node dissection (Fig. 4.1).

Level I   Submental (Ia) and submandibular (Ib) lymph nodes.

Level II   Lymph nodes in relation to upper third of internal jugular vein – jugulo-digastric nodes.

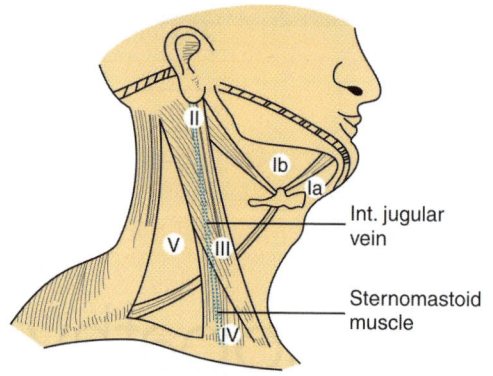

Fig. 4.1: Different levels of cervical lymph nodes.

Level III   Lymph nodes in relation to middle third of internal jugular vein – jugulo-omohyoid nodes.
Level IV   Lymph nodes in relation to lower third of internal jugular vein.
Level V   Lymph nodes in the posterior triangle of the neck. *Supraclavicular nodes* are included in this group.
Level VI   Pre- and paratracheal nodes.
Level VII   Superior mediastinal nodes.

EXAMINATION OF ENLARGED LYMPH NODE

Patients presenting with enlarged lymph node(s) are a common clinical problem. They usually present with a lump in any particular area, e.g. neck, axilla or groin.

First take the history of the lump(s). Then examine the lump or lymph nodes.

History:

1. Site and duration of the lump or enlarged lymph nodes.
2. Painful or painless.
3. History of fever:
   • evening rise of fever (Koch's)
   • fever occurring in a periodic fashion – Pel-Ebstein fever (Hodgkin)
4. Pruritis
5. Alcohol-induced nodal pain
6. Bone pain (lymphomatous infiltration)
7. Pallor
8. Weakness and loss of appetite, loss of weight
9. Family history of similar illness or leukaemia.

History from 3 to 9 are better confirmed at the end of the clinical examination to arrive at the suspected causes of lymphadenitis.

Then *examine the lump or lymph nodes in the following sequence.*

1. Site, i.e. anatomical region affected, e.g. neck, axilla, groin, abdomen.
2. Size and number.
3. Discrete or matted.
4. Tenderness.
5. Consistency of the lymph nodes
   (a) Soft – abscess
   (b) Firm – in cases of reactive hyperplasia and tuberculosis
   (c) Firm, discrete and shotty – in syphilis
   (d) Rubbery and elastic – in cases of Hodgkin's lymphoma
   (e) Hard – in secondary neoplasms
6. Surface – smooth or uneven.
7. Rise of local temperature – increased in bacterial infection/pyogenic inflammation.
8. Tenderness – in pyogenic inflammation.
9. Mobility – fixity to skin and surrounding structures (like muscles, vessels, nerves or with any viscus)
10. Skin changes – any sign of inflammation, any discharge, sinus, peau d'orange (orange skin appearance)
11. Lymphangitis – red, linear, tender lymph vessels radiating proximally – inflammation.

Note

How to examine the cervical lymph nodes in the neck
• Examine lymph nodes on both sides of the neck.
• By standing in front of the patient first and then by standing behind the patient.
• *Circular groups/horizontal groups:* Submental, submandibular, occipital.
• *Vertical groups: Anterior to the sternomastoid muscle,* i.e. nodes on the anterior triangle. *Posterior to the sternomastoid muscle,* i.e. nodes on the posterior triangle.

When one suspects that the lump is of lymph node origin, then one must complete the examination by fulfilling the following five requirements in addition to an examination of the lump proper.

1. *Examine the drainage area of the lymph nodes for any possible primary lesion, either infection or malignancy*, e.g.
   - *for enlarged lymph nodes in the neck* – examine the scalp, ear, nose, mouth cavity and tongue, larynx and pharynx, arms and breast;
   - *for enlarged lymph nodes in the axilla* – examine the arms, breasts, upper abdominal wall above the umbilicus;
   - *for enlarged lymph nodes in the groin* – examine the skin of the leg, buttock and lower abdominal wall below the umbilicus and the external genitalia and anus.

2. *Examine the other lymph node areas*, e.g. contralateral neck, axilla, groin, abdomen particularly where no primary source has been detected.

   In generalised lymphadenopathy enlarged lymph nodes are also found at other sites.

3. *Examine the abdomen* for:
   - *Liver and spleen*: If enlarged, suggest a reticulosis, sarcoid or glandular fever.
   - Any mass:
     - the mass may be enlarged retroperitoneal nodes, e.g. in seminoma testis.
     - the mass may be primary carcinoma of any intra-abdominal viscus, e.g. cancer stomach or pancreas causing left supra-clavicular lymph node enlargement (Virchow's gland).

4. *Examine the testis*, e.g. testicular tumour.

5. *Rectal and vaginal examination* – to exclude any rectal or prostatic growth, or ovarian tumour.

6. *Examine for anaemia, jaundice.*

7. *Look for venous congestion of the neck and upper chest* – superior vena caval obstruction produced by mediastinal mass.

8. *Look for oedema of both legs* – abdominal masses obstruct the inferior vena cava.

9. *Examine the skin for scaly elevated red patches of skin: Mycosis fungoides* – dermatological manifestation of lymphoma.

Investigations

1. *Blood:*
   - *Routine examination:* Hb%, WBC count, ESR may give clues to infection, malignancy or reticuloses.
   - *Examination of blood film* may give a clue to leukaemia or glandular fever.
   - *Examination of blood* for WR and Kahn – if syphilis is suspected.

2. *Chest X-ray:* To note
   - A primary lesion of the lung $\Big\langle$ Koch's / Tumour
   - Evidence of any secondary metastasis in the lung.
   - Evidence of enlarged mediastinal nodes.

3. *X-ray of the neck: Enlarged painless cervical nodes may show typical spotty calcification in tuberculous nodes.*

   Further investigations will depend on the clinical findings and the routine investigations.

4. *Biopsy of one enlarged lymph node* may be necessary for a definite histological proof of the diagnosis, e.g. tuberculosis, Hodgkin's disease, lymphosarcoma, or metastases for knowing the nature of a hidden primary lesion.

5. *Biopsy of any visible primary lesion in the drainage area of the lymph nodes* should be performed before planning an attack on the enlarged node or nodes.

6. *Laryngoscopy:* In the presence of enlarged hard nodes in the neck, when no visible primary lesion is evident, one should perform laryngoscopy to exclude any growth in the posterior one-third of the tongue, larynx and pharynx. *Posterior third growth of the tongue usually presents with enlarged neck nodes.*

CERVICAL LYMPHADENOPATHY

Enlargement of the cervical lymph node (or nodes) is by far the commonest swelling in the neck.

Causes

Acute

1. Acute pyogenic lymphadenitis
2. Acute lymphatic leukaemia
3. Acute infectious mononucleosis – caused by EB virus.

Chronic

I. Inflammatory

1. *Non-specific:* Chronic pyogenic lymph-adenitis
2. *Specific:*
   - Tuberculosis
   - Syphilis – in secondary stage
   - Sarcoidosis
   - Brucellosis
   - Fungal diseases like blastomycosis.
   - Parasitological – filariasis

II. Neoplastic

Almost always malignant.

1. *Primary:*
   - Lymphoma – Hodgkin's disease
   - Lymphosarcoma
   - Reticulum cell sarcoma
   - Chronic lymphatic leukaemia
   - Burkitt's lymphoma.
2. *Secondary:* Metastatic lymph node from a primary growth, mostly from carcinoma or melanoma.

III. Autoimmune disorders

1. Systemic lupus erythematosus
2. Juvenile rheumatoid arthritis (Still's disease).

Causes of generalised lymphadenopathy

I. Inflammatory

- Acute
  - Infectious mononucleosis
  - Septicaemia
- Chronic
  - Tuberculosis
  - Syphilis in secondary stage.

II. Reticuloses

- Hodgkin's disease
- Lymphosarcoma
- Lymphatic leukaemia

III. Sarcoidosis

Differential diagnosis of chronic cervical lymphadenopathy

I. Chronic pyogenic lymphadenitis

1. *Lymph nodes: Firm and tender but not matted.*
2. Chronic infection in the drainage area particularly in the oral cavity.
3. *Blood examination:* Leucocytosis with increased polymorphs.
4. Lymph node biopsy shows sinus hyperplasia.

II. Tuberculous lymphadenitis

1. Common in children, but may occur at any age.
2. *Painless enlargement of the lymph nodes.*
3. *Features of tuberculous toxaemia: Mild degree fever with evening rise, anorexia, anaemia, loss of weight, cough, etc.*
4. *Characteristics of enlarged nodes:*
   - Cervical group is enlarged earliest.
   - Occasionally the enlargement may be generalised.
   - *The enlarged glands are firm in feel and initially discrete* but *later matted (due to periadenitis)* and often slightly tender. There is no sign of inflammation unless secondarily infected.

     In the late stage, there may be *cold abscess* formation due to caseation and liquefaction, or there may be *sinus* or *ulcer formation* over the enlarged nodes which refuses to heal (Figs 4.2 and 4.3).
   - Mediastinal group may be enlarged in children and, therefore, may cause features of mediastinal compression.
5. Evidence of tuberculosis in the lung may be present.
6. *Investigations:*
   - *Blood examination:* Anaemia, leucocytosis with lymphocytosis and high ESR.
   - *Mantoux test:* Positive (Koch's).
   - *Chest X-ray:* May show evidence of primary complex with enlarged mediastinal lymph node.
   - *X-ray of the neck:* May show calcified lymph node.
   - *Sputum* may or may not show acid-fast bacilli.

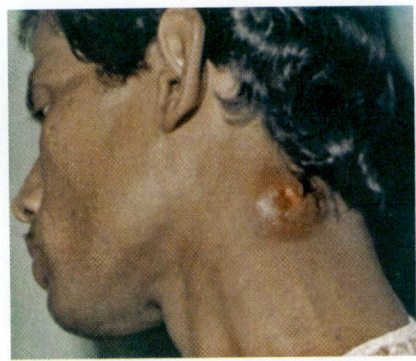

Fig. 4.2: Koch's ulcer with lymphadenitis.

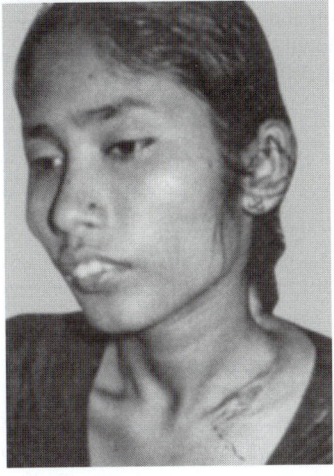

Fig. 4.3: Tubercular sinus left supraclavicular region. Also note the adjacent lymph node swelling.

- **Biopsy of the lymph node:** Confirms the diagnosis by showing the central area of caseation, surrounded by epithelioid cells, lymphocytes and giant cells.

III. Secondary metastatic lymph node

1. *Age:* Common in elderly individuals since cancers mostly occur in patients over the age of 50.

   The exception is papillary carcinoma of thyroid which occurs in adolescents and young adults.

   Metastatic cervical nodes in children are usually due to primary thyroid carcinoma or neuroblastoma.

2. *Sex:* Mostly common in men.

3. The patient presents with *a painless enlarged lump in the neck.* The lump usually grows slowly and new crops of lump may appear.

4. *General symptoms* of anorexia, weight loss, weakness may be present, but these are usually late and rare with head and neck cancers.

5. *The patient may have symptoms of the primary lesion* such as ulcer in the tongue, sore throat, hoarseness of voice, cough, haemoptysis, dysphagia, etc.

Examination:

6. *Site: Metastatic nodes are more common in the nodes of the anterior triangle.* These are deep to the anterior edge of the sterno-mastoid muscle.

7. *Characteristics of enlarged lymph nodes:* The enlarged nodes are *stony hard, mobile or fixed, not tender.* In the early stage, the nodes are smooth and discrete and of variable sizes. As they grow, they may coalesce into one large mass with *irregular* or *bosselated* surface. *The overlying skin usually looks normal unless infiltrated.*

8. *Evidence of primary growth is almost always present commonly in one of the following sites.*

   (a) Scalp, face, neck (e.g. thyroid, parotid), ear.

   (b) Buccal cavity: Lips, tongue, buccal mucous membrane, tonsils.

   (c) Nasal cavity and maxillary antrum.

   (d) Pharynx, larynx: *So, examine with mirrors.*

   (e) Upper limb and chest wall.

   (f) Thorax: Lungs, oesophagus.

   (g) Breast.

   (h) Abdomen: Stomach, pancreas, ovaries.

   (i) External genitalia: Testes.

   (So, the above mentioned sites should be examined in each case to detect the site of the primary lesion. Nature of the primary tumour is commonly either carcinoma or melanoma).

9. Presence of enlarged metastatic lymph nodes in the left supraclavicular fossa lying between

two heads of sternomastoid muscle is known as *Virchow's gland*. Its presence in association with abdominal malignant growths is called *Troisier's sign*.

10. *Investigation:* Apart from routine investigations the nature of the special investigations will be mostly dictated by the primary site of the lesion.

11. Biopsy of the enlarged lymph nodes occasionally may be helpful in detecting the hidden primary lesion.

IV. Hodgkin's disease (Fig. 4.4)

1. *Age:* It may occur at any age, but is common in the young between 15 and 30 years and in the old age above 40 years (bimodal peaks).

2. *Sex:* Common in males.

3. The patient usually presents with *slowly growing, discrete, painless, non-tender, rubbery enlargement of accessible nodes commonly in the neck.*

   The *superficial groups of cervical lymph nodes are enlarged first* which then increase progressively to involve the other groups to become generalised in nature.

4. *Presence of constitutional symptoms* as follows.

   (a) *Fever* with or without rigors occurring in a periodic fashion, i.e. a period of pyrexia for 5 to 10 days alternating with nearly a similar period of apyrexia which goes on for several months – *Pel-Ebstein fever.* Rarely, in advanced cases the temperature may be nearly continuous.

   (b) *Weight loss.*

   (c) *Night sweats.*

   (d) *Anaemia or pallor.*

   (e) *Itching of the skin (pruritus):* An unexplained but distinctive complaint.

   (f) *Pain in the abdomen.*

   (g) *Pain in the bones* due to lymphomatous infiltration of the skeleton.

These pains or itching may be induced or enhanced by drinking alcohol – *a peculiar and unexplained feature.*

5. There may be dyspnoea, hoarseness of voice with *features of mediastinal compression*

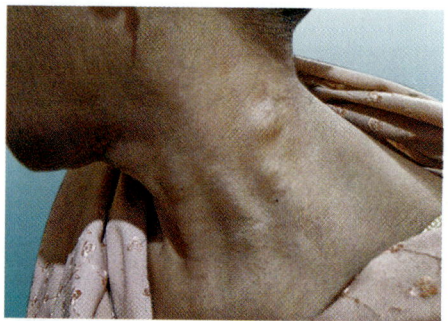

Fig. 4.4: Multiple enlarged neck lymph nodes: *Not matted.* Slowly growing in sizes over the last 8 months with h/o low grade fever suggestive of Hodgkin's lymphoma. Examine the abdomen for enlarged liver and spleen. Note also for constitutional symptoms referred to as B symptoms. Lymph node biopsy is essential.

syndrome like venous congestion in the neck with the development of collateral veins across the chest wall due to enlarged mediastinal nodes.

   Rarely, the patient may present with oedema of both legs *due to obstructions of inferior vena cava with large mass in the abdomen.*

Local examination:

6. *Site:* Any of the cervical lymph nodes can be affected but *lymphoma often causes lymphadenopathy in the posterior triangle, commonly in the supraclavicular fossa.*

7. *Characteristics of enlarged lymph nodes:* Usually painless, asymmetrical, moderate-to-severe degrees of enlargement. The nodes are ovoid, smooth and discrete. *These are solid, firm and rubbery in consistence and are not tender.* Usually mobile, but rarely, completely fixed. Occasionally, the lymph nodes may be matted in late stages (pseudo-matting). *The surrounding structures and the overlying skin are usually normal* (cf. Koch's lymphadenitis).

8. *General examination:*
   • The patient *may be anaemic* with peculiar pallor like white-coffee, and *may be jaundiced.*
   • Other groups of lymph nodes may be enlarged. (*So, palpate the lymph nodes in*

other areas of the body as well, e.g. axilla, abdomen and groin.)

- Moderate degree enlargement of spleen and liver, with or without enlarged abdominal lymph nodes. (*So, palpate the abdomen in each case. Testes should also be palpated*).
- Evidence of mediastinal compressions, pleural effusion may be present.
- *Enlarged mediastinal nodes may occlude the superior vena cava and cause venous congestion in the neck and the development of collateral veins across the chest wall.*
- Oedema of the legs due to obstruction of the inferior vena cava by large masses in the abdomen.
- Rarely, there may be elevated, reddened, scaly patches of the skin, known as *mycosis fungoides* due to spread of tumour cells in the skin (dermatological manifestations of lymphoma).

9. *Investigations:*
  - *Blood examination:*
    · Anaemia
    · Pancytopenia
    · Leucocytosis with lymphopenia but eosinophilia.
  - *Chest X-ray* may show enlarged mediastinal shadow and pleural effusion.
  - CT scan and MRI may be helpful to detect involvement of the retroperitoneal and mediastinal lymph nodes, liver and spleen.
  - Lymph node biopsy confirms the diagnosis.
    · *Macroscopic examination:* Enlarged node without any evidence of periadenitis. *Cut section shows fish-flesh appearance.*
    · *Microscopic examination: Cellular pleomorphism is the characteristic feature.* Central area of necrosis surrounded by various types of cells like eosinophils, polymorphs, lymphocytes, plasma cells, reticulum cells and characteristic giant cells popularly known as '*Reed–Sternberg's giant cells*'.

- *Gordon's test:* Intracerebral injection of an emulsion of the human gland extract into the rabbit causes encephalitis.
- Exploratory laparotomy may be helpful to detect involvement of retroperitoneal lymph nodes, liver and spleen.
- Recently CT/MRI-guided biopsy before laparotomy provides useful information.

V. Lymphosarcoma and reticulum cell sarcoma (non-Hodgkin's lymphoma)

The features are more or less the same as in Hodgkin's disease except *that prolonged duration is against lymphosarcoma and reticulum cell sarcoma.*

1. *Age:* Common in *children or younger age group.*
2. *Presence of constitutional symptoms* like loss of weight, anaemia, anorexia, gross weakness. Unexplained fever is present in 25% cases.
3. *Rapidly growing swelling in the neck.*
4. The swelling rapidly loses its normal ovoid outline.
5. The overlying skin is tense and shiny, and shows engorged veins.
6. Surface is irregular and consistence is heterogeneous, i.e. some are soft to firm and some are hard.
7. Chest X-ray may show enlarged mediastinal nodes.
8. Lymph node biopsy confirms the diagnosis.

VI. Chronic lymphatic leukaemia

1. *Age:* Usually *above 50 years,* commonly in males.
2. Presence of constitutional symptoms like fever, gross weakness, loss of weight, and recurrent upper respiratory tract infection.
3. There is painless, slowly growing progressive enlargement of the cervical lymph nodes and it ultimately becomes generalised.
4. *On examination:*
  - *Anaemia:* Moderate.
  - *Lymph nodes:* Either localised or generalised enlargement, discrete, firm in feel, mobile and not tender.

- Skin may show nodules or thickening of skin due to leukaemic tissue infiltration.
- *Spleen and liver:* Moderately enlarged, firm, smooth and not tender.

5. *Investigations:*
   - *Blood examination:* WBC count 80,000/mm^3 to 1 lakh/mm^3 with 90% lymphocytes.
   - *Lymph node biopsy:* Confirms the diagnosis and shows proliferation of the lymphocytes and the germinal centre.

VII. Syphilis in the secondary stage

1. *Age:* 20 to 25 years.
2. *History of exposure:* Present.
3. *Symptoms:* Ulcers in the mouth or genitalia, fever, arthritis and various skin rash.
4. *On examination:*
   - *Mucocutaneous lesion:* Ulcers on the dorsum of the tongue, angular fissure and condyloma.
   - Pleomorphic type of skin rash.
   - *Lymph nodes:* Generalised enlargement of the superficial group, mild degree, *firm in feel, discrete and shotty, not tender.* Most characteristically there is *enlargement of epitrochlear and suboccipital groups.*
5. *Investigation:*
   - *WR and Kahn test:* Strongly positive.
   - *Treponema pallidum:* May be demonstrated in the exudate collected from the mucocutaneous lesion.

VIII. Sarcoidosis

1. *Age:* Common in young adults and middle-aged persons.
2. (a) Presence of constitutional symptoms which are extremely variable – fever, pain in the bones, paroxysmal dyspnoea due to bronchospasm, pain in the eyes with redness, dysphagia. May present with Raynaud's phenomenon.
   (b) May present with enlarged superficial groups of lymph nodes.
3. *On examination:*
   - Uveitis and conjunctivitis.
   - Enlargement of salivary gland, particularly the parotid gland.

- *Lymph nodes:* Superficial groups are enlarged as a whole and *most characteristically the preauricular groups.* The qualities of the lymph nodes are like those of Hodgkin's, i.e. firm, discrete, not tender.
- Facial nerve paralysis is the characteristic feature.

4. *Investigation:*
   - *Blood examination* shows hyperglobulinaemia and hypercalcaemia.
   - *X-ray of the phalanges* shows punched out appearance.
   - *Chest X-ray* shows enlarged mediastinal lymph nodes.
   - *Kveim test* – positive and diagnostic.
   - *Lymph node biopsy* may add further diagnostic information. Histology shows follicles of epithelioid cells and giant cells in the acute stage which may eventually progress to irreversible hyaline fibrosis.

▌LYMPHOMAS

Lymphomas are malignant neoplasms of the lymphoreticular system that includes lymph nodes, spleen, liver, thymus gland and bone marrow; all are parts of the lymphatic system. *They arise from the lymphocytes.* They are characterised by proliferation of lymphocytes, histiocytes and their precursors and derivatives.

Aetiology

Exact aetiology is not known. Following have been implicated:

1. *Virus:* Epstein-Barr (DNA) virus is associated with Burkitt's lymphoma.
2. *Immunodeficiency diseases:* Inherited or acquired.
   - Associated with a primary immune disorder.
   - Associated with the human immunodeficiency virus (HIV).
   - Associated with post-transplant.
3. *Drugs:* Phenytoin induces lymphoma-like syndrome.
4. Ionising radiation.

Note

Lymphomas are more common in Western countries than in India.

Classification of malignant lymphoma

Rapport classification

1. Hodgkin's lymphoma (HL) characterised by cellular pleomorphism and *the presence of Reed-Sternberg giant cells (RS cells): Better prognosis than NHL.*
2. Non-Hodgkin's lymphoma (NHL) characterised by cellular pleomorphism *but RS cells are absent.*

Organ involved	HL	NHL
Nodal	90%	60%
Extranodal	10%	40%
Cells of origin	B lympho-cytes	B lymphocytes, T lympho-cytes, null cells, histio-cytes (rare)

- *B lymphocytes become plasma cells which in turn produce antibodies that neutralise foreign invaders.*
- *T lymphocytes are derived from the thymus.*
- *T cells kill the foreign invaders directly.*
- *B cells normally work with T cells.*

HODGKIN'S LYMPHOMA (HL)

The disease was described by Thomas Hodgkin in 1982. This is malignant neoplasm of the lymphoreticular system and *arises from B lymphocytes.* This is the commonest type of lymphoma and can occur wherever there is lymphoid tissue.

Pathology

- The disease *usually begins in a single lymph node as a painless mass* and then spreads to adjacent lymph nodes which are also enlarged but *without matting* (cf. Koch's lymphadenitis).
- *Commonly involves the node(s) in the left supraclavicular region.*
- Spread then may occur to the other groups of lymph nodes in an orderly fashion, i.e. progressing from one group of lymph nodes to next group. *The involvement of the nodes in*

Hodgkin's disease generally follows the following order: Cervical → Mediastinal → Para-aortic.

- The axial lymphatic system is almost always affected, i.e. mediastinal and para-aortic lymph nodes.
- Cut surfaces of the lymph nodes are smooth, homogenous and pink-grey in colour – *fish flesh appearance.*
- Microscopically, *cellular pleomorphism* is noted with lymphocytes, histiocytes, eosinophils and Reed-Sternberg cells (RS cells). *RS cells are the hallmark of Hodgkin's lymphoma.*

Reed-Sternberg cell: A giant cell derived from the abnormal B lymphocytes. It contains two large nuclei which are mirror images of each other – *looks like owl's eye.*

Presence of RS cells confirms the diagnosis of HL though absence of RS cells does not exclude the diagnosis. Presence of RS cells signifies worse prognosis.

The disease can involve the spleen, liver, bone marrow in the vertebral column and pelvis. Rarely, it may be confined to a single organ such as stomach.

RS cells are absent in NHL.

New histological classification

- Rye classification (histologic classification) is no longer used.
- REAL (**R**evised **E**uropean **A**merican **L**ymphoma) classification is in use *which divides HL in two groups:*

(a) *Lymphocyte predominant:* Prognosis very good.

(b) *Classic Hodgkin's lymphoma:*

  (i) *Nodular sclerosis:* Most common type. More common in young adult females; cervical and supraclavicular nodes are predominantly involved; prognosis good.

  (ii) *Mixed cellularity:* Predominantly affects elderly; abdominal nodes commonly involved; prognosis fair.

  (iii) *Lymphocyte depleted:* Prognosis poor.

  (iv) *Lymphocyte-rich:* A new entity; *carries best prognosis.*

(c) In about 50% of patients who have both Hodgkin's and non-Hodgkin's lymphomas, *the mediastinum may be the primary site* (Schwartz).

Clinical features

1. *Age:* HL has a *bimodal age-specific incidence rate*; one mode occurring at ages between 15 and 30 years and the other mode above age 50.
   HL in children under 10 years of age is seen more frequently in underdeveloped countries.
2. *Sex:* Common in males.
3. The patient usually presents with *a slowly growing, painless, non-tender lump in the neck, commonly supraclavicular region.*
   The lump may be *a single enlarged node* or *multiple but discrete enlarged nodes (not matted:* cf. Koch's lymphadenitis).
4. The patient may present with generalised lymphadenopathy when more than one group of lymph nodes are enlarged, e.g. neck, axillary, inguinal, mediastinal and para-aortic nodes are involved.
5. In addition to lymphadenopathy, the patient may present with *systemic symptoms* of fever, drenching night sweats, weight loss, malaise, anaemia and pruritus, these are known as '**B symptoms**': *Indicate poor prognosis.* Absence of B symptoms indicates A, which signifies good prognosis.

B symptoms are:

(a) *Fever* with or without night sweats is *usually remittent.* Occasionally, the fever occurs in a cyclical pattern called *Pel-Ebstein fever*, which is characterised by a period of pyrexia for 5 to 10 days alternating with nearly similar period of apyrexia which goes on for several months. Rarely, in advanced cases, the fever may be nearly continuous. *Fever is not accompanied by chill and rigor.*
(b) *Drenching night sweats.*
(c) *Weight loss* more than 10% of body weight in the previous 6 months.
(d) *Pruritus:* Itching of the skin. An unexplained but distinctive complaint due

to heavy eosinophilic infiltration at the sites involved by the tumour.

(e) *Alcohol-induced pain or pruritus after drinking alcohol –* a peculiar feature of HL.
(f) *Pain in the bones* due to bone involvement which are usually osteoblastic/osteosclerotic. *Pathological fractures are rare.*

6. Patient may also present with symptoms due to pathological compression.
   (i) Dyspnoea, hoarseness of voice, *features of mediastinal compression like* venous congestion and engorgement in the neck, with the development of collateral veins across the chest wall due to superior venacaval obstruction by the enlarged mediastinal nodes.
   (ii) Rarely, the patient may present with oedema of the legs due to lymphatic and/or inferior venacaval obstruction by large masses of para-aortic nodes in the abdomen. May present with paraplegia due to vertebral involvements.

Examination

1. Local examination:

(a) The lump in the neck may be an enlarged *single lymph node* more than 2 cm in diameter.
(b) The lump may be moderate-to-severe degrees enlarged lymph nodes with a '*bunch of grapes*' appearance.
   The nodes are ovoid, smooth, discrete, solid, firm and rubbery and *non-tender.* Usually mobile from side-to-side, neither fixed to deeper structures nor to the overlying skin. *The enlarged nodes remain discrete till the late stage* when the nodes may be matted – *pseudomatting* (cf. Koch's lymphadenitis).
(c) The surrounding structures and overlying skin are usually normal (cf. local signs of inflammation with or without abscess in septic lymphadenitis; cold abscess, sinus or ulcers in Koch's lymphadenitis).
(d) The enlarged nodes are neither warm nor tender.

2. General examination:
(a) Progressive anaemia with peculiar pallor— *coffee white pallor*.
(b) Jaundice due to excessive haemolysis of the red cells or involvement of liver or compression of CBD by enlarged glands at porta hepatis.
(c) Enlargement of other groups of lymph nodes – *generalised lymphadenopathy*; so palpate for lymphadenopathy in other parts of the body, e.g. opposite neck, axillae, groins and abdomen.
(d) Enlargement of spleen, liver and para-aortic lymph nodes may be noted on abdominal palpation.
(e) Venous congestion in the neck, engorged collateral veins across the chest wall due to mediastinal compression by enlarged mediastinal nodes causing superior venacaval obstruction.
(f) Presence of sternal and bony tenderness due to bone marrow involvement.
(g) Rarely, elevated, reddened scaly patches on the skin known as *mycosis fungoides* may be noted. *It is not a fungal infection* but is caused due to infiltration of the skin with malignant deposits.

Investigations
1. *Complete blood count, ESR.*
   (i) Anaemia – normocytic normochromic.
   (ii) Leukaemoid reaction (common in Hodgkin's disease).
   (iii) Eosinophilia.
   (iv) *Lymphocytopenia* indicates bad prognosis.
   (v) *High ESR* indicates persistent disease activity.
2. *Excision biopsy of the lymph node*
   (i) To establish diagnosis.
   (ii) To do accurate histological grading.
   (iii) To test the immune markers.
      Before proceeding to any sophisticated investigations biopsy of the lymph node(s) is essential.
      Biopsy of the lymph nodes: Cellular pleomorphism and *typical mirror image nucleated 'Reed Sternberg (RS) giant cells'*

are the important hallmark of Hodgkin's disease. RS cells are not actual cancer cells but represent local tissue response to malignant cells. *More the RS cells, worse the prognosis.*

For modern classification, LN biopsy material may be sent for immunophenotyping and cytogenic/molecular analysis.
- FNAC may give the diagnosis but fails to provide definite histological pattern.
- Core biopsy with a spring-loaded Trucut needle under image control can provide sufficient tissue for histological grading.
- *Excision biopsy is preferred* whenever possible to provide both diagnosis and histological pattern.
- *CT-guided FNAC may be performed in abdominal lymphoma and thus to avoid laparotomy.*

3. *Chest X-ray* to look for
   (i) Widening of mediastinum due to enlarged mediastinal nodes.
   (ii) Pleural effusion.
   (iii) Lung parenchymal infiltration.
4. *U/S, CT, MRI of chest and abdomen* to look for
   (i) Mediastinal lymph node enlargement.
   (ii) Para-aortic lymph node enlargement.
   (iii) Liver secondaries.
   (iv) Splenomegaly.
5. *PET scan* can detect small deposits as low as 0.2 cm, that do not show on CT scan.
6. *X-rays* of thoracic and lumbar vertebrae, pelvis and any other areas of bone tenderness.
7. *IVU* to note any distortion or compression of the renal calyces or pelvis by the enlarged para-aortic lymph nodes: Rarely performed.
8. *Lymphangiography:* Rarely performed.
9. *Gallium scan:* Sensitivity is approximately 80%.
10. *Other blood investigations*
    - LFT, serum calcium, serum alkaline phosphatase – *increased levels indicate* liver and bone involvement.
    - Urea, creatinine – *increased levels indicate* renal involvement.

- Uric acid – *increased levels indicate aggressive NHL.*
- HIV testing – positive high grade NHL may be associated with AIDS.
11. Skeletal survey and/or gallium bone scan:
    - To include thoracic and lumbar vertebrae, pelvis, proximal limbs and any other bone which may be tender.
    - Usually *osteosclerotic lesion (ivory vertebrae) with HL* and *osteolytic lesion with NHL.*
12. Bone marrow aspiration or trephine biopsy in presence of
    - ↑ Serum alkaline phosphatase
    - Abnormal skeletal survey
    - Unexplained anaemia

    Bone marrow involvement indicates stage IV disease.
13. *Staging laparotomy: Staging laparotomy followed by splenectomy and liver and lymph node biopsy are not performed routinely nowadays to stage the lymphoma because of:*
    - the availability and accuracy of the imaging techniques such as USG, CT and MRI;
    - the accuracy of the CT-guided FNAC of the liver and lymph nodes;
    - the significant morbidity from laparotomy (about 10%) from wound infection, subphrenic abscess, pulmonary infection and embolism, gastrointestinal haemorrhage;
    - Splenectomy increases the risk of overwhelming bacterial sepsis in children below 15 years of age;
    - the association between splenectomy and acute myeloid leukaemia noted in patients receiving chemotherapy;
    - the increased morbidity which is up to 6%.

    Staging laparotomy is also not justified in stage III and IV Hodgkin's lymphoma and in most cases of non-Hodgkin's lymphoma as they are treated by combination chemotherapy in most centres.
14. HIV testing, as high grade NHL may be associated with AIDS.

Clinical staging (Ann Arbor staging)

Stage I
- Involvement of a single lymph node region, e.g. palpable left supraclavicular nodes.

    OR

- Involvement of a single extralymphatic organ or site (IE).

Stage II
- Involvement of two or more lymph node regions on the same side of the diaphragm – above or below, e.g. left supraclavicular and left axillary nodes or left supraclavicular, left axillary and right supraclavicular nodes.

    OR

- Involvement of one extralymphatic organ or site with one or more lymph node regions on the same side of the diaphragm (IIE).

Stage III
- Involvement of lymph node regions on both sides of diaphragm, e.g. left supraclavicular and left inguinal nodes.

    ±

- Involvement of spleen (IIIS) or involvement of one extralymphatic organ or site (IIIE) or both (IIIE and IIIS).

Stage IV
- Diffuse or disseminated involvement of extralymphatic organs or sites.

    ±

- Lymph node involvement.

    The suffix (E) *indicates an extralymphatic site or organ. The suffix* (S) *indicates splenic disease.*

    Extralymphatic site or organ involves lung, pleura, liver, bone and bone marrow, skin and subcutaneous tissue.

    All stages are further subdivided into groups A or B on the basis of the absence (A) *or presence* (B) *of the associated generalised symptoms such as weight loss, fever, night sweats, anaemia.*

    The clinical staging of HL is required to determine accurately the extent of the disease, the subsequent treatment and prognosis.

The treatment and prognosis in HD depend largely on the clinical stage of the disease whereas in NHL the therapy is usually based on its histological type.

Differential diagnosis

From other causes of generalised or localised lymphadenopathy:

1. Tuberculosis (commonest cause of lymphadenopathy in our country)
2. Secondaries (second most common cause of lymphadenopathy in elderly people)
3. Brucellosis
4. Toxoplasmosis
5. Sarcoidosis
6. Infectious mononucleosis
7. Leukaemias

Treatment

Two forms of treatments are available and they are stage and site dependent: *Radiotherapy* and *combination chemotherapy.*

Surgery has no role except lymph node biopsy to confirm the diagnosis, the stage and grade of the tumour.

Staging laparotomy is less frequently used nowadays because of increased morbidity. Instead **CT/MRI** *gives sufficient information* regarding the status of lymph nodes, spleen, liver and any other lump.

Radiotherapy is the treatment of choice in stage I, II, and IIIA diseases.

Combination chemotherapy *is used* in stage IIIB and IV diseases.

Blood transfusions are required in severely anaemic patients before radiotherapy and chemotherapy.

Note

Staging of lymphoma – presence of constitutional symptoms

- *Stage A:* Absence of constitutional or generalised symptoms
- *Stage B:* Presence of constitutional or generalised symptoms

Radiotherapy

Indications

- Stage I, II and IIIA diseases.

- For lesions causing serious pressure symptoms, e.g. SVC pressure syndrome.

Type of machine

- Linear accelerator is preferred than cobalt 60, because *it provides sharply localised radiation.*

Dose

- Total dose of 35–40 centigray (cGy) given over a period of 4 weeks (5 days each week).

Mode of delivery (Fig. 4.5)

- *IF:* Involved field, e.g. mantle field or inverted Y-field
- *EF:* Extended field or
- *TANI:* Both mantle and inverted Y-fields

Differs in various stages:

(a) *Stage IA with lymphocyte predominant can be treated by involved field (IF) radiotherapy.*

(b) *Stage IA with other histology*
Stage IIA with any histology
Treated by extended field (EF) radiotherapy

(c) *Stage IB, IIB and IIIA:* Treated by a technique called 'total axial nodal irradiation (TANI)' which includes a combination of mantle field and inverted Y field.

Extended Field (EF) radiotherapy can be given as:

(a) *Mantle field* which covered both cervicals, both axillary regions, the mediastinal and upper para-aortic nodes down to the level of L2 – *used for supradiaphragmatic disease.*

(b) *Inverted Y field* which covers para-aortic, both iliacs, inguinal and femoral areas – *used for infradiaphragmatic disease.*

(c) *TANI* includes irradiation of both mantle and inverted Y fields – first the mantle field followed by inverted Y field after an interval of 4–6 weeks.

Chemotherapy

Indications

All patients with B symptoms:

1. Stage IIIB and IV diseases, because these are considered systemic diseases.
2. Stage IIIA has also been treated at some centres by chemotherapy with equal success.
3. Usually combination chemotherapy is used.

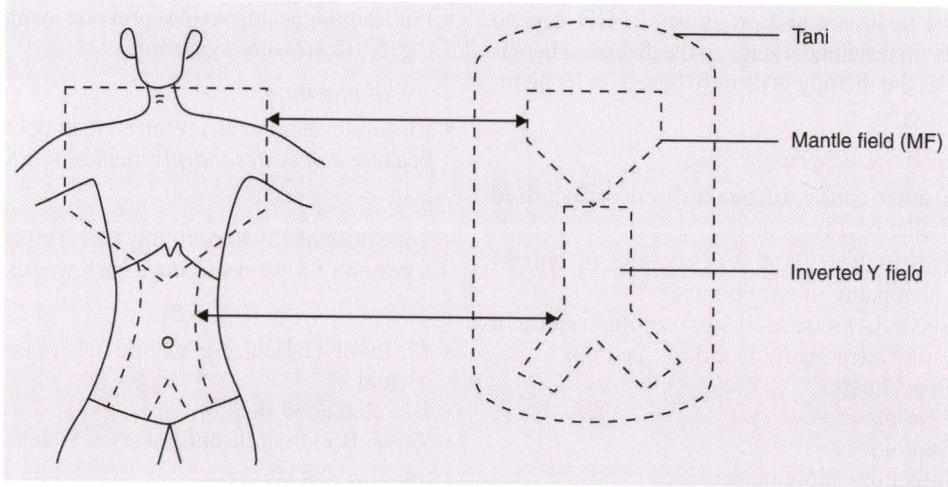

Fig. 4.5: Mode of delivery of radiotherapy in lymphoma.

Regimens of chemotherapy

1. *Chlorambucil*, as a single drug oral therapy in low grade NHL
2. *MOPP regime* is used in low risk patients
   - Includes **M**echlorethamine, **O**ncovin (Vincristine), **P**rocarbazine, **P**rednisolone.
   - *MOPP* is administered for six *two weeks* cycles of chemotherapy with two weeks rest between each period of drugs administration.
   - *Basic regimen* but is highly toxic.
   - *Side effects:*
     (i) Development of acute myeloid leukaemia.
     (ii) Bone marrow suppression.
     (iii) Infertility both in men and women.
3. *ABVD regime* is used mainly in high risk patients: Stage IIIB and IV
   - Includes **A**driamycin, **B**leomycin, **V**inblastine, **D**acarbazine (ABVD).
   - Less leukomogenic.
   - Causes less infertility.
   - Currently the preferred treatment.
4. Other regimens available are:
   - BEACOPP, COPPABVD, Stanford V, MOPPBV.

Prognosis

Depends on:

- *Extent of disease* (Stages I, II, III, IV)

- *Presence of symptoms* (B – presence of symptoms; A – absence of symptoms)
- *Histology* (REAL classification) – treatment and prognosis of NHL are *largely dependant upon histological or morphological type*

5 years survival rates for HL

1. 85% for stage I and II
2. 70% for stage IIIA (A – absence of symptoms)
3. 50% for stage IIIB (B – presence of symptoms
4. 40% for stage IV

Cause of death

Usually from

1. Systemic infection like respiratory tract infection, fungal, bacterial, e.g. tuberculosis because of immunosuppression.
2. Systemic failure.
3. Bone marrow failure.
4. Acute spinal cord compression leading to paraplegia.
5. Multiple bone metastasis, pathological fracture.

NON-HODGKIN'S LYMPHOMAS (NHL)

The non-Hodgkin's lymphomas are solid tumours arising in the peripheral lymphoreticular tissues particularly of the lymph nodes *but also of the oropharynx, the gut, skin and other sites.*

65% to 70% arise from the B lymphocytes (B cell NHL) and the rest arise from the T lymphocytes (T cell NHL):

- Rarely NHL arises from histiocytes.
- *RS cells are absent in NHL.*

Rappaport classified NHL morphologically into four types, each of which can be nodular (follicular) or diffuse.

1. Well-differentiated lymphocytic.
2. Poorly differentiated lymphocytic.
3. Mixed lymphocytic and histiocytic.
4. Histiocytic (reticulum cells).

- Prognostically these are conveniently divided into:

Morphological type	Degree of malignancy
1. Small lymphocytes and a nodular structure	Low grade tumour
2. Large lymphocytes with small lymphocytes, histiocytes and a diffuse structure	High grade tumour

- *NHL has a non-continuous spread* while HL has an orderly continuous spread.
- NHL has a *more frequent involvement of multiple peripheral nodes compared to HL which often remains localised to one group of nodes.*
- The Waldeyer's ring, epitrochlear nodes, and mesenteric nodes involvement are common in NHL, while their involvement is rare in HL.
- B symptoms described for HL are less common in patients with NHL.
- Prognosis and curability of NHL – poorer than HL.

Clinical presentation

1. Usually occurs in the 60–80 years age group.
2. Lymphadenopathy is a common presenting feature and usually generalised.

Enlargement of lymph nodes may affect any area initially. May present as enlarged, non-tender (rarely tender) with firm or variegated feel with smooth or nodular surface. Neither softening nor any suppuration will be noted. Local skin temperature may be elevated.

There is more chance of involvement of epitrochlear and Waldeyer's ring.
3. Extranodal tissue is frequently involved such as orbit, intestine, breast, testis.
4. There may be generalised spread to involve many organs, e.g. CNS, kidney, liver, lungs and heart.

Treatment

Chemotherapy

- *Chemotherapy is the mainstay of treatment in NHL.* Regimens of chemotherapy in use are:
- COP regimen includes **C**yclophosphamide, **O**ncovin (vincristine) and **P**rednisolone.
- CHOP regimen includes **C**yclophosphamide, **H**ydroxydaunorubicin, **O**ncovin and **P**rednisolone.
- Other regimens include BACOP (**B**leomycin **A**driamycin + **COP**).
- *Chlorambucil as a single drug oral therapy* may be used in low grade NHL.

Radiotherapy

- In some centres, *patients with low grade stages I and II NHL have also been treated with involved field (IF) radiation.*
- Following radiotherapy, the local recurrence rate is nearly nil with nodular lymphoma and around 15% with diffuse lymphoma.
- Whole body radiation (WBR) may be used in cases after failure of chemotherapy.

Monoclonal antibody therapy

- Recently being used in some centres with improved success rates.
- *It is the use of monoclonal antibodies (mAb) to specific target cells (antigens). The main objective is stimulating the patient's immune system to attack the malignant tumour cells (antigens)* and thus prevention of tumour growth by blocking specific cell receptors. Following *FDA approved therapeutic antibodies are in use for non-Hodgkin's lymphoma:* tositumomab, ibritumomab, rituximab.

BURKITT'S LYMPHOMA

- It is a type of *high grade non-Hodgkin's lymphoma.*

- It is named after Burkitt, a surgeon who first described the disease while working in Africa.
- It is caused by Epstein-Barr virus (EBV).
- It is believed that *impaired immunity* provides an opening for development of EB virus infection.
  (*EBV also causes glandular fever* – infectious mononucleosis, a non-malignant condition in young adults in Western societies).
- Clinically Burkitt's lymphoma can be divided into three clinical varieties: Endemic, sporadic and immunodeficiency associated variants.

(a) Endemic variety

- Occurs in Equatorial Africa, Nigeria, New Guinea and South America, *where malaria is endemic*. Where malaria has been eradicated the incidence of Burkitt's lymphoma falls *suggesting a possible insect vector of an infective origin*.
- *Males* are predominantly affected.
- *Young children are affected more* – over 80% of cases occur between the ages of 3 and 12 years. Involves body parts other than lymph nodes.
- *The tumour characteristically involves the jaw or the facial bones* (*about 60%*). Maxillary lesions may present as oral or orbital tumours (Fig. 4.6).

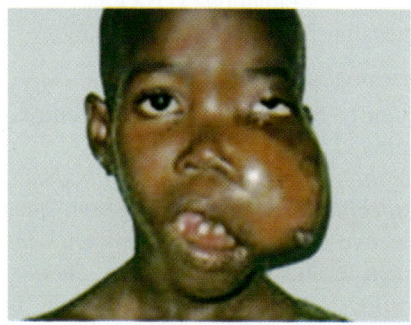

Fig. 4.6: Burkitt's lymphoma involving left maxilla.

- The tumour grows rapidly and is soft and painless.
- The disease may involve the distal ileum, caecum, ovaries, kidneys and breasts.
- *Endemic variety has a good prognosis.*

(b) Sporadic variety

- *Occurs throughout the world.*
- Jaw is less commonly involved compared to the endemic variety. *Ileocaecal region is the common site of involvement.*

(c) Immunodeficiency variety

Usually associated with HIV infection. Burkitt's lymphoma can be an initial manifestation of AIDS.

Histology: Histological appearance is typical and striking – presence of dense masses of lymphocytes interspersed with large histiocytes or macrophages containing debris derived from dead body of apoptotic tumour cells, contributing the '*starry-sky*' appearance.

Treatment

- *Endemic variety* responds well to chemotherapy.
  - (i) Single drug cyclophosphamide has been shown to be effective.
  - (ii) Long-term survival without maintenance therapy has been reported.
  - (iii) A number of spontaneous remissions have also been recorded.
- *Sporadic variety* needs to be treated with combination chemotherapy.
- Other treatments like immunotherapy, bone marrow transplants, surgery to remove the tumour, and radiotherapy may also be required.

Comparison between HL and NHL is summarised in Table 4.1.

Note

Lymph nodes are pathologically significant with the following features.

1. Usually greater than 1 cm in diameter.
2. Firm in consistency.
3. Round shaped.
4. Matted nodes become attached to each other – more common with Koch's lymphadenitis.
5. Tender on palpation in presence of infection.
6. Firm to solid and non-tender – lymphoma.

	Table 4.1: Comparison between HL and NHL	
Points	**Hodgkin's lymphoma (HL)**	**Non-Hodgkin's lymphoma (NHL)**
1. *Frequency*	Less common (30%)	More common (70%)
2. *Age*	Bimodal age: One in the younger and other in the elderly – between 15 and 30 years of life	Any age – more frequent after 50 years of age
3. *Cells of origin*	B lymphocytes 90%	B lymphocytes 60%, T lymphocytes, null cells, histiocytes
4. *Nodal involvement*	Common (90%) but localised to one group, commonly to cervical group; 10% extranodal	Common (60%) but involves multiple groups of nodes; 40% extranodal
• Mediastinal	Common	Common
• Abdominal	Uncommon	Common
• Epitrochlears	Uncommon	Common
• Waldeyer's	Uncommon	Common
5. *Nodal spread*	Contiguous	Non-contiguous
6. *Extranodal involvement*	Uncommon; *spleen may be involved*	Common; but *spleen less commonly involved*
7. *Systemic symptoms*	Common	Uncommon
• B symptoms	Early and prominent	Late and non-prominent
• Fluctuating fever	Present	Only in 20% cases
• Alcohol-induced pain or pruritus	Characteristic	Absent
8. *Anaemia*	Late	Early
9. *Dissemination*	Unifocal in origin	Multicentric in origin
10. *Nodal characteristics*	*Well located at diagnosis*	*Widespread at diagnosis*
• Size	Smaller	Larger
• Rate growth	Slow	Fast
• Consistency	*Rubbery elastic*	*Variegated or firm*
• Local temperature	Normal	May be raised
• Tenderness	Absent	May be present
• Epitrochlear nodes	Less common	Common
• Waldeyer's ring	Less common	Common
• Mediastinal LNS	More common	Less common
11. *Treatment*	*Radiotherapy for stages I and II diseases*; combination chemotherapy for stages III and IV diseases	Radiotherapy response poorer than HL; *combination chemotherapy mainly for all stages*
12. *Prognosis*	Better than NHL	Poorer than HL

Note

Lymphoma

1. Most patients with palpable lymphadeno-pathy – *the lymph nodes are non-tender.*

2. In most of these patients enlarged nodes are in the neck, supraclavicular area and axilla. Most of these patients will also have mediastinal lymphadenopathy at diagnosis.

3. Subdiaphragmatic presentation of Hodgkin's lymphoma is rare and more common in older people.

4. In more than 50% of patients who have both Hodgkin's and non-Hodgkin's lymphoma, the mediastinum is the primary site.

5. Nodular sclerosis is the most common sub-type in developed countries.

6. Mixed cellularity is most common in developing countries.
7. *Varieties of Hodgkin's lymphoma with best prognosis are of lymphocytic predominance.*
8. *Stomach is the most frequent extranodal site for lymphomas.* Vast majority of gastric lymphomas are non-Hodgkin's lymphomas of B lymphocytes. Hodgkin's disease involving stomach is extremely uncommon.

Note

Drugs producing lymphadenopathy (*pseudo-lymphoma*):

1. Phenytoin
2. Cyclosporin A (used during organ trans-plantation)
3. Carbamezapine
4. Cephalidin
5. PAS (used in multidrug-resistant tuber-culosis)
6. Primidone
7. Hydralazine
8. Allopurinol

Note

Markers of worse prognosis in lymphomas

(a) Tumour bulk
(b) Clinical stage
(c) Histopathology (grade)
  • Lymphocyte depleted – poor prognosis
  • Lymphocyte rich – good prognosis
(d) Presence of constitutional symptoms (B symptoms) – poor prognosis
(e) Low haematocrit at presentation (severe anaemia) due to bone marrow involvement
(f) High LDH (liver involvement)

Note

The treatment and prognosis in HL depend on *the stage of the disease* whereas in NHL therapy is usually based on *its histopathological and morphological types – low or high grade.*

Note

Prognosis of NHL depends on morphological types of lymphocytes:
• Small lymphocytes – low grade tumour
• Large lymphocytes – high grade tumour

Note

Virchow's gland

Medial group of left supraclavicular group of lymph glands lying between two heads of sternomastoid.

Note

Virchow's triad – thrombosis of deep veins (DVT) produced by:
  1. Stasis of the blood
  2. Hypercoagulability
  3. Intimal damage
All the three causes may not exist together in every case.

Salivary Glands

SURGICAL ANATOMY

There are three pairs of major salivary glands – the parotid, the submandibular and the sublingual glands. Besides these main salivary glands, small accessory glands are found scattered over the palate, lips, cheek, and tongue. These glands are occasional sites for development of mixed salivary tumour.

Note

- Parotid gland is ectodermal in origin (from first branchial cleft), hence dermoid cyst can develop in it.
- Submandibular and sublingual glands are endo-dermal in origin.

Parotid gland (Fig. 5.1)

It is the largest of the three paired salivary glands. It is situated *in the parotid mould* located on the side of the face between the zygomatic arch and the edge of the mandible in front of the ear lobule. The mould presents the following boundaries.

- *Anteriorly:* Posterior border of the ramus of the mandible and the muscles attached to it – superficially, the masseter, and on the deeper aspect, the medial pterygoid muscle.
- *Posteriorly:* Mastoid process and sterno-mastoid muscle.

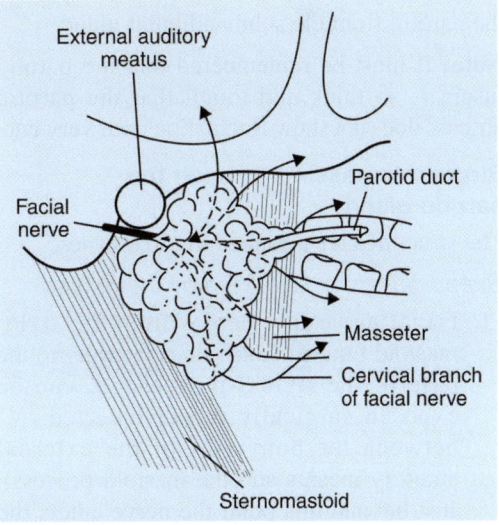

Fig. 5.1: Parotid mould with the gland. Note that the parotid duct opens into the cheek opposite the crown of the upper second molar tooth. Note the branches of facial nerve.

- *Above:* By the zygomatic arch.
- *Below:* Posterior belly of digastric muscle.
- *Medially:* Styloid process and the styloid groups of muscles.

Some parts of the gland extend beyond the mould and produce various processes of the gland.

Coverings: The gland is covered by inner true capsule and outer false capsule of parotido-masseteric fascia.

True capsule is formed by condensation of the fibrous stroma of the gland.

False capsule is known as *parotid sheath* and is formed by the splitting of the investing layer of deep cervical fascia. The superficial lamella of the sheath is strong and attached above to the zygomatic arch; and anteriorly it extends forward over the masseter muscle to form the parotido-masseteric fascia which is dense and tough.

The deep lamella is thin. It passes deep to the gland and is attached to the tympanic plate and styloid process of the temporal bone. *Antero-inferiorly this deep lamella is thickened and known as stylomandibular ligament.* It separates the parotid from the submandibular gland.

Note: It must be remembered that the parotid fascia is so thick and tough that the parotid abscess does not show fluctuation until very late.

Structures passing through the parotid gland

The structures are arranged in three zones.

Superficial zone: Occupied by the nerves

1. Facial nerve: It emerges from the stylo-mastoid foramen, and winds laterally to the base of the styloid process (so, can be exposed surgically in the inverted 'V' between the bony part of the external auditory meatus and the mastoid process). Just beyond this point the nerve enters the parotid gland at its posteromedial surface.

   Within the gland, the nerve divides and rejoins to form a plexus known as *pes anserinus* (pes anserinus means goose foot). Ultimately 5 branches come out of this plexus and emerge through the upper pole, anterior border and lower pole of the gland. The branches from above downwards are (Figs 5.1 and 5.3):

   - Temporal
   - Zygomatic — Upper
   - Buccal
   - Mandibular — Lower
   - Cervical

   Supply all the muscles of facial expression

2. Great auricular nerve
3. Auriculotemporal nerve

Intermediate zone: Occupied by the veins

1. Retromandibular vein which is formed by the union of superficial temporal and maxillary veins. *Immediately deep to facial nerve runs the retromandibular vein.*
2. Anterior division of retromandibular vein which joins the anterior facial vein to form the common facial vein.
3. Posterior division of retromandibular vein which joins the posterior auricular vein to form the external jugular vein.

Deep zone: Occupied by the arteries

1. *External carotid artery* dividing into super-ficial temporal and maxillary arteries.
2. Transverse facial artery, a branch of super-ficial temporal artery.
3. Sometimes posterior auricular artery arises within the gland, from the external carotid artery.

Note

Marginal mandibular nerve lies superficial to the facial vein above the inferior border of the mandible. *Injury to this nerve causes paralysis of the lower lip muscles* and so causes cons-picuous deformity of the mouth during smiling or grimacing.

Patey's faciovenous plane
(Figs 5.2 and 5.3)

Within the gland the facial nerve and its branches lie with remarkable constancy in one plane *super-ficial to the retromandibular vein*. The plane in which the nerve and the vein lie, has been designated by *Patey as the faciovenous plane.* In this plane the gland can be split sagittally into two parts – superficial and deep. *Along this plane superficial parotidectomy is carried out without injuring the nerve.* Pes anserinus (a description of arrangement of facial nerve) lies inside the parotid gland.

The parotid duct (Stensen's duct) emerges from the anterior border of the gland and runs horizontally across the masseter *a finger breadth below the zygomatic arch* and it makes a right-

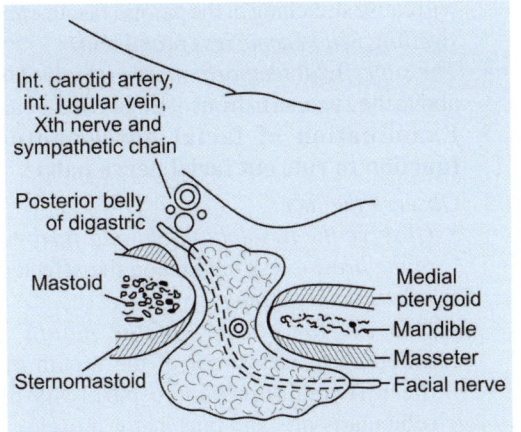

Fig. 5.2: Zones of parotid gland and its surrounding structures. Note that the facial nerve is the most superficial of the structures traversing the gland.

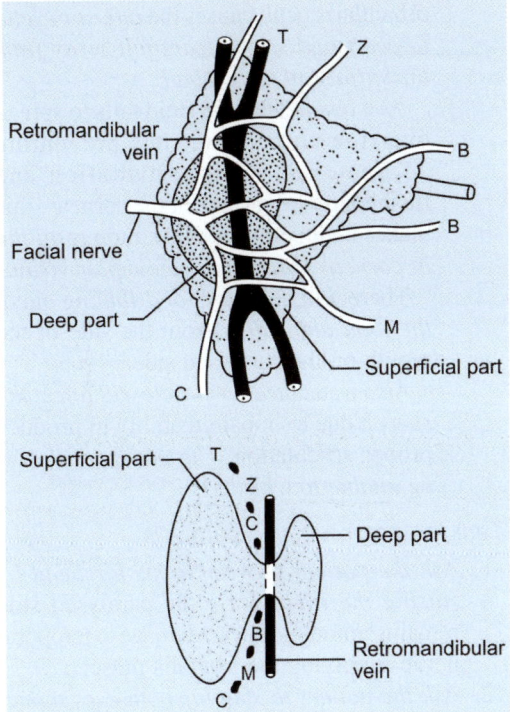

Fig. 5.3: Patey's faciovenous plane. Facial nerve and its branches are superficial to retromandibular vein.

angled turn at the anterior border of masseter to pierce the buccinator *to open in the vestibule of the mouth (buccal aspect of the cheek) via a small*

papilla opposite to the crown of the upper second molar tooth.

The Stensen's duct can be felt by bidigital palpation by index finger in the mouth and thumb over the cheek. Accessory parotid lobe arises from the horizontal part of the parotid duct as it extends beyond the anterior border of masseter. Any disease of main parotid gland can also involve the accessory lobe.

Nerve supply of parotid gland

Secretomotor supply via the auriculotemporal nerve carrying the parasympathetic fibres from the inferior salivary nucleus via the otic ganglion.

Submandibular gland

The gland is situated in the submandibular region partly below the mandible and partly deep to it. Each gland consists of a *larger superficial part* and a *smaller deep part:* Both the parts are continuous around the posterior border of mylohyoid muscle. *Superficial part of the gland lies on* the mylohyoid, hyoglossus and the middle constrictor muscle from before backwards. *The deep part extends* in the interval between mylohyoid and hyoglossus up to the sublingual salivary gland.

The gland is enclosed in a loose sheath derived from the investing layer of deep cervical fascia.

Relations of the deep part

- *Laterally:* Mylohyoid.
- *Medially:* Hyoglossus.
- *Below:* Hypoglossal nerve accompanied by a pair of veins.
- *Above:* Lingual nerve and the submandibular ganglia. The lingual nerve hooks the submandibular duct from superficial to deep at its lower border.

Superficially the gland is covered by the platysma and it is crossed by the cervical branch of the facial nerve and by the anterior facial vein.

The facial artery comes in close relationship with the gland. It approaches the gland posteriorly and then arches over the superficial aspect (which it indents) to attain the inferior border of the mandible and thence to ascend onto the face in front of the masseter.

The submandibular duct (Wharton's duct) emerges from the medial surface of the gland and runs forward under the cover of mylohyoid beneath the mucosa of the floor of the mouth along the side of the tongue to open on the sublingual papilla at the side of the frenum. Here its orifice is readily visible and saliva can be seen trickling from it.

The sublingual gland lies in the submucous plane immediately lateral to Wharton's duct in the floor of the mouth. They secrete mucoid discharge.

The submandibular lymph nodes lie superficial to the submandibular gland. They may lie partly embedded within the gland.

PAROTID SWELLING

Characteristic features

1. *Site of the swelling:* Swelling is in the parotid region or mould. *Swelling appears below, in front of and behind the lobule of ear.*
2. It obliterates the furrow behind the ramus of the mandible just below the lobule of the ear, between the mandible and mastoid process.
3. In many cases where the swelling is big, the lobule of the ear is pushed up (Figs 5.6 and 5.9).
4. Shape of the swelling may look like parotid gland if it is a larger one.
5. *The swelling does not extend above the zygoma.*
6. Tumours of the parotid gland are usually common at the tail of the gland.

Clinical examination of parotid swelling

In addition, to note the site, size, shape, consistency, etc., of the swelling, the following points must be examined.

1. *Relation of the swelling to the skin: Free or fixed.*
2. *Relation of the swelling with relaxed* and taut masseter (*the patient is asked to clinch the teeth thus making the masseter taut*) – *Mobile or fixed.*
3. *Relation of the swelling to the parotid fascia:* The patient is asked to open the mouth which

will cause stretching of the parotid fascia – *the swelling will become less prominent.*
4. *The superficial temporal artery is palpable* above the zygoma in front of tragus of the ear.
5. **Examination of facial nerve motor function to rule out facial nerve palsy:**
   Observe the face:
   - *Observe the nasolabial fold and furrows of the brow* – less marked on the affected side: *Facial asymmetry.*
   - *Observe the corners of the mouth* – drooping of the corner of the mouth on the affected side due to paralysis of orbicularis oris and buccinator muscle.

      Above two conditions make facial expression distorted making it appear passive or *sad-looking* appearance.
   - *Observe the eyes* – the loss of tonus of the orbicularis oculi causes the *inferior eyelid to evert and so the tears fall away from the surface of the eyeball.*

      As a result, lacrimal fluid fails to spread over the cornea and thus preventing adequate lubrication, hydration and flushing of the surface of the cornea – this makes it vulnerable to ulceration *resulting in corneal scar which can impair vision.*

      There will be *history of dribbling out of the food and saliva* from the side of the mouth on the paralysed side.

      Also weakened lip muscle will affect the speech due to impaired ability to produce proper articulation. *The patient will also be unable to whistle.*

Test for motor function paralysis

1. *Ask the patient to wrinkle his forehead by raising the eyebrows* – the paralysed side remains immobile due to damage to temporal nerve supplying the frontalis muscle.
2. *Ask the patient to shut his both eyes tightly* – the patient will not be able to close his eyelids tightly on the affected side. *Moreover, the eyeball will be seen to roll upwards* – due to damage to the zygomatic branch supplying orbicularis oculi muscle.
3. *Ask the patient to whistle* – inability to whistle suggests damage to the buccal

branch supplying buccinator and part of orbicularis oris muscle.

4. *Ask the patient to puff out cheeks* – the paralysed side bellows out more than the normal side due to damage to the buccal branch.

5. *Ask the patient to smile* – the patient is unable to smile as the lips do not separate on the affected side and *there will also be drooping of the angle of the mouth on the affected side* – due to damage to the marginal mandibular branch which supplies the muscles around the mouth including orbicularis oris muscle. *This branch is the thinnest and has the largest course through the parotid gland and, therefore, is most likely to be injured.*

6. *Ask the patient to pull down corners of the mouth* – the patient will be unable to do this on the affected side due to damage to the cervical branch which supplies platysma.

Note

The facial nerve is never involved in benign parotid tumours.

7. **Intraoral examination:**
   - Approximately 10% of parotid tumours develop in the deep lobe and lie beneath the facial nerve.
   - So, examine the oral cavity. *The deep lobe tumour presents with a parapharyngeal mass which pushes the pharyngeal wall, tonsil and soft palate medially.*
   - Deep lobe tumours may present with the complaints of dysphagia.
   - Deep lobe tumours usually do not appear as a gross swelling on the surface of the face until it is too large or both the superficial and deep lobes are involved.
   - *Bimanual palpation of the parotid gland for deep lobe tumour.* One finger externally behind the ramus of the mandible and one finger inside the mouth just in front of the tonsil and behind the 3rd molar tooth internally to assess the deep lobe tumour.
   - Parotid duct and its orifice – for redness, oedema of the duct, or exudation of pus or blood. *The orifice of the parotid duct*

(Stensen's duct) is situated opposite the crown of the second upper molar tooth.

8. Movements of the temporomandibular joint.
9. Lymph nodes of the neck.

Differential diagnosis of the swelling in the neighbourhood of parotid region

I. **Preauricular lymphadenitis**
   Diagnostic points:
   1. Ovoid, firm, smooth, swelling is situated just in front of the tragus.
   2. The furrow behind the ramus of the mandible is not obliterated.
   3. Presence of some primary focus of infection or tumour in the drainage area – forehead and temporal region of the scalp, auditory meatus, eyelids, cheek.
   4. The swelling is very mobile, *as the node is outside the capsule of the parotid gland* – the most distinctive physical sign. (Most tumours of the parotid gland are tethered to the gland. So, they are less mobile.)

II. **Swelling in connection with masseter muscle**
   1. Fibroma
   2. Lipoma
   3. Rhabdomyoma
   4. Idiopathic hypertrophy of the masseter muscle.
   Diagnostic points: The swelling becomes fixed and hard beneath the fingers when the masseter is contracted (*by clinching the teeth*) and free and relatively soft when the masseter is relaxed.

III. **Swelling in relation to the overlying skin**, e.g. sebaceous cyst, lipoma and haemangioma.

IV. **Neuroma of the facial nerve**.

V. **Adamantinoma of the mandible**.

NEOPLASMS OF THE SALIVARY GLANDS

Approximately 75% of the neoplasms of the salivary gland occur in the parotid glands. *80% of parotid tumours are benign and of these, pleomorphic adenoma is the commonest (80%) and Warthin's tumour is the second most common benign tumour.* The remaining 20% are malignant.

About 15% of salivary gland tumours occur in the submandibular salivary glands, 60% of which are benign. Of the benign tumours 90% are pleomorphic adenomas.

10% of the salivary tumours occur in the sublingual salivary glands and minor salivary glands situated in the palate, lips and cheeks. Of these 40% are benign and virtually all these benign tumours are pleomorphic adenomas.

Note

Most salivary gland neoplasms are benign and even the malignant tumours are relatively slow growing.

PAROTID TUMOUR

International classification

1. Epithelial tumours.
2. Non-epithelial tumours.
3. Metastatic carcinoma.

I. Epithelial tumours

A. Adenomas
  (a) Pleomorphic adenoma (myoepithelial origin) also known as mixed parotid tumour – potentially malignant.
      Note: Pleomorphic means many forms.
  (b) Monomorphic adenomas (duct cell origin):
      1. Adenolymphoma or Warthin's tumour
      2. Oxyphilic adenoma
      3. Other types, e.g. basal cell carcinoma
  (c) Acinic cell tumour (arising from acinar cells)
B. Carcinoma:
  (a) Mucoepidermoid tumour or squamous cell carcinoma (arising from duct cells) – low grade malignancy and very slowly growing tumour. *Most common malignant salivary gland tumour. Most common in parotid gland.*
  (b) Adenoid cystic carcinoma or cylindroma (arising from glandular cells) – relatively

radiosensitive. *Second most common malignant salivary neoplasm.* Most common in the submandibular and other salivary glands. *Perineural invasion is common with this lesion.*
  (c) Adenocarcinoma (arising from glandular cells) – polymorphous low grade type in Indian scenario.
  (d) Undifferentiated carcinoma:
      • Carcinoma ex pleomorphic adenoma.
      • Anaplastic carcinoma.

II. Non-epithelial tumours

• Benign
  (a) Haemangioma
  (b) Lymphangioma
  (c) Neurofibroma.
  (d) Oncocytoma.
• Malignant – lymphoma

III. Metastatic carcinoma

• Secondary to the epidermoid carcinoma and malignant melanoma.

Characteristic features of parotid tumour

1. Most salivary gland tumours are benign (80%) and even the malignant tumours are relatively slow growing.
2. Parotid tumours usually occur in the tail of the gland lying over the angle of the mandible.
3. In 10% cases, the parotid tumours are bilateral.
4. *Commonest tumour of the parotid is the pleomorphic adenoma.*
   Second common is Warthin's tumour. Usually occurs in the tail of the gland.
5. Most benign adenomas (90%) are superficial to facial nerve.
6. Like benign tumours, malignant tumours also *usually present as painless, slowly growing tumours.*
7. Presence of pain, facial nerve involvement or fixation of lump to adjacent structures, secondary skin changes indicate a more advanced stage with a worse prognosis.
8. *High grade mucoepidermoid and squamous cell carcinoma have very high degree incidence of nodal metastasis.*

9. No formal biopsy should be performed in parotid tumour, except in tumour of ectopic salivary glands, e.g. palatal salivary gland.

10. *Recently FNAC using 23G needle is advocated as it does not cause tumour cell implantation in the needle tract. Ultrasound guidance may also help.*

11. *For deep lobe tumour,* FNAB through intraoral route is recommended and it does not cause skin infiltration.

12. *Technetium (Tc-99) scans are effective in the diagnosis of Warthin's tumour.* Most malignancies form a cold spot with technetium scan; but *Warthin's tumour is unique as it produces a hot spot.* Thus, a firm preoperative diagnosis is possible without biopsy.

13. CT or MRI is used if the lesion is large or involves deep lobe or adjacent structures or recurrent tumours.

14. *All parotid neoplasms are radioresistant.* So, complete excision with negative margin is the treatment of choice.

15. Knowledge of the anatomy and variations of the branches of the facial nerve is critical to the safe dissection and resection of the gland.

16. *Warthin's tumour and pleomorphic adenomas are usually treated by partial parotidectomy.*

17. Rarely a tumour may arise in the deep lobe *which then presents as parapharyngeal mass* – symptoms include difficulty in swallowing and snoring. *Clinical examination of oral cavity reveals a diffuse, firm swelling in the soft palate and tonsil.*

18. In 10% of cases, parotid tumours are bilateral.

19. *CT findings of inoperability – involvement of masseteric space.* It is divided by zygomatic bone into supratemporal space (contains temporalis muscle) and infratemporal space (contains lateral and medial pterygoid muscles).

Causes for bilateral parotid tumours

(i) Warthin's tumour, (ii) acinic cell tumour.

PLEOMORPHIC ADENOMA

Syn. Mixed parotid tumour. *It is the most common benign tumour of the parotid gland. It is called mixed tumour because it contains pleomorphic stroma, e.g. cartilaginous tissue (mesodermal origin) beside epithelial tissue. Pleomorphic means many forms.* (For pleomorphic adenoma, *see* Figs 5.4 to 5.6.

It is a benign tumour but may change into malignancy at any time and hence should be considered as *potentially malignant.*

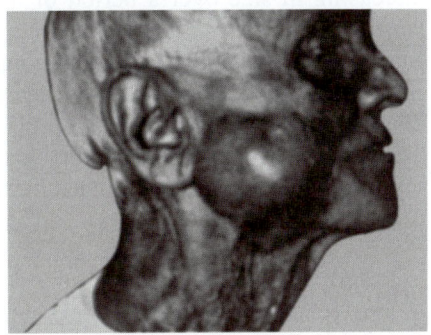

Fig. 5.4: Mixed parotid tumour right side (typical location) extending below and behind the ear lobule—the ear lobule is raised and everted over the swelling. No facial nerve involvement.

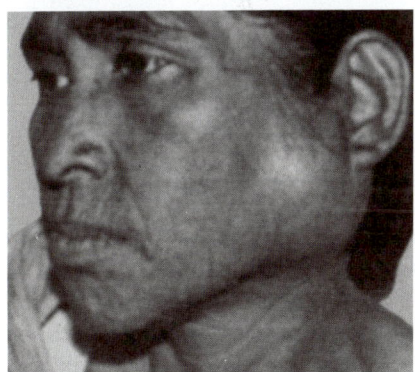

Fig. 5.5: Swelling over the left parotid region extending below and behind the ear lobule (typical location). No facial nerve involvement—mixed parotid tumour.

Pathology

1. *Origin:* Regarding its origin there are two views:

(i) According to some, the mixed parotid tumours arise from the embryonic rests due to invagination of the oral ectoderm along with the salivary and oral glands.

(ii) According to others, the tumours are true adenomas of the salivary glands rather than true mixed tumours.

2. It is called mixed parotid tumour *because it has got both epithelial and mesodermal elements*.

3. Slowly growing benign tumour, gradually increasing in size over a period of many years.

4. *Unicentric in origin*. But *recurrence is multicentric when the tumour will have extension*.

5. The tumour possesses a pseudocapsule but the tumour may have extension beyond the capsule. The tumour tissue juts out if incision is made on the capsule.

6. *Potentially malignant*, therefore, malignancy can supervene at any time.

7. In long-standing pleomorphic adenoma, an adenocarcinoma may develop which is known as *carcinoma ex pleomorphic adenoma*.

8. Some fringe of the tumour mass may protrude through the thinned out capsule and invade the adjoining areas. These protrusions through the capsular deficiencies may give rise to recurrence after removal of the tumour.

9. *The tumour is radioresistant*.

Histological picture

It is adenoma of the salivary gland with a *pleomorphic stroma* containing fibrous, lymphoid, myxomatous, pseudocartilaginous elements *in addition to epithelial elements*. It is believed that the cartilage it contains is not mesodermal in origin but is mucin or pseudomucin secreted by the epithelial cells which when stained resemble cartilage.

Diagnostic criteria

1. *Age:* Usually first appears in adult life – usually in the 5th decade.

2. *Sex:* More common in females.

3. The patient presents with *a slowly growing painless swelling on a side of the face*, which has been existent for months or years without any appreciable change in size.

4. *Site:* The swelling is situated in the parotid region, usually commences in the part of the parotid gland overlying the angle of the mandible. It often obliterates the hollow just below the lobule of the ear, between the mandible and mastoid process.

5. *Shape:* Rounded swelling with well-defined margins.

6. *Size:* Varies from a pea-sized nodule to a large, almost pendulous mass.

7. Surface is smooth, sometimes lobulated.

8. *Consistence: Firm elastic to rubbery hard, not fluctuant, not translucent.*

9. *Not tender*.

10. *Overlying skin is free from the swelling*, and looks and feels normal. There is *no venous prominence*.

11. *Mobility:* Not fixed to the deeper structure, e.g. masseter. It is mobile in both axes over both the relaxed and taut masseter.

12. *No evidence of involvement of the facial nerve.*

13. Cervical lymph nodes are not enlarged.

14. *Examination of the oral cavity:* A pleomorphic adenoma arising in the deep part of the parotid gland may push the tonsil and the pillar of the fauces towards the midline.

Differential diagnosis

1. Adenolymphoma.
2. Carcinoma parotid.

Investigation

FNAC is diagnostic.

Complications

1. *Malignant changes*
    • Occasionally, the variegated epithelial elements may burst into mitotic activity giving rise to pleomorphic carcinoma. Develops 15 years after the original swelling.
    • On rare occasions, one epithelial component alone runs a riot resulting in highly

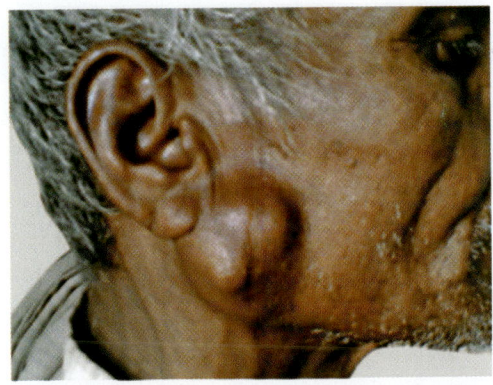

Fig. 5.6: Right parotid tumour with multiple nodules over the angle of the mandible (a typical location); no facial nerve involvement—mixed parotid tumour. (*Courtesy:* Professor Sudeb Saha, MS, FAMS)

malignant anaplastic carcinoma – an adenocarcinoma known as *carcinoma ex pleomorphic adenoma.*
- High incidence of metastases.
- 5-year survival is less than 40%.

2. *Recurrence:* Particularly after enucleation. *Recurrence is multicentric and may be malignant.*
Causes of recurrence may be:
- Incomplete surgical excision.
- Implantation of the tumour cells during manipulation.
- Multicentric growth potentiality of the tumour.

Investigations

See characteristic features of parotid tumour on page 160.

Treatment

The tumour is *radioresistant.*

So, treatment of choice is surgery. The surgical procedure includes *superficial parotidectomy with preservation of the facial nerve,* because most of the tumours lie in the superficial lobe. The operation is known as *Patey's superficial parotidectomy.*

The dissection is made in the Patey's faciovenous plane, and *commenced at the posteroinferior border of the parotid gland, where the main trunk of the facial nerve is found out.*

Incidence of transient facial nerve palsy leading to neuropraxia may occur in up to 30% cases but usually recovers within 6 weeks.

Indications for postoperative adjuvant radiotherapy for major and minor malignant salivary tumours

1. High grade cancer.
2. Recurrent cancer.
3. Unresectable/inoperable/gross residual tumour.
4. Tumour spillage during operation.
5. Large tumour requiring radical excision.
6. Lymph node metastasis.
7. Microscopically positive margin.
8. Close surgical margin deep lobe tumours that are surrounded by little or no glandular parenchyma (facial nerve sparing resection).
9. Involvement of skin, bone, nerve and extension beyond the capsule of the gland with periglandular soft tissue invasion.
10. Perineural invasion.
11. If deep lobe is involved.

Criteria of malignant change in a mixed parotid tumour

1. Sudden and rapid increase in the size of a swelling which is present for long times.
2. Painless tumour becomes painful and so tender.
3. Feels stony hard. Surface may be nodular.
4. Overlying skin may become fixed to the swelling and looks and feels reddish-blue and hot. There may be fungation and ulceration of the skin.
5. The growth becomes fixed to the deeper structures, e.g. masseter, mandible.
6. Evidence of facial nerve involvement causing asymmetry of the face and difficulty in closing the eyes.
7. Areas of anaesthesia over the skin.
8. Jaw movements may become restricted.
9. Veins over the swelling become prominent.
10. Enlargement of cervical lymph nodes may be present.
11. There may be evidence of disseminated blood-borne metastases.

Note

There is no place of incisional biopsy in parotid tumour as chances of seedling and recurrence are high and also there is chance of injury to the facial nerve while doing the biopsy. *Recently* fine needle aspiration cytology (FNAC) using 23G needle has been advocated by few surgeons. *For deep lobe tumours* FNAB through intraoral route is advocated.

Note

80% of benign salivary tumours are pleomorphic adenomas.

Note

Pleomorphic adenoma can arise in submandibular gland also.

ADENOLYMPHOMA

Syn. Papillary cystadenoma lymphomatosum; Warthin's tumour. Adenolymphoma is not a lymphoma. It is a misnomer. It is a *benign epithelial tumour* arising *within a periparotid lymph node containing ectopic salivary tissue.* (For adenolymphoma see Figs 5.7 to 5.9.)

During development of the parotid gland, the ductal structures from the primary parotid bud (*containing epithelial cells*) may grow into the developing juxtaparotid lymph nodes. These epithelial cells later may proliferate in an acinar form and give rise to a swelling called adenolymphoma.

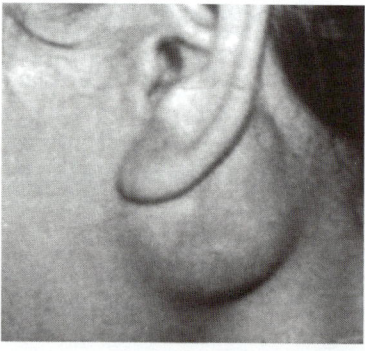

Fig. 5.7: Parotid swelling left side. Smooth, soft swelling below and behind the lobule of the ear (typical site)—adenolymphoma.

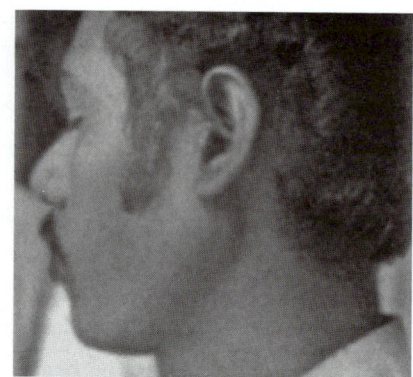

Fig. 5.8: Adenolymphoma. A smooth, soft swelling in the parotid region over the angle of the mandible. No fixity to the overlying or underlying structures. D/D: 1. Mixed parotid tumour—can be differentiated by ^{99m}Tc pertechnetate scan. *Adenolymphoma produces a 'hot spot'.* 2. Parotid cyst—aspiration will confirm fluid.

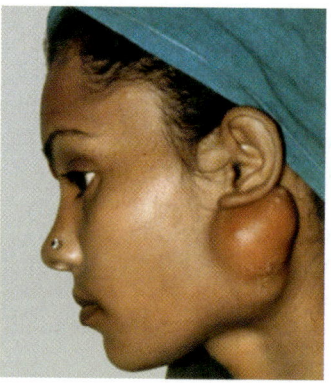

Fig. 5.9: Left parotid tumour. Smooth, soft swelling below and behind the lobule of the ear over the angle of the mandible (a typical location); the ear lobule is elevated—adenolymphoma. No evidence of facial palsy noted. (*Courtesy:* Professor Sudeb Saha, MS, FAMS)

It is usually limited to the area of the parotid gland because lymph node containing ectopic salivary tissue is usually found in the parotid gland but not in other submaxillary salivary glands.

Pathology

1. This is a cystic tumour containing epithelial and lymphoid tissues thus known as adenolymphoma.

2. The neoplasm is situated just beneath the capsule embedded in the superficial lobe.
3. Benign, slowly growing, encapsulated tumour. Does not undergo malignant change.
4. May be multiple or bilateral.
5. Though developmental in origin, it does not appear before the age of 40 years.
6. Second most common benign tumour of parotid.

Macroscopy: Multiple cysts are revealed varying in size from pinhead to hazel nut. The cyst usually contains glairy brown mucus.

Microscopy: Papillary epithelium embedded in a lymphoid stroma – an extremely characteristic feature.

Diagnostic criteria

1. *Age:* Commonly in elderly people after 40 years.
2. *Sex:* Males are more commonly affected.
3. *Race:* Mostly confined to White races. *It has never been recorded in Blacks.*
4. The patient presents with *a slowly growing painless swelling on the side of the face.*
5. *Site:* The swelling is situated in the parotid region commonly at or above the level of the lower border of the mandible over the angle of the mandible.
6. *Shape and size:* Oval or circular, and usually 1–3 cm in diameter.
7. *Surface:* Smooth with well-defined margins.
8. *Consistence: Soft to cystic*, so often fluctuating. *Not translucent.*
9. Not tender.
10. Overlying skin is free from the swelling and looks and feels normal. There is no evidence of venous prominence.
11. *Mobility:* Not fixed to the deeper structures, i.e. masseter, so mobile in both axes.
12. *No evidence of involvement of the facial nerve.*
13. Cervical lymph nodes are not enlarged.

Differential diagnosis

1. Sometimes adenolymphoma may be confused with mixed parotid tumour because

of presentation at the same age group. *So they can be differentiated by* ^{99m}*Tc pertechnetate scan –* **the adenolymphoma produces a 'hot spot'** *while all other neoplasms form* 'cold spot', so that a firm preoperative diagnosis is possible without biopsy. However, *the treatment of both the conditions is superficial parotidectomy.*
2. Sometimes the swelling may be situated in the neck below the angle of the mandible when it is to be differentiated from:
   (a) Branchial cyst (aspirated material will show cholesterol crystals).
   (b) Enlarged cervical lymph node.
3. Parotid cyst.

Treatment

Superficial parotidectomy.

CARCINOMA OF THE PAROTID GLAND

Types of malignant tumours in order of frequency

See International classification of parotid tumours on page 160.

Characteristic features

1. Malignancy may start *de novo* in the parotid gland with a rapidly increasing swelling from the onset.
2. Malignant change may occur in a mixed parotid tumour which has pursued an apparently benign course for many years (10–15 years) with history of recent rapid increase of a preexisting benign swelling.
3. Usually arises in elderly persons.
4. Men and women are equally affected.
5. *Evidence of facial nerve palsy is most likely.* So, perform examination for the facial nerve palsy.
6. The lymph nodes are involved in 15% cases. Regional node spread: Periparotid node → Submandibular node → Upper and mid-jugular nodes
7. *The tumour is radioresistant.*
8. *Five years survival rate is less than 15%.*

Note

Mucoepidermoid carcinoma of parotid arises from secretory cells.

Diagnostic criteria (Fig. 5.10)

1. Vide before (malignant change in a mixed parotid tumour, *see* page 161).
2. FNAC from the swelling to confirm diagnosis.
3. *High frequency U/S, CT scan or MRI of parotid region* to assess the tumour extent, its relations to the adjacent structures, involvement of deep lobe – helps to plan definite surgical margins and therapy.

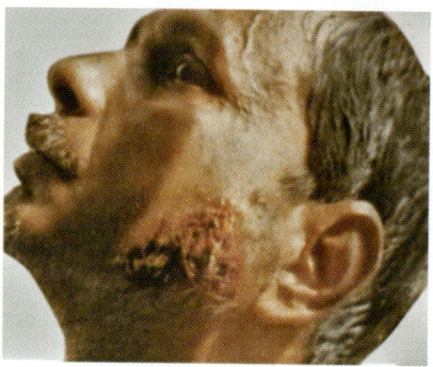

Fig. 5.10: Carcinoma of the parotid gland infiltrating the overlying skin—the facial nerve was not involved.

Treatment

Malignant parotid tumour is radioresistant. So, treatment of choice is surgery. The procedures include:

I. **Complete parotidectomy** which may be either:
1. *Radical parotidectomy* (i.e. where the facial nerve is sacrificed, particularly if there is a reasonable prospect of cure. It is otherwise certain that nerve function will eventually be destroyed by the tumour).
2. *Total conservative parotidectomy,* i.e. total parotidectomy *with preservation of facial nerve.* Superficial parotidectomy is done first preserving the facial nerve; the deep part of the gland is then removed preserving the facial nerve branches.

Postoperative radiotherapy is advocated by some to minimise the chances of local recurrence.
3. Block dissection of the lymph nodes usually on the side of the tumour is occasionally of value when operable metastatic lymph nodes are present after successful treatment of primary.

II. **Other procedures:**
A. *Role of radiotherapy:*
1. When the tumour is as a whole irremovable, particularly in presence of the deep lobe tumour – partial excision combined with radium implantation may give the best prospect of palliation.
2. If the margins of excised specimen are positive of malignancy.
3. Perineural invasion.
4. Lymphovascular invasion.
5. If the deep lobe tumour is fixed to the deeper structures and found to be inoperable – *only palliative radiotherapy is advocated.*
6. *Postoperative radiotherapy* routinely following primary or first operation helps to minimise chances of local recurrence.
B. *Role of chemotherapy: Chemotherapy has limited role.* Methotrexate or 5-fluorouracil therapy may cause limited regression, but its efficacy is not established for long-term palliation.
   Perfusion with cyclophosphamide through the superficial temporal artery has produced marked regression in certain cases of advanced parotid carcinoma.

Peculiarities of adenoid cystic carcinomas

1. Slowly growing malignant epithelial tumour.
2. *Propensity for perineural invasion.*
3. *Malignancy will start as pain in the parotid swelling.*
4. Infiltrate locally along submucosal and perineural tissue planes often far beyond the boundaries of gross tumour.

5. Regional lymph node metastasis is rare.
6. Distant metastasis occurs within 5 years. However, they remain asymptomatic for years.
7. Lung metastasis may also present.
8. Relatively radiosensitive.
9. Most common malignant tumours of sub-mandibular salivary gland.

Peculiarities of carcinoma arising in ex-pleomorphic adenoma

1. Carcinoma ex-pleomorphic adenoma.
2. Develops 15 years after the original swelling appeared – incidence 9.5%.
3. Accelerated recurrence rates.
4. High incidence of metastasis.
5. 5 years survival is less than 15%.

Note

Indication of radiotherapy in salivary gland tumour

- High grade tumour
- Large primary lesion
- Perineural invasion
- Bone invasion
- Cervical lymph node metastases
- Positive surgical margin in a postoperative specimen

▎PAROTID FISTULA

A salivary gland fistula may be *internal or external*. An internal fistula which opens inside the mouth does not give rise to symptoms, and hence is not of much clinical importance.

An external fistula of the submandibular salivary gland is very rare and, if it occurs, can be cured readily by removal of the gland. But *an external fistula of parotid causes troublesome condition*, and hence is of much importance.

Parotid fistula may be gland fistula or duct fistula.

Causes

1. Rupture of parotid abscess.
2. Inadvertent incision during drainage of parotid abscess.

3. Penetrating injury, especially by glass splinters.
4. Aftermath of operations on the gland, e.g. superficial parotidectomy – a persistent fistula is rare, though some leakage of saliva occurs for several days.

Diagnostic criteria

1. *When the external fistula is connected with the gland:*
   - There will be little moisture on the face at the time of eating.
   - The external opening is pinpoint.
   - It produces little inconvenience.
   - Though there is discharge for several months, it usually closes spontaneously.
2. *When the external fistula is connected with the duct, particularly a major duct:*
   - There is outpouring of parotid secretions onto the cheek every time during eating, smelling of food, thought of taking food.
   - Excoriation of the neighbourhood skin.
   - So, there will be extreme discomfort.

Investigation

A sialogram with a watery solution of lipiodol must be done in these cases to assess *whether the fistula is in relation to the main duct or a ductule*. This information will indicate the proper line of treatment.

Treatment

A. *If the fistula is connected with the main duct:* Reconstruction of the duct after the method of Newman and Seabrook's operation.

   Steps of reconstruction:
   1. One probe is introduced through the orifice of the parotid duct in the vestibule of the mouth.
   2. Another probe is introduced through the external fistula.
   3. With the probes in position, a suitable horizontal incision is made over the cheek.
   4. The ducts are dissected out and the severed ends of the duct are identified and made free.

5. A twisted tantalum wire (No. 10 size) is negotiated in both the distal and proximal parts of the duct.
6. Any portion of the twisted wire that lies exposed is buried with the adjacent connective tissue by catgut sutures.
7. The skin is closed.
8. The distal end of the wire is suitably bent around the angle of the mouth and anchored there by adhesive plaster.

Postoperative management:

- Antibiotic to be given for several days.
- Maintenance of oral hygiene.
- *Each day the wire splint is moved very gently.*
- The wire is to be kept *in situ* for about 3 to 4 weeks.

B. *If the reconstruction fails,* resection of the auriculotemporal nerve which carries secretomotor fibres to the gland.
C. *If the above method fails,* complete parotidectomy should be performed preserving the facial nerve intact.
D. *If the fistula is connected with the minor branch of the parotid gland:*
  - Conservative treatment with propantheline bromide (parasympatholytic) 50 mg 6 hourly for a week to diminish the parotid secretion.
  - Excision of the fistulous tract may also be tried.

AURICULOTEMPORAL SYNDROME

(*Syn.* Frey's syndrome)

This syndrome usually *follows the injury to the auriculotemporal nerve due to inadvertent incision* during operation for parotidectomy, parotid abscess or suppurative parotitis.

   This syndrome is characterised by the following.

- *Painful sweating and flushing on the cheek near the ear of the operated side while eating (gustatory sweating).*
- Sometimes *cutaneous hyperaesthesia* in front of and above the ear particularly during shaving.

Explanation of the syndrome

Explanations are not very satisfactory. A satisfying hypothesis is that during regeneration of the nerve after its division, there is regrowth of parasympathetic motor nerve fibres of the auriculotemporal nerve into the cutaneous nerve fibres of the skin flap. *Such crossed innervation of the sweat glands produces uncomfortable gustatory sweating and hyperaesthesia.*

Clinical test to demonstrate Frey's syndrome

Starch iodine test: The affected area is first painted with iodine and allowed to dry. Apply dry starch over it. *The starch turns blue on exposure to iodine in the presence of sweat.*

Management

Prevention

- Proper placement of incision during parotidectomy.
- *Placement of –*
  - artificial membrane
  - sternomastoid muscle flap
  - temporalis fascial flap
  between the skin and the parotid bed following parotidectomy.
- Resection of a segment of auriculotemporal nerve during parotidectomy.

Treatment

- *Reassurance:* Usually the symptoms pass off spontaneously in few months.
- *Local application:* Antiperspirant – aluminium chloride is a useful astringent.
- *Injection of botulinum toxin* into the affected skin may help.
- *Avulsion of the auriculotemporal nerve* will result in effective treatment.
- Denervation by tympanic neurectomy.

Note

Auriculotemporal nerve runs with the superficial temporal artery and vein.

Note

Auriculotemporal nerve ascends upwards on the temple *just behind and deep to the superficial temporal artery in front of the tragus.* One can palpate the superficial temporal artery in front of the tragus. *So, dissection of the facial nerve branches should be done in front of the superficial temporal artery.*

Auriculotemporal nerve supplies *cutaneous sensory innervation* to the skin of the cheek over the parotid gland and temple *and also the secretomotor to the parotid gland. Injury to this nerve causes gustatory sweating and hyper-aesthesia over the parotid region.*

Note

- *Bell's palsy:* The facial nerve is commonly involved in Bell's palsy following exposure to extreme cold or draught. Rarely, it may be involved in viral infection.
- *Bell's phenomenon:* The eyeball rolls upwards on the paralysed side during attempted closure of both the eyes and becomes conspicuous since the patient is unable to close the eyelids on the paralysed side when asked for. The fore-head does not wrinkle. The angle of the mouth also droops on the affected side. *Failure to close the eyelids may result in exposure keratitis.*

DISEASES OF SUBMANDIBULAR SALIVARY GLAND

CALCULUS DISEASE OF THE GLAND (SIALOLITHIASIS)

Site

Common sites are:
- Within the submandibular salivary gland substance.
- Within its duct (Wharton's duct) deep to the mucous membrane of the floor of the mouth – more common.

Submandibular salivary calculi are 80 times more common than the parotid calculi, because:

1. Submandibular duct (Wharton's duct) has a long curved and upward course and is hooked by the lingual nerve. The secretion of the submandibular salivary gland starts down in the neck and drains up in the floor of the mouth *so non-dependent drainage.* So,

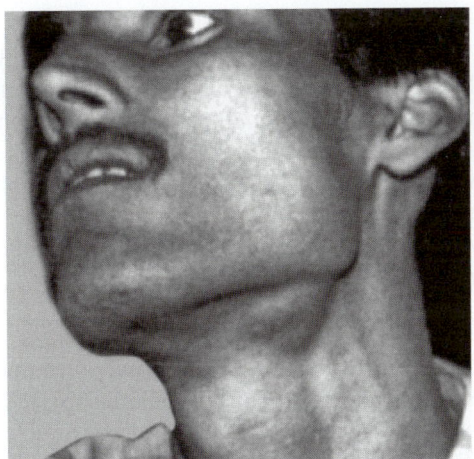

Fig. 5.11: Enlargement of the submandibular salivary gland. On bidigital palpation, there was stone in the gland itself but no stone in Wharton's duct—a case of sialolithiasis.

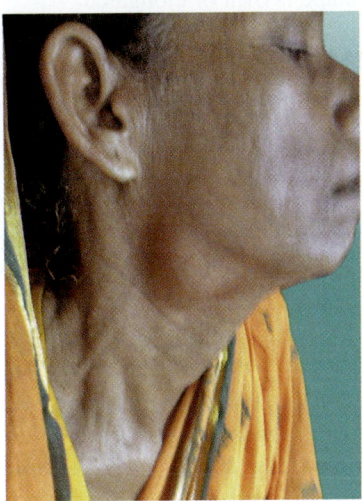

Fig. 5.12: Right-sided enlarged submandibular gland—bimanually palpable and non-tender.

there is inadequate drainage and therefore stasis which precipitates salt deposition.

2. The secretion of submandibular salivary gland is more viscid and rich in salt content than parotid gland secretion.

Note

Parotid duct (Stensen's duct) has a straight course and has dependent drainage.

Composition of stone

The calculus is composed mainly of the phosphate and carbonate of calcium and magnesium, with a small percentage of organic matter, i.e. dried secretions of cellular debris or intraductal bacterial clumps. It closely resembles that of tartar that collects upon the teeth. *Due to deposition of calcium salts the stone is radio-opaque.*

Cause of stone formation

Chronic inflammation of the gland – retention of secretions which later become inspissated – deposition of inorganic calcium salts on a nucleus of degenerated epithelium and inspissated secretions.

Size and shape of the stone

- The size varies from a millet to a pea.
- The shape is oval or elongated.

SUBMANDIBULAR CALCULI

Diagnostic criteria

1. *Age:* Mostly common in young and middle-aged adults.
2. *Sex:* Both sexes are equally affected.
3. The patient complains of pain and swelling at the submandibular region (i.e. beneath and in front of the angle of the jaw), aggravated by food, classically by sucking a lemon. *The gland gets tense and tender.*

   At first the attacks are transient and the gland quickly resumes its normal size, *but in course of time it tends to remain permanently enlarged. Salivary colic sometimes occurs*, typically at the commencement of a meal, and it is *described by the patient as toothache* (for which the patient is sometimes referred to a dental surgeon).

   A stone impacted in the duct may produce the referred pain in the tongue due to irritation of the lingual nerve as it hooks around the submandibular duct.

4. *Site:* The lump is situated beneath the horizontal ramus of the mandible, 1 to 2 cm in front of the anterior border of sterno-mastoid muscle.

5. *Shape:* A flattened ovoid or almond-shaped.
6. *Surface:* Usually smooth but may be bosselated. The overlying skin is usually normal and freely mobile over the swollen gland.
7. *Margin:* Anterior, posterior and inferior margins of the gland are easily defined but the upper margin is impalpable as it is wedged between the mandible and the mylohyoid muscle.
8. *Consistence:* A distended submandibular gland feels firm to rubbery hard.
9. *Mobility:* The gland can be moved a little from side-to-side. The gland becomes less mobile when the muscles of the floor of the mouth are taut by asking the patient to push his tongue against the palate.
10. *Bidigital palpation:* One index finger is inserted inside the mouth between the side of the tongue and the inner surface of the alveolus. The finger of the other hand is placed under the jaw. *Now first the gland and next the duct are palpated from behind forward.*

    By this method one can appreciate that the lump is outside the structures forming the floor of the mouth – both the submandibular and sublingual glands are palpable for swelling and tenderness.

    One can palpate also a stone in the deeper part of the gland or in the Wharton's duct.

    Bidigital palpation also helps to differentiate an enlarged submandibular gland from enlarged submandibular lymph node because the finger inside the mouth can feel the deep part of the submandibular salivary gland as it lies above the mylohyoid muscle. *But, the inner finger cannot palpate the lymph node as it lies below the mylohyoid muscle.*

11. *Examination of the floor of the mouth:* The patient should be asked to show the under-surface of the tongue, this will display the orifices of submandibular duct on their small papillae on either side of the frenum of the tongue. *Swollen, oedematous and congested orifice indicates the impaction of the stone. Occasionally, the stone impacted in the ampulla could be observed and palpated.*

If some lemon juice is poured in the tongue and mouth, there will be outpouring of saliva from one orifice while there will be absence of saliva flowing from the other orifice, *which indicates that this duct is obstructed.* At the same time one may notice the prominence or increase of the swelling in the submandibular region. *Bidigital palpation also* confirms the stone by the tip of inner finger. It also helps to detect the enlargement of entire submandibular salivary gland.

Differential diagnosis

- Submandibular lymphadenitis.
- Salivary gland neoplasm.

Investigation

All cases should be X-rayed before operation.

Submandibular salivary calculi either in the duct or in the gland substance *will cast a clear radiopaque shadow due to presence of calcium.* About 80% calculi are radiopaque and can be identified in plain X-ray. Sometimes, the stone may be non-opaque due to poor mineral content.

Treatment

Surgical

1. *When the stone is in the duct:* Removal of the stone is done intraorally.
   - General or local anaesthesia.
   - Tissues immediately behind the stone are grasped by the forceps which steady the stone and, thus, prevent it from slipping backwards in the gland substance.
   - An incision is made on the mucous membrane and duct directly over the stone in the long axis of the duct.
   - The stone is removed.
   - The cut ends of the mucous membrane and the duct wall are left unsutured.
2. *When the stone is in the gland substance:* Excision of submandibular salivary gland is done by external skin crease incision.

Care to be taken during excision of sub-mandibular gland.

- A skin crease incision is made directly over the gland.
- The posterior part of the incision should lie at least 3 cm below and in front of the angle of the mandible—*to avoid injury to the mandibular branch of the facial nerve to avoid drooping of the angle of the mouth on the paralysed side and inability to smile.*
- The facial vein and facial artery should be divided in between the ligatures twice.
- *The lingual nerve and the hypoglossal nerve lying between the deep surface of the gland and mylohyoid muscle and hyoglossus muscle, should be identified and preserved.* Mylohyoid muscle is retracted to remove the deep portion of the gland.

TUMOURS OF THE SUBMANDIBULAR GLAND

All the tumours involving the parotid gland may be found in the submandibular salivary gland but they are comparatively rare.

If diagnosed early, the treatment is satisfactory, because the excision of the submandibular salivary gland in toto is rather easy.

ECTOPIC SALIVARY TUMOURS

The tumours of the salivary gland may involve the tiny, unnamed minor salivary glands situated in the buccopharyngeal cavity or other uncommon sites.

Minor, unnamed salivary glands are present in the following sites.
- Hard palate
- Lips and cheeks – at retromolar area
- Tongue
- Fauces
- Pharynx
- Larynx

Migrant (ectopic) salivary gland may be present in the following sites.
- Eyelids
- Lacrimal gland
- Ear – middle ear
- Paranasal sinuses

- Nose
- Jaws
- Skin of the face and neck.

The commonest site is the hard palate.

These tumours make up some 10% of all salivary gland tumours, 40% of which are benign and virtually all these benign tumours are pleomorphic adenoma.

Characteristic features

1. The great majority of these tumours is quite symptomless.
2. More commonly found in children below the age of 5 years.
3. These tumours may be pigmented (cf. Peutz–Jeghers syndrome).
4. Unless the tumour is excised early and widely, local recurrence is relentless.
5. *During recurrence,* metastases of the regional lymph nodes and occasionally of the viscera and skeleton may occur.
6. These tumours are radioresistant.
7. Excision of these tumours may be followed by radiotherapy.

SJOGREN'S DISEASE

It is regarded as *an autoimmune disorder* – the antibodies arise in response to antigen derived from the nuclei and cytoplasm of the cells of the parotid gland. It involves the *salivary glands,* mucous glands and is *associated with some other systemic manifestations like scleroderma, rheumatoid arthritis, SLE.*

Histology reveals replacement of salivary tissue by lymphoid tissue containing islets of epithelial tissue.

Some pathologists consider this condition to be due to an obscure chronic inflammation.

Characteristic features

1. Commonly found in women above the age of 40 years.
2. The condition is usually *bilateral.*
3. There will be *symmetrical enlargement of the salivary glands (commonly parotid glands).*

4. *Dryness of the mouth (xerostomia) and eyes (keratoconjunctivitis sicca).*
5. *Systemic manifestations:* There will be generalised arthritis particularly of the small joints (rheumatoid type), keratoconjunctivitis, scleroderma, polyarteritis nodosa.
6. The condition develops slowly and painlessly.

Plain X-ray occasionally reveals small areas of calcification throughout the involved gland.

MIKULICZ DISEASE

It is also *an autoimmune disorder* and is regarded as a variety of Sjogren's disease where in addition to bilateral enlargement of all the salivary glands, *the lacrimal glands are also enlarged causing bulges below the outer ends of the eyebrows leading to narrowing of the palpebral fissures. But, there are no systemic manifestations as noted in Sjogren's disease.*

Treatment

1. Spontaneous cure may occur after several weeks or several years.
2. Steroid therapy may be of help.
3. Radiotherapy may be employed when the diagnosis is confirmed.

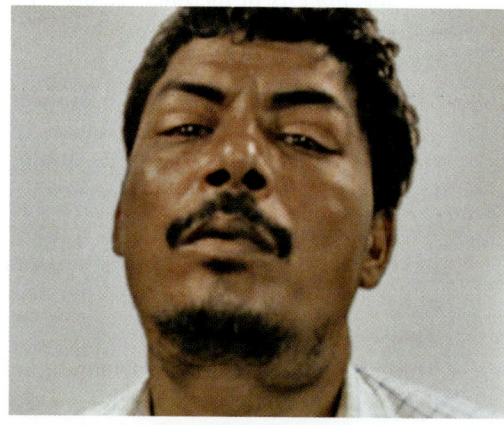

Fig. 5.13: Mikulicz disease. Note bilateral enlarged submandibular salivary glands and bilateral enlarged lacrimal glands causing narrowing of the palpable fissures. (*Courtesy:* Professor Tarun Chatterjee, MS)

4. *Surgery:* If there are cases of massive deformity then removal of submandibular salivary glands and bilateral superficial lobectomy of the parotids are advocated. *The lacrimal glands are better left alone.*

The surgery should be followed by either steroid therapy or radiotherapy.

Note

When Mikulicz disease is associated with any systemic manifestations like rheumatoid arthritis the condition is addressed as Sjogren's disease.

Note

Minor salivary glands: There are about 450 minor salivary glands which are present in the oral cavity and distributed in the lips, cheeks and floor of the mouth. Glands may also be present in the oropharynx, larynx, trachea and paranasal sinuses. They contribute up to 10% of total salivary secretions *to keep the oral cavity soft.*

Note

Causes of facial nerve palsy:

1. Malignant parotid tumour.
2. Complication of parotidectomy – inadvertent injury or deliberately sacrificed during surgery of malignant parotid tumour.
3. Inflammation of stylomastoid foramen – viral infection which causes oedema and compression of the nerve in the facial canal at its exit point.
4. Compression of facial nerve within the intraosseus part of the petrous temporal bone – by fracture of the base of the skull.
5. *Exposure to extreme cold* as occurs when riding or driving a car or sleeping *with the window open*, e.g. during a train journey particularly *in cold weather* or *draught* without a muffler on – **Bell's palsy**.
6. Idiopathic occurring without a known cause.

Note

80% of benign salivary tumours are pleomorphic adenomas.

Note

Pleomorphic adenoma can arise in submandibular gland also.

Note

Stafne's bone cyst: *Most common ectopic salivary tissue in a bone*, near the angle of mandible below the mandibular canal.

Note

Chorda tympani nerve is a branch of the facial nerve. It exits from the facial nerve at the stylomastoid foramen. It is secretomotor to the submandibular and sublingual salivary glands and it carries also the taste sensation from the anterior two-thirds of the tongue via the lingual nerve.

Compression of facial nerve within the interosseous part of temporal bone by fracture of the base of the skull causes facial nerve palsy and *also* loss of taste sensation of the anterior two-thirds of the tongue on the same side due to chorda tympani nerve injury.

Swellings in the Jaw

Swellings of the jaw are caused by innumerable lesions and they may arise from the muco-periosteum or from the tooth-germs or from the bones.

I. Arising from the mucoperiosteum, i.e. epulis

Epulis – may be:

1. Fibrous
2. Granulomatous
3. Myeloid
4. Sarcomatous
5. Carcinomatous.

II. Arising from the tooth germs, i.e. odontomes (after McGregor)

Odontomes – may be:

1. Epithelial odontomes, i.e. arising from epithelial elements:
   • Dental cyst
   • Dentigerous cyst
   • Adamantinoma.
2. Mesothelial odontomes, i.e. arising from connective tissue elements:
   • Fibrous odontomes
   • Cementomes
   • Osseous or sarcomatous odontomes } Rare
3. Composite odontomes, i.e. arising from both epithelial and mesothelial elements:

• Radicular odontomes
• Osseous or sarcomatous odontomes } Extremely rare

III. Arising from the bones

1. Traumatic
2. Inflammatory
   • Specific, e.g. actinomycosis
   • Non-specific, e.g. osteomyelitis, alveolar abscess
3. Neoplastic
   • Benign
   • Malignant.

Benign:
(a) Arising from fibrous tissue – fibrous dysplasia.
(b) Arising from osteoblasts –
   • Osteoma — localised or diffused
   • Osteoclastoma.

Malignant:
(a) Primary – carcinoma and sarcoma.
(b) Secondary, i.e. by extension from an adjacent growth, e.g. carcinoma of the tongue involving the lower jaw.

EPULIS

The word 'epulis' means upon the gum. It is a solid swelling situated on the gum and arises from the alveolar margin of the jaw. *It can originate from the mucous membrane, periosteum, or bone.* Usually it occurs *secondary to chronic inflammation* and sometimes it is considered as hamartoma.

Following varieties of epulis are commonly encountered:

1. Fibrous
2. Granulomatous } Benign
3. Myeloid
4. Sarcomatous } Malignant
5. Carcinomatous

FIBROUS EPULIS

Commonest variety. *It arises from the periosteum or from the periodontal membrane* and forms a firm nodule at the junction of the gum and tooth. *Chronic dental sepsis* is considered to be an important predisposing factor.

Histologically, it is *whorled fibroma*, and is composed of fusiform cells with many new blood vessels.

Diagnostic criteria

1. More common in women and in young adults.
2. Lower gum is commonly affected.
3. More commonly found on the external aspect of the gum, *at the neck of canine or premolar tooth.*
4. It may be sessile or pedunculated.
5. It is a slowly growing, firm swelling and non-tender.
6. *Overlying mucous membrane is healthy but it is grey or slightly brighter pink than that of the normal gum.*
7. The adjacent teeth are irregularly displaced and loosened and the tumour may protrude between the irregular teeth.
8. Draining lymph nodes are not enlarged.

Complications

1. Although it is benign, *it has a tendency to recur after operation*, if its root is not thoroughly excised.
2. Malignant change—fibrosarcoma, rare.

Treatment

Excision of the swelling. *Adjacent tooth and a wedge of bone around its root may be removed to prevent recurrence.*

GRANULOMATOUS EPULIS

It consists of *a mass of granulation tissue which forms around a carious tooth or at the site of chronic irritation by a denture.* This is not a true epulis and hence *considered false epulis* (Fig. 6.1).

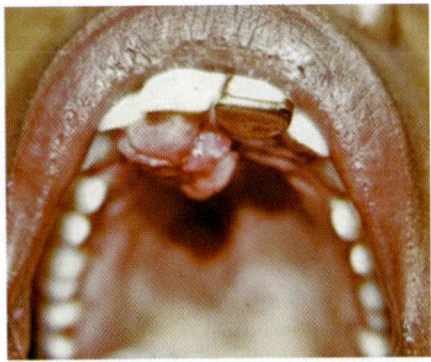

Fig. 6.1: Epulis of the upper inner margin of the gum in relation to right incisor tooth. (*Courtesy:* Dr Arun Anand, MS General Surgery)

Sometimes, a similar condition may be found temporarily during pregnancy which is known as *gingivitis gravidarum.*

Diagnostic criteria

1. Rapidly growing soft swelling, bright red in colour.
2. *The overlying mucous membrane is granular, persistently ulcerated. It bleeds on touch or during brushing of the teeth.*
3. *Offensive smell due to infection.*
4. Presence of adjacent carious tooth or ill-fitting denture.
5. *Draining lymph nodes (submental or submandibular) are enlarged and tender.*

Treatment

1. Scraping of the granulation tissue.
2. Extraction of the carious tooth.
3. Pre- and postoperative antibiotics to combat infection.
4. Maintenance of oral hygiene.
5. Any ill-fitting denture should be replaced.

MYELOID EPULIS (*Syn.* Giant cell epulis)

Pathologically, *it is an **osteoclastoma**, arising from the mucoperiosteum of the gum.*

Histologically, it consists of fibrocellular tissue scattered through which are *multinucleated giant cells.*

Diagnostic criteria

1. Commonly occurs between the ages of 10 and 25 years.
2. *Common in the lower jaw, near the angle of the mandible.*
3. It is a *rapidly growing painless tumour* presenting under the gum.
4. The swelling is soft and sessile, surface is smooth and lobulated. The overlying mucous membrane of the gum becomes hyperaemic and oedematous. *It looks dark-red or plum-coloured and may bleed and ulcerate.*
5. *Expansion of the bone occurs – both externally and internally* (cf. *adamantinoma*).
6. In a well developed case there may be the presence of eggshell cracking.
7. Draining lymph nodes are not enlarged.
8. *Confirmation by X-ray: Soap-bubble or honeycomb appearance due to bone destruction with ridging of the walls (pseudotrabeculation).*

Complications

1. Ulceration.
2. Haemorrhage which may be severe.

Treatment

1. *If the swelling is small,* curettage of the tumour followed by cauterisation and filling up of the remaining cavity by cancellous bone chips taken from the iliac crest.
2. *When the swelling is of a big size,* radical excision of the tumour with adjacent margin of healthy bone followed by grafting for the mandible. The graft is taken usually from a rib or iliac crest.

CARCINOMATOUS EPULIS

It is an *epithelioma of the gum arising from the mucosa of the alveolar margin.* It may start around a tooth, or in a socket, giving rise to a painful, infected and infiltrating lesion. Later on the lesion becomes frankly fungating and ulcerating and invades the bone. *Cervical lymph nodes are enlarged.*

Biopsy should be performed to confirm the diagnosis.

Treatment

1. *Radical resection* followed by grafting for the mandible. When it occurs in relation to upper jaw, adequate resection of the maxilla should be done.
2. Radiotherapy may be of help in selected cases.

ODONTOMES

Odontomes are cysts, tooth malformations, or tumours *arising from the tooth germs. Truly they are hamartomatous malformations but not tumours* (Willis). They *usually arise from the epithelial or mesothelial elements of the teeth, or sometimes from both.*

In human beings epithelial odontomes are commonly encountered and there are three important epithelial odontomes, namely:

1. Dental cyst
2. Dentigerous cyst
3. Adamantinoma.

Basis of origin of epithelial odontomes

During development of tooth there occurs an ingrowth of epithelium (ectoderm) lining the mouth over the site of the future gums. *This epithelial element later forms the enamel organ of tooth and is called ameloblast.* Clusters of this epithelium may persist as *epithelial debris or epithelial rest* and later may grow into cysts or tumours.

DENTAL CYST (*Syn.* Radicular cyst, periodontal cyst or epitheliated granuloma)

This is a *unilocular cyst* arising in connection with *the root of a normally erupted, but chronically infected* and usually pulpless tooth (Fig. 6.2).

The continued irritation of infection appears to stimulate the epithelial cells, believed to be

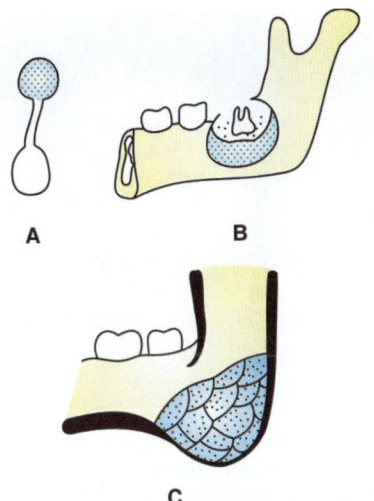

Figs 6.2 A to C: Common types of odontomes. (A) dental cyst; (B) dentigerous cyst; (C) adamantinoma.

derived from the enamel organ. As a result these epithelial cells proliferate and degenerate to form a cyst.

Pathology
- *Lining of the cyst wall:* Squamous epithelium.
- *Contents:* The contents of the cyst may be fluid or semisolid in nature, containing cellular debris with cholesterol crystals and foreign body giant cells. As a rule, the content is sterile on culture but secondary infection can occur.

The cyst enlarges slowly causing expansion of the alveolus, and eventually most of the epithelial lining is destroyed, if infection remains active.

Diagnostic criteria
1. It can appear at any age, but commonly in or after middle age.
2. Usually painless swelling unless secondarily infected.
3. It commonly affects the upper jaw, in association with a carious tooth or pulpless tooth – incisor or canine tooth.
4. It causes an expansion of the bone as it grows, and in advanced cases there may be eggshell crackling.
5. There may be fluctuation, if the bone is completely destroyed.

X-ray: An oval or circular radio-translucent area in relation to the root of a tooth. The margin of the translucent area is clear but sclerosed.

DENTIGEROUS CYST
(*Syn.* Follicular odontome or cyst)

This is a *unilocular cyst* arising in *connection with a non-erupted but permanent tooth* (cf. dental cyst). The lesion arises from the follicle of the developing tooth. The follicle consists of an inner epithelial lining and an outer connective tissue covering.

Pathology
- *Lining of the cyst wall:* Usually fibrous, but may be lined by squamous cell epithelium derived from the enamel producing cells.
  The crown of the tooth inside the cyst lacks the dental cuticle.
- *Contents:* The contents of the cyst may be glairy and viscid fluid or semisolid in nature, with cholesterol crystals and giant cells. It also contains unerupted tooth, *commonly an upper or lower third molar tooth, with truncated root.* The tooth lies either free in the cavity lying obliquely or, rarely, the tooth lies embedded in the wall of the cyst (Fig. 6.2).

Diagnostic criteria
1. Any age may be affected but more common in teens.
2. A painless, slowly growing swelling at the site of an unerupted tooth.
3. *More commonly occurring in the lower jaw in the third molar tooth region.*
4. The tooth is missing at the site of a dentigerous cyst (but on counting during examination the tooth may be found normal, because the milk tooth may persist).
5. There is an *expansion of the outer table of the jaw even causing eggshell crackling.* The inner table remains strong and prevents pathological fracture.

X-ray or orthopantomogram: A well circumscribed radiotranslucent area with the crown of the tooth inside it. Similar X-ray findings may be noticed in other lesion of the jaw like adenomatoid odontogenic tumour. There may be pseudotrabeculation or soap-bubble appearance due to ridges of bone on the side walls.

Treatment of dental and dentigerous cyst
Operative
1. *Total excision of the cyst wall.* The steps are:
   Intraoral approach: Two types of incision are in use:
   (a) A transversely placed curved incision is made over the mucoperiosteum at the maximum point of convexity of the swelling. Then the mucoperiosteal flaps are raised.
   (b) Three-sided flap incision with broader base at the mucobuccal junction is made to raise the mucoperiosteal flap.
   • An opening is made in the thin outer shell of the bone; the cyst is entered.
   • The cyst is thoroughly scooped out along with its whole epithelial lining and the related tooth.
   • After thorough excision, the bone cavity is obliterated by soft tissue 'push-in' or with the bone chips.
   • The mucoperiosteal flap is approximated and sutured.
2. If the cyst is too big and total excision is not possible, then the cyst is deroofed, scooped out as much as possible and marsupialized.
3. *Any carious tooth should be removed.*
4. Pre- and postoperative dental hygiene, and control of infection.

ADAMANTINOMA

Syn. Ameloblastoma; multicystic disease of the jaw; fibrocystic disease of the jaw; eve's disease.

Origin of the lesion
Regarding its origin there are two views:

1. It is an *epithelial tumour arising from the ameloblast* which is the primitive enamel forming epithelial cells of the tooth.

2. According to Willis, *it is a basal cell carcinoma arising from the ectodermal epithelium of the stomodeum.* It behaves pathologically and looks histologically like a basal-

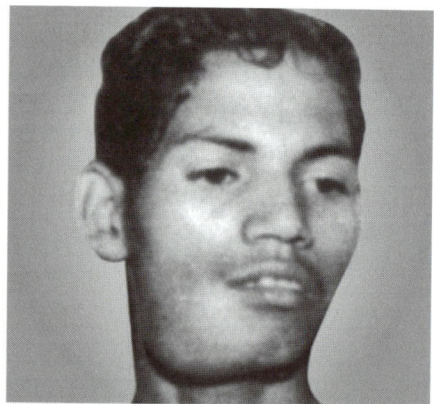

Fig. 6.3: Adamantinoma lower jaw—a slowly growing, painless, firm tumour involving the lower end of mandible near the angle of the jaw.

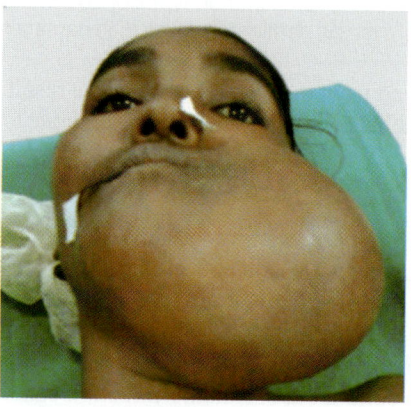

Fig. 6.4: Large-sized adamantinoma of the left lower jaw. (*Courtesy:* Professor RN Poddar, R Ahmed Dental College, Kolkata)

celled carcinoma. The histological picture and recurrence of the tumour after incomplete removal supports the view of basal cell carcinoma.

Pathology

It is *a painless slowly growing, benign, solid tumour. Subsequently, it undergoes multicentric cystic degeneration,* causing simultaneous resorption of the bone and expansion of the jaw – *mostly of the outer table in the region of molar tooth,* with thinning of the cortex and deposition of periosteal new bone. Some of the loculi are separated by bony trabeculae.

Although benign, it may infiltrate the bone further than what is apparent to the naked eye, so that *removal of the tumour by curettage may be followed by recurrence. But it does not metastasize to lymph nodes.*

- *Lining of the cyst wall:* Either squamous or columnar cell epithelium with areas of fibrous and osseous tissue.
- *Contents:* Yellowish mucoid material. Very rarely adamantinoma may contain melanin pigment.

Histological picture

Usually it consists of an outer layer of deeply basophilic columnar cells – *the enameloblasts,* and a central core of '*star cells*', i.e. cells with large vacuoles in the cytoplasm and connecting cytoplasmic bridges.

In other cases, there is presence of sheets of epidermoid cells resembling a basal cell carcinoma, but presence of isolated clumps of columnar enameloblasts will usually indicate the true nature of the lesion.

Diagnostic criteria

1. *Age:* Majority of the tumours occur between 10 and 35 years, and after 50 years they are rare.
2. *Sex:* Females are commonly affected.
3. It is a slowly growing, painless, firm tumour.
4. *Commonly affecting the mandible in the region of the molar teeth* (i.e. near the angle of the jaw).
5. It causes expansion *with thinning out mostly of the outer table* (cf. *osteoclastoma*) and so gives rise to a swelling more often on the cheek than within the mouth. With a marked expansion of the bone, there may be eggshell crackling on palpation.
6. Occasionally due to gross cystic degeneration, the tumour may be soft and fluctuant.
7. Generally there is no missing tooth. There may be malalignment and malocclusion of the neighbouring teeth.
8. The tumour may attain a large size to produce an ugly deformity of the face.
9. Cervical lymph nodes are not enlarged.

X-ray or orthopantomogram: *Soap-bubble appearance, or honeycomb appearance,* i.e. multiple small translucent areas separated by well-formed bony trabeculae (Fig. 6.2C). There is expansion of the outer table of the mandible. *Skiagraphy is very often simulated with that of osteoclastoma.*

Differential diagnosis

1. Osteoclastoma or giant cell tumour.
2. Giant cell reparative granuloma of the jaw.

Treatment

1. *Evacuation and curettage of the cyst with or without bone grafting: There is every chance of recurrence, showing up even many years after excision and hence earned the name adamantinoma.* Though recurrence does not cause any lymph node metastasis.
2. *Selective block excision of the bone along with tumour:* If the basal bone of the mandible is not affected by the tumour, the tumour is excised with a generous amount of surrounding healthy bone *leaving the lower border of the mandible intact to maintain the continuity of the jaw.* The remaining cavity is electrocauterised and may be filled with marrow cancellous bone graft.
3. *Partial resection of the segment of the jaw bearing the tumour,* together with a margin of surrounding healthy bone.
4. *If the tumour is too large in size, affecting the ramus of the mandible, or is of advanced stage, hemimandibulectomy is necessary.* Following resection of the segment of the jaw or hemimandibulectomy, the defect can be filled up by an immediate bone graft. Failure of immediate bone graft is substituted by a holding prosthesis such as that of Bowerman and Conroy, or a silastic rod carved to the design and skewed over a K-wire. After a period of 3 to 6 months the holding prosthesis is dissected and replaced by a block bone graft, or marrow cancellous bone graft put in a tray of tantalum mesh bone implant.
5. *Radiotherapy:* Not of much value.

Can adamantinoma occur elsewhere other than the jaw?

Yes, in the following situations.

1. *In the stalk of the pituitary gland (suprasellar tumour):* The reason being that both the pituitary stalk and the enamel organ of the tooth arise from the same source, viz., oral epithelium.

2. *In the tibia:* The exact reason is not known. There are three hypothesis.

   (a) Abnormal embryonic inclusion of tooth-germ epithelium within the developing tibia giving rise to neoplasm many years later.

   (b) Traumatic separation of the epithelium of the skin and implantation beneath the periosteum, even in the absence of any history of a penetrating wound, though history of trauma is often present.

   (c) The lesion may be an apparent atypical synovioma.

GIANT-CELLED REPARATIVE GRANULOMA

This is a condition arising due to occurrence of haemorrhage within the bone marrow causing an expansion of the bony wall.

Pathology

• *Naked eye appearance:* During operation found to be consisting of opaque, semisolid, dark-red material.

• *Histologically*, consisting of small multinuclear cells which are sparsely and unevenly distributed.

Diagnostic criteria

1. *Age:* Nearly always between the ages of 10 and 25 years.

2. More common in females.

3. A *painless swelling of the jaw*, situated more frequently in the mandible. It may occur in the maxilla.

   X-ray: Rounded or oval area of trans-lucency with expansion and thinning out of the cortex.

Differential diagnosis

1. *Osteoclastoma:* By age, osteoclastoma appears in patients between 25 and 40 years of age.

2. *Adamantinoma:* At operation found to contain transparent yellowish mucoid material in contrast to opaque, dark-red semisolid material.

3. *Brown tumour or pseudotumour of hyper-parathyroidism:* Histologically, it is very difficult to differentiate between the two.

   Brown tumour of hyperparathyroidism should be suspected if:

• there is *the rise of serum calcium, fall of serum phosphorus*, and rise of serum alkaline phosphatase;

• X-ray of other parts of the skeleton will show *subperiosteal bone resorption giving rise to small clear cystic spaces.*

Treatment

1. *Thorough curettage of the cavity through external approach* without opening the bone cavity into the mouth to avoid chronic osteomyelitis from intraoral microbes.

   If there is recurrence after operation, hyperparathyroidism must be excluded.

2. Recent reports of success with calcitonin therapy, achieving near total regression, have appeared.

Inflammatory swelling of the jaw

1. Alveolar abscess
2. Osteomyelitis
3. Actinomycosis

OSTEOMYELITIS OF THE JAW

Syn. Necrosis of the jaw. This may be:

1. Acute (suppurative) – very rare.
2. Subacute.
3. Chronic – suppurative or chronic sclerosing (Fig. 6.5).

Predisposing factors

1. Spread of apical dental infection following infection of a dental root.

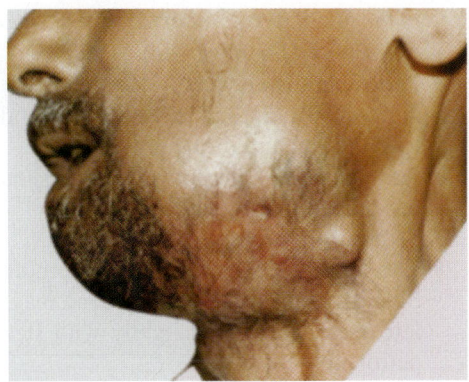

Fig. 6.5: Chronic suppurative osteomyelitis of the mandible. (*Courtesy:* Dr S Jayachandran, MDS)

2. Inadequate drainage of an alveolar abscess.
3. Compound fracture of the jaw.
4. Radiation necrosis.
5. Buccal carcinoma involving the jaw.
6. Cancrum oris.
7. Chemical:
   - Phosphate (leading to phossy jaw/ necrosis)
   - Arsenic
   - Mercury.
8. Actinomycosis, syphilis and tuberculosis rarely.
9. Malnutrition, diabetes mellitus, immuno-suppression.

Organism

Staphylococcus aureus.

Which jaw is commonly affected?

The lower jaw, i.e. the mandible is commonly affected, *because it has a single, rather tenuous blood supply (inferior alveolar artery)* running along the long axis of the bone. Therefore, it is easily obstructed by infection or trauma, leading to necrosis of the bone, which is the essence of osteomyelitis of the jaw.

The upper jaw, i.e. the maxilla is less commonly affected, because the blood supply of the upper jaw is segmental and vertical with anastomoses with each other. Therefore, it is not dependent on a single vessel and thus infection or trauma is most unlikely to cause complete cutting off of the blood supply to the bone.

Diagnostic criteria

1. Commonly, the mandible is affected.
2. History of any predisposing factors, e.g. dental extraction or incompletely treated alveolar abscess, etc.
3. Insidious onset of a painful swelling with or without fever. The pain is due to tension within the bone.
4. *Presence of either internal or external discharging sinus –* may be due to spontaneous bursting which may relieve tension within the bone, and so pain is relieved on discharge of pus. The sinus is usually fixed to the underlying bone with sprouting granulation tissue in its opening suggesting the presence of sequestrum inside.
5. *History of extrusion of bone chips may be there.*
6. *On palpation:* The bone thickening is not a prominent feature, because reparative bone formation is poor (as opposed to osteomyelitis of the other sites).
7. The swelling is tender.
8. The draining lymph nodes are enlarged and tender.
9. Paraesthesia or numbness of the chin in the distribution of the mental nerve may be present (because increased tension within the dental canal compresses the inferior alveolar nerve as well as the vessels).

X-ray: One of the following pictures is evident.

- Evidence of local osteitis with periosteal reaction.
- A small cavity (due to bone destruction) with surrounding sclerosis with or without a sequestrum. The sequestrum formation is late as the jaw bones are developed from membrane. Sometimes the sequestrum may be a massive one and *the lower jaw may collapse leading to an ugly deformity of the face.*

Occasionally, the offending broken root of a tooth may be seen within the cavity.

Radiological evidence of bone necrosis takes at least 3 weeks to become manifest.

Treatment

1. When osteomyelitis is suspected clinically but not confirmed radiologically, *X-rays*

must be taken at regular intervals (weekly). As soon as the bone necrosis will be evident, operation should be done to relieve tension and remove the diseased materials.

2. If there is a discharging sinus, pus should be sent for culture and sensitivity to antibiotics.

3. Both pre- and postoperative suitable antibiotics should be given according to sensitivity test.

4. In a well proved case, dependent drainage gives the best result.

Steps of operation:

• Incision is made about 1/4″ below the lower border of mandible. It should not extend beyond the point one inch below and in front of the angle of the mandible (*to avoid injury to the mandibular division*

of the facial nerve, otherwise there will be paralysis of the lower lip).

• Periosteum is elevated.
• A trough is chiselled in the bone carefully to avoid fracture of the jaw.
• Any unhealthy granulation tissue should be scraped thoroughly.
• Sequestrum, if present, is removed.
• The sclerosed cavity should be deroofed.
• Skin may be closed, or the wound may be left open and packed lightly with sterile petroleum jelly gauze.

5. Infected tooth, if any remaining, should be extracted.

Differential diagnoses of adamantinoma, giant-celled reparative granuloma and osteoclastoma

See Table 6.1.

Table 6.1: Differential diagnoses of adamantinoma, giant-celled reparative granuloma and osteoclastoma affecting the jaw

Points	Adamantinoma	Giant-celled reparative granuloma	Osteoclastoma
Frequency	More common	Less common	Less common
Age	Commonly between 10 and 35 years	Between 10 and 25 years	Commonly between 25 and 40 years
Sex	Females – more common	Females – more common	Males – more common
Rate of growth	Slowly growing	Slowly growing	Relatively rapidly growing
Expansion of bony walls	Outer table is expanded	Both the tables are expanded	Both the inner and outer tables are expanded
Eggshell crackling	Less frequent	Frequent	More frequent
Pathological fracture	Very rare	Rare	Not uncommon
Fungation	Very unusual	Very unusual	May occur
Sinus/fistula	May occur externally or internally	Rare	Rare
Radiography	Same appearance but the cysts are smaller in size with well-marked trabeculations	Rounded or oval translucent cystic area with or without faint trabeculations	Soap-bubble or honeycomb appearance – the cysts are larger in size with fine and ill-defined trabeculations (pseudo-trabeculations)
Histology	Presence of peripheral columnar cells – the enameloblasts, with a central core of star cells	Presence of small multinucleated cells which are sparsely and unevenly distributed	Features of osteoclastoma – presence of multinucleated giant cells in fibrocellular stroma
Radiosensitivity	Non-radiosensitive	Does not arise	Radiosensitive
Recurrence	Common – particularly when evacuation and curettage is done	Nil. If it at all occurs, hyperparathyroidism should be suspected and investigated	Common
Malignancy	Very uncommon	Nil	May occur in 10% cases

ACTINOMYCOSIS OF THE JAW

Vide actinomycosis (Chapter 7).

Note

Stafne's bone cyst

Most commonly noted near the angle of the mandible below the mandibular canal *due to* *inclusion of ectopic lingual or submandibular salivary gland tissue within the bone* leading to swelling of the angle of the mandible on the floor of the mouth below the molar teeth.

X-ray will show a well circumscribed round radiolucent defect in the said area of the bone. CT will confirm the diagnosis.

Actinomycosis and Maduramycosis

ACTINOMYCOSIS

Actinomycosis is a chronic, suppurative granulomatous disease occurring *particularly in the region of the lower jaw*. The causal organism is potentially pathogenic *fungus-like* organism *Actinomyces israelii*.

Actinomycosis is a common infection in the West, but not in the East.

Bacteriology

A. israelii is an *anaerobic gram-positive organism*. This organism is now considered to be a bacterium in the family Actinomycetaceae which also includes the genus *Nocardia*. The *Actinomyces* is non-acid-fast and *Nocardia* is relatively acid-fast.

In the tissues, the *Actinomyces* grow in the form of complete colonies which can be recognised in the pus by the naked eye as *pinhead granules, greyish yellow in colour*. These are called '*sulphur granules*' or '*fish-roe*' bodies. When teased out on a microscopic slide and examined unstained they are seen to consist of branching mycelial filaments. Each filament ends in a terminal club.

The clubs are gram-negative, and are not formed in artificial culture. It is believed that they

are produced as the result of deposition of the colony of lipid material derived from the host tissues. *The filaments are gram-positive.*

These organisms are found in the colonies in characteristic radial arrangement and hence popularly known as '*ray-fungus*'.

Natural habitat

A. israelii is a normal commensal of the mouth and it is found in the tonsils and carious teeth and infected gum without any clinical manifestations of the disease.

It may also be found in the large intestine.

Mode of infection

Actinomycosis is *an endogenous infection*. It gains access to the tissue planes through the crypts or defects in the mucous membrane as a result of ulceration or trauma (e.g. following dental extraction).

The actinomycotic lesion starts as an acute suppurative inflammation which ultimately progresses to chronicity. *A granulomatous mass is produced and it comprises multiple nodules of fibrocellular tissue*. Some of the nodules liquefy to form multiple small chronic abscesses. Some of them fuse together but others remain discrete owing to the persistence of fibrous septa. This produces a characteristically loculated appearance (*honeycomb appearance*).

Some of the abscesses burst to the surface to discharge necrotic yellowish material through multiple sinuses. *Thus a hard brawny painless swelling with multiple discharging sinuses is developed.*

Predisposing factors

- Trauma, presence of carious tooth
- Secondary bacterial infection
- Hypersensitivity

Clinical types of actinomycosis

Cervicofacial	65%
Ileocaecal	25%
Pulmonary	10%

Spread

Infection spreads by continuity and contiguity. In cervicofacial actinomycosis there is a direct spread to the adjacent connective tissue, the muscle and the bone which are replaced by granulation tissue with an abundance of fibrous tissue reaction. There is also progressive cutaneous involvement resulting in *multiple discharging sinuses.*

Lymphatic spread does not occur in actinomycosis, because the filaments cannot pass through the lymphatic channels. *Any regional lymphadenitis, if it occurs, is due to secondary bacterial infection.*

Blood spread may occur. Liver may be involved either via the hepatic artery from cervicofacial lesion, or via the portal vein from ileocaecal lesion.

Pulmonary actinomycosis may disseminate into the systemic circulation and thus produce lesion in the kidney, brain, bone and other parts.

Prognosis

The prognosis of cervicofacial actinomycosis is good, but the abdominal and pulmonary infections are sometimes fatal.

Note

Actinomycosis infection is not contagious.

CERVICOFACIAL (NECK) ACTINOMYCOSIS

Diagnostic criteria

1. *Common site:* In the region of the lower jaw (angle of mandible), often adjacent to a carious tooth.
2. Insidious in onset. Very slowly growing.
3. *A hard brawny indurated painless swelling of the mandible (known as lumpy jaw).*
4. The hard indurated swelling ultimately becomes soft and fluctuant due to central suppuration leading to multiple discharging sinuses.
5. Bluish discoloration of the overlying skin.
6. Characteristic *yellow sulphur granules* can be demonstrated in the discharging sinuses.
7. *X-ray may reveal* multiple sclerosed bony cavities *with sequestra in the lower jaw.*
8. *On microscopic examination*, granules consisting of branching mycelial filaments with terminal clubs are seen.

Treatment

1. Medical treatment
2. Surgical treatment
3. Radiotherapy.

Medical treatment

Actinomycin is usually sensitive to penicillin, tetracycline, lincomycin, erythromycin.

A massive dose of penicillin – to start with 10 mega units, then reducing it to 4 mega units IM daily, is administered for a prolonged period and the treatment should be continued at least for 3 months after clinical cure with oral penicillin.

In resistant cases broad-spectrum antibiotics should be tried after antibiotic sensitivity test.

Iodides: The penicillin therapy is supplemented with *oral administration of tincture iodine* in the dose of m X to XV in a glass of milk 3 times a day. *The iodides are supposed to help in the resolution of fibrosis.*

Antifibroblastic agent: Stanozolol is also helpful in resolving fibrosis.

Antimycotic drugs such as nystatin, clotrimazole, fluconazole, miconidazole, amphotericin-A, may be used in various combinations to eradicate actinomycosis.

Surgical treatment

Incision and drainage: Under the cover of anti-biotic the abscesses and sinuses should better be widely opened up and drained and the wound is then loosely packed up with roller gauze soaked in tincture iodine (2%). *Excision of the granulo-matous tissue is very difficult.*

If there is osteomyelitis of the jaw, the bony cavity should be drained and sequestra, when present, be removed.

Radiotherapy

In resistant cases radiotherapy may be tried.

Note

Punch actinomycosis (Fig. 7.1)

Rarely there may be actinomycotic infection in a hand wound caused by hitting an assailant in the teeth. *The infection develops from the organism from the mouth cavity of the assailant* – exogenous infection.

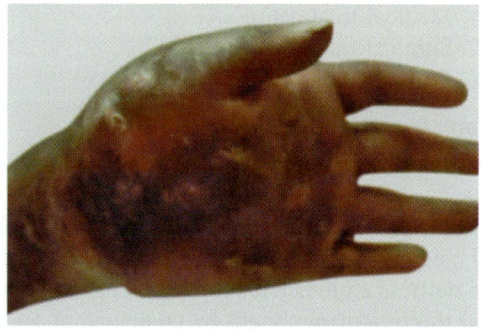

Fig. 7.1: Punch actinomycosis of the left hand. A hard brawny indurated painless swelling with multiple discharging sinuses over the palmar aspect of the hand. The discharge was yellowish in colour. (*Courtesy:* Dr Yogesh Salphale)

Note

Pelvic actinomycosis

Presents as a hard mass with infiltration into surrounding structures commonly ileocaecal region with discharging sinuses at the right iliac fossa. May mimic inflammatory pseudotumour or carcinomatosis with discharging sinuses. *The discharge from the sinuses will reveal the organisms on microscopic examination.*

Note

Actinomycotic bone lesions are also seen in vertebrae (spreading from lung or gut), and in pelvis (spreading from caecum or colon).

MADURAMYCOSIS

It is a chronic infective granulomatous condition affecting the subcutaneous tissues of the foot caused by the filamentous organism known as '*aerobic streptothrix*'. There are two types of organisms:

1. Bacterial known as *Nocardia madurae.*
2. Fungal known as *Madurella mycetomi.*

Nocardia infection is common. Nocardia are aerobic, gram-positive, and often acid-fast.

These organisms are usually found in the soil and they are introduced into the skin and subcutaneous tissue of the soles of the foot through minute abrasions caused by trivial injury – so, *exogenous infection* (cf. *Actinomycosis israelii*).

The condition is common in tropical countries, and is endemic in Madura district of South India, hence it is named *Madura foot.* It was first described from Madurai in South India.

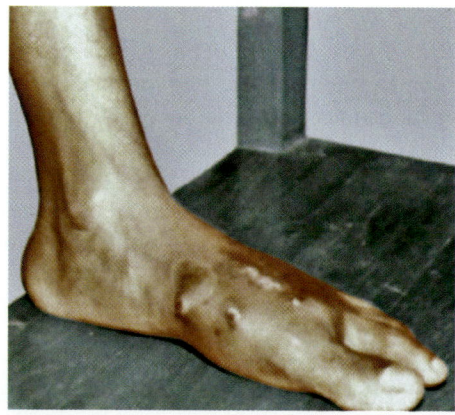

Fig. 7.2: A hard, brawny, indurated swelling with multiple discharging sinuses in the left foot of a farmer. The discharge was black in colour—Madura foot. D/D: Koch's osteomyelitis.

Most of the patients are farmers who walk barefooted. The condition may also occur in other parts of the body besides the foot.

In the early stage, pale, firm nodules appear. The nodules are surrounded with vesicles. Some of the nodules liquefy and result in chronic abscess formation. *Some of the abscess burst and multiple discharging sinuses develop over the top of the nodules.* The discharging granules may be yellow, black or red in colour. *In the late stage, there will be invasion of deeper structures like tendon, muscles, and also bones leading to osteo-myelitis.*

Spread

1. Spreads by direct continuity and contiguity.
2. Lymphatic spread does not occur.
3. Blood spread does not occur.

Diagnostic criteria

1. *Common in farmers who walk barefooted.*
2. *Common in southern part of India.*
3. A chronic, firm to hard, brawny, indurated *painless swelling of the foot and ankle with nodules and multiple discharging sinuses.* The foot is oedematous with a bulge on the dorsum and flattening of the concavity of the sole.
4. The overlying skin shows bluish discoloration.
5. Discharging granules may be yellow, black or red in colour.
6. In the late stage, the swelling may be fixed to the underlying bone and adjacent tendon sheaths, and becomes thick and tender.
7. Significant limb disability and limping is common.
8. Secondary infection, which is invariably present, may lead to enlarged lymph nodes and sometimes lymphangitic streaks.
9. *X-ray: In actinomycosis Nocardia type, X-ray reveals erosion of bones with sclerosis but no sequestra.*

   In Madura mycosis type, X-ray reveals multiple rarefied circular areas in the bones looking like a honeycomb.

10. Microscopic examination of the granules and biopsy reveal characteristic organisms and mixed infections. Acid-fast bacilli (*Nocardia*) may be detected by Ziehl-Neelsen stain.
11. Madura mycosis may involve the hand also – common in gardeners.

Complications

1. Spreading cellulitis, pyemic abscess.
2. Reactive arthritis.
3. Amyloidosis.
4. Rarely STS in long-standing disease.

Treatment

1. Medical treatment
2. Surgical treatment

Medical treatment

1. All cases should be treated *with massive dosage of penicillin.* Rifampicin and third generation cephalosporins may also be used.
2. *Dapsone* (diaminodiphenylsulfone) – drugs of sulphone group are useful in Nocardia infection (bacterial), but are of little or no value against Madura mycotic type (fungal). Dose is 100 mg twice a day for a period of 2 years.
3. *Oral iodides* may be given to help the resolution of fibrosis.

Surgical treatment

1. Multiple incisions and drainage under the cover of penicillin and dapsone.
2. In resistant cases, amputation is required at a suitable level, which depends on the site and spread of the disease.

Prognosis

The prognosis is poor and unfortunately the disease recurs in about 20 to 30% of cases because of continuing with the same job – may involve the other foot also.

Note

Madura mycosis may also occur in the hand specially in the gardeners who work with bare hands.

The Mouth and the Tongue

CYSTS IN THE MOUTH

The following cysts may be encountered.

1. Mucous cysts.
2. Dermoid, *see* Chapter 2.
3. Ranula, *see* Chapter 2.

MUCOUS CYSTS

The inner surface of the lips and the cheek is covered with *non-keratinised stratified squamous epithelium* that contains many tiny mucus-secreting glands. Obstruction of the duct of one of the glands causes *mucus-retention cyst*. Often mucus escapes into the tissues following rupture of the duct and causes mucus-extravasation cyst.

Diagnostic criteria

1. *Age:* These cysts can occur at all ages.
2. The patient complains of a slowly growing lump on the inside of the lips or cheek. *The lump may interfere with eating and get bitten through.*
3. *Site: Commonly present on the lower lip.* It may occur on the buccal mucous membrane.
4. Spherical or globular in shape, and the size varies from 0.5 to 2 cm in diameter.

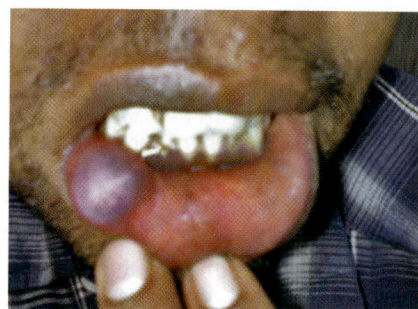

Fig. 8.1: Mucous cyst—lower lip.

5. *Translucent, soft cystic swelling* having a pale pink colour with a smooth surface (Fig. 8.1). The overlying epithelium may be white and scarred if the cyst has been frequently damaged by biting.

Complications

1. Spontaneous rupture
2. Recurrence
3. Gets bitten through.

Treatment

1. Excision under local anaesthesia.
2. Injections of boiling water when the cysts are multiple.
3. Cryosurgery.

ANKYLOGLOSSIA (*Syn.* Tongue tie)

It is a congenital lesion *due to long frenulum adhering to the ventral aspect of the tongue almost from its tip to the floor of the mouth which prevents full protrusion of tongue.*

It causes problems of phonation and pronunciation of certain letters (consonants).

Treatment

Frenuloplasty – dividing the frenulum transversely and suturing longitudinally, usually around 12 months of age to allow the development of normal phonation and articulation.

Note

Ankyloglossia may be acquired due to cancer infiltration of the floor of the mouth and tongue.

MACROGLOSSIA (Fig. 8.2)

It is a painless, diffuse enlargement of the tongue which interferes with phonation, articulation of letters, and swallowing. It may get bitten through – *prone to recurrent trauma.*

Causes are:

1. Hamartomas – haemangioma, lymphangioma, neurofibroma.
2. Arteriovenous malformation (AVM).
3. Muscle hypertrophy in cretins.

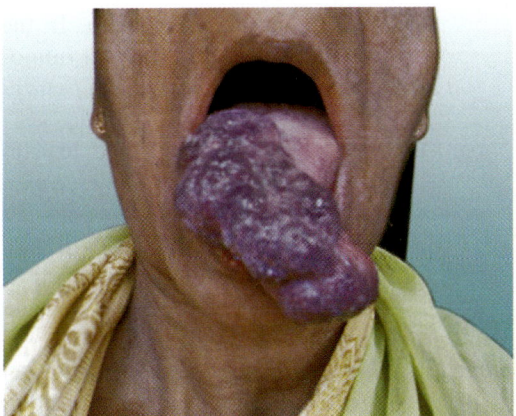

Fig. 8.2: Macroglossia of tongue. Cavernous haemangioma over the dorsum, right anterolateral part and tip of the tongue. (*Courtesy:* Dr Gurusaday Bhattacharya, MS, FRCS, Professor and Head of Department, KPC Medical College, Kolkata)

4. Myxoedema.
5. Amyloidosis (rare).
6. Diffuse infiltrating carcinoma (rare).

Prone to recurrent trauma and bleeding from bite – commonly with haemangioma and arteriovenous malformation.

BENIGN TUMOURS OF THE CHEEK, LIP AND FLOOR OF THE MOUTH

Papilloma

1. It is usually uncommon.
2. *It appears as a soft, fleshy mass.*
3. Chance of malignancy is remote.
4. Gets bitten through while chewing food causing pain and/or bleeding.
5. *Treatment:* Excision with an adequate margin of tissue followed by histopathology examination of the excised tissue.

Fibroepithelial polyp

1. *It appears as a firm pale swelling on the inner surface of the cheek.*
2. It arises after repeated trauma to mucous membrane of the cheek after getting bitten during chewing of food.
3. Histologically, it contains a dense core of fibrous tissue.
4. Treated by excision.

Lipoma

It can arise in any part of the fatty supporting structures of the mouth. Features are the same as with other lipomas. Treated by excision.

Neurofibroma

Rare. Treated by excision.

Haemangioma/Lymphangioma

It can arise under the mucous membrane of the cheek and floor of the mouth, lips and tongue. Features are the same as with other haemangiomas or lymphangiomas.

Soft, compressible swelling with or without bluish hue. Recurrent bleeding after getting bitten through is common.

Treatment

• Sclerotherapy.

- Injection of boiling water, polidocanol alone or in combination with 10% glucose.
- Cryosurgery.
- Excision – preferably with cryo or Nd:YAG laser knife to obtain a bloodless field.

Note

During excision of medium or larger lesion of haemangioma/lymphangioma *preliminary bilateral control of external carotid arteries is preferred for extensive lesion, before excision.*

Ectopic salivary tumours

See Chapter 5, pages 171–172.

LEUKOPLAKIA (Fig. 8.3)

This is a descriptive term meaning sharply outlined *white patches* on a squamous epithelium *in or near a mucous surface.* This condition may occur anywhere within the mouth, commonly on the tongue and cheek. *It is basically an increased keratinising process (hyperkeratosis) of the superficial cells of the squamous epithelium* which occurs *in response to a chronic irritant,* e.g. sharp tooth or ill-fitting dentures, smoking, sepsis, spirits and spices, syphilis (well known list of *Six S's*). **In India** – *Gutka, pan masala* and *khainy* are predominant causes of leukoplakia and cancer of cheek and tongue.

Macroscopically, the affected area of mucous membrane appears as *a thickened grey-white plaque* with/without cracks or fissures. The

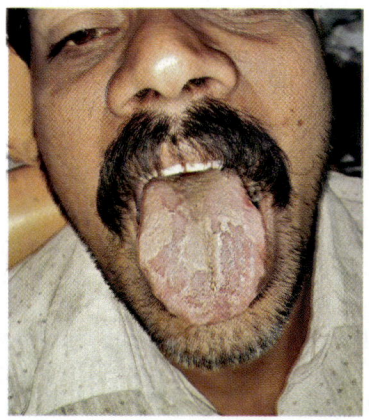

Fig. 8.3: Leukoplakia on the dorsum of the tongue—geographical tongue: Precancerous.

plaque is without induration and pain. *The plaque is difficult to rub-off or peel.*

Microscopically, there is hyperplasia of superficial layers of squamous epithelium with hyperkeratosis, swelling and vacuolation of cells of the middle layer, and hyperplasia and hyperchromasia of the basal layers of cells. There may be *dyskeratosis* which is most serious because of its association with malignancy.

The importance of the lesion is that *it is premalignant* and the frequency of the neoplastic change is about 25%. *The neoplastic change usually occurs within the fissures* and should be suspected if there is local thickening, bleeding, area of erythema, appearance of nodules, induration around the white patch, or local pain.

Diagnostic criteria

1. *Age:* Usually found in middle-aged or elderly subjects.
2. *Sex:* Men are more affected.
3. Patient may present with one of the following features which are divided into 4 clinical stages:

Stage I   Appearance of *thin grey transparent patch* on the tongue and/or cheek which may be localised or widespread.

Stage II   This thin patch gradually turns into *sharply outlined white or opaque plaque.* This is *leukoplakia.* In the beginning it looks soft and homogeneous *but later cracks and fissures appear.*

Stage III Gradually hyperplasia will lead to *small nodules or warty excrescences.* The warty nodular leukoplakias are the most likely ones that will turn malignant. Desquamation may follow which leaves areas of smooth, red and shiny patches.

Stage IV   *This is the stage of appearance of carcinoma.* The lesion possesses all the characteristic features of carcinoma. *The carcinomatous change usually occurs within the fissures* and should be suspected, if there is local thickening, bleeding, or pain.

Note

Clinical features of malignancy in leukoplakia

- Indurated area
- Nodularity and increase in thickness
- Ulceration – leading to pain or bleeding
- Growths
- Rolled margins

Treatment

1. Removal of any underlying cause, e.g. removal of the sharp tooth causing chronic irritation, care of oral hygiene. *Smoking, chewing tobacco and alcohol should be stopped immediately and forever.*
2. *Any indurated white patch suspicious of malignancy should be biopsied at once.*
3. (a) *Small superficial patches of leukoplakia* may be satisfactorily treated by excision.
   (b) *Larger lesion requires excision followed by closure* with mobilisation of local flaps or skin grafting. *Rarely, the raw area after excision may be left for spontaneous epithelialisation.*
4. Patients should be examined at regular intervals of not longer than 3 months *to note the appearance of any area of warty excrescence or any doubtful area* which must be removed and examined histologically.
5. *Radiotherapy: Its role is intricate.* Although it improves the condition initially, it increases the chance of malignancy. Moreover such malignant lesions become resistant to further radiotherapy.

Note

Other sites of leukoplakia are the larynx, the perianal region, glans penis, and the vulva.

Note

Hairy leukoplakia – a white patch on the side of the tongue with corrugated or hairy appearance – a condition *triggered by Epstein-Barr virus.* Requires oral therapy with acyclovir in high doses.

ERYTHROPLAKIA (Fig. 8.4)

A type of lesion of the oral mucosa that presents as *bright red velvety plaques in the oral cavity commonly over soft palate or tonsillar pillars due to severe cellular dysplasia of unknown cause.*

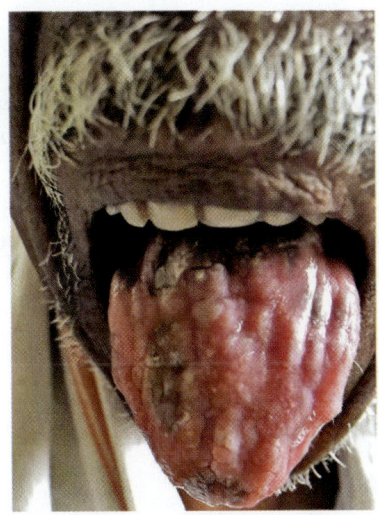

Fig. 8.4: Erythroplakia on the dorsum of the tongue.

This lesion has *a high incidence of malignancy* (17 times higher than that of leukoplakia) and should be excised either by surgery or CO_2 or Nd:YAG laser knife.

ULCERS OF THE TONGUE

Types

Non-specific

1. Dyspeptic or aphthous ulcer
2. Traumatic or dental ulcer
3. Infective and allied:
   - Chronic non-specific ulcer
   - Post-pertussis ulcer
   - Simple ulcer due to glossitis
   - Herpetic and pseudo-herpetic ulcer.

Specific

1. Tubercular ulcer
2. Syphilitic ulcer
3. Malignant ulcer

Differential diagnosis of tongue ulcers

See Table 8.1 (pages 206 and 207).

Management of tongue ulcer in elderly persons

After thorough clinical examination and investigation, *biopsy of the ulcer is a must* in every case and the tissue should be sent for histopathological examination to exclude carcinoma.

TUMOURS OF THE TONGUE
Benign and malignant

Benign tumours of the tongue are very un-common. The following may be encountered rarely.

- *Papilloma:* Sessile or pedunculated (Fig. 8.5)
- *Haemangioma:* Usually cavernous type
- *Lymphangioma*
- *Neurofibroma, plexiform neuroma*
- *Lipoma*
- *Lingual thyroid*
- *Mixed salivary gland tumour*
- *Osteoma*

Malignant tumours

- Carcinoma
- Sarcoma.

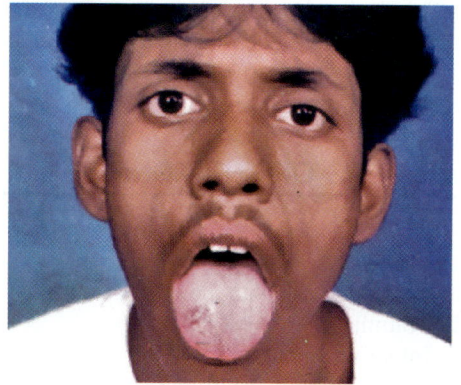

Fig. 8.5: Papilloma of the tongue. Treatment: Excision biopsy.

CARCINOMA OF THE TONGUE

The squamous-cell mucous membrane lining the buccal cavity, including the lip, the gum, the inner aspect of the cheek, the tongue, and the floor of the mouth, is a rare site for benign tumours; *but it is comparatively a common site for carcinoma.*

Carcinoma of the tongue is a common lesion and accounts for more than a half of all intraoral carcinomas.

Aetiopathogenesis of oral/tongue cancers
Remember SLAVE (SLAVE means a bonded labour)

S. **S**harp tooth, **S**moking (tobacco), **S**pirits, **S**pices (tobacco or pan chewing with betel nut and lime) – all lead to **S**uperficial glossitis which ultimately leads to chronic irritation → leukoplakia → cancer; **S**yphilis (tertiary syphilis can cause leukoplakia, cancer; syphilis and carcinoma often coexist); **S**ubmucous fibrosis of oral cavity: more common with the use of tobacco or zarda with lime and betel nut (supari). So, '**7S**'s lead to chronic irritation → leukoplakia → cancer.

L. Leukoplakia – a precancerous condition.

A. Avitaminosis
  - *Vitamin A deficiency:* β-carotene or carotenoid (antioxidant nutrients) is precursor of vitamin A. Source of β-carotene is spinach.
  - *Vitamin C and E deficiency.*
  Normally they prevent damage to DNA.

V. Viral infection: HPV genomes 16 and 18 and HSV genomes 1 and 2 have been implicated following oral sex – particularly base of the tongue and lingual and palatine tonsils.

E. Erythroplakia – a precancerous condition.

Note

Iron deficiency can cause Plummer-Vinson syndrome – a sideropenic dysphagia characterised by anaemia, glossitis, cheilosis and eso-phageal webs and cancer.

Note

HPV genome-induced cancer is associated with favourable prognosis.

Precancerous conditions of oral cavity

1. Sessile papilloma of tongue
2. Leukoplakia
3. Erythroplakia
4. Oral submucous fibrosis – surgical division of bands and skin grafting may help. Postoperatively patient is advised to stop pan with betel nut and lime, tobacco with lime chewing and smoking for rest of life.
5. Hyperkeratosis – leading to leukoplakia.
6. Dyskeratosis congenita – a congenital

disorder: Abnormal keratinisation occurring prematurely lead to leukoplakia.

7. Chronic hyperplastic candidiasis of oral cavity can lead to leukoplakia → cancer, particularly in immunocompromised patients.
8. Oral lichen planus – painful erythematous erosive lesion in the oral cavity – an auto-immune disorder.
9. Plummer-Vinson syndrome or Kelly-Paterson syndrome – sideropenic dysphagia due to iron deficiency anaemia, glossitis, cheilosis and oesophageal web leading to dysphagia to both solids and liquids: Treatment with iron supplementation and mechanical widening (dilatation) of oesophagus provides excellent outcome.

Note

Most common oral precancerous conditions:

• Leukoplakia
• Submucous fibrosis
• Erythroplakia

Note

Daily use of raw tobacco with slacked lime (*Khainy*) and *Pan* and betel nut with lime, *Pan Bahar* – holding the quid between the gum and cheek in the mouth for some time (common in India) *is a major factor in predisposing to oral malignancy including tongue – common in India.*

Note

Nearly two-thirds of oral cancers are located in the lateral margin of the tongue and gingivo-buccal complex where the betel quids or tobacco (*Khainy*) is kept for a prolonged time – very common in India.

Note

Cancer of the palate is also common amongst the Europeans who smoked pipe for a prolonged time, while consuming alcohol and so under the influence of drowsiness.

Note

Chutta cancer – cancer of the roof of the mouth or palate – *who smoke with the reverse lighted end of the biri or cigarette keeping inside the mouth.*

Note

HPV16 & 18 and HSV1 & 2 are also responsible for genital cancer, cervical cancer, cancer around the *anus and rectus (following anal sex)* and mouth *(following oral sex)* – direct contact.

Note

Spinach is an edible flowering plant with excellent source of vitamins B_6 and B_2, riboflavin, vitamin E, β-carotene. **β-carotene is anticancer** and is converted to vitamin A in the body.

Surgical pathology

Site of election (Fig. 8.6)

1. Anterior two-thirds of the tongue at or near the lateral margin – 25% × 2.
2. Posterior one-third of the tongue – 20%.
3. Tip of the tongue – 10%.
4. Dorsal surface of anterior two-thirds of the tongue – 10%.
5. Ventral surface of anterior two-thirds of the tongue – 10%.

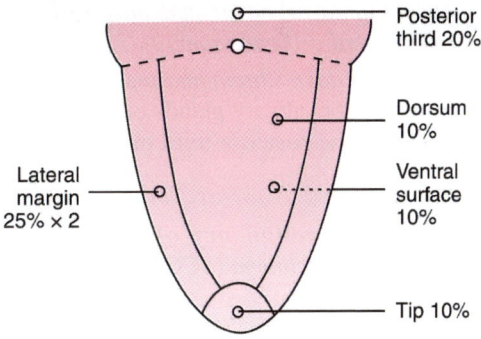

Fig. 8.6: Site of election for carcinoma of the tongue.

The tip or the centre of the tongue is less commonly affected by carcinoma unless it arises in gummatous (syphilitic) ulcer in the region.

Macroscopic features

The growth may appear as:

1. *Ulcerative type:* With raised, irregular, rolled or everted margin, and a sloughing yellow-

grey base and induration of the surrounding tissues.

2. *Papilliferous or warty type:* Varying from *a small papilloma* with broad and indurated base and covered with an excess of proliferating filiform epithelium to *a large verrucous* or cauliflower-like mass.

3. *Nodular type or plaque type:* A submucous nodule or plaque with diffuse infiltration.

4. *Fissured or cracked type with induration:* Chronic in nature with no signs of healing, usually follows chronic superficial glossitis or syphilis.

5. *Frozen type:* Here the tongue is transformed into an indurated mass with restricted mobility – *ankyloglossia.*

Microscopic features

Depend largely on which part of the tongue is affected:

1. *Anterior two-thirds of the tongue: Squamous cell carcinoma* with characteristic cell-nest formation with the inner older cells showing keratinization and the outer younger cells arranged in an 'onion-peel-like' manner.

2. *Posterior one-third of the tongue: Lymphoepithelioma or basal cell carcinoma or transitional cell carcinoma.*

3. *Rarely an adenocarcinoma* may also occur in the minor salivary glands or the mucous glands in the posterior third of tongue.

Note

Most common malignancy of the tongue – squamous cell carcinoma (SCC).

Spread

1. Local spread

• *Carcinoma of the anterior two-thirds of the tongue, which starts usually on the lateral margin* – invades the floor of the mouth early; but contiguous spread seldom extends across the midline.

• Invasion of the floor of the mouth causes thickening of local tissues and invasion to genioglossus muscle reduces mobility of the tongue. *Spread may extend to the mandible.*

• *Carcinoma of the posterior one-third of the tongue* – tends to spread to the corresponding tonsil, epiglottis, the soft palate, and even the vocal cord.

2. Lymphatic spread

Common: The lymph nodes are enlarged and very firm to hard. The lymph nodes are involved by embolic spread (due to squeezing off of the malignant cells by the activity of the tongue musculature), not by permeation, *so that the intervening tissue is not involved.*

The lymphatics drain in the following way.

• *From the tip,* drain into the submental lymph nodes of both the sides and then jugulo-omohyoid nodes.

• *From the anterior two-thirds,* drain unilaterally to the submandibular nodes and then to the lower deep cervical chain or jugulo-omohyoid nodes.

• *From the posterior one-third,* drain into the upper deep cervical chain or jugulodigastric nodes of both the sides.

Ultimately all the lymph drainage from the tongue reaches the jugulo-omohyoid lymph nodes in the deep cervical chain (Figs 8.7 A and B). *Jugulo-omohyoid nodes are known as the lymph nodes of the tongue.*

Points to Note

• It is important to note that in 50% of cases, the lymphatic vessels draining the anterior two-thirds of the tongue and the floor of the mouth *traverse the periosteum of the mandible on their way to submental and submandibular lymph nodes.*

• Lymphatics of the tongue are freely communicating and *so involvement of bilateral neck lymph nodes is common.*

• The lymph nodes of both sides of the neck must be examined even if the lesion is unilateral *since the lymphatic vessels are decussating.*

• It is also to be remembered that the septic infection which invariably occurs in the malignant ulcer, may cause a non-malignant enlargement of the lymph nodes under the jaw. *Such nodes are tender and firm and respond to antibiotics.*

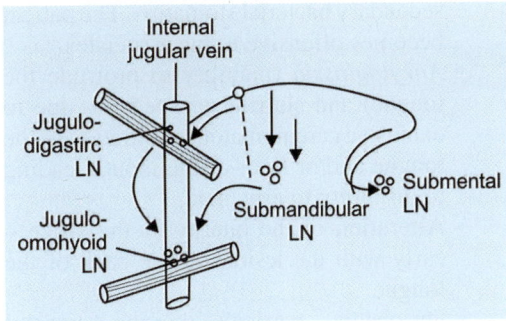

Fig. 8.7A: Lymph drainage of the tongue.

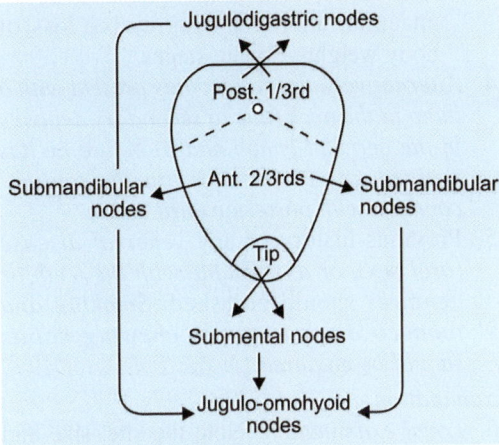

Fig. 8.7B: Lymph drainage of the tongue.

• *Because of the secluded position and consequent late diagnosis*, growths of the posterior third of the tongue show the highest incidence of cervical node metastases.

3. Blood spread

Very rare, occurs in only 2% of patients and in these cases the neoplasm is situated in the extreme posterior third of the tongue in almost every instance.

Diagnostic criteria

1. *Age:* Common in fifth or sixth decades (*Note:* But in India common in third and fourth decades because of use of 'Khainy' and 'betel quids').
2. *Sex:* Sex incidence is now equal.
3. *Symptoms:* In the early stage, the patient complains of a *painless lump, irregularity,*

or *non-healing ulcer on the surface of the tongue* (Figs 8.8 to 8.12).

The patient may experience burning, discomfort or numb feeling over the site of the lesion.

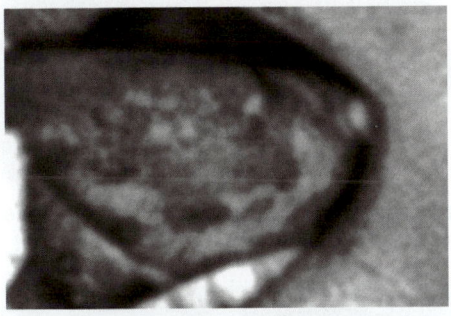

Fig. 8.8: Flat type of malignant growth on the left lateral margin of the tongue extending also on the undersurface of the tongue.

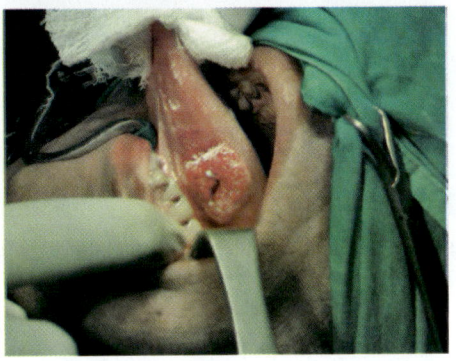

Fig. 8.9: Malignant ulcer on the left lateral margin of the tongue. (*Courtesy:* Professor Sudeb Saha, MS, FAMS)

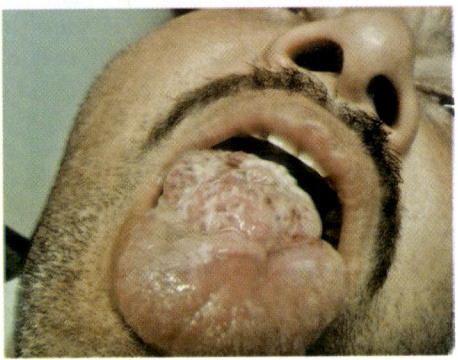

Fig. 8.10: Carcinoma dorsum of the tongue—mostly on the right side.

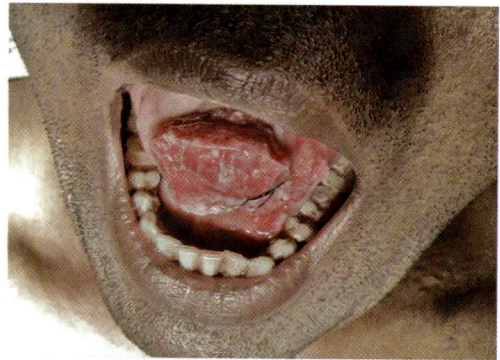

Fig. 8.11: Carcinoma dorsum of tongue near the tip of tongue.

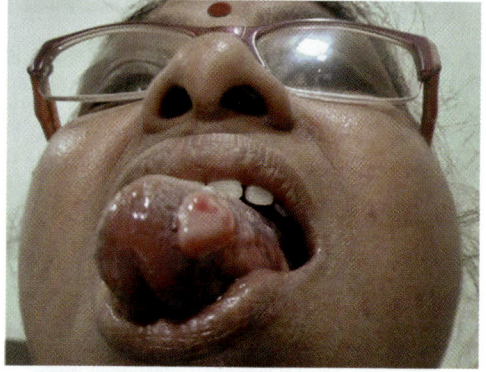

Fig. 8.12: Carcinoma of tongue—left lateral margin near the tip.

Sadly, many a patient fails to notice or else disregards the lesion in its early stage and may report to the doctor only because of one or more of the following symptoms.

• Enlarging ulcer causing local pain in the tongue; *the pain is burning in nature.*

• *Pain referred to the ear* (this is due to involvement of the lingual nerve and the pain is referred via the auriculotemporal nerve which is also a branch of the mandibular division of trigeminal nerve).

• *Excessive salivation:* The saliva may be bloodstained. Excessive salivation is due both to excessive secretion from irritative lesion of the tongue and to difficulty in swallowing.

• *Difficulty in mastication and swallowing.*

• *Foetor oris* due to bad oral hygiene and

secondary bacterial stomatitis. The patient becomes offensive to his associates.

• *Ankyloglossia* (inability to protrude the tongue) and slurring of speech – due to extensive carcinomatous infiltration of the tongue and/or floor of the mouth leading to disability to articulate.

• Alteration of the quality of the voice – early with the lesions at the back of the tongue.

• Dysphagia – particularly in the lesions at the back of the tongue.

• General features of malignant cachexia, anaemia, anorexia, progressive loss of body weight – in late stages.

4. *Alternatively, the patient may present with a lump in the neck (due to secondary deposits in the cervical lymph nodes) before he has noticed any abnormality in the tongue: common with posterior third lesion.*

5. Previous history of any *venereal disease (oral sex), or any trouble with the teeth or dentures* should be asked. *Smoking and tobacco or pan masala chewing habits should be enquired.*

Examination:

6. *Local examination:* Note the site, size and character of the lesion on the tongue (*see* macroscopic features).

   Palpate for the *induration* of the lesion. *Note the mobility* of the lesion, and of the tongue.

7. It is also important to examine the posterior part of the tongue, floor of the mouth, tonsils and fauces, gums and teeth, and jaw for a second lesion or infiltration.

8. *Examine the neck for lymph node enlargement,* i.e. submental, submandibular and deep cervical (upper, middle and lower) groups may be involved. *Check both sides for enlarged node (because of decussation of lymphatics of the tongue)* (Fig. 8.7B).

Note

Lesions in the posterior third of the tongue are difficult to diagnose in early stage. Usually presents when large in size causing *difficulty in swallowing. Change of voice* may be the earliest symptom. *Presence of multiple enlarged neck nodes (secondaries) is the commonest symptom. Early indirect laryngoscopy is the best way of early diagnosis.*

Special investigations

1. *Biopsy* must be performed before any treatment is planned.

    Wedge biopsy from the edge of the ulcer can be taken under local anaesthesia. In case of proliferative growth *punch biopsy is recommended. In case of posterior third growth, biopsy taken* under general anaesthesia with the help of laryngoscope.

    For doubtful lesions of the tongue, toluidine blue (a supravital dye that stains carcinoma in situ lesions) staining is an adjunct to early detection.
2. *Laryngoscopy* – to see the posterior one-third of the tongue, especially the region of the vallecula.
3. *Blood for WR and Kahn* – to be done in every case and, if positive, antisyphilitic treatment should be started.
4. *X-ray of the mandible* preferably orthopantomogram in every case to detect any bony involvement, erosion.
5. *Chest X-ray* to detect any rare pulmonary metastasis.
6. *In the presence of enlarged lymph nodes, a trial course of antibiotics is given* while awaiting for biopsy report of the lesion. Any further doubts about the lymph node status must be settled by an *FNAC of the node.*
7. *A fibreoptic endoscopy of oro-/laryngopharynx* may be needed for posterior third growth.

Differential diagnosis

1. From other types of ulcers of the tongue.
2. From the rare tumours of the tongue – papilloma, haemangioma, lymphangioma, neurofibroma, lingual thyroid.

Treatment

Either surgery or radiotherapy is the treatment of choice. *Results of surgery or radiotherapy for early carcinoma of tongue are equivalent.*

Preliminary measures

1. A swab from the ulcer and the mouth is taken for culture and antibiogram to determine the predominant organism, and the most suitable antibiotics to be used.
2. Suitable antibiotics (according to sensitivity test) to be given to control and prevent secondary infection for at least 3 weeks preoperatively.
3. Maintenance of oral hygiene by frequent antiseptic mouth washes.
4. Extraction of any sharp or carious tooth.

Radical treatment

It includes:

1. Management of the primary lesion.
2. Management of the involved neck glands.

Management of the primary lesion

(Fig. 8.13)

Management of the primary lesion depends on the site and stage of the tumour.

A. *Site of the tumour*
    Anterior two-thirds
    Posterior one-third

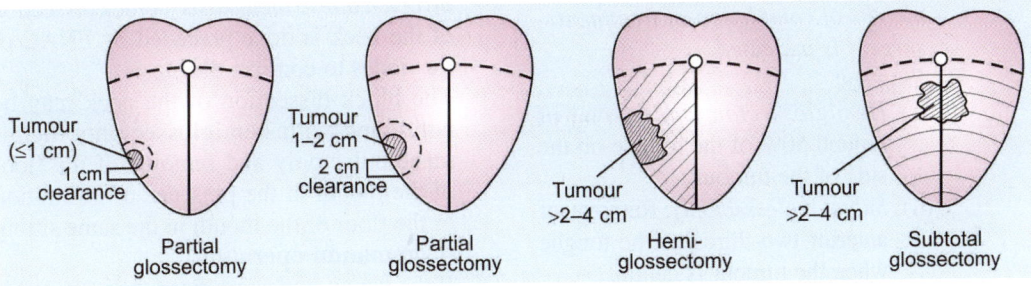

Fig. 8.13: Surgical management of primary tumour of the tongue.

B. *Early stages of tumour:* T_1 or T_2

T_1: Tumour 2 cm or less; in greatest dimension ≤2 cm.

T_2: Tumour more than 2 cm but not more than 4 cm; >2 to ≤4 cm.

I. *Growth in the anterior two-thirds of the tongue:* Wide excision is the preferred choice. *Three-dimensional excision is the treatment of choice for the primary lesion.*

1. *Carcinoma in situ (CIS) or the lesion is ≤1 cm in size: Wide excision of the growth with 1 cm clearance* both in margin and depth is to be performed. Reconstruction of the tongue is not necessary. The defect is left to granulate and epithelialize.

   The excised tissue should be sent for histopathological examination. *If it shows either a CIS or an early invasive carcinoma which has of course been adequately excised* – no further treatment is necessary but monthly follow-up is required up to 6 months.

2. *Growth is between >1 and 2 cm in size* (T_1): Treated by *partial glossectomy with 2 cm clearance* around the tumour. *The defect may be grafted with split skin. Morbidity of excising these T_1 lesions is less than a full course of radiotherapy.*

3. *Growth is between >2 to 4 cm in size* (T_2): Options are:

   A. *Primary radiotherapy:* Usually external beam irradiation (Teletherapy: Distant beam radiotherapy) is preferred. Radiotherapy is successful in majority of cases depending on the site and type of the tumour. *If radiotherapy fails to cure within 2 months of completion of treatment – surgery is indicated.*

   B. *Surgery:*

      (i) *Hemiglossectomy:* Removal of around 50% of the tongue on the side of the tumour.

      (ii) *Subtotal glossectomy:* Removal of anterior two-thirds of the tongue when the tumour is central.

   The defect may be grafted with split skin.

4. *When the growth is more than 4 cm or reaches or involves within 2 cm of the mandible:* Removal of that half of the mandible (hemimandibulectomy) is to be done in addition to hemiglossectomy. A stainless steel wire may be used to hold the remaining half of the jaw in position.

   In these cases radiotherapy may not be successful. Moreover, radiotherapy causes necrosis of the mandible.

II. *Any growth in the posterior third of the tongue,* whether less or more than 1 cm in diameter, is treated by *Teletherapy,* because this secluded position is anatomically difficult both for surgery and for interstitial irradiation therapy.

III. *When the carcinoma of the tongue is associated with syphilis, they should be treated with surgery because these cases are radioresistant due to endarteritis.*

Management of the lymph nodes

Depends upon *whether they are palpable or not. If palpable, whether mobile or fixed.*

I. *If the lymph nodes are impalpable or clinically normal* then prophylactic excision is unnecessary, but a careful regular monthly checkup is required.

II. *If the lymph nodes are palpable but mobile,* it may be due to infection, with or without metastasis.

   So, a course of antibiotics for 3 weeks is given preoperatively. If no response, block dissection of the neck is done preceded by FNAC of the nodes.

III. *If the lymph nodes are palpable, firm to hard, mobile and they are suspected of being involved due to metastasis* – block dissection of the neck is done preceded by FNAC of the nodes to confirm diagnosis.

   The block dissection of the neck may be combined with hemiglossectomy, hemimandibulectomy and removal of the floor of the mouth in the presence of infiltration of the floor of the mouth in the same sitting (**Commando operation**).

IV. *If the lymph nodes are fixed* then surgery is contraindicated and radiotherapy is used.

Radiotherapy

(a) *Brachytherapy* [interstitial (near beam) irradiation]: For small primary tumours ≤2 cm – may be curative.

For large primary tumours, initial radiotherapy may be given to reduce the tumour size so that the resection will be better performed later.

Radium needles, radon seeds, radio-active tantalum wires or ^{192}iridium wires are used. The average dose in carcinoma of the tongue is between 6,000 r and 8,000 r.

The needles are inserted vertically in the substance of the tongue in one plane at 1 cm apart. The eyes of the radium needles are placed below the mucous membrane and are tied with one another by a silk thread. The free end of the thread is fixed to the face by leucoplast. The needles are kept *in situ* for 7 to 10 days.

(b) *Teletherapy* (external beam radiation with a telecobalt or linear accelerator): The form usually used is *cobalt 60 unit*. It is *indicated particularly for the growth of the posterior third of the tongue and for recurrent growths after adequate excision as palliative mode.*

Note

- *Brachytherapy: Near beam or interstitial radiation* with radium needle insertion around the lesion.
- *Teletherapy: Distance or external beam radiation* with telecobalt or linear accelerator.

Role of chemotherapy in carcinoma of tongue

- Not of much help.
- Given in postoperative period after excisional surgery (adjuvant) and also for palliation for non-resectable or recurrent tumours.
- Price-Hill regimen is commonly used. Drugs used are methotrexate, vincristine, adriamycin, bleomycin and mercaptopurine.
- Regional intra-arterial administration (through external carotid artery using arterial pump) of *amethopterin* in the dose of 50 mg per day for 5 days can be used, either as a preliminary to excision or as a palliative measure.

Palliative treatment in carcinoma of tongue

1. In case of large and fixed primary growth – radiotherapy will be tried.
2. In case of recurrence after radiotherapy or surgery – cryosurgery may be tried.
3. In case of extreme pain due to advanced growth – blocking of the trigeminal nerve with 5% phenol may be tried.

Prognosis

This depends on the site and size of the tumour, nodal status and stage of the growth.

1. *Site:*
   - Growth in anterior two-thirds – 50% 5 years survival rate.
   - Growth in posterior one-third – 10% 5 years survival rate.

2. *Size of tumour:*
   - T_1 – tumour ≤2 cm; the cure rate is 90%.
   - T_2 – tumour >2 to 4 cm.
   - T_3 – tumour >4 cm; the cure rate falls to 10%.

3. *Nodes:*
   - If not involved – 60% 5 years survival rate.
   - If involved – 15% 5 years survival rate.

4. *Stage:*
   - Early stage – 60% 5 years survival rate.
   - Late stage – 15% 5 years survival rate.

Terminal events

If unsuccessfully treated, the disease turns inevitably to a fatal course. Death occurs usually in one of the following ways.

1. *Haemorrhage* from the primary growth and also from the carotid artery or internal jugular vein when eroded by metastatic lymph nodes.

2. *Combined malignant cachexia, starvation and exhaustion* from a combination of difficulty in swallowing and anorexia resulting from infected, foul-smelling fungating ulcer within the mouth.

3. *Aspiration bronchopneumonia*, from the superadded oral sepsis.
4. *Asphyxia* resulting either from pressure upon the upper air passages by metastatic lymph nodes, or from oedema of the glottis which is due to an extension of the lymphatic oedema around a growth at the back of the tongue.

Note

Osteoradionecrosis

It is a common complication of radiation when used for tumours very close to bone or involving the bone. In such cases radiation is preferred *after surgical excision of the tumour along with adjacent bone.*

Note

Patient with carcinoma of the tongue or oral carcinoma often have bilateral nodal metastases. A radical neck dissection on the ipsilateral (involved) side and a supramylohyoid dissection on the opposite (non-involved) side are advised. Internal jugular vein on one side, preferably non-involved side, should be preserved.

Note

Commando operation

Complicated operation for 1st degree malignancy of the tongue. It comprises hemiglossectomy and hemimandibulectomy, removal of the floor of the mouth together with block dissection of the cervical nodes. *Rarely done nowadays.*

LIPS

Pigmented lips

Causes

1. Peutz-Jeghers' syndrome
2. Addison's disease

Macrocheilia (permanent swelling of the lip)

Causes

1. Lymphangioma – commonest

2. Haemangioma
3. Chronic inflammation

Neoplasms

Benign

Usually uncommon and of following:

- Naevi
- Papilloma
- Fibroma
- Lipoma
- Haemangioma
- Lymphangioma
- Pyogenic granuloma
- Keratoacanthoma
- Leukoplakia
- Ectopic salivary tumour.

Malignant

1. Squamous cell carcinoma – commonest
2. Basal cell carcinoma
3. Melanoma } Rare
4. Adenocarcinoma.

CARCINOMA OF THE LIPS

Squamous cell carcinoma is common in the lip, affecting almost exclusively the lower lip.

Incidence (Fig. 8.14)

Lower lip	93%
Upper lip	5%
Angle of the mouth	2%

Site of lesion

The carcinoma may arise at:

- the junction of the skin and mucous membrane of the lip;

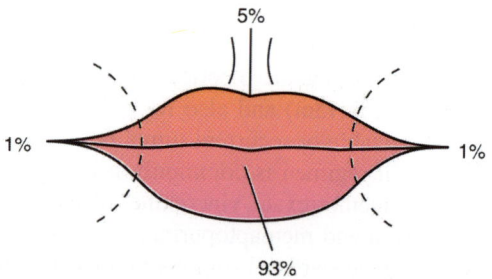

Fig. 8.14: Incidence of carcinoma lip.

- the mucous membrane of the 'true lip', i.e. the area between the red margin and the area of contact between the two lips;
- the mucous membrane covering the inner side of the lip – *so during examination the lip should be everted to expose the inner surface.*

Predisposing factors

1. Aged males between 60–70 years.
2. Usually an outdoor worker like farmers, who is continuously exposed to strong sunlight – exposed to actinic radiation, wind-drift and driving rain, known as *countrymen's lip.*
3. Recurrent blistering cheilitis (inflammation of the lips) – 40% cases.
4. *Addiction to 'Khainy'* – 'Khainy' is a mixture of raw tobacco and slaked lime. In many parts of India, people are *in the habit of keeping Khainy, Pan Bahar/pan masala between the lower lip and gum* and thus make the lower lip and inner side of buccal cavity especially vulnerable to carcinoma.
5. *Addiction to betel nut and pan with lime.*
6. *Chronic irritation from pipe smoking while consuming alcohol.*

With the last three predisposing factors 4, 5 and 6, the carcinoma developed in early age.

Origin

1. *De novo*
2. On some precancerous conditions, e.g.
   - Leukoplakia
   - Chronic fissures at the angle of the mouth
   - A sessile papilloma.

Macroscopic features

Carcinoma of the lip may present as:

- A nodule or fissure
- A typical malignant ulcer
- A warty papilliferous growth (Figs 8.15 and 8.16 A and B)
- An infiltrative induration – when carcinoma spreads deeply.

Microscopic features

Most of the carcinomas are *squamous cell carcinoma* with 'cell-nests' and prickle cells.

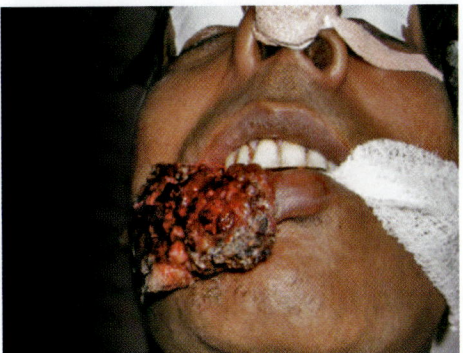

Fig. 8.15: Carcinoma lip involving the right half of the lower lip (*proliferative and spreading growth*) extending to the angle of the mouth. (*Courtesy:* Professor Diptendra Sarkar, MS, DNB, FRCS)

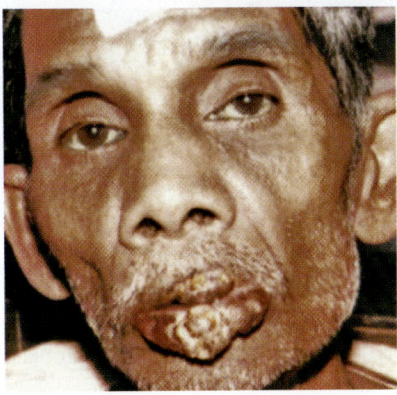

Fig. 8.16A: Carcinoma lip involving both the lower lip and upper lip. The upper lip lesion becomes more visible on everting the upper lip—'Kissing ulcer'. No lymph node metastases were noted in the neck.

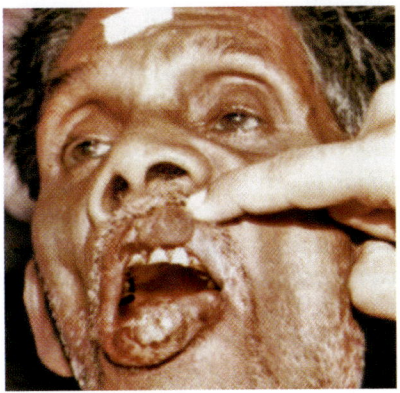

Fig. 8.16B: Same patient. The upper lip everted.

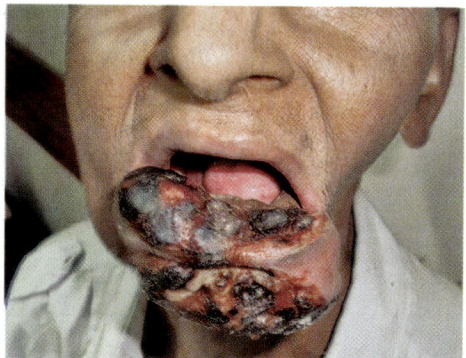

Fig. 8.17: Carcinoma lower lip extending to chin and upper neck.

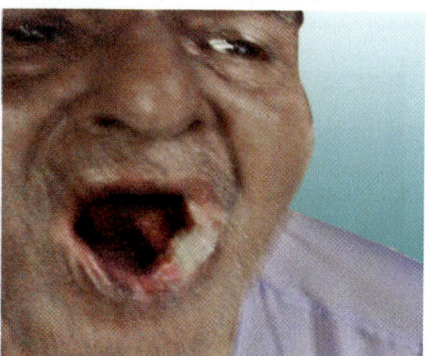

Fig. 8.18: Carcinoma of the angle of the mouth and lower lip—left side, developing over chronic fissure.

Rarely basal-cell carcinoma, adenocarcinoma or malignant melanoma may occur.

Spread

Local spread

It may occur and it is more on the surface than in the substance of the lip. Because of close contiguity, the jaws may be invaded directly.

Lymphatic spread

- *From the lower lip* to the submental and submandibular lymph nodes, and later to the jugulodigastric lymph nodes.
- *From the upper lip,* spread occurs early to the preauricular, submandibular and later to the deep cervical lymph nodes.
- *From the angle of the mouth,* spread occurs both above and down, and *so carcinoma situated at this site is more malignant.*

Metastasis, however, is slow, and 80 to 85% patients show no sign of lymph node metastasis within the first year.

Blood spread

Very rare.

Special investigation

- Blood for WR and Kahn, to exclude syphilis, because carcinoma may supervene on preexisting syphilitic sore. *Carcinoma supervening on a syphilitic sore is almost always radioresistant.*
- Edge biopsy.
- FNAC of lymph nodes.

Differential diagnosis

1. Simple papilliferous wart which may itself be a premalignant condition.
2. Keratoacanthoma.
3. *Chancre (syphilitic sore): The lip is the commonest extragenital site for a chancre.* It is accompanied by local oedema and enlarged regional lymph nodes. Carcinoma may supervene on preexisting syphilitic sore.
4. Haemangioma.
5. Lymphangioma.
6. Herpes simplex.
7. Mucous cyst.

Treatment

It includes:
1. Management of the primary lesion
2. Management of the lymph nodes.

Management of the primary lesion

1. In early cases without glandular metastasis, *radiotherapy is the treatment of choice* and the prognosis is extremely favourable. *If commissure is involved* radiotherapy is preferred due to better functional and cosmetic results.
2. *Excisional surgery is indicated:*
   - If radiotherapy is not available.
   - When the patient is unable to attend the radiotherapy clinic regularly as he resides in a place which is far away from the clinic.
   - In late cases.

- Recurrence after irradiation.
- Carcinoma lip invading the lower jaw.
- Carcinoma supervening on a leukoplakic patch.
- Carcinoma supervening on syphilitic sore.

Principle

The tumour is removed together *with a 1 cm margin of surrounding healthy tissue,* by means of a 'V' shaped incision which includes the full thickness of the lip.

When a more radical excision is indicated some form of plastic surgery are adopted for construction of a new lip (swinging or rotation flaps from the cheek or neck).

Management of the lymph nodes

1. *If not palpable,* only observe at a regular interval of one month.
2. *If palpable, mobile, but not hard,* it may be due to infection. So, a course of antibiotics for 3 weeks is given. If no response, block dissection of the neck.
3. *If palpable, hard and mobile,* and suspected to be due to metastasis – block dissection.
4. *If palpable and fixed* – radiotherapy.

Prognosis

80% 5 years survival rate with surgery or radio-therapy *when cervical lymph nodes are not involved.*

Note

CA tongue <2 cm – excision
CA lip <1 cm – excision $\Big]$ Better choice

CARCINOMA OF THE CHEEK

- Squamous cell carcinoma can occur in any part of the mucous membrane of the mouth including the inner aspects of the cheek.
- More common in males than in females.
- Commonly found in Indian subcontinent, mostly Eastern races who are in the habit of chewing the betel nut with lime and store the squid thereof in the cheek. Also common in people who use 'Khainy' – a mixture of roasted tobacco with lime.
- In Western countries, it is more common among the people who smoke heavily (specially pipe) while drinking alcohol.
- Chutta cancers inside the mouth – common in persons who smoke with the lightened end of the Biri or cigarette keeping inside the mouth while drinking alcohol.
- The early symptoms are minimal and so are frequently ignored until there is pain and difficulty in speaking or eating.
- *The patient may present with:*
  · A non-healing fissure mostly at the angle of the mouth

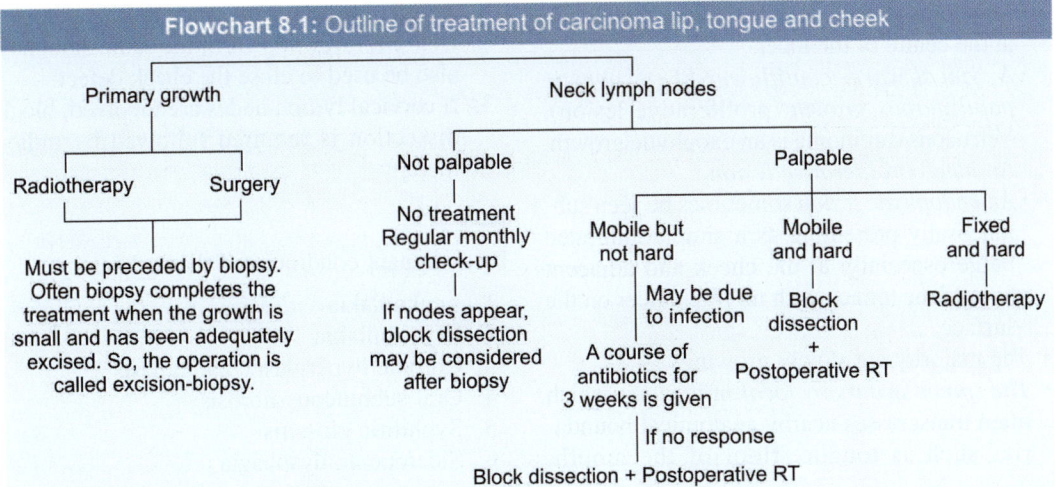

Flowchart 8.1: Outline of treatment of carcinoma lip, tongue and cheek

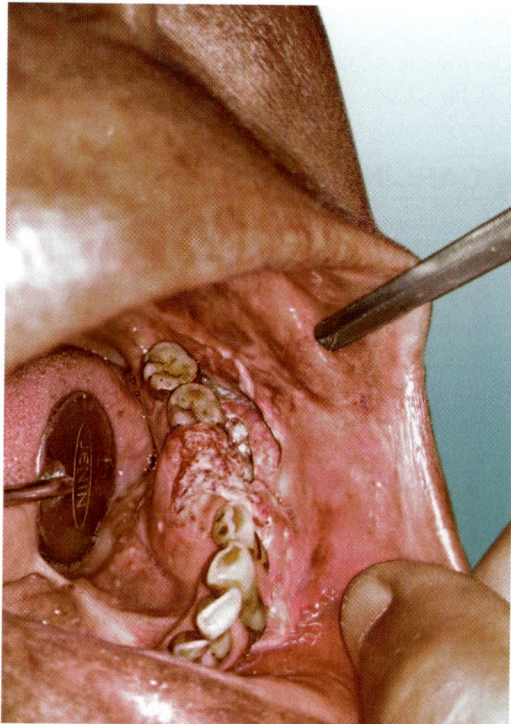

Fig. 8.19: Leukoplakia near the angle of the mouth over the left buccal cavity with growth below the left inner gum extending to the floor of the mouth: Carcinoma developing on leukoplakia. Bimanual palpation will confirm the site, size, consistency and extension of growth.

- A typical non-healing malignant ulcer with everted edge and induration both at the base as well as at the edge. There may be slough at the centre of the ulcer.
- *A typical warty cauliflower-like exophytic papilliferous growth* (proliferative lesion). Verrucous carcinoma is an exophytic growth.
- *An ulceroproliferative lesion.*
- *An endophytic lesion* sometimes be seen submucosally presenting as a simple indurated bulge especially at the cheek and adjacent base of the tongue with no frank ulcer on the surface.
- The majority are slowly growing.
- *The spread occurs by local infiltration* which often transgresses nearby anatomical boundaries such as tongue, floor of the mouth,

mandible and overlying skin. The skin may fungate with multiple sinuses.
- Cervical lymph nodes are commonly involved following a secondary spread.

Distant metastasis is rare and late, but *local recurrence rate is high.*

Treatment

1. *Radiotherapy:* Squamous cell carcinoma of cheek is radiosensitive. *In early cases without lymph node metastasis,* radiotherapy may be tried first after confirmation of biopsy.
   - *Interstitial irradiation* may be given by Iridium wire – brachytherapy.
   - *External irradiation* is given by megavoltage machines – teletherapy.
2. *Surgery:* Excisional surgery is indicated in:
   - Meagre facilities of radiotherapy
   - Late cases
   - Recurrence after radiotherapy
   - Residual tumours.

   Wide excision of the tumour which includes removal of tumour with 2 cm of the normal tissues around, with or without bone.

   The resulting defect following excisional surgery is made good *by rotational flap,* reflecting a *flap of skin from the temporal region* or *by pedicle grafts.* When the skin from the temporal region is taken the *buccal aspect of the cheek becomes lined by the skin. Deltopectoral flap* from the same side may also be used to close the cheek defect.
3. If cervical lymph nodes are involved, block dissection is required followed by radiotherapy.

Note

Premalignant conditions of the oral cavity:

1. Leukoplakia
2. Erythroplakia
3. Chronic hyperplastic candidiasis
4. Oral submucous fibrosis
5. Syphilitic glossitis
6. Sideropenic dysphagia

7. Oral lichen planus
8. Discoid lupus erythematosus
9. Dyskeratosis congenita

Note

Treatment of premalignant lesion:

- Leukoplakia:
  · Early lesion – stop all the predisposing factors
  · Antioxidants – retinoids and β-carotene orally for a prolonged period
  · If not improved within 6 months, cryo or laser total excision biopsy is advised.
- Erythroplakia:
  · Highly premalignant.
  · Early cryo or laser excisional biopsy is advised.
- Submucous fibrosis:
  · Surgical division of the bands and skin grafting.

Note

Chronic hyperplastic candidiasis is a fungal infection leading to *multiple dense white plaques* at the angle of the mouth and inner aspect of cheek just beneath the labial corner. This plaque can be partially rubbed off, *thus differentiating this condition from leukoplakia.*

Note

Oral submucous fibrosis – endemic in Asia due to hypersensitivity to spices: Pan with betel/areca nut with lime or tobacco (Khainy with lime) keeping inside the mouth for prolonged time during walking and working hours.

Note

Lingual thyroid: Characteristic features

- A round reddish swelling may be seen at the back of the tongue at and around the foramen caecum of the tongue containing thyroid tissue *– the thyroid diverticulum starts at the foramen caecum.*
- It may be enlarged in size and causes impairment of speech, dysphagia, respiratory obstruction and haemorrhage.
- *When doubt arises*, L-thyroxine replacement therapy can be given to reduce the size of the swelling.

Note

During excision of a medium or large lesion, e.g. haemangioma or carcinoma of tongue/oral cavity: *Preliminary bilateral control of external carotid arteries are preferred before excision to control haemorrhage.*

Table 8.1: Common ulcers of the tongue and their differential diagnosis

Points	Dyspeptic	Traumatic	Tuberculous	Syphilitic (tertiary)	Malignant
1. Age	Any age	Any age	Young adults	Young adults	Elderly
2. Site	Usually at the tip but may occur at any site with or without ulcers in the lip or cheek	Usually at the margin of the tongue, commonly towards the back	May occur at any site – margin, tip or dorsum of the tongue	Dorsum of the tongue mostly towards the base usually in the midline	Usually at the margin, common in anterior two-thirds of the tongue. May occur on the dorsum when super-imposed on chronic superficial glossitis
3. Symptoms	Features of dyspepsia	Presence of a sharp tooth or ill-fitted denture causing repeated trauma	Features of tuberculous toxaemia	History of exposure, abortion or miscarriage	Excessive salivation, difficulty in articulation and speech, ankylo-glossia, lump in the neck
4. Pain and tenderness	Exquisite	Marked	Exquisite	Painless	Early – painless. Late – painful and may be referred to ear
5. Shape	Small and circular	Any shape according to the shape of traumatic agent	Oval or circular	Oval or circular	Irregular
6. Number	Single or multiple	Single	Multiple	Single	Usually single; may be multiple when super-imposed on chronic superficial glossitis
7. Depth and size	Shallow and small	Moderate	Shallow and moderate	Deep and may be large	Early – shallow and small. Late – moderate
8. Edge of the ulcer	Oedematous	Oedematous	Undermined	Punched out	Rolled out and everted
9. Floor	Covered by red granulation tissue	Covered with slough	Covered with pale granulation tissue	Covered with washed leather slough	Covered with necrotic debris and looks dirty grey

(Contd.)

	Dyspeptic	Traumatic	Tuberculous	Syphilitic (tertiary)	Malignant
10. Discharge	Thin and watery	Often purulent	Thin and watery	Greyish white	Products of necrosis, thick and sometimes purulent. The discharge is offensive
11. Induration in the base and in the wall	Nil	Very slight	Nil	Very slight	Marked
12. Neck lymph nodes	Nil	Nil unless secondarily infected when the lymph nodes are firm and tender	Enlarged and matted with or without cold abscess	Enlarged, shotty and discrete. There may be enlarged epitrochlear and occipital lymph nodes	Early – nil. Late – enlarged and stony hard, may be fixed
13. Investigation	Stool – to exclude amoebiasis, irritable bowel syndrome	For presence of sharp tooth or ill-fitted denture	1. Routine blood for Hb% TC, DC and fasting ESR 2. Chest X-ray 3. Sputum for AFB 4. Mantoux test 5. Examination of the ulcer under magnifying glass – ulcer appears to be surrounded by minute sentinel tubercles	Blood for W.R. and Kahn	Blood for WR and Kahn Cancer may develop over a syphilitic sore
14. Response to	Responds to treatment of dyspepsia	Usually heals after removal of source of irritation, e.g. sharp tooth	Responds to anti-Koch's treatment	Responds to anti-syphilitic treatment	No response to conservative treatment. Surgery is the method of choice in most cases

Postpertussis ulcer:
1. Occurs in children following whooping cough.
2. Ulcer is confined mostly on the frenum linguae.

Herpetic ulcer:
1. Common in children and young adults
2. Occurs due to herpetic affection of the lingual nerve.
3. To start with there is unilateral acute neuralgic pain on the affected side.
4. Followed a few hours later by appearance of a vesicle which later on bursts to form *a very painful superficial ulcer.*

Simple ulcers due to glossitis:
1. Ulcer is usually single, known as smoker's patch.
2. Occurs in chronic superficial glossitis.
3. *Burning pain during taking of food.*

Umbilicus and Abdominal Wall

UMBILICUS

The umbilicus is represented by a depressed scar in the midline of the anterior abdominal wall. It is a deficiency formed due to meeting of the four folds of embryo – head-fold, tail-fold and two lateral folds. Through this deficiency, the umbilical cord connects the foetus with the mother. This deficiency transmits two sets of structures:

1. Vitelline components
2. Body stalk components.

Vitelline components consist of:
- the vitelline duct;
- the vitelline vessels;
- the splanchnic layer of the intra-embryonic mesoderm forming the coverings of the vitelline structures.

Body stalk components consist of:
- allantoic diverticulum – which later becomes urachus;
- umbilical vessels;
- extra-embryonic mesoderm of the connecting stalk which gives rise to Wharton's jelly by mucoid degeneration.

VITELLOINTESTINAL DUCT

It is a tubular outgrowth of the yolk sac which connects the extra-embryonic part of the yolk sac

with primitive midgut. During the 12th week of the intrauterine life when the gut returns from the extra-embryonic coelom the vitellointestinal duct separates from the intestinal loop and ultimately gets obliterated and disappears.

Anomalies

The vitellointestinal duct occasionally persists and gives rise to one of the following complications (Fig. 9.1).

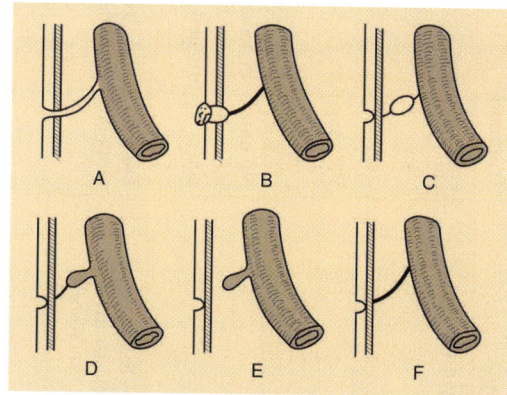

Figs 9.1 A to F: Different anomalies of vitello-intestinal component of umbilicus. A, intestinal fistula; B, umbilical adenoma; C, enterocystoma; D and E, Meckel's diverticulum; F, remnant of V.I. duct persists as intraperitoneal fibrous band—vitello-intestinal band.

1. It remains patent throughout its whole length giving rise to *umbilical fistula* – intestinal fistula (Fig. 9.1A) due to patent vitello-intestinal duct.
   - The fistula discharges mucous, and rarely faeces – ***umbilical faecal fistula***. The discharge is usually noticed in the first few weeks or months of life.
   - Occasionally, intestinal parasites such as *Ascaris lumbricoides* may extrude from the umbilicus.
   - It may be possible to cannulate the fistula. The catheter goes into the intestines.
   - There could be double intussusception through the umbilicus rarely.
   - The fistula may close spontaneously when the lumen of the communicating tract is narrow.
   - *Sometimes the fistula persists, when the abdomen should be explored at the age of 6 months, and the patent duct should be excised in toto along with a segment of ileum.*

2. Sometimes small portions of the duct near the umbilicus remain patent, the rest being obliterated towards the intestinal end. This gives rise to a sinus that discharges mucous. The epithelial lining of this patent sinus may be everted to form an **adenoma or raspberry tumour** (Fig. 9.1B).

3. Sometimes both the umbilical and the intestinal ends of the duct become obliterated, but the central portion remains patent and continues to secrete mucus giving rise to an intra-abdominal cyst – **enterocystoma** (Fig. 9.1C).

4. Sometimes the patency of the intestinal end of the vitellointestinal duct gives rise to **Meckel's diverticulum** at the antimesenteric border of intestine usually 20–35 cm above the ileocaecal junction. This diverticulum may or may not be attached to the umbilicus (Figs 9.1 D and E).

5. With its lumen obliterated or unobliterated the vitellointestinal duct provides an **intra-peritoneal band** which is a potential danger, for intestinal obstruction is liable to occur. The obstruction results from a coil of small intestine passing under or over, or becoming twisted around, the band (Fig. 9.1F).

6. Such a band may contract and pull a Meckel's diverticulum into a congenital umbilical hernia.

7. Rarely the vitellointestinal remnant connected to the Meckel's diverticulum, but not attached to the umbilicus, become adherent to, or knotted around another loop of small intestine, and so causes intestinal obstruction.

8. Very rarely a cord-like structure may stretch from the umbilicus across the ileum to end in the mesentery. This is an obliterated vitelline artery but not the vitellointestinal duct.

9. Very rarely, there may be stenosis/atresia of the ileum at the site of attachment of the duct.

Note

Causes of faecal fistula through the umbilicus:
- Patent vitellointestinal duct
- Neoplastic disease – carcinoma of colon or small gut infiltrating the umbilicus
- Abdominal tuberculosis
- Crohn's disease
- Intra-abdominal abscess may point to the umbilicus resulting in faecal fistula

ALLANTOIS

It is a tubular diverticulum from the yolk sac passing from the cloaca through the umbilicus and the umbilical cord to end blindly at the placenta. *The part within the body forms the urachus and the bladder except the trigone.* The remainder disappears.

As the bladder descends into the pelvis the urachus becomes obliterated and turns into a fibrous remnant which is known as median umbilical ligament. This ligament lies between the transversalis fascia and the peritoneum.

Anomalies (Fig. 9.2)

1. The urachus occasionally remains patent and communicates with the umbilicus leading to umbilical fistula through which the urine is discharged – *urinary fistula*. Though the patent urachus is a congenital lesion, *urinary*

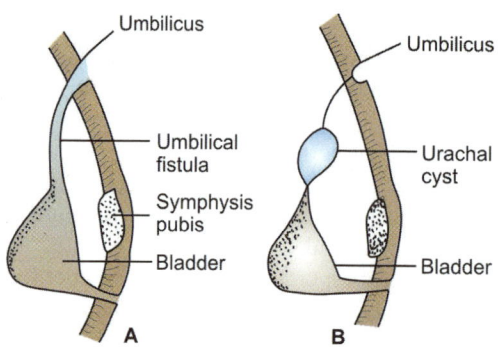

Figs 9.2 A and B: Various anomalies of the allantois.

fistula develops only when there is obstruction to the flow of urine in the distal urinary passage, i.e. the neck of the bladder to downwards, e.g. posterior urethral valve. A fistulogram will confirm the diagnosis. *The treatment is directed to remove the distal obstruction, e.g. posterior urethral valve first, which helps in the spontaneous closure of the fistula.* If the leak still continues, umbilectomy and excision of the urachus down to the apex of the bladder are performed.

2. Rarely, the central portion of the urachus remains patent with the umbilical and vesical ends obliterated. This is a *urachal cyst.*

DISEASES OF THE UMBILICUS

1. *Umbilical hernia* – commonest.
   - Congenital
     – Exomphalos
     – Congenital umbilical hernia
   - Acquired
     – Infantile umbilical hernia
     – Adult umbilical hernia (*see* Chapter 10)
2. *Anomalies of vitelline components*
3. *Anomalies of body stalk components*
4. *Umbilical fistula*
5. *Umbilical sinus* – pilonidal sinus
6. *Inflammation*
   - Umbilical granuloma
   - Umbilical dermatitis or omphalitis
7. *Neoplasm*
   - Benign
     – Umbilical adenoma
     – Endometrioma

- Malignant
  – Primary carcinoma
  – Secondary carcinoma
8. *Umbilical calculus*
9. *Eversion* (e.g. *in ascites*)

ENTEROCYSTOMA

Arising from the vitelline component, it is a pathological condition arising from the patent central portion of the vitellointestinal duct (Fig. 9.1C). It gives rise to *intra-abdominal cyst.* Through a band it is fixed to the umbilicus and to the small intestine when the small intestine may wind around this band and cause intestinal obstruction.

The patient presents with a small, spherical, mobile swelling deep to the umbilicus.

Treatment

Excision of the cyst along with the band *to avoid future intestinal obstruction.*

URACHAL CYST

Arising from the body stalk components, it is a rare pathological condition *arising from the patent central portion of the urachus* with the umbilical and vesical ends obliterated. It also gives rise to intra-abdominal swelling.

The patient presents with a small immobile swelling in the hypogastrium deep to the umbilicus. The small intestine can twist around the cyst and causes intestinal obstruction.

Treatment

Excision of the cyst to avoid future intestinal obstruction.

UMBILICAL FISTULAE

Causes

1. *Faecal:*
   - Patent vitellointestinal duct – already discussed – *resulting in serous/faecal fistula. This should be operated at 6 months of age.*
   - Neoplastic ulceration due to direct infiltration by carcinoma of the transverse colon – resulting in faecal fistula.

- Neoplastic ulceration infiltrating the underlying bowel – faecal fistula.
- Tuberculous peritonitis which may give rise to serous discharge.
- Crohn's disease.
- Actinomycosis.

2. *Urinary:* Patent urachus – urinary discharge – already discussed.
3. *Biliary:* Gallbladder perforating at the fundus and *sometimes discharging stone and bile* also – biliary discharge.
4. *Iatrogenic:* If a gauze piece and/or an instrument was accidentally left behind in the abdomen during abdominal operation.

UMBILICAL GRANULOMA (Fig. 9.3)

It is a chronic infection of the umbilical cicatrix following severance and tying off of the umbilical cord. By the end of first week after birth, the dry umbilical cord separates following tying off. Either delay in separation or inadequate desiccation, the cord remnant can permit infection at the base and *lead to granuloma formation.* This granuloma prevents the raw area from becoming epithelialised.

The baby presents with a pouting umbilicus surmounted by a red or pink, moist mass of granulation tissue. The granuloma discharges serous fluid. It is friable and bleeds on touch (Fig. 9.3).

Differential diagnosis
Umbilical adenoma or raspberry tumour.

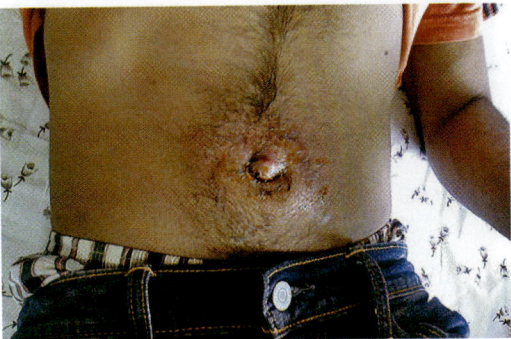

Fig. 9.4: Pyogenic granuloma at umbilicus. Note inflammatory changes around the umbilicus.

Treatment
Cauterisation: Either chemical cauterisation with silver nitrate stick or copper sulphate or diathermy cauterisation followed by dry dressing usually destroys the umbilical granuloma. *Excision is rarely necessary.*

If the granuloma persists or recurs in spite of the above treatment, one should suspect an umbilical adenoma or a sinus/fistula.

RASPBERRY TUMOUR (Figs 9.5 and 9.6)
(*Syn.* Umbilical adenoma; enteroteratoma)

It is a pathological condition arising from the patent distal segment (i.e. near the umbilicus) of the vitellointestinal duct (Fig. 9.1B). The majority of the proximal duct disappears.

The mucosa of the patent duct prolapses through the umbilicus and gives rise to a soft

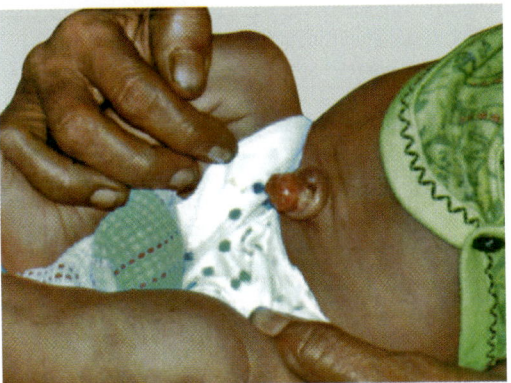

Fig. 9.3: Umbilical granuloma in a child.

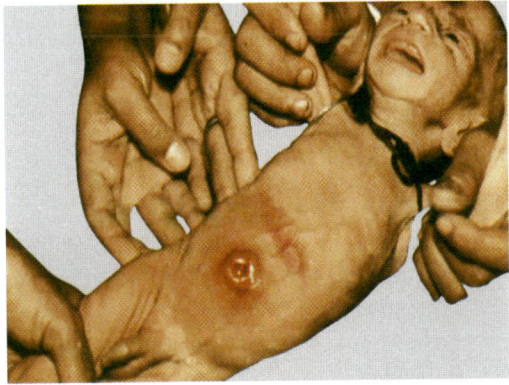

Fig. 9.5: Raspberry tumour. D/D: umbilical granuloma

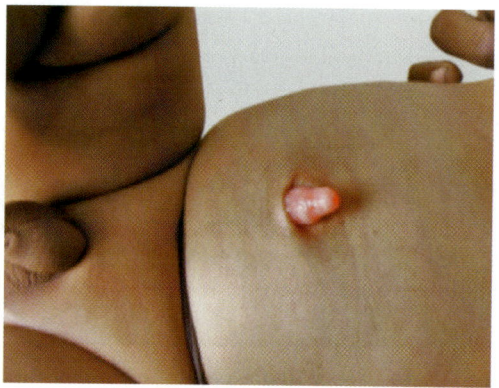

Fig. 9.6: *Raspberry tumour—note the excessive prolapse of the mucosa from the patent distal segment.*

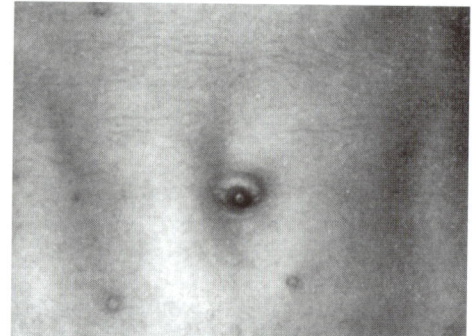

Fig. 9.7: Umbilical fistula discharging watery discharge—? urachal fistula. This patient gave history of good urinary outflow.

pink tumour which looks like a raspberry, hence the name. Histological picture usually consists of small bowel mucosa, i.e. columnar epithelium rich in goblet cells.

Diagnostic criteria

1. *Age: Infancy*, rarely it may occur in later life.
2. A soft fleshy mass, pinkish in colour (raspberry-like), situated at the pit of umbilicus.
3. The mass may be pedunculated or sessile.
4. The mass is moist with mucus and tends to bleed.
5. There may be serosanguineous discharge from the umbilicus.
6. Intestinal obstruction may occur, if there is an associated intra-abdominal band.
7. Meckel's diverticulum may be coexistent and should be excluded by a barium meal, if possible.

Differential diagnosis

Umbilical granuloma.

Treatment

1. If the tumour is pedunculated, a ligature is tied around its base. In a few days the polypus drops off.
   If there is recurrence, umbilectomy is indicated.
2. Some groups advocate umbilectomy as the first choice of treatment.

3. Others advocate exploration of the abdomen routinely, because the tumour sometimes is associated with a patent vitellointestinal duct or a vitellointestinal band along with the Meckel's diverticulum.

So, *after exploration of the abdomen*, umbilectomy, total excision of vitellointestinal duct, Meckel's diverticulum along with wedge resection of adjacent ileum followed by end-to-end anastomosis of the resected margin of ileum may be required.

Causes of discharge from umbilicus

Nature of the discharge	Cause
Serous/purulent discharge	Umbilical granuloma Umbilical adenoma
Faeculent discharge (usually with faeculent smell)	Patent vitellointestinal duct
Clear fluid (smells of urine)	Patent urachus
Blood discharge	Raspberry tumour; endometrioma of the umbilicus; umbilical granuloma; umbilical calculus; secondary carcinoma of the umbilicus

ENDOMETRIOMA OF THE UMBILICUS

It is a pathological condition where there is presence of ectopic endometrial glands in the umbilicus.

Diagnostic features

1. It occurs in women between 20 and 45 years of age.
2. There is a small fleshy mass at the umbilicus.
3. The mass becomes painful and *bleeds at each menstruation* – a typical history which clinches the diagnosis.
4. Occasionally, an umbilical endometrioma is associated with endometriomas in the uterus or ovary.

Treatment

When solitary, umbilectomy will cure the condition.

UMBILICAL CALCULUS

It is inspissated desquamated epithelium which collects in a deep recess of the umbilicus and gives rise to inflammation and often bloodstained discharge. The calculus is black in colour.

Treatment is to dilate the orifice and extract the calculus. If recurrence or there is persistent umbilical sepsis or abscess – umbilectomy.

NEOPLASMS OF THE ABDOMINAL WALL

• Benign
• Malignant

Benign tumours of the abdominal wall may arise from any of the anatomical structures contained in it. Examples are lipoma, fibroma, neurofibroma, haemangioma etc. These are treated in the same manner as in other locations.

The most characteristic benign tumour of abdominal wall is the Desmoid tumour.

Primary malignant tumours of the abdominal wall are extremely uncommon. However, rarely one may come across fibrosarcoma of the abdominal wall.

DESMOID TUMOUR

Greek: *desmos* = tendon; *eidos* = appearance

The tumour is so called because it looks like a tendon in its appearance and texture.

It is a *benign, non-capsulated fibrous tumour* arising in the fibroblasts of the musculoapo-neurotic structures of the abdominal wall,

especially below the level of umbilicus (*particularly in the sheath of the rectus abdominis muscle*). It is notorious for recurrence in spite of apparently adequate excision. So, it is also known as '*recurrent fibroid of Paget*'.

The tumour may also be *extra-abdominal* when it can involve the musculoaponeurotic structures in the region of the shoulder, neck, the medial side of the thigh, buttocks and chest.

Aetiology

Exact aetiology is not known.

1. *Common in women (80%):* Particularly middle-aged multiparous women, the reason being repeated trauma caused by stretching of the muscle fibres during pregnancy. *Estrogen stimulates desmoid growth.*
2. May occur in the scars of old hernial or other abdominal operation scar – *recurrent fibroma*.
3. A small haematoma of the abdominal wall due to trauma may be a precipitating factor. However, haemosiderin pigment is absent in this lesion.
4. In certain cases of familial polyposis coli this condition may be noted along with sebaceous cysts and frontal osteoma (*Gardner's syndrome*).

Pathology

1. It is essentially a benign, hard fibroma. It is composed of fibrous tissue and multi-nucleated plasmodial masses resembling foreign body giant cells.
2. It may appear as circumscribed – yet un-capsulated or diffusely infiltrating fibroma.
3. It may be so hard that it cracks when it is cut.
4. It is a slowly growing, non-capsulated tumour, but it infiltrates the surrounding muscle. Rarely it may extend through the muscles of the anterior abdominal wall to involve the bowel or bladder.
5. There may be myxomatous change when the tumour increases in size rapidly.
6. *Recurrence is very common* even after wide excision – particularly high after excision of the extra-abdominal desmoids.

7. But there is *no tendency to metastasize.*
8. *Spontaneous regression may occur with chemical or surgical menopause.*
9. Very rarely may undergo low grade sarcomatous change.

Diagnostic criteria

1. *Subject:* Common in middle-aged women.
2. Presents with lower abdominal lump, commonly in relation to rectus sheath – *painless hard parietal lump below the umbilicus.* Common after caesarean section.
3. The lump is present on one side of abdomen and *does not cross the midline.*
4. The lump may be well circumscribed or diffusely infiltrating.
5. The mass is firm to hard, smooth, discrete, non-tender and unattached to the skin. *The mass is irreducible.*
6. Parietal swelling as confirmed by *rising test* when the tumour becomes more prominent.
7. Clinically, it may be difficult to differentiate a desmoid tumour from a fibrosarcoma.
8. Diagnosis is confirmed by excision biopsy.
9. Rarely, there may be osteoma over the forehead – *examine head for bony lump.*

Differential diagnosis

- Interparietal hernia
- Spigelian hernia
- Incisional hernia
- Lipoma
- Neurofibroma
- Foreign body granuloma
- Abdominal wall sarcoma

Investigations

1. MRI provides information regarding the extent of the lesion and its relationship to the adjacent neurovascular structures and the underlying abdominal organs.
2. Trucut core biopsy with wide bore needle or incisional wedge biopsy – done at a site which can be included in the future elliptical incision during definitive surgery. *Tumour composed of spindle cells with variable amounts of collagen. The fibroblasts are highly differentiated but with no mitotic activity.*

3. *Oestrogen receptor status may be positive in this tumour.*

Treatment

1. *Wide excision* including a margin of surrounding healthy tissue of *at least 2.5 cm of normal aponeurosis all around.* The resulting defect is made good by using tantalum gauze or nylon, prolene or PTFE mesh in the repair.
2. *Radiotherapy is of controversial value*; may be of value to downstage the tumour before surgery – neoadjuvant.
3. *Drug therapy:*
   - Theophylline and chlorothiazide may be given as an adjunct to surgery to promote tumour shrinkage.
   - *Indomethacin,* a non-steroidal, antiinflammatory drug, which inhibits prostaglandin synthesis, *together with ascorbic acid* may be given. *It retards the tumour growth.*
   - *Chemotherapy is of no value.* It is reserved for unresectable clinically aggressive disease. Drugs are sulindac, antiestrogen (tamoxifen).

Note

Spontaneous regression of desmoid tumour may occur with chemical or surgical menopause.

SECONDARY CARCINOMA OF THE UMBILICUS

Secondary carcinoma at the umbilicus is not very common but its presence indicates an advanced, widespread malignant disease. *The primary tumour is commonly in the abdomen,* e.g. in the stomach, colon, pancreas or ovary or uterus. *Occasionally, a metastasis from the breast may be located here.*

The tumour cells reach the umbilicus by transperitoneal spread or via the lymphatics that run in the edge of the falciform ligament of the liver. *Umbilical metastasis is usually associated with multiple peritoneal metastases.*

Umbilical metastasis is present as a nodule at the umbilicus, in a patient who is losing weight and feels sick. *The metastatic nodule may ulcerate, bleed and become infected.* It may become attached to and infiltrate the underlying bowel. Ascites may develop. *Necrosis of the tumour then can cause an acquired umbilical fistula – intestinal fistula discharging faecal matter.*

Note

Sister Mary Joseph's nodule: Sister Mary observed this sign first *in a patient with a nodule(s) at the umbilicus* who was sick and losing weight due to intra-abdominal cancer. *This indicates poor prognosis.* There may be associated ascites (Fig. 9.8).

Causes of Sister Mary Joseph's nodule:

- Gastric cancer – commonest
- Colonic cancer
- Pancreatic cancer
- Ovarian cancer
- Uterine cancer

Note

Cullen sign: Bluish ecchymotic discoloration seen around the umbilicus due to diffusion of blood pigments – *methaemalbumin* from digested

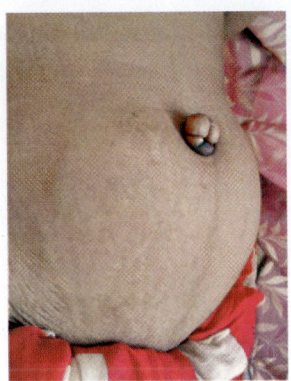

Fig. 9.8: Nodules at umbilicus—'Sister Mary Joseph nodules'. Secondary metastases from primary malignant tumour in the abdomen: Examine the abdomen for primary lesion and ascites. Examine the breasts also for any primary malignant lesion.

blood – typically noticed *following haemorrhagic pancreatitis.*

Similar discoloration is seen around the flanks – **Grey Turner's sign**.

These signs may also be noticed following retroperitoneal haemorrhage due to *blunt trauma, leaking aortic aneurysm* and may take 24 to 48 hours to appear.

Hernia

Hernia is an abnormal protrusion of the whole or a part of a viscus, commonly intestines, through a normal or abnormal opening in the wall of the cavity in which it is contained.

Internal hernia

Also known as concealed hernia, it is due to the protrusion of the viscus, commonly intestine, through *an internal defect* or *into a peritoneal recess* within the abdomen. *The different types are:*

1. Diaphragmatic hernia
    (a) *Hiatus hernia* – most common type
    (b) *Bochdalek hernia – posterolateral hernia.* It occurs through the pleuroperitoneal hiatus due to defective formation or failure of fusion of pleuroperitoneal membrane, which provides free communication between the pleural and peritoneal cavities. *It is more common on the left side.* It is the most common type of congenital hernia of diaphragm. The lung on the affected side is small and hypoplastic due to compression by bowel protruding into the chest.

    On the right side presence of right lobe of the liver under right diaphragm prevents development of diaphragmatic hernia on the right side.

    (c) *Retrosternal hernia* occurs through the space between xiphoid and costal margin of diaphragm.
    (d) *Congenital paraesophageal hernia – rolling hernia* through a defect in the diaphragm around the hiatus.
2. Hernia through the foramen of Winslow
3. Hernia through the peritoneal recess around:
    (a) Duodenojejunal junctions – *paraduodenal hernia*
        (i) Superior
        (ii) Inferior
        (iii) Lateral
        (iv) Medial – rare
    (b) Caecum-*paracaecal hernia – usually in association with malrotation*
        (i) Superior ileocaecal
        (ii) Inferior ileocaecal
        (iii) Retrocaecal
    (c) Sigmoid colon – *usually in association with malrotation.*
        A loop of small bowel may also pass through a defect in the sigmoid mesocolon.
    (d) *Hernia through a defect in the mesentery* following bowel resection and anastomosis when mesenteric defect is not closed properly.

4. Sliding hernia (*hernia en-glissade*) – *in which posterior wall of the sac is formed by a viscus. More common on the left side* with sigmoid colon sliding down along the sac. Often urinary bladder slides along with hernia. *Viscus is labile to be injured if the hernia sac is resected during surgery.*
5. Obturator hernia – common in females.

   Most of the internal herniae are present with intestinal obstruction – so, exploratory laparotomy can confirm the nature and site of the defect.

External hernia

An external abdominal hernia (Fig. 10.1) is protrusion of a peritoneal sac with or without a viscus from the peritoneal cavity through a weak part of the abdominal wall, *either congenital or acquired – accounting for 75% of hernias.*

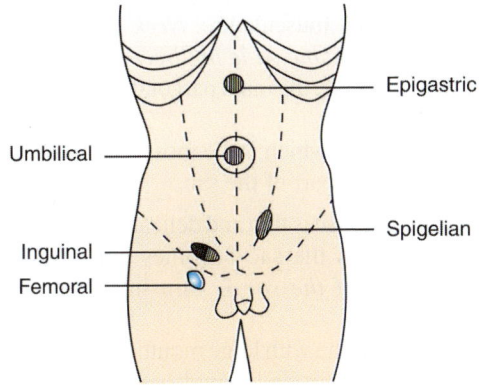

Fig. 10.1: External abdominal hernia.

Common external herniae are:

1. Inguinal
2. Incisional
3. Umbilical
4. Femoral

   Inguinal and femoral herniae are considered as groin hernia.

Less common types are:

1. Epigastric
2. Paraumbilical
3. Lumbar.

Rare types are:

1. Spigelian

2. Obturator – a herniation of peritoneal sac into the medial thigh through the obturator foramen.
3. Gluteal – between levator ani and coccygeous muscles.

Note

Cystocele, urethrocele and rectocele are also kinds of hernia common in females. These are herniations of urinary bladder, urethra and rectum into the vagina through the introitus.

Precipitating factors of abdominal wall hernia

Two factors are responsible for the production of a hernia:

A. Weakness of the abdominal wall, and
B. Continued or repeated increase in intra-abdominal pressure.

A. Weakness of the abdominal wall

It may be congenital or acquired.

Congenital weakness: Due to persistence of congenital peritoneal sac, e.g.

1. Persistence of patent processus vaginalis may lead to indirect inguinal hernia in males.
2. Patent canal of Nuck may lead to indirect inguinal hernia in females.
3. Incomplete obliteration of umbilicus may lead to umbilical hernia.
4. Congenital connective tissue disorders:
   - Prune belly syndrome (also presents with exstrophy of bladder).
   - Ehlers-Danlos syndrome.

   Both these conditions (*at 4*) *cause weakness of the abdominal wall.*

Acquired weakness: Weakness of the abdominal wall can result from:

1. Muscle weakness following obesity with fatty infiltration of the flat muscles, repeated pregnancy, wasting disease.
2. Poor wound healing leading to weakened wound due to inadequate closure with or without infection in the early postoperative period – *incisional hernia.*
3. Iatrogenic – surgical incision may cause division of the nerves which causes muscle

weakness, e.g. McBurney's incision for appendicectomy may cause divisions of the iliohypogastric or ilioinguinal nerve leading to right sided direct inguinal hernia.

4. Advancing age and chronic debilitating diseases. A significant number of men develop hernia at the age of 50 to 60 years.

B. The increased intra-abdominal pressure

It becomes continued or repeated in following conditions:

1. Chronic cough, e.g. bronchitis, bronchial asthma, COPD, emphysema, smoking, whooping cough in children.
2. Constipation – chronic straining during defaecation.
3. Bladder neck or urethral obstruction, e.g. enlarged prostate or stricture urethra – chronic straining during micturition.
4. Severe muscular effort, e.g. weight lifting or work-related physical exertion.
5. Parturition – multiple pregnancy.
6. Vomiting.
7. Ascites.
8. Obesity.
9. Other risk factors:
   • Family history of inguinal hernia
   • Sex – *indirect hernia more common in males*
   • Pre-term babies
   • History of hernia on one side is a risk factor for the other side – *so, also examine the opposite side which appears normal to exclude presence of an early hernia.*
   • Hernias are more common in smokers which may be a result of an acquired collagen deficiency and chronic cough.

Surgical pathology

An external abdominal hernia consists of:

1. A peritoneal sac
2. The coverings of the sac
3. The contents of the sac.

The sac is a pouch of stretched peritoneum which comes out through a gap in the abdominal musculature. *The sac consists of four parts* (Fig. 10.2).

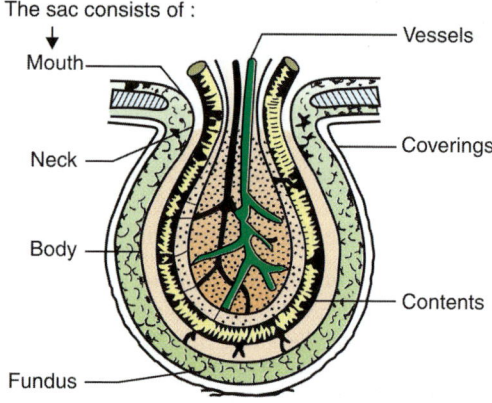

The sac consists of :

Fig. 10.2: Different parts of the hernial sac.

1. *The mouth,* i.e. the opening of the sac through which the contents enter the sac.
2. *The neck of the sac* which is the most constricted part and passes through the abdominal musculature. *Neck is narrow in indirect sac but wide in direct sac.*
3. *The body,* i.e. the main part of the sac holding the contents.
4. *The fundus* which is the most redundant and dependent part of the sac.

At first the sac is thin and delicate, but in long-standing cases the sac becomes considerably thick. *Body of the sac is thin in infants and children.*

Those herniae with large mouth lack the neck, e.g. direct hernia, incisional hernia – *usually reduced spontaneously on lying down.*

The *coverings* are the layers of the abdominal wall which cover the hernial sac. These depend on the site and type of hernia and usually include skin and muscles of the abdomen.

The *contents* may comprise one of the following.

1. Omentum (omentocele/epiplocele)
2. A loop of intestine commonly small (entero-cele)
3. Meckel's diverticulum (Littre's hernia)
4. A part of the circumference of intestinal wall (Richter's hernia)
5. Two loops of intestine in the manner of 'W' (Maydl's hernia)

6. A part of bladder wall (direct/femoral hernia)
7. Ovary with or without fallopian tube
8. Fluid – slight amount of fluid almost always present but it increases in presence of ascites. The fluid may be blood stained and infected when the hernia is strangulated.
9. Only a lobule of extraperitoneal fat – epigastric hernia without any sac.

Basic features of all herniae

1. They occur *through a weak spot* of the abdominal wall.
2. They have an *expansile impulse on coughing* (both visible and palpable).
3. They are *reducible – either on lying down or with manual pressure*. A reducible hernia is one in which the contained viscus can be returned to its original cavity.
4. A reducible hernia expands on coughing or straining – *cough impulse positive*.
   In irreducible hernia – cough impulse is absent.
5. *The contents of the hernia* are commonly gut or omentum. *In presence of gut*, the hernia will feel soft and it may gurgle during reduction. *In presence of omentum*, the hernia feels doughy.

Complications of the hernia

1. *Irreducibility or incarceration:* When the contents of the sac cannot be completely reduced and returned to its original domain because of:
   • adhesion formed between the contents and the sac wall or between the contents themselves;
   • growth of the omentum within the sac;
   • narrowing of the neck of the sac because of fibrosis, e.g. following continuous pressure of truss;
   • retention of faeces in the large intestine occupying the sac.
   Indirect inguinal hernia has higher incidence of incarceration than direct hernia.
   In a *simple irreducible hernia*, though the contents cannot be reduced, the blood supply

remains intact, and there are no symptoms of intestinal obstruction. So the operation is not very urgent.

2. *Obstruction:* Irreducibility + obstruction of the lumen of the contained bowel leading to intestinal obstruction. The features are:
   • The hernia is *irreducible* but *painless*.
   • The sac is *lax and not tender*.
   • *Cough impulse may be present.*
   • *Features of intestinal obstruction are present.*
   • Can precipitate strangulation if not treated early.
   Hernia is one of the commonest causes of intestinal obstruction. So, hernial sites should always be examined in a patient presenting with intestinal obstruction.
   Features of intestinal obstruction may be absent in case of omentocele, Richter's hernia, Littre's hernia.

3. *Strangulation:* Irreducibility + features of intestinal obstruction + arrest of blood supply to the contained intestine leading to gangrene. The features are:
   • The hernia is *irreducible* and *painful*.
   • The sac is *tense and tender*.
   • *Cough impulse absent.*
   • *Features of intestinal obstruction present* – pain abdomen, vomiting, abdominal distension, *rebound tenderness*.
   Strangulation is more likely to happen in a hernia with a narrow neck. Most strangulated herniae are therefore either inguinal or femoral, because these herniae have narrow necks. *Often, the sac contains the greater omentum* which may become gangrenous due to arrest of blood supply showing the features of strangulation but without the features of intestinal obstruction. *Strangulation without obstruction also noted in Richter's hernia.*
   Strangulation is a serious complication with a *chance of time-bound bowel gangrene and necrosis, unless relieved within 6 hours.*
   Both obstruction and strangulation are serious conditions and require urgent

operation. Bile vomiting, brownish or faeculent vomitus are *sinister signs.*

4. *Reduction-en-masse:* Sometimes, during forceful manual reduction of irreducible hernia, *the contents together with the covering sac gets pushed forcibly back into the abdominal cavity;* the bowel within the sac may be strangulated by the neck of the sac. Thus the symptoms of obstruction or strangulation may not be relieved.

5. *Incarceration:* Incarcerated hernia is *a variety of irreducible hernia where the content of the sac is large gut containing faeces.* The large gut is fixed in the sac because of its size or adhesions. Here, *the hernia can be indented like putty with the finger tip pressure* because of the scybalous content of the gut. Though the hernia is irreducible, obstruction or strangulation rarely occur. The chances of incarceration are greater with sacs with a narrow neck; thus, indirect herniae have higher incidence of incarceration than the direct herniae.

6. *Inflammation,* e.g. sepsis of the sac; when inflamed appendix or Meckel's diverticulum or salpinx become the contents of the sac.

7. *Compression or torsion of the omentum within the sac.* The omentum may become gangrenous due to arrest of blood supply showing the features of strangulation but without features of intestinal obstruction.

8. *Collection of fluid in the hernial sac –* hydrocele of the hernial sac.

9. Maydl's hernia.

10. *Sliding hernia: A hernia in which a portion of the wall of the hernia is comprised of an organ,* commonly the caecum, sigmoid colon or urinary bladder.

11. Recurrent hernia.

12. Bar to join the services or sports – particularly military, police, athletes or players.

Note

Intraparietal hernia – a groin hernia in which *the sac spreads out between the layers of the* *abdominal wall* instead of following the inguinal canal.

INGUINAL HERNIA

This is the most common type of abdominal hernia in both males and females. There are two types.

1. Indirect or oblique inguinal hernia.
2. Direct inguinal hernia.

Surgical anatomy

Inguinal canal

The inguinal canal (Fig. 10.3) is an oblique fibromuscular tunnel about 4 cm long in the lower part of the anterior abdominal wall, a little above and parallel to the inner half of the inguinal ligament. It passes downward and medially and extends from the deep inguinal ring to the superficial inguinal ring. The canal transmits the spermatic cord in males and the round ligament of uterus in females.

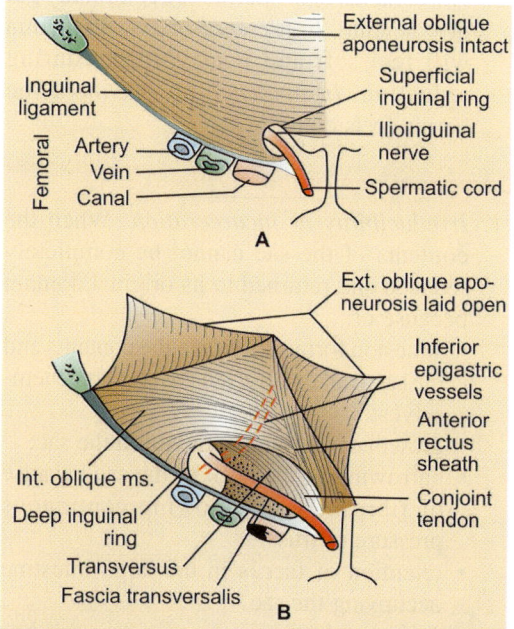

Figs 10.3 A and B: Anatomy of the inguinal canal. (A) External oblique aponeurosis intact; (B) External oblique aponeurosis laid open.

In infants, the superficial and deep inguinal rings are almost superimposed and the obliquity of the canal is only slight.

Boundaries

Anterior wall

1. Skin
2. Superficial fascia
3. External oblique aponeurosis – in its whole length
4. Internal oblique muscle – in its lateral third.

Posterior wall

1. Fascia transversalis – in its whole length
2. Conjoint tendon – in its medial half
3. Reflected part of inguinal ligament – in its medial third.

Conjoint tendon is the common tendon of insertion of internal oblique and transversus abdominis muscles.

Roof

The arched fibres of the internal oblique and transversus abdominis muscles.

Floor

1. Upper grooved surface of the inguinal ligament.
2. Upper surface of the lacunar ligament – at the medial end.

Superficial inguinal ring

It is a triangular aperture or slit in the external oblique aponeurosis situated 1 cm above and lateral to the pubic tubercle. It transmits the spermatic cord or round ligament, the ilioinguinal nerve, the genital branch of the genitofemoral nerve and the processus vaginalis when it persists. The external oblique aponeurosis extends over the spermatic cord as external spermatic fascia.

Deep inguinal ring

It is a U-shaped condensation of the fascia transversalis being incomplete above. It is situated 1 cm above the midpoint between the anterior superior iliac spine and symphysis pubis. *Clinically the ring lies 1 cm above the point where the femoral artery passes under the inguinal ligament, i.e. 1 cm above the femoral pulse felt.*

It transmits the spermatic cord or the round ligament, and the processus vaginalis when it persists. The fascia transversalis extends into the spermatic cord as internal spermatic fascia. The inferior epigastric artery courses up along the medial side of the ring.

The deep ring is the site through which indirect inguinal hernia occurs.

Hesselbach's triangle

This triangle is situated in the posterior wall of the inguinal canal. The triangle is bounded:

1. *medially* by the outer border of rectus abdominis muscle;
2. *laterally* by the inferior epigastric vessels;
3. *below* by the inner half of the inguinal ligament;
4. *floor* is formed by the fascia transversalis.

The triangle is almost bisected by the lateral umbilical ligament which is obliterated hypogastric artery. *Hesselbach's triangle is the site through which direct inguinal hernia occurs.*

Contents

1. *In male:* The spermatic cord.
2. *In female:* The round ligament of the uterus.
3. *Ilioinguinal nerve in both sexes:* It passes through the superficial inguinal ring along with the contents of the inguinal canal and it supplies the scrotum and mons pubis in males and labia majora and mons pubis in females.

Natural mechanisms preventing hernia

1. Obliquity of the canal.
2. Internal oblique muscle opposite the deep ring.
3. Shutter action of the arched fibres of internal oblique and transversus abdominis.
4. Plugging action of the spermatic cord due to contraction of the cremasteric muscle.
5. Sliding valve action of the U-shaped internal ring.
6. Pinch-cock mechanism by the arching fibres of the conjoint tendon, encircling the internal ring, shutting off any gap in the fascia transversalis.

7. Strong conjoint tendon in front of Hessel-bach's triangle also prevents direct inguinal hernia.
8. Both crura of external ring come together during muscular contraction.

INDIRECT INGUINAL HERNIA

The hernia sac associated with a patent processus vaginalis enters the inguinal canal through the weak deep inguinal ring lateral to the inferior epigastric artery. *The neck of the sac is lateral to the inferior epigastric artery.*

Indirect hernia is *usually congenital in origin* due to persistence of patent processus vaginalis; it appears at or soon after birth or may appear in adolescence.

Indirect hernia *may be acquired* when the sac is formed as an outpushing of the abdominal peri-toneum through the deep ring. *The acquired variety may occur at any age in adult life due to increased intra-abdominal pressure* following strenuous exercises, heavy weight lifting, straining at defaecation (chronic constipation) or at micturition (enlarged prostate, stricture urethra) or at coughing (chronic bronchitis).

An indirect hernia is covered by the layers of the spermatic cord.

Note

- The deep inguinal ring lies above and midway between the pubic tubercle and anterior superior iliac spine.
- A line which begins at a point midway between the symphysis pubis and the anterior superior iliac spine and extends to the umbilicus demarcates the path of the inferior epigastric artery as it arises from the external iliac artery and courses behind the rectus muscle.

Types of indirect inguinal hernia

The indirect hernia may be subdivided into:

- Bubonocele ⎫
- Funicular ⎬ Incomplete hernia
- Vaginal or complete hernia

Bubonocele (Fig. 10.4A)

The processus vaginalis is closed proximal to the superficial inguinal ring. The hernia is limited in the inguinal canal and so *appears as an inguinal swelling and appears like a bubo.* The knuckle of intestine has not yet emerged from the internal inguinal ring.

Funicular (Fig. 10.4B)

Here the processus vaginalis is closed at its lower end, so the sac of the hernia is separate from the sac of tunica vaginalis. The sac is closed and extends beyond the superficial inguinal ring but stops above the testis. *The testis lies below the hernia and can be felt separately from the contents of the hernial sac.*

Most of the indirect inguinal herniae belong to this category and are commonly seen in adults. *It is usually acquired but may be congenital.*

Vaginal hernia (Fig. 10.4C)

Also known as complete hernia. Here the processus vaginalis is patent throughout. Hence *the sac is continuous with the tunica vaginalis of the testis.* The hernia descends down to the bottom of the scrotum covering the testis in front and at the sides, *so the testis cannot be felt separately before reduction of hernial contents.*

Both the funicular and vaginal herniae appear as inguinoscrotal swellings. Bubonocele appears as an inguinal swelling.

Coverings of indirect inguinal hernia

From superficial to deep:

1. Skin
2. Superficial fascia. When the hernia comes out through superficial ring and descends into the scrotum – dartos muscle of the scrotum.
3. External spermatic fascia when the hernia comes out through the superficial inguinal ring.
4. Cremaster muscle/fascia.
5. Internal spermatic fascia.
6. Processus vaginalis or peritoneum – the sac.

Note

- Indirect inguinal hernia – most common of all forms of hernia.

- Indirect inguinal hernia is the most common hernia in children, adult men and women.
- Most common in the young male (~ 20 times).
- Laterality: Right side – 60%
                  Left side – 30%
                  Bilateral – 10%

Note

An inguinal hernia in a child is indirect type as it occurs in a patent processus vaginalis. Sometimes it may be incarcerated, obstructed or even strangulated. *So, inguinal hernia in a child should be repaired as early as possible once it comes to notice.*

Note

Hernia or cyst of the canal of the Nuck: *If the processus vaginalis persists in females*, it forms a small peritoneal pouch, known as *canal of Nuck, in the inguinal canal that may extend to labium majus. In female infants, such remnants can enlarge to form cysts in the inguinal canal.* This cyst may produce a bulge in the anterior aspect of labium majus and the potential to develop into an indirect inguinal hernia.

DIRECT INGUINAL HERNIA

The hernia protrudes directly through the weakness of fascia transversalis in the posterior wall of the inguinal canal in the Hesselbach's triangle. The direct hernial sac lies outside the cord (cf. indirect inguinal hernia) – behind, above or below the cord. *The neck of the sac lies medial to the inferior epigastric artery* – a differentiating point at operation from indirect hernial sac where the neck of the sac lies lateral to the artery. *The neck of the direct sac is wide.*

Direct herniae are mostly acquired in nature. It is found predominantly in the elderly males *due to increased intra-abdominal pressure leading to increased wear and tear of the conjoined tendon.*

A direct inguinal hernia seldom comes out through the superficial inguinal ring and thus it is unusual for the sac to descend into the scrotum (Fig. 10.7).

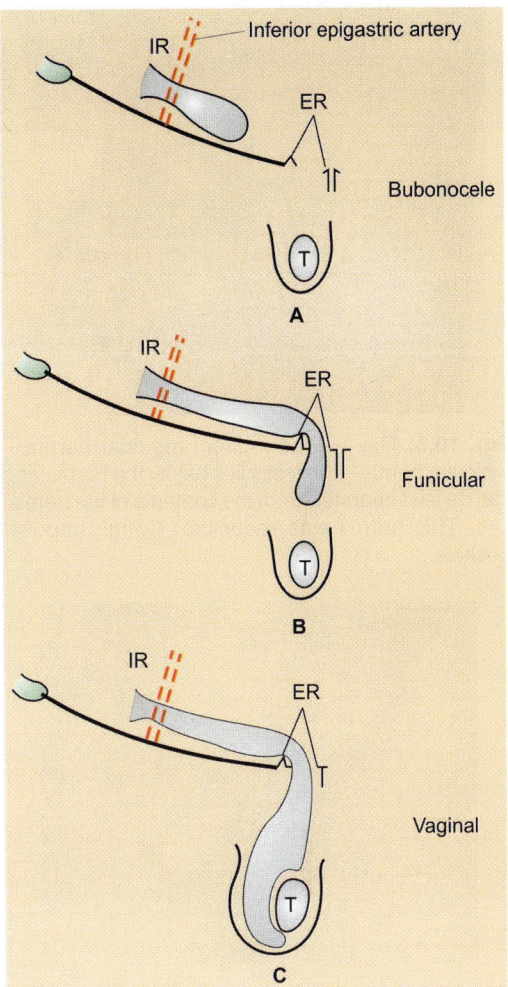

Figs 10.4 A to C: Different types of indirect inguinal hernia. IR, internal or deep ring; ER, external or superficial ring.

The neck of the direct hernial sac is wide and therefore the hernia appears immediately on standing and disappears again immediately when the patient lies down. *Moreover, because of this wide neck obstruction or strangulation is extremely rare.*

Note

Criteria of direct inguinal hernia

- Direct hernia is always acquired due to increased intra-abdominal pressure.

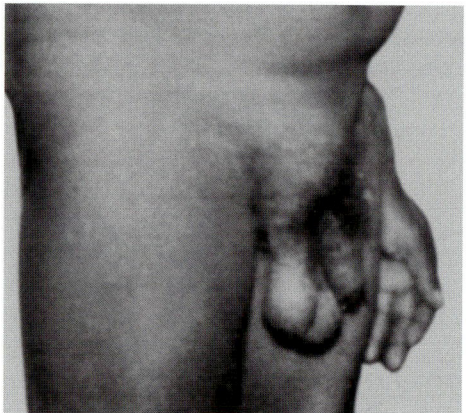

Fig. 10.5: Right-sided indirect inguinal hernia—funicular hernia—the testis lies below the hernia and can be felt separately from the contents of the hernial sac. This hernia was reducible. Cough impulse positive.

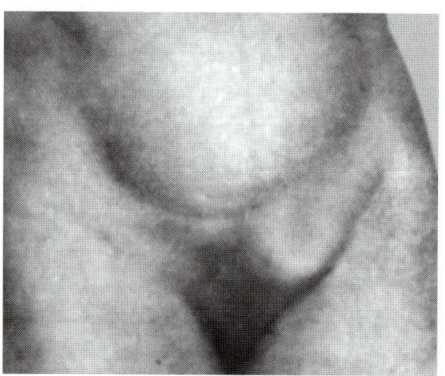

Fig. 10.6: Left incomplete indirect inguinal hernia in female: Bubonocele looks like a lymph node. Note the site of the swelling—this is in the inguinal region above the groin crease, i.e. above the inguinal ligament. On palpation the swelling will be found above and medial to the pubic tubercle (cf. femoral hernia). The swelling was reducible. Cough impulse positive. *Note:* Bubo is the swelling of the lymph node.

- Appears in elderly groups.
- May appear as bubonocele also.
- Very rare in women.
- Do not occur in children.
- Has no side predilection. Bilateral only in 12% cases.
- Less likely to undergo strangulation as the neck is wide.

Note

Causes of increased intra-abdominal pressure in old age are chronic constipation, difficulty in passing urine due to enlarged prostate, chronic cough due to bronchitis/asthma.

Coverings of direct inguinal hernia

From superficial to deep:

1. Skin
2. Superficial fascia
3. External oblique aponeurosis
4. Conjoint tendon when the sac passes medial to the lateral umbilical ligament
5. Fascia transversalis
6. Peritoneum – the sac. The sac may be thick and often the medial wall or the content may be urinary bladder.

The direct inguinal hernia lies behind the spermatic cord.

Diagnostic criteria of an uncomplicated inguinal hernia

1. *Age:* It occurs in all ages, from birth to elderly. *Indirect hernia* is more common in younger and adult life. *Direct hernia* is more common in elderly people.

    Indirect hernia is the most common of all forms of hernia. M : F = 20 : 1. More common on the right side.

2. *Sex:* Common in males.

3. *Symptoms:*
    - History of swellings in the groin – *inguinal swelling* which is gradually increasing in size. The swelling becomes more prominent on standing or straining and gets smaller or disappears on lying or on manipulation, unless it is complicated.
    - The swelling may expand and extend down to the scrotum – *inguinoscrotal swelling*.
    - Local discomfort or pain which gets worsened on strenuous effort. The pain may be aching sensation in the groin due to the stretching of the deep inguinal ring by the protruding viscus.
    - The pain may be dragging indicating omentocele. As the omentum is attached

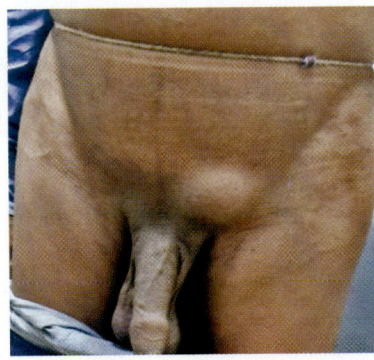

Fig. 10.7: Left-sided direct inguinal hernia in a young adult. Note the history of difficulty in passing urine common with stricture urethra.

to stomach and supplied by T12 nerve, *the pain may be referred to the umbilicus.*

- The swelling may be asymptomatic – the hernia may be accidentally discovered during a medical checkup.
- *Sudden severe pain in the hernia with vomiting and irreducibility indicates obstruction of the hernia.*
- History of chronic strain causing increased intra-abdominal pressure, e.g. cough, constipation and difficulty in passing urine should be enquired as these may be the cause of hernia formation.

Examination

The patient should be examined first in the standing (erect) position and then in lying down position (supine), if necessary.

1. (a) *Inguinal swelling* – indirect hernia: bubonocele or direct hernia (Fig. 10.4A).
   (b) Inguinoscrotal swelling – indirect hernia: funicular or vaginal hernia (Figs 10.4 B and C).
   (c) Inguinal hernia in females appears as *increased thickness of labium majus on palpation* when compared with the contralateral side (Fig. 10.6).
   The swelling may be unilateral or bilateral.
2. *Shape:* A bubonocele or direct hernia is globular in shape. A funicular or vaginal hernia is usually pyriform in shape.
3. *Expansile impulse on coughing at the root of the scrotum* (felt between the fingers and

the thumb) or *at the superficial inguinal ring* (felt with the thumb) when the patient is asked to cough – *visible and palpable in uncomplicated hernia.*

4. Non-tender if uncomplicated.
5. Consistency – depends on the contents of the sac: *soft, elastic and fluctuant, resonant on percussion* – if it contains gut.
   Firm and doughy, non-fluctuant and dull on percussion – if it contains omentum.
6. ***Getting above the swelling in presence of inguinoscrotal swelling.***
   - *To differentiate a scrotal swelling from inguinoscrotal swelling.*
   - With the patient standing, normally the spermatic cord is palpated between the thumb and the fingers at the root of the scrotum.
     (i) In case of scrotal swelling, e.g. hydrocele, the spermatic cord can also be felt easily, above the swelling – *so, getting above the swelling is possible.*
     (ii) In inguinoscrotal swelling, funicular and complete indirect hernia, *the spermatic cord cannot be felt nakedly or easily*, because it is covered antero-laterally by the sac, *so getting above the swelling is not possible.*
     On complete reduction of swelling, one can feel the cord at the root of the scrotum.
7. *Relation of the sac with pubic tubercle:* It is the *most important landmark* to differentiate inguinal hernia from femoral hernia.
   - *Inguinal hernia:* The neck of the sac is situated above and medial to the pubic tubercle.
   - *Femoral hernia:* The neck of the sac is situated below and lateral to the pubic tubercle.
8. *Reducibility:* All herniae are reducible unless complicated.
   - *On lying down*, the direct hernia usually reduces immediately and spontaneously, *but indirect hernia usually requires manipulation.*
   - A direct hernia reduces directly backwards.
   - An indirect hernia reduces in an upward,

backward and lateral direction on manipulation.

- *During reduction confirm the contents of the sac* – if there is gurgling sound, it is an enterocele; if the sac feels doughy, it is omentocele.
- *In enterocele*, during reduction the first part of the content is difficult to reduce but the latter part is easy to reduce. *It reduces with gurgle.*
- *In omentocele*, during reduction the first part is easy to reduce while the latter part is difficult to reduce.

  The comparison of enterocele and omentocele is summarised in Table 10.2.
- *After reduction:*
  – *Note the relation of the neck of the sac with the pubic tubercle.*

    In inguinal hernia, the neck of the sac lies medial to pubic tubercle.

    In femoral hernia, the neck of the sac lies lateral to pubic tubercle.
  – *Note the reappearance of the swelling on straining or coughing:*
    - In indirect hernia, the swelling reappears gradually and steadily in medial and downward directions.
    - In direct hernia, the swelling reappears immediately straightforward exactly where it was observed before.

9. *Deep ring occlusion test:*
   - *Anatomically,* deep ring is located *1 cm above the mid-inguinal point* – centre point between the anterior superior iliac spine and symphysis pubis.
   - **Identification of deep inguinal ring:** *Clinically it lies 1 inch above the femoral pulse felt below the inguinal ligament.*
   - After the reduction of hernia, the deep ring is occluded by the pressure of the thumb and the patient is asked to cough:
     (i) Indirect hernia: The swelling does not reappear, so the test is positive.
     (ii) Direct hernia: The swelling reappears immediately, so the test is negative.

10. *Invagination test:* After the hernia is reduced, the tip of the index finger can be invaginated into the neck of the scrotum and then pushed inside the inguinal canal through the superficial inguinal ring – *the patient is then asked to cough:*
    (i) Indirect hernia: A thrust will be felt at the tip of the finger.
    (ii) Direct hernia: A thrust will be felt at the pulp of the finger.

    Invagination test helps to diagnose an early case of incomplete hernia. It also helps to differentiate bubonocele and direct hernia from femoral hernia.

    Invagination test is not a must. When necessary, it should be performed very gently *not to cause any pain to the patient.*

    This test *cannot be done in female* as the labial skin is thick and not lax.

11. Examine the opposite side also to exclude hernia. *Direct hernia is often bilateral.*
12. Examine the testis, epididymis and spermatic cord after reduction of hernia.
13. Examine the tone of abdominal muscles by *head or leg rising test.* Also look for Malgaigne bulgings. Valsalva manoeuvre may be used to check the tone of the abdominal muscles.
14. Note for any evidence of chronic straining like chronic bronchitis, chronic constipation, enlarged prostate (per rectal examination), stricture urethra (palpation of bulbar urethra for thickening) with history of difficulty in passing urine.

Differential diagnosis

Depends on whether the swelling is *incomplete* or *complete.*

A. When the swelling is incomplete, i.e. *inguinal or groin swelling.*
B. When the swelling is complete, i.e. *inguino-scrotal swelling.*

Differential diagnosis of groin swellings

1. Inguinal hernia
2. Femoral hernia
3. Enlarged inguinal lymph nodes
4. Saphena varix
5. Femoral aneurysm

Table 10.1: Differences between indirect and direct inguinal herniae

Points	Indirect	Direct
• Age	At any age but common in infants and young adults.	Usually in the elderly persons. Does not occur in children. Rare in women.
• Site	Usually unilateral (30% bilateral).	Usually bilateral.
• Extent	May be incomplete or complete.	Usually incomplete. Does not descend into the scrotum.
• Entrance	Through the deep inguinal ring.	Through the floor of the Hesselbach's triangle.
• Exit	May be through the superficial inguinal ring. Can descend into the scrotum.	Rarely through the superficial inguinal ring.
• Relation with the inferior epigastric vessels	*Inferior epigastric vessels lie close to the medial site of the neck of the sac.*	*Inferior epigastric vessels lie lateral to the neck of the sac.*
• Relation with the spermatic cord	The sac lies within the coverings of the spermatic cord. The sac is anterior to the cord.	The sac lies outside the coverings of the spermatic cord. The sac is either behind, below or above the cord.
• Shape of the swelling	Usually pyriform shape, with the narrow end above and the broad base below.	Usually globular with the broad base above.
• Appearance of the swelling	Slowly appears on straining or coughing.	Easily pops out on standing, straining or coughing.
• Reducibility	Gradually reduces, may need manipulation.	Usually reduces immediately and spontaneously on lying down.
• Direction of reduction	Reduces upwards, then laterally and backwards.	Reduces upwards and backwards.
• Deep ring occlusion test after reduction	Positive, i.e. the swelling does not appear when the patient coughs.	Negative, i.e. the swelling reappears.
• Release of occlusion followed by coughing	The swelling appears first in the middle of inguinal region and then flows medially and ultimately turns down to the neck of the scrotum.	The swelling reappears straight forward exactly where it was before.
• Obstruction/strangulation	Common due to narrow neck of the sac.	Rare due to wide neck of the sac.

Table 10.2: Differences between enterocele and omentocele

Points	Enterocele (presence of intestine in the sac)	Omentocele (presence of omentum in the sac)
Inspection	Visible peristalsis is usually seen.	Peristalsis is never seen.
Palpation	Consistence is soft, elastic and fluctuant.	Consistence is firm, doughy and non-fluctuant.
Percussion	Usually resonant on percussion.	Dull on percussion.
Reducibility	Reduction is easy. The first part is difficult to reduce than the last part which slips in easily. Gurgling sounds can be heard during reduction.	Reduction is usually difficult. The first part reduces easily but the last part resents to be reduced. No gurgling sound is heard.
Auscultation	One may hear peristaltic sound.	No peristaltic sound can be heard.

6. Lipoma of the cord
7. Encysted hydrocele of the cord
8. Undescended or ectopic testis
9. Psoas abscess
10. Malgaigne's bulge.
11. Hydrocele of the canal of Nuck (in female).
12. Groin abscess.

Femoral hernia

The globular swelling is *below the inguinal ligament* and *below and lateral to the pubic tubercle.* Also the swelling is just medial to the femoral vessels. *In inguinal hernia* the swelling is above the inguinal ligament and *above and medial to the pubic tubercle.*

In femoral hernia the inguinal canal remains empty when invagination test through the superficial ring is performed. *The landmark to differentiate between inguinal hernia and femoral hernia is pubic tubercle.*

Enlarged inguinal lymph nodes

Enlarged lymph nodes are found below the inguinal ligament, usually multiple with irregular consistency. *Cough impulse is absent.* When tender and inflamed look for a septic focus on his leg, his lower abdomen, or his buttock. If suspected look for evidence of tuberculosis elsewhere.

Saphena varix

The swelling is below the inguinal ligament and associated with varicosities of the long saphenous vein. The swelling is soft and easily compressible (unless it is thrombosed), which fills up again when the pressure is released. On coughing the swelling imparts a fluid thrill. The swelling disappears on elevation of the limb with the patient lying down. *On auscultation a venous hum may be heard.*

Femoral aneurysm

Swelling is below the inguinal ligament and on palpation there is *expansile impulse corresponding with the radial pulse.* On auscultation a bruit may be heard.

Encysted hydrocele of the cord

A smooth elongated, tense cystic swelling. Not reducible. Cough impulse absent. *On traction of the testis the swelling comes down and becomes fixed. Transillumination is positive.*

Lipoma of the cord

Features are the same as those of the hydrocele of the cord but *transillumination is negative.*

Undescended or ectopic testis

Ipsilateral scrotum is empty. Cough impulse is absent unless there is a coexistent hernia. *Characteristic testicular sensation is present on pressure over the swelling.*

Psoas abscess

A fluctuant swelling below the inguinal ligament. Cross fluctuation positive when the swelling is associated with iliopsoas abscess. *The swelling may be partially reducible but there is no true expansile impulse on coughing.* There will be evidence of tuberculosis of the spine or hip on clinical and/or radiological examination.

Malgaigne's bulge

Malgaigne described a bulge in the inguinal region which occurs in old people with poor physique *but it has no cough impulse. Bulge is usually bilateral.* It may be the precursor of a direct inguinal hernia.

Differential diagnosis of inguinoscrotal swelling

1. Congenital hydrocele
2. Infantile hydrocele
3. Encysted hydrocele of the cord
4. Hydrocele of the canal of Nuck (in female)
5. Lipoma of the cord
6. Lymph varix or lymphangiectasis of the spermatic cord: Dilated, tortuous lymphatics of the cord.
7. Funiculitis
8. Varicocele

Infantile hydrocele

The swelling appears as inguinoscrotal swelling. The swelling is fluctuant, also cross fluctuation positive (*bilocular hydrocele*), translucent and irreducible. Cough impulse is absent.

Varicocele

Presence of characteristic feel like 'Bag of worms': On coughing, it imparts a fluid thrill. *On lying down* when the scrotum is elevated the swelling reduces gradually and disappears. *On standing* the swelling reappears – fills up from the bottom of the scrotum, whereas the hernia descends from above and the descent can be prevented on deep ring occlusion test.

Funiculitis

A thickened oedematous, tender spermatic cord can be felt with no cough impulse.

Congenital hydrocele

Occurs commonly in children. The swelling is fluctuant and translucent. it reduces very slowly.

Encysted hydrocele of the cord

Already discussed – see above (groin swelling).

Complications of hernia

1. *Irreducibility, incarceration:* Chances are greater with sacs with narrow necks. *Indirect hernia has higher incidence of incarceration.*
2. *Obstruction:* More common in femoral, umbilical herniae and inguinal hernia.
3. *Strangulation:* Most strangulated herniae are indirect inguinal herniae.
   • Strangulation of small bowels commonly.
   • About 20% become gangrenous.
4. Barred from joining the military or police services.
5. Cryptorchidism is associated with indirect inguinal hernia due to patent processus vaginalis.

Note

• Any hernia which is *chronically irreducible or poorly incarcerated* must get urgent notice.
• Short history of irreducibility should be viewed with suspicion and treated as an emergency because it is not possible to reliably exclude strangulation, e.g. Richter's hernia.
• Moreover, *infection of the contents of the sac*, e.g. acute appendicitis, acute salpingitis or from external causes such as a trophic ulcer developing on the dependent areas of a large hernia may cause inflammation.

Note

Direct inguinal hernia rarely descends into the scrotum. *So, complications are not as common as in indirect hernia.* But, rarely, in long-standing cases in an elderly patient with poor musculature, it can descend down to scrotum and may lead to obstruction.

Note

Right inguinal hernia may occur following a grid iron (McBurney's) incision for appendicectomy and is due to injury to the iliohypogastric nerve which causes weakness of the conjoin tendon *leading to direct inguinal hernia.* Iliohypogastric nerve supplies the internal oblique and transverse abdominis muscles which form the conjoint tendon.

Treatment of inguinal hernia

• Conservative
• Operative

Conservative

A. No treatment

In a patient with severe medical comorbidities with a short life expectancy.

Old patients with chronic bronchitis should not be considered unsuitable for operation because they are in danger of getting herniae strangulated. With modern anaesthesia surgery can be undertaken safely in all ages. *If necessary the operation can be performed under local anaesthesia and using a laryngeal mask airway* (which does not control the patient's respiration).

B. Truss treatment

A truss never cures a hernia. It is an appliance which is designed to prevent descent of the contents into the sac.

A truss cannot prevent progression of sliding hernia.

Mode of action

(a) The truss acts by pressing the anterior wall against the posterior wall of the inguinal canal. It also compresses the deep inguinal ring.
(b) By repeated friction it causes adhesion of the sac with the wall of the canal. This might cause difficulty during operation when necessary.

Indication

• *In infants:* A truss often helps in spontaneous cure. *But when the hernia is associated with undescended testis, a truss should never be used*, rather early operation is indicated.
• *In old patients:* When surgery is contra-indicated because of associated general disease, e.g. severe cardiorespiratory disorder.
• *Those who refuse treatment: Truss may be advised on request only*, but they must be informed about the problem of truss.

Contraindications

• Irreducible hernia.
• Patients with source of chronic strain, e.g.

chronic constipation, prostatism, chronic bronchitis; patient doing strenuous job.
- Patients with poor intelligence and perseverance as the wearing of the truss needs careful attention to its positioning and to cleanliness in the area.
- Hernia with huge hydrocele.
- Hernia associated with undescended testis.

Problems of truss
- Improper use can lead to obstruction or strangulation of the hernia. This occurs frequently to patient with poor intelligence or with a persistent source of chronic strain.
- Improper cleanliness causes unhealthy skin which may result in poor wound healing when operation is necessary.
- Prolonged use causes attenuation of the musculature which interferes with subsequent repair and this might be a factor for failure of operation.
- Adhesion due to repeated friction can cause difficulty during operation when necessary.
- But remember control of truss is usually difficult to manage by an infant. *So, not advised.*

   For these disadvantages of truss operation should be insisted upon whenever possible.

Types of truss
'Rat-tailed' or 'Adder-headed' truss. The truss must fit snugly over the inguinal canal.

Method of use
- Cumbersome in nature.
- The truss should be applied in lying down position after reduction of hernia completely.
- It should be used constantly except when the patient is in bed. It should be worn again before getting up from the bed.
- The skin covered by the pad and the perineum should be kept clean by daily toilet.

Note
- *All indirect and sliding herniae should be repaired because of significant incidence of obstruction or strangulation.*
- Truss cannot prevent progression of sliding hernia.

- *Small, non-symptomatic direct inguinal herniae in elderly patients do not require surgery* because they almost never produce obstruction or strangulation.
- Infant hernia can be treated by herniotomy alone and as a day-care basis also.

C. Taxis
It implies vigorous manipulation in an attempt to reduce an acute obstructed hernia of short duration only *but without any feature of intestinal obstruction or strangulation.*

Procedure
- Should be done by an experienced surgeon.
- Should be done after admitting the patient in the hospital.
- Patient should lie down supine on a warm bed with the foot end of the bed raised by 9 inches block before taxis applied.
- Immediate IV/IM injection of pethidine is given to allay the pain and stress.
- Wait for 20–30 minutes. Then IV calmpose and IV baralgan/buscopan are given.
- Once the patient is well sedated, manipulation is tried to reduce the hernia.
   Manipulation is done with the patient in supine position with hip and knee flexed and hip internally rotated. Contents are pushed with one hand while directing with other hand.
- Patient should be observed for 24 to 48 hours, and examined repeatedly to exclude recurrence of hernia, and/or development of intestinal obstruction or strangulation.
- During this observation, patient is allowed plain water and electrolytes orally only. If necessary IV elementation and NPM are advised.
- Once the hernia remains in reduced position, plan for an early elective operation.

Dangers of taxis
Rarely attempted nowadays because of dangers:

(i) *Reduction-en-masse:* The sac together with its contents gets pushed back into the abdomen, without actually the contents being pushed out of the sac. As a result, constriction around the neck of the sac persists leading to obstruction and strangulation.

(ii) Reduction of contents into a loculus of the sac, so persistence of obstruction.

(iii) Contusion or rupture of the intestine contained within the sac.

(iv) *Extraperitoneal reduction:* The sac ruptures leading to reduction of contents extraperitoneally.

Operative

Operation is the treatment of choice and it should be advised whenever possible.

• *In indirect hernia and sliding hernia*, the elective operation *should be performed as early as possible* because chances of obstruction or strangulation are more common with them due to the narrow necks.

• Elective repair under controlled circumstances is far safe with low morbidity than to wait and then operate urgently in the face of the potential serious complications of bowel obstruction or strangulation.

• In direct hernia, as the chances of obstruction or strangulation are much less common due to its wide neck, one can delay the trial of operation.

• Elderly men with asymptomatic or minimal symptoms of inguinal hernia may also undergo a period of observation.

• In an uncomplicated hernia, the surgeon should treat first any chronic source of strain from constipation, prostatism, stricture urethra or chronic cough before an operation. In presence of any chronic strain the repair of hernia very often fails and results in recurrence. Correct chronic cough with stoppage of smoking, postural drainage, chest physiotherapy and antibiotics as necessary. Correct chronic constipation, prostatism or structure urethra first.

• Operation can be performed under local, regional, epidural anaesthesia or general anaesthesia.

• *Infant of only few days old: Wait until the baby is 6 months old.* Obstructions unlikely in infancy because the neck of the sac is fairly wide and the inguinal canal is straight and short. *Moreover*

it reduces the chances of injury to the vas which is very thin like a thread at this age.

Operative procedures

Basically three types of operations are available:

1. Herniotomy alone
2. Herniotomy + Herniorrhaphy – posterior wall repair using *in situ* structures
3. Herniotomy + Hernioplasty – with mesh strengthening of posterior wall

Suitability of any one of these methods depends on the age of the patient, type of hernia and the conditions of the musculature of the inguinal canal.

Herniotomy

Indications

1. In infants and children.
2. In adolescents and young adults with good musculature.
3. Prior to herniorrhaphy or hernioplasty in other ages of patients.

It consists of high ligation of the sac at the neck followed by excision of the sac only. The sac is isolated, opened and the contents are reduced. The neck of the sac is twisted and is transfixed and ligated high up near the deep ring followed by excision of the remaining distal portion of the sac.

However, it is to be noted that herniotomy is not performed in direct inguinal hernia; instead the sac is inverted here. In case of a large sac, after the inversion of the sac, the fascia transversalis may be plicated or imbricated over the reduced sac to keep the sac reduced.

In infants and children, it is not necessary to open the inguinal canal, as the internal and external rings are superimposed.

Herniotomy is employed either by itself or as a first step in a repair procedure – herniorrhaphy or hernioplasty. *By itself herniotomy alone is sufficient for the treatment of hernias in infants, adolescents and young adults.*

Note

Most important step in the repair of an indirect inguinal hernia is narrowing of the internal inguinal ring.

Herniorrhaphy

It consists of

1. Herniotomy after high ligation of hernia sac.
2. *Herniorrhaphy: Reconstruction of the posterior wall of inguinal canal* by approximating the conjoined muscle and tendon to the recurved edge of the inguinal ligament and the periosteum of the pubic tubercle *with non-absorbable suture* such as nylon or prolene. This is known as *Bassini's repair. Silk is better avoided*; if it becomes infected, it will lead to sinuses.

The aim of Bassini's repair is to strengthen the posterior wall of the inguinal canal by pulling down the conjoined muscle and tendon behind the spermatic cord and sutured to the inner shelving edge of the inguinal ligament, i.e. *transplantation of the spermatic cord over the conjoined tendon*; interrupted or continuous sutures are applied without tension as this will lead to cutting of the muscles and/or ligaments from the sutures.

Many modifications added to the Bassini's repair have been advocated to strengthen the repair further:

(a) *To avoid tension*, one may add *Tanner's slide operation:* Here a curved release incision is made on the anterior rectus sheath above the conjoined tendon so that the lower lateral leaf of the sheath at once retracts down and makes the conjoined tendon loose.

(b) *Lytle's repair in indirect hernia:* Tightening of the stretched internal inguinal ring on its medial side, if it is too wide, for which standard repair is not necessary. A figure of '8' stitch of non-absorbable suture material (prolene) is placed just medial to internal inguinal ring. The ring should not be tightened too much. The tip of the haemostat should slide easily.

Commonly done in children. In adults, this step may be used when the internal ring is abnormally patulous and has the advantage of displacing the spermatic cord laterally. *Most important step in the repair of indirect*

inguinal hernia is narrowing of the internal ring. So, Lytle's repair may be added to Bassini's repair.

(c) Lateralization of the ligated neck of the sac after excision.

(d) Plication of fascia transversalis: In direct hernia.

(e) *McVay's repair* involves herniotomy after high ligation of the hernia sac followed by *suturing of the conjoined tendon to the Cooper's ligament medial to the femoral vein and to the iliopubic tract*, above and lateral to the femoral vein. *Because the femoral ring is also closed during this procedure this is a good method of repair when an associated femoral hernia is noted during repair of an inguinal hernia.*

McVay's repair covers all the three groin defects – indirect, direct and femoral. However, the chances of femoral vein injury are common.

(f) *Shouldice repair:* It is a modification of Bassini's repair developed at the Shouldice clinic in Toronto. It is *basically a multi-layered (Four layers) Bassini's repair* using prolene (non-absorbable sutures). *No mesh is used.*

- *First two layers* involve *double-breasting of the fascia transversalis.*
- *3rd layer* involves suturing of the conjoined tendon to the inguinal ligament.
- *4th layer* involves suturing the anterior rectus sheath and the conjoined tendon to the inner surface of lower leaf of external oblique muscle.

(g) *Halstead modifications: Here the spermatic cord is exteriorised* by suturing both the flaps of external oblique aponeurosis behind it, thus the cord remains in subcutaneous plane.

(h) *Willy-Andrew's modifications:* Here the upper flap of external oblique aponeurosis is brought down behind the cord and is sutured to the inguinal ligament and the lower flap is brought over the cord and sutured to the upper flap, *so that the cord remains sandwiched between the two flaps of external oblique.*

Indication: In middle aged or elderly patient with weak abdominal musculature.

(i) *Kuntz operation:* In elderly patient with large scrotal hernia and weak abdominal musculature Kuntz operation is advocated. *Here orchidectomy along with excision of spermatic cord distal to the deep ring* is carried out followed by obliteration of the inguinal canal. This will guard against recurrence. *So, in old men permission for orchidectomy should be taken in writing before operation.*

(j) *In women, it is advisable to remove the round ligament.*

Hernioplasty

Indications

(a) In elderly patients with grossly weak abdominal musculatures.

(b) Recurrent hernia.

It consists of

1. Herniotomy +
2. *Reinforcement of the weak posterior wall of the inguinal canal by filling the defect of the posterior wall with some material* – autogenous or heterogenous.

Uses of autogenous materials (i.e. patient's own tissues) are obsolete now.

Heterogenous materials such as prolene, nylon or stainless steel wire, or a *prolene or Marlex mesh* may be used.

(a) *Darning:* After herniotomy (in indirect hernia) or inversion of the sac (in direct hernia) the gap between the conjoined tendon and the inguinal ligament is *covered with the prolene suture without tension in criss-cross manner* to strengthen the posterior wall. *The procedure is called darning.* The fibroblasts and capillaries grow in between the interstices of the darn, thus converting it into a thick fibrous sheath.

(b) *Lichtenstein tension-free mesh repair:* The gap in the posterior wall of the inguinal canal and the internal ring is covered by a prolene mesh (size 8 cm × 6 cm), *in a tension-free manner without closing the gap by direct suturing. The conjoint tendon is not sutured to the inguinal ligament. The mesh is sutured to the conjoint tendon with transversalis fascia, pubic tubercle,*

lacunar ligament and the shelving edge of the inguinal ligament deep to the spermatic cord with a window placed laterally permitting the spermatic cord to traverse. Recurrence rate is quite low.

Operation for direct inguinal hernia

Herniotomy is not performed; instead the sac is inverted after reduction of the contents followed by plication of the fascia transversalis. This is then followed by some form of repair of the posterior wall as mentioned in herniorrhaphy or hernioplasty.

Complications of hernia operation

Complications during the operation:

1. Injury to the external iliac or femoral vessels during suturing too deeply through the iliopubic or inguinal ligament during the lateral part of the repair.
2. Injury to the vas deferens especially in children.
3. Injury to the urinary bladder and colon especially with sliding hernia. *Whenever a bulky indirect inguinal hernia is not accompanied by a thin-walled transparent sac, suspect a sliding component.*
4. Injury to the inferior epigastric vessels.
5. Injury to the contents of the sac.
6. Injury to the testicular artery.
7. Injury to the nerves – ilioinguinal nerve, iliohypogastric nerve, genitofemoral nerve.

Early postoperative complications:

1. Retention of urine.
2. Haematoma of the cord and scrotum.
3. Wound infection.

Late postoperative complications:

1. Recurrence. *Causes of recurrence* – (a) absorbable suture used; (b) sliding hernia; (c) missed sac; and (d) infection.
2. Sinuses.
3. *Neuralgic pain due to inclusion of ilioinguinal nerve in the suture* – causes hyperaesthesia over the medial side of inguinal canal – chronic groin pain or inguinodynia.
4. Painless scar. *If the nerve is severed,* there will be loss of sensation over the mons pubis,

and the scrotum in male or labium majus in female.

5. Atrophy of the testis due to injury to testicular artery or due to compression of the spermatic cord following narrowing of the internal ring too tight.
6. Injury to the vas in children.
7. Osteitis pubis.
8. Mesh extrusion with or without foreign body reaction.
9. *Seroma formation:* U/S helps in the diagnosis and aspiration.
10. *Epidermoid cysts:* When the skin flap is used for plastic repair.

Recurrence rate after inguinal hernia repair

• Bassini's repair   10%
• Shouldice repair   1%
• Hernioplasty   1–3%
• Other methods   1–5%

Causes of recurrence after inguinal hernia repair

• Most of the recurrences occur by the end of the first year.
• A recurrent hernia may be direct or indirect.

   The following factors are responsible for the recurrence.

   (i) Weak abdominal muscles most common in elderly and obese people.
   (ii) Persistence or recurrence of chronic straining factors leading to chronic or recurrent raised intra-abdominal pressure, e.g. chronic straining at micturition (e.g. enlarged prostate/stricture urethra), chronic constipation, chronic bronchitis – *these problems should be taken care of first before hernia operation and also after operation.*
   (iii) Missed sac – presence of both indirect and direct sacs, i.e. *saddle hernia* but failure to recognise either of them during operation.
   (iv) Failure to dissect the sac right up to the neck and to perform high ligation and inadequate removal of sac in indirect hernia.
   (v) Inadequate closure of the internal ring.

   (vi) Inadequate repair of the posterior wall of the inguinal canal – either too tight or too loose.
   (vii) Failure to repair with nylon or prolene (*non-absorbable suture material*).
   (viii) Inadequate haemostasis.
   (ix) Wound infection which destroys the repair.
   (x) *Too early resumption of strenuous labour.* A patient should be advised to avoid strenuous activity or games/weightlifting following hernia repair for a period of 6 months at least.
   (xi) Metabolic problems or collagen disorders of the tissues of the groin leading to continuing failure of the floor of the canal.
   (xii) In women, it is advisable to remove the round ligament.
   (xiii) *Kuntz operation:* In elderly patient with large scrotal hernia and weak abdominal musculature Kuntz operation is advocated, *Here, orchidectomy along with excision of spermatic cord distal to the deep ring* is carried out followed by obliteration of the inguinal canal. This will guard against recurrence. *So, in old men, permission for orchidectomy should be taken in writing before operation.*

Management of recurrent hernia

1. Exclude or correct any persistent source of chronic strain, e.g. chronic cough, constipation, straining at micturition. *Ultrasound of KUB is useful to exclude enlarged prostate or bladder neck obstruction.*
2. Following operations may be helpful.
   (a) Lichtenstein tension-free mesh repair is preferable.
   (b) In an elderly patient, Kuntz operation may be added to Lichtenstein repair.
   (c) Shouldice repair.
   (d) Stoppa's preperitoneal mesh placement repair (hernioplasty).
   (e) Laparoscopic repair with preperitoneal mesh replacement.

Note

All indirect and sliding hernias should be repaired because of the significant incidence of strangulation.

Small, non-symptomatic direct inguinal hernias in elderly patients do not require surgery because they almost never develop obstruction or strangulation. Direct hernias that produce symptoms, on the other hand, should be repaired.

Laparoscopic repair of inguinal hernia

Inguinal hernia may be repaired laparoscopically by preperitoneal placement of mesh.

Two methods are in wide use:

1. *Totally extraperitoneal approach* (TEP)
2. *Transabdominal preperitoneal approach* (TAPP)

These are based on *Stoppa's method of reconstruction of the weakened anterior abdominal wall by preperitoneal placement of the mesh between the posterior surface of the anterior abdominal wall and the peritoneum.* The mesh may or may not require any fixation by anchoring sutures or tacker. *In absence of fixation, the mesh is kept in place by Pascal's principle of hydrostatic pressure:* The intra-abdominal pressure acting via the anterior peritoneal layer keeps the mesh steadily against the abdominal wall.

Both the methods of repair are similar in principle in actual repair but *differ in the manner by which the preperitoneal space is accessed.*

In TEP repair, the preperitoneal space is accessed without entering the peritoneal cavity.

Indications

1. Both indirect and direct inguinal herniae
2. Bilateral inguinal herniae
3. Recurrent hernia.

Advantages

1. Minimal access surgery.
2. *Laparoscopic mesh repair also takes consideration of coverage of femoral ring and obturator ring in addition to direct and indirect inguinal rings.*
3. If fixation of mesh repair is preferred, two point fixations are performed – one at the pubic bone and the other at the Cooper's ligament by tackers/staplers.
4. Patient can be discharged within 48 hours.
5. Early return to work.

RARE VARIETIES OF INGUINAL HERNIA

Dual hernia (Romberg hernia)

- Also known as *saddle bag* or *pantaloon hernia.*
- It has two sacs – one direct and another indirect sac lying on either side of the inferior epigastric vessels; both are connected by an isthmus which lies behind the inferior epigastric vessels.
- Most common overlooked hernia during surgery.

Significance:

1. Deep ring occlusion test may be confusing as it only controls the indirect sac.
2. *One of the causes of recurrence if one sac, particularly the indirect sac, is missed during operation. So, during direct hernia repair one should explore the internal ring and the coverings of the spermatic cord to exclude indirect hernia.*

Sliding hernia (Fig. 10.8)

- Also known as *Hernia-en-glissade.*
- It is a type of hernia in which a portion of extraperitoneal bowel, e.g. caecum, sigmoid colon or urinary bladder, may slide down into the inguinal canal pulling a peritoneal sac with it. *Thus the posterior wall of the sac is formed by both the peritoneum of the sac and by the wall of a viscus which lies beneath the peritoneum.*
- *The sac may contain other loops of bowel or omentum.* But if the caecum and appendix on

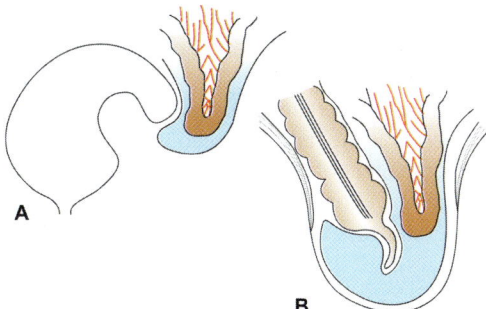

Figs 10.8 A and B: Sliding hernia. (A) Posterior wall of the hernial sac is formed by the part of the urinary bladder wall which lies behind the peritoneum of the sac; (B) Posterior wall of the hernial sac is formed by the part of the caecal wall which lies behind the peritoneum of the sac.

the right side or a part of left colon on left side are the contents of the hernial sac, it is not a sliding hernia. *It is to be remembered that these structures are not within the sac but actually forming part of sac wall.*

- These viscera must form a wall of the sac to be termed as sliding hernia.
- Sliding component of a large direct hernia may be urinary bladder.

Wall of the sliding hernia include:

- On the left side – sigmoid colon and its mesentery
- On the right side – caecum with appendix
- On either side – urinary bladder

Contents of the sliding hernia include:

- Small intestine or omentum

Clinical features:

1. Most commonly seen in elderly men.
2. Particularly occurs in long-standing cases.
3. Left-sided hernia is more common than right-sided.
4. *This hernia is suspected when a large globular hernia descends down into the scrotum.*
5. Complete reduction is not possible.
6. After reduction, sliding hernia reappears very slowly.

Significance:

1. *This hernia can easily be strangulated.* There may be strangulation of small bowel inside the sac. Rarely, large bowel forming the wall of the sac may be strangulated when a large globular swelling descends down into the scrotum.
2. *The real danger associated with a sliding hernia* is the failure to recognise the visceral component of the hernia sac before injury to the bowel or bladder during operation if the hernial sac is resected during surgery.

Treatment:

1. Truss treatment is absolutely contraindicated.
2. The hernial sac should be dissected carefully *to avoid injury to colon or bladder.*
3. Once the hernial sac is opened and the contents are reduced back in the abdomen, *the sac should not be twisted to avoid*

inclusion of colon wall or bladder wall. Instead the distal sac is removed and the proximal part of the sac is closed with a purse-string suture. The hernia repair is then completed. *A mesh enforcement repair is preferable.*

4. In elderly patient, orchidectomy is advised to furnish complete closure of the inguinal canal and thus to avoid recurrence. *Hence, prior consent for orchidectomy should be taken.*

Note

Sliding component of large direct hernia:

- Urinary bladder.
- Sigmoid colon and caecum slide into indirect sac; not in direct sac.
- Rarely, the contents may be uterus, fallopian tube or ovary within the sliding hernial sac in females.

Interstitial hernia

- In this hernia, the hernial sac instead of being present in the inguinal canal, may lie in the musculofascial layers of the abdominal wall.
- The hernia is usually *intraparietal and in-complete.*
- Following varieties may be encountered.
  (i) *Preperitoneal:* The hernia sac lies between the peritoneum and the fascia trans-versalis.
  (ii) *Intraparietal:* The hernia sac lies between the internal oblique and the external oblique aponeurosis – most common.
  (iii) *Extraparietal:* The hernia sac lies outside the external oblique aponeurosis in the subcutaneous fat.
- *Hernia in association with undescended testis is commonly one of interstitial variety.*

Ogilvie hernia

- This is a rare variety of direct inguinal hernia. Occurs in elderly persons.
- Here the hernia sac *protrudes through an oval defect in the conjoined tendon just lateral to where it inserts into the rectus sheath.*
- So it is also known as funicular direct inguinal

hernia (cf. funicular indirect inguinal hernia, prevesical hernia).
- Chances of obstruction are common than usual direct hernia.

Prevesical hernia

- It is also called funicular direct hernia.
- Rare variety. Occurs principally in elderly men.
- The hernia sac containing a portion of bladder wall and prevesical fat protrudes *through a small oval defect in the conjoined tendon* just above the pubic tubercle.
- *A history of swelling in the groin becoming less prominent or disappear after micturition is present.*
- Operation should always be advised except in patients with significant medical comorbidities.
- Chances of obstruction are more common than usual direct hernia.
- Chances of bladder injury are frequent during operation if not careful.

Richter's hernia

- In this hernia, *only a portion of the circumference of bowel wall becomes protruded in the hernia sac.*
- This condition often complicates a femoral hernia and rarely an obturator hernia.
- *Chances of strangulation without complete obstruction of bowel lumen is common.* So, absolute constipation is rare.
- But the diagnosis is frequently delayed, because the patient may present with gastroenteritis, i.e. diarrhoea and often blood in the stools with or without vomiting. *The intestinal colic may be present but the bowels open normally.*
- Intestinal obstruction may develop late when half of the circumference of the bowel is involved. Absolute constipation is delayed until strangulation and/or paralytic ileus develops.
- *Often, diagnosis is established after exploratory laparotomy in a case of intestinal obstruction.*

Maydl's hernia

- Also known as hernia-en-W.

- In this condition, two adjacent loops of bowel remain in the sac, the connecting portion remains inside the abdomen. The bowel loops in the hernial sac looks like W.
- *This connecting portion of W loop is more vulnerable to become strangulated early in an obstructed hernia.* Thus the strangulated piece of the gut remains inside the abdomen (Fig. 10.9).
- The patient presents with obstructed hernia with intestinal obstruction.
- On examination, there are no signs of gangrene over the scrotum and groin, but tenderness and rebound tenderness will be elicited over the lower abdomen above the inguinal ligament.
- *On exploration:* After examining the bowels inside the sac, the intra-abdominal segment of bowel is to be examined for gangrene and the gangrenous part should be excised.

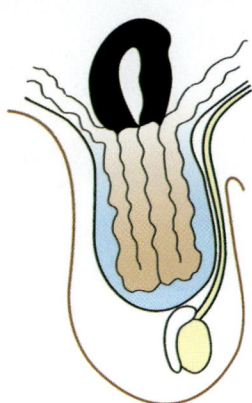

Fig. 10.9: Maydl's hernia.

Littre's hernia

- In this condition, Meckel's diverticulum is the content of the sac. If the diverticulum gets

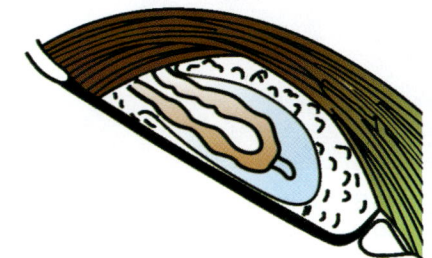

Fig. 10.10: Littre's hernia.

infected, hernia becomes inflamed. The cause of infection may be precipitated by partial obstruction to the diverticulum.

Amyand's hernia

In this condition appendix along with caecum descends into the right hernial sac (cf. sliding hernia, Fig. 10.8).

CONGENITAL INGUINAL HERNIA

• *A type of paediatric hernia.* Develops due to failure of obliteration of processus vaginalis. Patent processus vaginalis admits a small indirect sac.

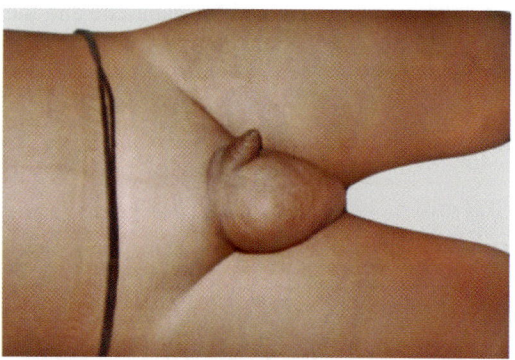

Fig. 10.11A: Congenital right inguinal hernia.

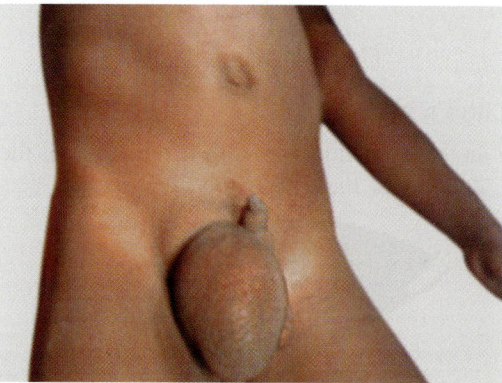

Fig. 10.11B: Congenital right inguinal hernia—presented with intestinal obstruction. Note the dilated small bowel loops right upper abdomen—step ladder pattern.

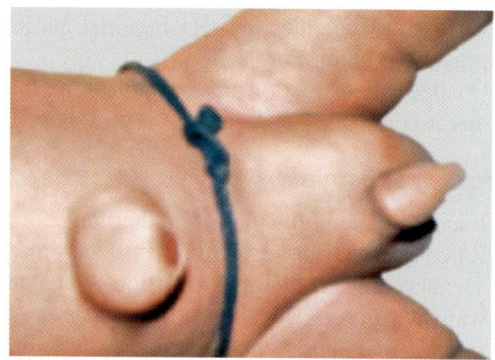

Fig. 10.12: Congenital umbilical hernia with left inguinoscrotal hernia.

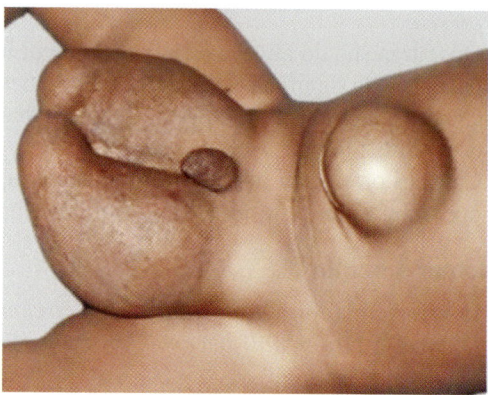

Fig. 10.13: Congenital umbilical and bilateral inguinal herniae. Both are reducible.

• *Always indirect type. Usually appears as an inguinoscrotal swelling since birth.* It gradually increases in size.
• The swelling appears on straining or crying, on crawling, sitting and standing.
• The swelling disappears when the child lies down.
• The swelling may transilluminate (cf. congenital hydrocele).
• Reducible with or without gurgling sound.
• The swelling will reappear, if the child is induced to cry.
• In newborn infant, the inguinal canal is not developed and the deep and superficial inguinal rings lie close or superimposed to each other.
• By the age of 2 years, as the deep ring moves laterally, the inguinal canal is formed with wide separation of the two rings.

- *Early operation is advocated in infants and children* because of high chance of obstruction or incarceration though strangulation is rare.
- *Only simple herniotomy is required.* No herniorrhaphy is attempted. Because the inguinal canal is short and straight and the external ring lies directly over the internal ring, opening of inguinal canal is not required.

Problems of inguinal hernia in children:

- It is very difficult to distinguish congenital hernia from a congenital hydrocele because they both transmit light of a torch. The distinction is not critical because most hydroceles require operation.
- Operation is delayed until the baby is 6 months old when anaesthesia will be easier. In a rare fortunate baby, his hernia may resolve spontaneously during this 6 months period of waiting.
- In young children the hernial sac is thin, delicate and difficult to find.
- *The baby vas is thin like a thread only and liable to injury easily.*
- Post-op follow up should be continued for 5 years at least to detect recurrent or contralateral hernia.
- Chances of developing hernia on opposite side – *Around 5–10% of children may develop hernia on contralateral side during follow up.* In children, if inguinal hernia (indirect) is present on one side, then the processus vaginalis is patent on other side in 60% cases.
- But, routine contralateral exploration which was advocated earlier is not advised nowadays.
- Laparoscopic suturing of the internal ring is a less traumatic operation. Moreover, *both the internal rings are inspected from inside at the same time and tackled accordingly at the same sitting.*

Note

The left testicle precedes the right testicle in descent. Thus, if a hernia is present in the left side, there almost always will be a hernia on the right side. So, *justifying a bilateral exploration of inguinal canal and repair especially in children.*

█ FEMORAL HERNIA

It is the protrusion of the extraperitoneal fat and peritoneum with or without abdominal contents into the femoral canal. In this hernia the sac passes through the femoral ring medial to the femoral vein and lateral to the lacunar ligament and enters the femoral canal (Fig. 10.14).

Surgical anatomy

Femoral sheath

This is a funnel shaped fascial prolongation around the femoral vessels below the medial half of the inguinal ligament. The anterior wall of the sheath is formed by the fascia transversalis and the posterior wall by the fascia iliaca. *The sheath has got three compartments separated by fibrous septae:*

1. Lateral compartment, contains femoral artery and femoral branch of genitofemoral nerve.
2. Intermediate compartment, contains femoral vein.
3. Medial compartment, femoral canal containing Cloquet's lymph node.

Femoral nerve lies outside the femoral sheath lateral to the artery.

Femoral canal

It is the innermost compartment of the femoral sheath. The canal is about 2 cm long and is conical in shape with the base directed upwards and the apex directed downwards. *At the base*

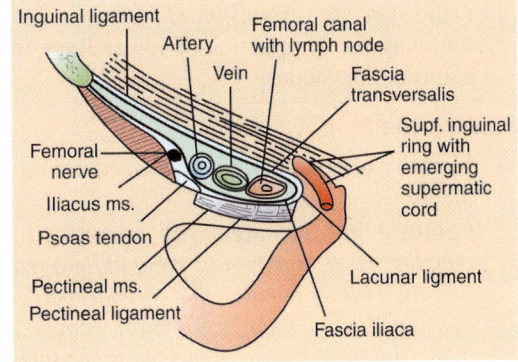

Fig. 10.14: Femoral canal—its boundaries and relations.

lies the femoral ring which is the mouth of the canal. The canal extends from the femoral ring above up to the saphenous ring below.

Boundaries of the femoral ring
- *Anteriorly:* Inguinal ligament.
- *Posteriorly:* Pectineal line of the horizontal ramus of the pubic and the pectineal ligament.
- *Medially:* Crescentic edge of the lacunar ligament.
- *Laterally:* Fibrous septum separating the canal from the femoral vein.

All these boundaries are rigid except the fibrous septum laterally.

The ring is closed above by the septum crurale – a condensed extraperitoneal tissue pierced by the lymphatic vessels.

The femoral hernia is related to the femoral vein laterally and the lacunar ligament medially.

In 20% cases, the obturator artery is replaced by the pubic branch of the inferior epigastric artery which, when present, courses along the crescentic margin of the lacunar ligament. This abnormal artery is vulnerable – if the lacunar ligament needs division for release of the constricted ring for reduction of the femoral hernia.

Contents of the femoral canal
1. Fibrofatty tissue.
2. Lymph nodes and lymphatics. Lymph node situated at the ring is known as Cloquet's node.

Functions of the femoral canal
1. *Dead space for expansion of femoral vein.*
2. Pathway for lymphatics of lower limb to external iliac nodes.

Surgical pathology
1. Majority of femoral herniae are acquired in nature.
2. Femoral herniae are *more common in females. More common in the middle-aged and the elderly females due to wide pelvis and repeated pregnancy*; so, *more common in multiparous women.* Repeated pregnancy causes increased abdominal pressure which is probably an initiating factor.
   - *Less common in nulliparous women.*
   - However, inguinal hernia is more common than femoral hernia in females.
   - Femoral hernia is rare in men.
   - Femoral hernia is almost unknown in infants.
3. *Right-sided hernia is more common* than the left-sided one. The hernia may be bilateral.
4. *Sites of constriction:*
   - Lacunar ligament
   - Neck of the sac
5. *Course of the hernia:* The hernial sac enters through the femoral ring and descends vertically down along the femoral canal up to the lower border of fossa ovalis where it lies in close relation to the long saphenous vein. Due to attachment of the superficial fascia of the abdomen (fascia of Scarpa) to the fascia lata of the thigh at the lower border of the fossa ovalis, the sac cannot pass down in the thigh. So the sac courses forward, and when enlarging it courses upward over the inguinal ligament and external oblique apo-neurosis and *thus the distal part of the sac overlies the inguinal ligament and occupies the inguinal region*. The shape of the sac then becomes retort-shaped. *The neck of the sac lies below and lateral to the pubic tubercle* (cf. *inguinal hernia* – the neck of the sac lies above and medial to the pubic tubercle).

Contents of the sac
May contain:
1. A part of the omentum.
2. A loop of small bowel.
3. A part of the circumference of small bowel (Richter's hernia).

Coverings of the sac
From superficial to deep:
1. Skin.
2. Superficial fascia.
3. Cribriform fascia covering the saphenous opening.
4. Fascia transversalis – representing the anterior femoral sheath.
5. Extraperitoneal fat.
6. Peritoneum – the hernial sac.

Table 10.3: Differences between inguinal and femoral herniae

Points	Inguinal	Femoral
• *Age*	Any age	Middle-aged or elderly persons commonly
• *Sex*	More common in males	More common in females
• *Side*	Unilateral; common on the right side	Unilateral; common on the right side
• *Relation with the pubic tubercle*	The sac lies above and medial to pubic tubercle	The sac lies below and lateral to pubic tubercle
• *Cough impulse*	Usually present	Usually absent
• *Reducibility*	Usually reducible; the hernia reduces in an upward, backward and lateral direction	Often partial; when complete, the hernia reduces directly upward and backwards
• *Invagination test after reduction*	On coughing, a thrust will be felt at the tip of the finger	On coughing, no thrust will be felt; the inguinal canal found to be empty

Diagnostic criteria

1. *Age:* Middle-aged or elderly persons commonly.
2. *Sex:* More common in females (particularly after repeated pregnancies). F : M = 4 : 1.
3. *Symptoms:*
   - The patient complains of dragging pain in the groin.
   - Usually she or he presents with a small globular swelling in the groin. It becomes more prominent on standing or straining but may disappear on lying down.
   - An obese lady may present with the features of intestinal obstruction or strangulation of an unnoticed femoral hernia.

   Examination:
   - The femoral hernia should be examined in the similar manner as in inguinal hernia. Ask the patient to stand up, note the exact position of the lump, *try to determine the exact anatomical relations of the lump to the inguinal ligament and pubic tubercle* and *then note if the lump has a cough impulse and whether it is reducible.*
4. *Position:* A round or oval swelling below the medial end of the inguinal ligament – at or below the groin crease.
5. *Palpation:* The neck of the lump (or sac) is situated below and lateral to the pubic tubercle (cf. *inguinal hernia* where the neck of the sac lies above and medial to the pubic tubercle).

6. *Cough impulse:* Both visible and palpable, may be absent in many femoral hernia because the contents are adherent to the peritoneal sac.
7. *Reducibility: Often partial.* When complete it reduces directly upwards and backwards.
8. *Inguinal canal examination, e.g. invagination test – empty.*

Note

In the female, pelvis is wider and the opening of the canal is, therefore, larger. *Femoral hernia is consequently more common in females.*

Complications

1. Irreducibility
2. Obstruction
3. *Strangulation:* Femoral hernias have the highest incidence of strangulation (15%) of all hernias.

These are commoner in femoral hernia than in inguinal hernia or any other hernia *because the neck of the femoral canal is narrow and has a sharp and rigid medial border formed by lacunar ligament. Strangulation without obstruction of gut lumen is also possible in femoral hernia – Richter's hernia. In fact, strangulation is the initial presentation of 40% femoral hernias. That is why femoral hernia should be operated upon as soon as possible at the time of discovery and should not be controlled by a truss.*

The overriding importance is that femoral hernia should not be controlled by truss and it has an increased tendency to get strangulated (Figs 10.15 and 10.16).

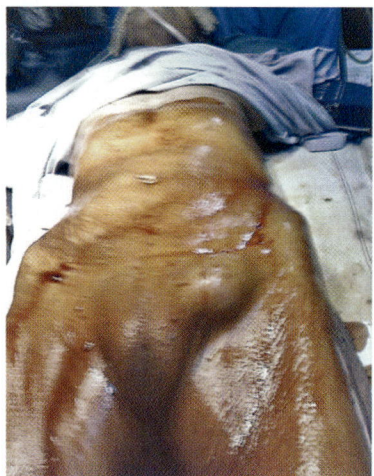

Fig. 10.15: Obstructed *left femoral hernia* with stepladder pattern of distended small bowel.

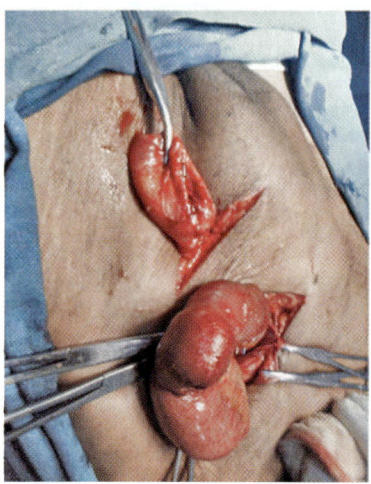

Fig. 10.16: Same patient. On exploration first through subinguinal followed by lower abdominal approach the distended bowel reduced to abdominal cavity when the hernia was found to be Richter's hernia.

Differential diagnosis

1. Incomplete inguinal hernia or bubonocele
2. Saphena varix
3. Enlarged lymph node
4. Lipoma
5. Aneurysm of the femoral artery
6. Psoas abscess
7. Rupture of the adductor longus muscle.

Incomplete inguinal hernia

The swelling is in the inguinal region above the inguinal ligament, *above and medial to the pubic tubercle.* Invagination test through the superficial ring will confirm that the swelling is inside the inguinal canal. The swelling has a cough impulse and is usually reducible.

Saphena varix

- *Saphena varix is usually associated with varicosity of long saphenous vein.*
- Saphena varix is softer than the femoral hernia.
- Blue discoloration of the skin over the saphena varix may be noted particularly in people of fair complexion.

Enlarged lymph node

An enlarged deep inguinal lymph node (Cloquet's node) may be almost always impossible to distinguish from a femoral hernia. For a suspected enlarged Cloquet's node, *search for a focus of infection in the following sites* – lower limb, buttocks, perineum, anus, glans penis. If with antibiotics and rest the swelling does not get smaller it should be explored. *If suspicion of strangulated hernia arises* – operation should be done immediately without delay.

Lipoma

It is a soft lobulated swelling and mobile. It can never be reducible. Cough impulse absent. If suspicion arises, it should always be explored.

Rupture of the adductor longus muscle

Common in athletes, so history of injury is present. *Patient presents with an oval swelling on the medial side of the femoral triangle.* Cough impulse absent. Reducibility absent. *When the patient is asked to adduct the thigh against resistance* – the swelling becomes more prominent, well-defined, painful and tender.

Others

See under D/D of inguinal hernia.

Treatment of femoral hernia

Always operative.

   Conservative treatment has no role in femoral hernia because:

- No truss can be fitted to control the femoral ring.
- *Risk of obstruction or strangulation is very common in femoral hernia* due to narrow and tight femoral ring.
- So, early operation is always recommended.

Operations

Essentials of operation: Herniotomy + closure of the femoral ring either by suturing the inguinal ligament to the pectineal ligament, or the conjoint tendon to the pectineal ligament.

There are *three avenues of approach* to the femoral hernia:

1. Low or subinguinal – Lockwood's operation.
2. Inguinal – Lotheissen's operation.
3. High or suprainguinal – McEvedy's operation.

Lockwood's operation (sublingual or groin approach)

The sac is approached below the inguinal ligament through groin crease incision over the swelling, *so that the fundus of the sac is approached and dissected by direct vision.* The repair is done from below – *inguinal ligament is sutured to Cooper's ligament.*

Advantage:

A direct approach to the swelling and hence the sac. Speedy and simple method, so suitable for small and uncomplicated femoral hernia.

Disadvantage:

- Difficult to resect a gangrenous bowel so not suitable for the operation of a strangulated hernia.
- Difficult to repair the femoral ring.

Lotheissen's operation (inguinal approach)

The sac is approached through inguinal canal (just like for inguinal hernia repair), fascia transversalis opened and the neck of the sac is identified at the femoral ring. The sac is dissected from above and neck is ligated. After herniotomy, *conjoined tendon is sutured to the pectineal ligament* by interrupted non-absorbable monofilament sutures.

Advantage:

Easy to deal with gangrenous bowel.

Disadvantage:

It causes weakening of the inguinal canal and its posterior wall.

McEvedy's operation (combined inguinofemoral approach)

An incision is made over the femoral canal extending vertically above the inguinal ligament. Sac is dissected from below to approach the neck above and then ligate the neck. It gives a very good exposure of both the fundus of the sac and the neck.

Advantage:

- Easy to deal with gangrenous bowel and to repair the femoral ring.
- It does not damage the inguinal canal.

Disadvantage:

Access to the fundus of the sac is not sufficient, so removal is difficult.

Note

Danger during operation: Injury to abnormal obturator artery which lies close to the inner ring – so, chance of trauma during stretching or incising the inner border to enlarge the ring for easy reduction. This will cause haemorrhage which may be difficult to control.

RARE TYPES OF FEMORAL HERNIA

1. Prevascular hernia (Narath hernia)

- In this case, the femoral hernia sac lies behind the femoral vessels.
- Occurs in patient with congenital dislocation of hip.

2. Pectineal hernia (Cloquet's hernia)

The femoral hernia sac passes between the pectineal muscle and fascia, behind the femoral vessels.

3. External femoral hernia (Hesselbach's hernia)

The femoral hernial sac lies lateral to the femoral artery.

4. Lacunar hernia (Laugier's hernia)

In this case, the femoral hernia sac passes through a small defect in the lacunar ligament.

5. Serafini's hernia

The hernial sac lies behind the femoral vessels.

Note

Among all the types of hernia, femoral hernia is most liable to become strangulated, mainly because of the narrowness of the neck and rigidity of the femoral ring. In fact, strangulation is the initial presentation of 40% of femoral herniae. *That is why femoral hernia should not be tried to control by truss.* When diagnosed, operation is a must and urgent.

Note

Most common hernia in female is inguinal hernia.

INCISIONAL HERNIA

Syn. Postoperative hernia, ventral hernia. An abdominal incisional hernia is one *where the peritoneal sac herniates through an acquired scar* in the abdominal wall, usually caused by a previous laparotomy or an accidental trauma leading to separation of the edges of a muscular aponeurotic suture line – partial or total disruption. *Scar tissue is inelastic and can be stretched easily if subjected to constant strain.*

2–10% of all abdominal operations result in incisional hernia due to failure of fascial tissues to heal and close following laparotomy. *Contents of such hernia* are usually bowel and/or omentum.

Predisposing factors

1. *Some subjects:*
   (a) Obese individuals with poor musculature.
   (b) Diabetic patients – more with obesity.
   (c) Malnutrition:
      • Patients with severe anaemia.
      • Patients with hypoproteinaemia.
      • Patients with avitaminosis, e.g. vitamin C deficiency.
      • Patients with diabetes, jaundice, uremia, immune suppression and cancer.
      • Patients with cachexia and advanced malignant disease.
   (d) Patients with any chronic source of straining *leading to increased intra-abdominal pressure*, e.g. chronic cough, chronic constipation, chronic straining at micturition due to enlarged prostate, or any other factors which lead to increase in intra-abdominal pressure, e.g. ascites, distended bowel or recurrent vomiting.
   (e) Old age is a risk factor for incisional hernia, but not for wound dehiscence.

2. *Some operations:*
   (a) Operation for peptic perforation or appendicular perforation which causes infection.
   (b) Operation in case of peritonitis: Infection or sepsis.
   (c) Operation in a case of strangulated bowel where intraperitoneal infection is the rule.
   (d) Operation for visceral cancer.
   (e) Pancreatic resection operation.
   (f) Operation in a case of bowel obstruction where decompression of the grossly distended bowel is not properly done.
   (g) Operation in a jaundice/diabetic patient.

3. *Some incisions:*
   (a) Kocher's subcostal incision for cholecystectomy causing injury to the ninth and tenth thoracic nerves.
   (b) McBurney's incision for appendicectomy causing injury to the iliohypogastric nerve.
   (c) *Battle's pararectal incision for appendicectomy causing nerve injury to rectus.*
   (d) *Midline infraumbilical incision,* e.g. during caesarean section.
   (e) *Midline vertical incisions are more prone to burst than transverse incisions. Highest incidence is seen with midline vertical incisions.* Transverse incisions are associated with reduced incidence.

4. *Some faults during operation:*
   (a) Division of motor nerves supplying the muscles around the wound.
   (b) Defective or inadequate closure of the laparotomy wound, e.g. failure of suturing the abdominal wounds in anatomical layers; suturing under tension causes pressure necrosis of intervening tissues. Interrupted sutures are better than continuous sutures.
   (c) Inadequate haemostasis during operation leading to wound haematoma which becomes more vulnerable if infected.
   (d) *Wound closed with non-absorbable monofilament suture materials like nylon, prolene are followed by a lesser incidence of incisional hernia* than the wound closed with absorbable suture like catgut as it gets quickly absorbed.
   (e) Drainage tubes brought directly through the main laparotomy wound and left behind for a long time. *Intraperitoneal drains should always be brought out through a separate stab incision.*

5. *Some postoperative complications leading to burst abdomen:*
   (a) Severe postoperative abdominal distensions causing tension over the suture line (due to raised intra-abdominal pressure).
   (b) Persistent postoperative cough causing tension over the suture line (causes raised intra-abdominal pressure).
   (c) Postoperative peritonitis, because there is a *chance of wound infection* and *abdominal distension* (causes raised intra-abdominal pressure).
   (d) Wound infection – most important.
   (e) Wound haematoma/seroma.
   (f) Too early removal of sutures.
   (g) Too early resumption of strenuous labour.
   (h) Steroid therapy in postoperative period.
   (i) Persistence of diabetes, vitamin C deficiency, hypoproteinaemia, malnutrition, etc.

   (j) Failure of proper tissue healing due to abnormal collagen production and maintenance causes weak scar tissue which may lead to late development of incisional hernia after 5 to 10 years of operation.

6. *Suture material:* Repair with chromic catgut is associated with higher incidence of burst abdomen as it gets absorbed very quickly (in 8 to 10 days). Suture with non-absorbable monofilament sutures, nylon or prolene, are found to be good.

Note
- All the above-mentioned factors may lead to burst abdomen.
- Burst abdomen commonly occurs on the seventh postoperative day.
- *2–10% of all abdominal operations result in incisional hernia.*

Pathology
Wound dehiscence: Partial or total disruption of all the layers of the operative wound is commonly observed between the third and fifth postoperative days. *Serous or serosanguinous discharge from the wound is the first sign of dehiscence.*

Extrusion of abdominal viscera after rupture of all layers is known as *evisceration.*

Aetiopathology
Can be discussed under two headings:
A. Without infection.
B. With infection.

A. Without infection

There is a partial and quiet disruption of the deeper layers of a laparotomy wound occurring immediately after operation or around 3rd postoperative day; but such an event usually passes unnoticed because the skin edges remain apposed with intact sutures. *Early sign of wound disruption is a serosanguinous discharge through laparotomy wound around third postoperative day and it should be regarded as a red signal of wound dehiscence or burst abdomen. This signal demands immediate examination of the laparo-*

tomy wound and, *if necessary*, resuture of the deeper disrupted layers of the wound. In case of failure of this urgent attention and action, there is separation of both sheath and muscles resulting in healing by weak scar tissue.

Burst abdomen more commonly occurs on the fifth to seventh postoperative day.

Extrusion of abdominal viscera after rupture of all layers is known as *evisceration*.

B. With infection

Wound suppuration – disruptions of the sutures leading to wound dehiscence – separations of sheath and muscles – healing by weak scar tissue.

In both cases herniation occurs through this weak scar tissue.

Structural changes

1. Skin over the hernial protuberance is thinned out, stretched and often shows a wide irregular scar. *The scar is devoid of subcutaneous fat and is very often adherent to peritoneal sac.*
2. The sac is usually big and multiloculated.
3. *Contents:* The bowel and/or the omentum which are often matted together and may be adherent to the loculated peritoneal sac.

Types of defect

Incisional hernia may be of two types:

1. *One type occurs through the midline upper abdominal incision or midline lower abdominal incision* where the muscular defect is wide with smooth and regular margins. More frequently this type of hernia takes the form of a diffuse bulge along the whole length of the incision and usually reduces spontaneously as soon as the patient lies down. *With this type the risk of strangulation is remote.*

   Battle's pararectal incision is also prone to incision hernia *because of nerve injuries.*
2. In the second type, the hernia occurs mainly through the defect in the lateral part of the abdomen *specially after transverse incision* where the muscular defect is relatively small and irregular; there may be presence of two

or more such defects in the same scar. *Risk of strangulation is very common with this type.*

3. Size of the defect:
   • Large and wide defect
   • Small defect
   • Multiple defects

Why the midline infraumbilical abdominal incision is frequently followed by an incisional hernia?

Because of the following reasons.

1. The posterior rectus sheath is complete only up to a point midway between umbilicus and symphysis pubis, where it ends in a free border, the linea semicircularis. *Below this level the posterior sheath is deficient because all the three aponeurosis pass in front of the rectus muscle.* The rectus abdominis muscle here is separated from the peritoneum by the fascia transversalis alone.
2. Below the linea semicircularis the linea alba is thin and narrow and it lies mainly in front of the recti muscles *as the posterior sheath is deficient.*

So, midline infraumbilical incision results in a weakly supported scar which is likely to be followed by hernia.

Immediate management of wound dehiscence with evisceration

Prompt elective closure of the wound.

• Immediately cover the wound with moist towel soaked in normal saline followed by transfer to OT.
• Under GA, any exposed bowel or omentum is rinsed with NS or RL mixed with antibiotics and lavage of abdominal cavity. Then return the exposed structures back into the abdominal cavity.
• Previous sutures are removed. *Wound is closed with monofilament prolene/nylon sutures. Tension sutures may also be applied.*
• If necessary, closed suction drainage may be used.
• Wound collections to be sent for C&S and antibiogram study.

In the mean time, antibiotics and metrogyl infusion started.

- Ryle's tube suction is also started to decompress the abdomen.

Diagnostic criteria of established incisional hernia (Figs 10.17 and 10.18)

1. *The patient usually presents with a bulging in the vicinity of an incisional scar.*

2. The bulging may be *either localised* occurring through a small portion of the scar, mostly at the lower end appears as a globular swelling, or *diffuse swelling* along the whole length of the scar.

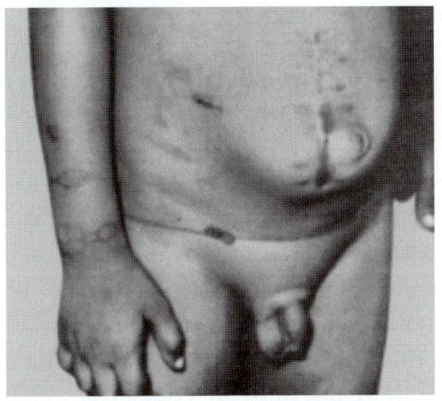

Fig. 10.17: Incisional hernia. Note the swelling with overlying scar. This hernia was reducible. Cough impulse positive.

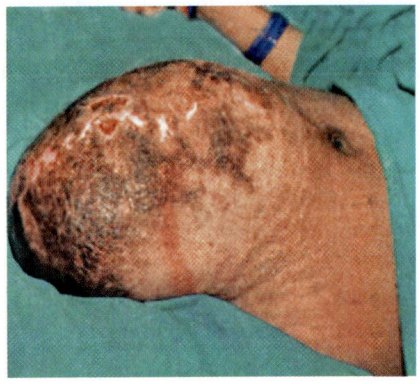

Fig. 10.18: Large incisional hernia. Note the overlying stretched skin, depigmented irregular scar, ulcers and pigmented areas. This hernia was reducible. Cough impulse positive.

3. *The bulge becomes more marked on standing and coughing. Usually it reduces spontaneously* as soon as the patient lies down.

   The reducibility may be partial or complete. Very often the hernia may be completely irreducible.

4. *Expansile impulse on coughing is present.*

5. *The skin over the hernia is thin and atrophic* and sometimes through this atrophic skin *the peristaltic wave of the small intestine may be visible. The overlying skin may be unhealthy, infected or ulcerated.*

6. *On palpation*, the edge of the defect can be delineated.

   After reduction of the reducible hernia the size of *the defect should be assessed by insinuating the fingers through the gap* – this should be done both when the abdominal musculature is *relaxed fully and when the musculature becomes taut after applying the method of head and/or leg rising test.*

   The rising test also determines the tone of the abdominal muscles. If the margins of the fascial defect come together jamming against the insinuating fingers, a comfortable herniorrhaphy can be accomplished. *But if a wide gap remains even after putting the abdominal muscles to contract, hernioplasty with a synthetic mesh is essential.*

   Divarication of the recti is also to be noted.

7. *The patient may be symptomless, except for the obvious bulge.* Sometimes the patient may suffer from recurrent attacks of subacute intestinal obstruction, or strangulation when the neck of the sac is narrow.

8. *History of previous operation noted from the scar mark*, wound infection with or without discharge requiring prolonged dressing, history of postoperative cough, vomiting and abdominal distension are to be enquired.

Complications

1. Often patient complains of *discomfort or pain around the scar of the hernia*, mostly after strenuous jobs. The pain is dragging in nature and due to stretching of the gut or omentum adherent to the sac underneath the

scar. Often, this pain may incapacitate the patient from his/her regular jobs; so the patient seeks early consultation of the doctor.

2. *Irreducibility.*
3. *Obstruction:* Adhesions of the contents, bowel and omentum, with the sac may lead to angulation and subacute obstruction.
4. *Strangulation,* particularly when the neck of the sac is narrow – more common at the ends of transverse scar.
5. Ulceration and depigmentation over the scar.
6. *Spontaneous rupture may rarely occur.* It is surprisingly benign and peritonitis is rare because adhesions and oedema at the neck of the sac probably prevent immediate peritoneal contamination (Figs 10.19 and 10.20).

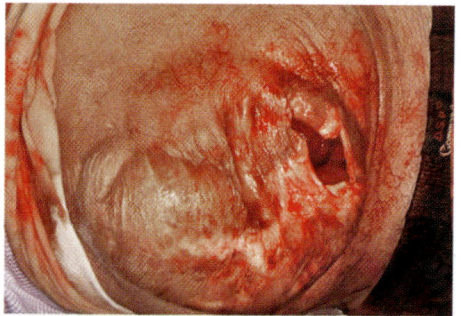

Fig. 10.19: Spontaneous rupture of incisional hernia.

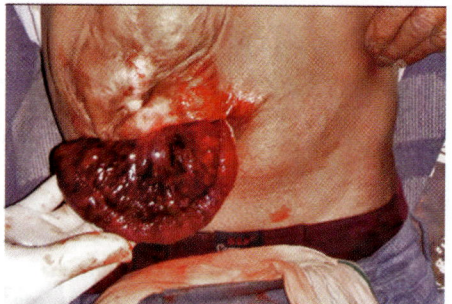

Fig. 10.20: Same patient with spontaneous rupture—with extrusion of small intestine with mesentery.

Treatment

- Preventive
- Palliative
- Operative

Preventive

The incidence of incisional hernia can be reduced by eliminating, where possible, the predisposing factors mentioned above.

Postoperatively, convalescence should be gradual and all sorts of strain be avoided. *Heavy weightlifting or any strenuous work should be avoided for at least 3 months.* The wound must be checked one month after operation, and *any suspected weakness is supported by abdominal corset for a few months.*

Palliative

By using abdominal corset fitted with suitable pad, providing that there are no complications within the hernia.

Although truss (an external support) is generally not successful, the patient with a large ventral hernia where surgical repair is delayed for medical reasons, or may be difficult, can be successfully managed non-operatively with properly fitted corset and close follow up.

Operative

Indications:

1. Discomfort in the hernia.
2. Hernia with complications such as irreducibility, intermittent attacks of subacute obstruction or complete obstruction.
3. Cosmetic reasons.

Preoperative measures:

1. Correction of obesity and weight reduction by proper controlled diet.
2. Correction of any other contributory factor as already mentioned (e.g. cough, anaemia, hypoproteinaemia, diabetes, etc.).
3. If chronic bronchitis, asthma, urinary obstruction or constipation are present, they should be corrected preoperatively.
4. Preoperative colonic lavage is given to prepare the bowel in the event of inadvertent injury, if extensive adhesions are anticipated during operation.
5. *Induction of artificial pneumoperitoneum:* In patients with very large ventral hernia containing nearly half the abdominal content, replacement of the contents within

the abdominal cavity, is either impossible, or dangerous as it will raise the intra-abdominal pressure greatly (*abdominal compartment syndrome*) to cause elevation of the diaphragm and thereby respiratory embarrassment, compression of inferior vena cava and venous congestion, paralytic ileus due to mesenteric oedema followed by stasis in the splanchnic bed leading to shock. Any repair under such excessive tension is also likely to give way. *To avoid these*, it is advisable to prepare these patients by producing *preoperative artificial pneumo-peritoneum at frequent intervals* and with increasing pressure to stretch the abdominal wall gradually to increase the abdominal capacity.

Methods of repair of incisional hernia:

The following methods of operative repair are available, which can be remembered by the mnemonics 'MILK'.

M • Repair by **M**ayo's technique (double-breast technique).
   • Repair by **M**uscle pedicle flap.
I • **I**nlay patch/mesh grafting.
L • **L**attice or darning.
   • Repair in **L**ayers – Cattle's technique.
   • **L**aparoscopic inlay mesh repair.
K • **K**eel operation.

Cattle's operation – repair in layers

Principle

The hernia is repaired in layers, which aims at anatomical restoration. The method is particularly suitable in small hernia where scarring is minimal.

Essentials of operation

After dealing with the sac and its contents the repair is done in multiple layers.

• *First layer:* Neck of the sack with an interlocking suture of thick vicryl which is a braided synthetic long-lasting absorbable suture material.
• *Second layer:* The cut edges of the base of the sac with unabsorbable sutures like prolene.

• *Third layer:* Matted tissue and fascia around the peritoneal sac with prolene.
• *Fourth layer:* Muscles are apposed with prolene.
• *Fifth layer:* Anterior rectus sheath with prolene.
• *Last layer:* Skin.

Keel operation

Principle

In this operation *the hernial sac is not opened and the repair is done by wide inversion of the sac.* In this repair the appearance of the inverted sac on cross section resembles the 'keel' of a ship (i.e. the bottom of the ship – Fig. 10.21); hence the name, *Keel operation* (Rodney Maingot). So it is an *extraperitoneal operation.* This method is particularly suitable for large ventral hernia.

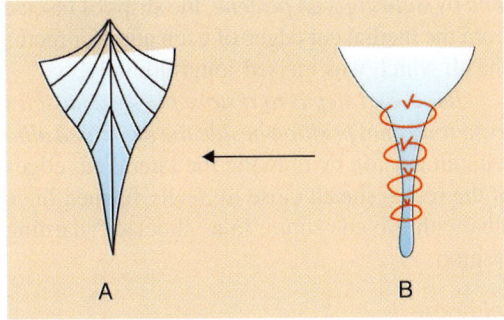

Figs 10.21 A and B: (A) Looking like the bottom of the ship; (B) Keel operation.

Essentials of operation

After dissecting and cleaning the neck of the sac, the sac is pushed back into the abdominal cavity by a series of inverting and pleating layers of unabsorbable sutures (3 to 4 layers of sutures). Lastly, the anterior sheath and skin are repaired.

Advantages

1. Chance of peritonitis, postoperative ileus and abdominal distension is nil.
2. Early feeding may be started.

Disadvantages

1. As it is a blind operation (the sac is not opened) and the intra-abdominal pathology (e.g. any adhesions of the bowel and omentum with the sac) cannot be corrected,

there may be a chance of subacute intestinal obstruction in late postoperative period.

2. During dissection of the sac and suturing of the sac after inversion, there is a chance of injuring the underneath bowel and omental vessels.

Lattice or darning

After dealing with the sac and its contents, the defect in the abdominal wall is closed with fascial sutures in an interlacing manner between muscle and aponeurosis of either side. *The interlacing suture is made in the form of lattice work or darning.*

Shoelace darning

There are two steps in this operation. *The first step is to reconstitute a strong midline new linea alba by suturing with prolene*, the strips of fasciae from the medial cut edges of each anterior rectus sheath which was incised longitudinally.

The second step is to restore the recti muscles to their normal position beside the new linea alba without tension by drawing the lateral cut edges of the rectus sheath close to newly formed linea alba with prolene suture in a 'shoelace' darning fashion.

Inlay graft

These are becoming increasingly popular particularly when the defect is very large and cannot be closed effectively by local tissues.

After dealing with the sac and its contents the peritoneum is sutured with PDS (poly-dioxanone suture), non-absorbable suture. Then *the defect in the abdominal wall is bridged across by implanting a sheet of tantalum gauze or dacron or marlex or polypropylene mesh.* The sheet of mesh should be tacked beneath the recti muscles and sutured all round with fine prolene sutures without tension – *inlay graft. The recti muscles and anterior rectus sheath should then cover the mesh completely.*

This repair may be supplemented with onlay graft which is placed on the outer aspect of musculoaponeurotic sheath wall deep to the skin and subcutaneous tissue – *combined inlay and onlay graft.*

Recently, dual mesh is available which allows an improved placement of inner mesh deep to the abdominal wall and the hernial defect. This type of mesh presents an *intraperitoneal sheet with non-adherent surface* (expanded polytetra-fluoroethylene – PTFE), to the bowel side and *an outer polypropylene mesh* grid or screen for adherence and incorporation both into the peritoneum and the posterior or deeper surface of abdominal wall fascia.

Postoperative measures

1. Gastric suction to avoid distension.
2. Intravenous infusion of fluid and electrolytes till flatus is passed.
3. Avoid prolonged retention of urine and any other strain (e.g. cough, constipation).
4. Adequate antibiotic therapy.
5. Adequate nutrition and vitamins.
6. Early ambulation should be discouraged.
7. No strenuous work for 3 months at least.
8. Use of abdominal corset for 3 months.
9. *Avoid weight gain and obesity strictly.*

Incidence of recurrence after mesh repair

- Without mesh repair, incidence of recurrence is 30–40%.
- With mesh repair, the recurrence rate comes down to 10%.

Muscle pedicle flap

Many advocates the use of muscle pedicle flap to reconstruct the *defect in the lower abdominal wall below the umbilicus. Two muscles are particularly suitable for this purpose* – tensor fascia lata and rectus femoris.

Laparoscopic repair

Recently, laparoscopic repair of incisional hernia is being tried in some centres for small reducible hernia. After creation of pneumoperitoneum the adherent contents from the sac, omentum or intestine, in the gap/gaps are released. *Then the gap/gaps are covered intraperitoneally* with an appropriate size ($\geq 15 \times 15$ cm) mesh which is fixed to the abdominal wall with sutures and tackers: *IPOM* (intraperitoneal onlay mesh repair).

Complications of incisional hernia repair

Immediate complications:

1. Increased risk of paralytic ileus from visceral compression.
2. Pulmonary complications, as a result of elevation of the diaphragm due to reduction of contents.

Delayed complications:

1. Wound infection.
2. Seroma formation.
3. Wound sinus with discharge.
4. Recurrence.
5. Enterocutaneous fistula.
6. Infection of mesh – may require removal.

Note

Diverticulum of recti: The patient presents because of obvious bulge between the recti muscles. This is wide based and does not have a sac. Hence, it cannot be obstructed or strangulated and an operation is not required.

Note

Types of mesh used for hernia repair:

- Prolene
- Dacron
- Marlex
- ePTFE (Gortex)

Note

Placement of mesh in ventral hernia repair:

- Intraperitoneal onlay mesh repair (IPOM)
- Supraperitoneal onlay mesh repair (SPOM)

UMBILICAL HERNIA

It is the herniation through or around the weak umbilical scar (cicatrix). It may be congenital present at birth or acquired and is of four different types:

1. Exomphalos.
2. Gastroschisis.
3. Congenital umbilical hernia.
4. Infantile umbilical hernia.
5. Adult umbilical hernia.

EXOMPHALOS (Figs 10.22 and 10.23)
(*Syn.* Omphalocele)

It is a hernia *occurring through the umbilicus into a transparent sac* whose wall consists of peritoneum and amniotic membrane with intervening Wharton's jelly.

This rare hernia is due to failure of all or part of the midgut to return to the abdominal cavity during early part of intrauterine life (i.e. failure of second stage of gut rotation at about the beginning of the tenth week). *At the same time there is failure of migration and fusion of the lateral folds of the anterior abdominal wall.*

Pathology

The gut is found to be contained within a sac protruding through a defective umbilicus.

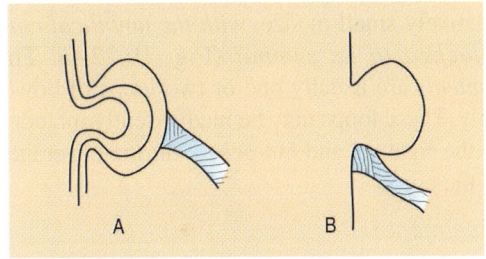

Fig. 10.22: Exomphalos: (A) Minor; (B) Major.

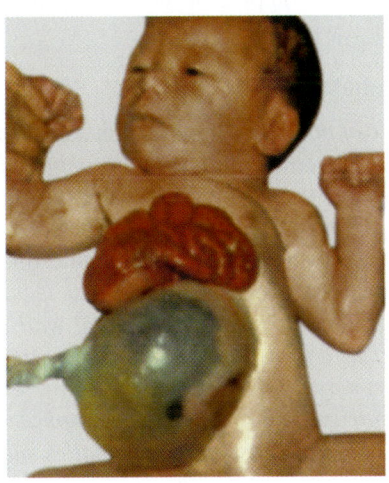

Fig. 10.23: Exomphalos major. The intestine prolapsed outside through a rupture of the sac at the upper part—just before taking the photo. (*Courtesy:* Dr Abinash Roy, MD)

The *covering sac* when remains intact, looks like a thin semitranslucent membrane and consists of three layers – an outer layer of amniotic membrane, an intermediate layer of Wharton's jelly, and an inner layer of peritoneum (Fig. 10.22).

The *base of the sac* is surrounded by skin.

The *contents of the sac* vary. *In the complete variety*, the whole of the midgut loop occupies the hernial sac. *In the partial variety*, only the caecum and/or lower ileum occupy the sac. The sac may occasionally be ruptured at delivery.

Depending on the size of the fascial defect at the umbilical ring, *exomphalos can be divided into minor and major.*

Exomphalos minor

The size of the defect is less than 5 cm. The sac is relatively small in size, *with the umbilical cord attached to its summit* (Fig. 10.22A). The *contents* are usually one or two loops of bowel only. These loops may be inadvertently included in the ligature and cut across during severance of the cord.

Treatment

Twisting of the umbilical cord (which reduces the contents of the sac into the peritoneal cavity) followed by strapping of the abdominal wall at least for 2 weeks.

Exomphalos major

The size of the defect is more than 5 cm. The sac is larger in size and thin, *with the umbilical cord attached to its base mostly near the inferior aspect* (Figs 10.22B and 10.23). The *contents* of the sac are always small and large intestines and occasionally a portion of liver.

On examination, the abdominal wall defect appears as a transparent veil through which the contents may be seen.

Majority of babies with exomphalos are reported to have associated anomalies such as:

(a) Trisomy 13 or 18
(b) Beckwith-Wiedemann syndrome
(c) Cloacal exstrophy
(d) Congenital heart disease.

Differential diagnosis
• Gastroschisis.

Treatment
• Conservative
• Operative

Conservative treatment
Indication:

1. In presence of associated other major congenital abnormalities.
2. *In absence of facilities of operative repair,* e.g. lack of experienced surgeon or well-equipped hospital.

Method:

Repeated application of 0.5% mercurochrome, or 0.25% silver nitrate and silver sulfadiazine cream over the intact sac is done followed by covering the sac with wet sterile gauge. *This local application aims at promoting escharification of the sac* which then shrinks and slowly gets epithelialised to form a ventral hernia. *This hernia is repaired at a later date.*

Operative treatment

Immediate surgical repair is preferable in presence of facilitates. Operation should be done within the first few hours of life, otherwise the sac will burst.

Different types of operations are available depending on the size of the defect, the general condition of the baby, and the presence or absence of other anomalies.

Preoperative measures:

1. No feeding by mouth. Intravenous transfusion should be started.
2. Ryle's tube suction.
3. Blood transfusion should be arranged.
4. Antibiotics to be started.
5. The sac is protected with wet sterile dressings soaked in mild antiseptic or normal saline.

Types of operation:
A. *Primary repair:* It consists of excision of the sac, reduction of the herniated viscera into the peritoneal cavity, and closure of abdomen in layers, all of which are *performed in one stage.*

B. *Staged skin flap closure:* In the first stage, the umbilical cord is excised. The skin flaps are created by undermining the subcutaneous tissue on either side in the flanks. These flaps are then mobilised to facilitate closure over the intact sac. If necessary, lateral release incisions may be made and they are left to heal secondarily. Skin closure over the defect is performed in two layers. If the patient survives this operation, this leaves the child with a large ventral hernia. This ventral hernia is then repaired as a second stage procedure months or years later.

C. *Staged silastic pouch closure:* In this procedure, a temporary closure of the abdominal wall is achieved by using Dacron reinforced silastic sheet in the form of a sac. At an interval of 2 days, the silastic sheet is shortened gradually, till it is finally removed when the approximated edges of the abdominal wall are sutured.

Whichever method of operation is adopted, the cardiopulmonary system must never be embarrassed by the tight closure of the abdominal wall. *A tight closure may cause:*

(a) decrease in cardiac output due to decrease in venous return;

(b) hypoxia following ventilatory insufficiency due to splinting of the diaphragm by the abdominal viscera.

The *survival rates in exomphalos major are about 50%* if there are no associated anomalies.

GASTROSCHISIS

1. In this condition there is a full-thickness defect in the abdominal wall either immediately adjacent to the umbilicus beside the insertion of umbilical cord or separated from it by a thin strip of skin. *There is no intervening sac* (cf. omphalocele).

2. In gastroschisis, anomalies of other systems are rare. *But chances of obstruction are common.*

3. Gastroschisis needs urgent surgical intervention to avoid obstruction.

4. *The survival rates in gastroschisis are better than exomphalos major*, ranging up to 90%.

5. Operative treatment:

(a) *Primary repair:* It consists of reduction of the herniated viscera into the peritoneal cavity and closure of abdomen in layers, all of which are performed in one stage.

(b) Occasionally, *staged silastic pouch closure* may be required, as in exomphalos major.

Clinical differences between exomphalos and gastroschisis are tabulated in Table 10.4.

Table 10.4: Clinical differences between exomphalos and gastroschisis

Feature	Exomphalos	Gastroschisis
Defect	At the umbilical ring	Adjacent to the umbilical ring
Size of defect	Variable	Usually less than 5 cm
Sac	Usually present unless ruptured	Absent
Umbilical cord	Attached to sac	Normal in position
Herniated bowel	Usually normal	Oedematous, thickened and shortened
Herniation of liver	Common	Uncommon

CONGENITAL UMBILICAL HERNIA

It is a rare variety of well-developed umbilical hernia occurring as a result of intrauterine epithelialisation of an exomphalos minor.

INFANTILE UMBILICAL HERNIA

It is the herniation through the weak umbilical cicatrix. It may be present since birth or may develop in the first few days of life usually following neonatal sepsis. *Most umbilical hernias close spontaneously by 2 years of age.* Even larger hernias are known to disappear spontaneously by 5–6 years of age.

Diagnostic criteria

1. Males are more frequently affected (M : F = 2 : 1).

2. There is fullness of the umbilicus with a redundant loose skin over the swelling – this causes parental distress and worry.

3. The bulge becomes more prominent when the infant or child cries or strains.

4. The hernia is usually symptomless, but increase in size because of crying causes pain which makes the baby cry more.

5. *On examination:* The hernia is reducible and a small gap can be palpated admitting the tip or tips of the fingers.

6. Obstruction or strangulation is very rare below the age of 3 years.

Treatment

Conservative

Most of the herniae close spontaneously without any treatment within 2 years of age. Even larger herniae are known to disappear spontaneously by 5 years of age. *So, the methods are:*

• Masterly inactivity.
• Reassurance to the parents.
• Customary strapping after reduction of the hernia: A coin covered with a pad is placed over the umbilicus, which is then fixed by adhesive strapping.

Operative

Indication for surgery:

The swelling:
• Presents beyond 2–4 years of age
• Progressively enlarging hernia after the age of 2 years
• Defect exceeding 2 cm
• Causing symptoms – frequent crying from pain due to distension after feeding
• Becoming incarcerated/strangulated

Essentials of operation:

1. The umbilicus should be preserved.

2. A small transverse curved incision is made immediately below the umbilicus with convexity towards the pubis.

3. The incision is deepened to expose the anterior rectus sheath.

4. After mobilisation of the skin flaps, the flaps with the umbilicus are retracted upwards.

5. The neck of the sac is identified and the sac is opened at the neck (cf. *inguinal hernia where the sac is opened at the fundus*).

6. Contents are reduced and the sac is ligatured and divided at the neck.

7. The hernial sac is usually tightly adherent to the umbilical skin. If the hernia is incarcerated, the sac should be carefully isolated. The umbilical ring should be incised.

8. *The defect in the linea alba is closed by overlapping the rectus sheath with two or three interrupted prolene mattress sutures.*

9. The skin edges are accurately apposed and sutured.

ADULT UMBILICAL HERNIA

There are two types: Umbilical hernia and paraumbilical hernia.

Umbilical hernia (Fig. 10.24)

The herniation occurs *through the umbilical scar* when the umbilical cicatrix is weak. The abdominal contents bulge through this weak spot and evert the umbilicus. *It is a congenital hernia due to incomplete closure of the umbilical ring at birth.*

Paraumbilical hernia (Fig. 10.25)

The herniation occurs *not through umbilical scar* but besides the margin of the umbilical scar.

Contributory factors

1. Commonly in middle-aged or elderly women.

2. Obesity.

3. Multiparous women causing weakness of the abdominal wall.

4. Persistent source of straining, e.g. chronic cough, constipation, bladder neck obstruction, etc., leading to increased intra-abdominal pressure.

5. More common in Blacks.

Pathology

The hernia occurs through the weak area in the linea alba which is the result of repeated

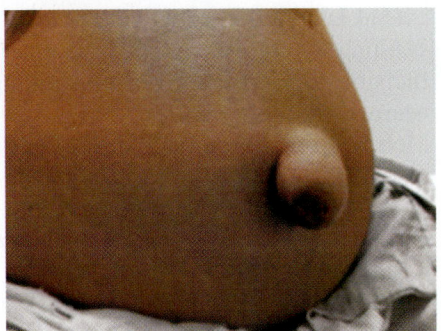

Fig. 10.24: Umbilical hernia through the umbilical cicatrix in 64 years aged male. No H/O constipation, urinary obstruction and asthma. The lump was reducible. Cough impulse positive. But in this patient the abdomen was distended with ascites. *In an aged patient with umbilical hernia* percussion for fluid thrill and shifting dullness should be performed to exclude ascitis. *Management of ascites should take consideration first.*

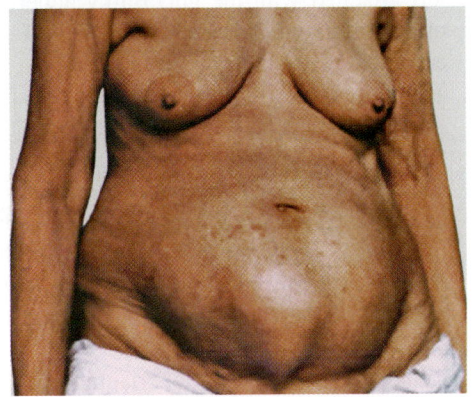

Fig. 10.25: Paraumbilical hernia. Swelling bulging through a defect in the linea alba below the umbilicus. Reducible. Cough impulse positive. No overlying scar.

stretching and thinning out of the linea alba leading to wide separation of the recti.

The sac is usually multiloculated. The neck of the sac is relatively narrower than the fundus because of its bulky contents. The superficial layer of the rectus sheath is stretched out over the protruding sac and is adherent to the sac. The overlying skin of the umbilical cicatrix may be adherent to the fundus of the sac in late cases.

Contents of the sac: Portions of small intestine, large intestine together with greater omentum. These contents are very often adherent to the fundus of the sac and also to one another.

Owing to the multiple loculi of the sac and to the presence of adhesions between the contents and the sac and the narrow neck, *the hernia is usually irreducible.*

Diagnostic criteria (Fig. 10.25)

1. *Common in the elderly, multiparous women,* usually obese with a persistent source of straining like chronic bronchitis, chronic constipation and difficulty in passing urine.
2. *The patient presents with a swelling round about the umbilicus* (Fig. 10.25).

   She also complains of pain or discomfort and tenderness around the umbilicus. Such pain gets worse by prolonged standing or strenuous work. The patient may present with intermittent attacks of intestinal colic or subacute intestinal obstruction.
3. The swelling appears as a firm, round, knobby and *pendulous mass.*
4. Skin with the umbilical cicatrix hangs over the swelling like a festoon. The skin beneath the swelling may be unhealthy, infected or ulcerated.
5. *Cough impulse is present in most cases.*
6. *Most of the herniae are reducible at least partially.* They may be irreducible when the contents are adherent to the sac, or the neck of the sac is very narrow.

   (The reducibility on lying down is not as early and easy as in incisional hernia because the neck of the sac in umbilical hernia is narrow whereas in incisional hernia it is wide.)
7. After reduction, a doughy mass due to adherent omentum may be felt.
8. *On palpation, the defect in the linea alba can be felt as firm fibrous edge, particularly in reducible hernia by insinuating the fingers along the margin of the swelling.*
9. The recti may feel divaricated.

Complications

1. Irreducibility.
2. Obstruction.
3. Incarceration – more common than obstruction.
4. Strangulation.

Treatment

Always operative because of the persistent risk of complications particularly when the hernia is irreducible. *The standard practice is herniotomy followed by repair of the gap in the linea alba by overlapping of the flaps of the anterior rectus sheath,* either from above and below (*Mayo*), or from side-to-side (*Wells*) and suturing them with interrupted stitches.

Preoperative measures

1. Correction of obesity.
2. Correction of any other contributory factors like chronic cough or constipation. Cardiac and renal functions are also to be investigated.
3. Careful skin preparation: *An important measure* because the skin creases below the swelling are very often infected or ulcerated.

Mayo's operation

Principle of operation:

1. *The incision should be made transversely across the abdomen* to deal with the umbilical hernia.
   Advantage: By the transverse incision, *the fibres of the rectus sheath can be simply separated and so the abdominal wall is not further weakened.* [If a vertical incision is made, the fibres of the rectus sheath are also divided, thus adding to the already existent weakness of the abdominal wall (McGregor)].

2. After dealing with the hernial sac and its contents, *the defective linea alba is repaired by overlapping of the flaps of the rectus sheath across a transverse axis (**Double-breasting technique**).*

   Advantages:
   • A satisfactory degree of overlapping is obtained without tension.
   • Tension to suture line is nil or minimum.

Essentials of operation:

1. A transverse elliptical incision is made encircling the umbilicus. The incision should extend laterally on either side beyond the swelling.
2. Incision is deepened to expose the aponeurotic sheath.
3. Mobilisation of upper and lower skin flaps to expose aponeurotic sheath adequately *for about 3 inches, both above and below, beyond the rim of the gap. Edge of the defect is made well-defined.*
4. The neck of the sac is identified and cleaned first.
5. *The neck of the sac should be opened first* because the contents are adherent to the fundus, and the neck remains free from adhesions (cf. inguinal hernia).
6. *Dealing with the contents of the sac:* Any adherent omentum and bowel are carefully dissected, freed and returned to the abdominal cavity. Small portion of sac may be left attached with the gut. Bulky adherent omentum may be excised taking care of the colon.
7. The redundant sac along with the overlying skin is excised, and the peritoneum of the neck is closed with catgut.
8. *Creation of upper and lower flaps of the anterior rectus sheath* by elongating the transverse incision on either side of the defect sufficiently to allow adequate overlapping of the flaps. The flaps should be cleared of any fatty tissue.
9. Repair of the defect by overlapping of the flaps including the peritoneum using four or five non-absorbable mattress sutures. *Usually the lower flap is placed underneath the upper flap.*

   Each suture should pass through all the layers of the flaps.

   The margin of the upper flap is next sutured with the lower flap by a continuous or interrupted stitches.
10. Skin is closed with a subcutaneous drain at each end of the wound, preferably a vacuum drain, which should be kept for 48 to 72 hours.

Postoperative measures

As discussed under incisional hernia.

Note

Recurrence rate of Mayo's repair is around 30%. So, recently prosthetic mesh repair is preferred – open or laparoscopic repair.

EPIGASTRIC HERNIA

Syn. Preperitoneal lipoma; epigastric lipoma; fatty hernia of linea alba. *It is the protrusion or herniation of extraperitoneal fat through a defect in the linea alba* anywhere between the xiphoid process and the umbilicus, usually midway between these structures.

Contributing factors

1. Always acquired.
2. More common in manual labourers between the ages of 30 and 45 years.
3. Sudden strain causes tearing of the interlacing fibres of the linea alba.

Pathological event

In the first stage there is protrusion of extraperitoneal fat through a defect in the linea alba, usually where the latter is pierced by a small blood vessel. At this stage there is no well-formed sac *but only the extruded extraperitoneal fat*, and so it is known as *preperitoneal lipoma*. This lipoma is attached by a pedicle to the underlying peritoneum. *Often it is called epigastric lipoma though it is misnomer.*

In the next stage this extruded extraperitoneal fat or lipoma grows bigger and bigger to come out of the defect and drags a pouch of peritoneum after it and thus gives rise to *a true epigastric hernia. The lipoma is attached to the apex of the peritoneal sac.* The mouth of the sac is very narrow and does not permit a part of hollow viscus to enter into it. The sac is usually empty or it may contain a small portion of the greater omentum.

Regardless of size, incarceration and strangulation are always a possibility.

Diagnostic criteria

1. *Subject:* Common in manual labourers.
2. *Age:* 30 to 45 years.

3. *Sex:* More common in men than women.
4. *Presenting symptoms:* May be:
   - *Symptomless:* No symptoms. Discovered only during routine abdominal palpation.
   - *Pain:* The patient complains of epigastric pain which is localised exactly to the site of the hernia and worsens on physical exertion but often he does not notice any lump.
   - *Lump in the epigastrium* is located above the umbilicus *between xiphisternum and umbilicus on either side of midline.* The lump is usually small and *contains pre- or extraperitoneal fat.* There is no risk of bowel strangulation, *but an operation is advised to ameliorate the pain.*

     Painless, or painful when the lump may be tender to touch or tight clothing. (It is possibly because the fatty contents become nipped sufficiently to produce incarceration or partial strangulation.)
   - *Referred pain:* Often the patient does not notice the epigastric lump. But he complains of epigastric pain suggestive of a peptic ulcer or gallbladder disease. In many cases of epigastric hernia there is coexistent upper abdominal disease. U/S upper abdomen may exclude gallbladder disease.
5. *On examination:*
   - *A firm swelling in the epigastrium.*
   - Does not usually have cough impulse.
   - Cannot be reduced even in uncomplicated cases.
   - May be tender if incarcerated.

Differential diagnosis

- Parietal swelling
- Subcutaneous lipoma
- Neurofibroma
- Fibroma
- Divarication of rectus abdominis

Complications

- Incarceration and strangulation of the extraperitoneal fat causing persistent pain. *But no risk of bowel obstruction or strangulation.*

Treatment

If small and no symptoms – the lump can be over-looked.

If there are symptoms – operation. If incarcerated, painful and tender, the ring may be enlarged surgically by superior or inferior incision of the anterior lamina of the rectus sheath – followed by excision of the incarcerated preperitoneal tissue and simple closure of the fascial defect.

But before undergoing any operation the patient should be thoroughly investigated *to exclude any other intra-abdominal pathology*, e.g. peptic ulcer or disease of gallbladder which can be dealt with same time.

In a large size hernia, mesh repair is performed.

LUMBAR HERNIA

Two types:

1. Primary
2. Secondary – acquired mostly:
   - Following an operation upon an infected kidney or drainage of psoas abscess, in which the wound gets infected post-operatively – *the example of incisional hernia.* So, *an incisional scar is noted in and around the swelling.*
   - Following local paralysis of the antero-lateral abdominal muscles, e.g. due to poliomyelitis – also known as *Phantom hernia.*

PRIMARY LUMBAR HERNIA (Fig. 10.26)

The hernia protrudes through the weak postero-lateral wall of the abdominal cavity (which becomes floor on lying down or supine position). *There are two triangles in the lumbar area – superior and inferior lumbar triangles.*

Boundary of superior lumbar triangle of Grynfeltt

- Above – 12th rib
- Medially – Sacrospinalis
- Laterally – Internal oblique

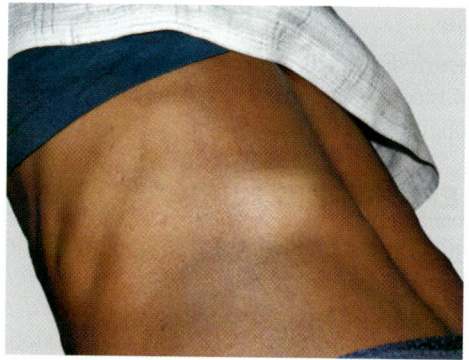

Fig. 10.26: Left-sided superior lumbar hernia in prone position—cough impulse positive and reducible—primary superior lumbar hernia.

Boundary of inferior lumbar triangle of Petit

- Below – Iliac crest
- Medially – Latissimus dorsi
- Laterally – External oblique

Floors of these two triangles are formed by the transversus abdominis muscle. *Floor must be weak or absent to allow hernia to occur.*

- The lumbar hernia is *more common on the left side.*
- The hernia sac has usually a wide neck.
- The sac may contain the left or right colon.

Diagnostic criteria

1. Swelling in the lumbar region of posterior abdominal wall – either below the 12th rib (superior) or above the iliac crest (inferior) – lumbar triangles.
2. *Most common on the left side.*
3. *More common in aged men.*
4. Soft swelling.
5. Cough impulse – present.
6. Reducible – on lying down or on pressure.

Differential diagnosis

1. *Lipoma:* Firm to solid swelling. Cough impulse absent. Not reducible.
2. *Paravertebral cold abscess* pointing to this position – soft cystic swelling, fluctuation positive. *Cough impulse absent. Not reducible. Both clinical and radiological examinations of the spine* will show evidence of tuberculosis of vertebrae.

3. *Incisional lumbar hernia:* Previous history of operation followed by wound infection and *local scar* is present.

Complications

Incarceration, strangulation.

Treatment

Operation: Herniotomy + Herniorrhaphy, or hernioplasty with a piece of tentalum gauze or dacron mesh.

Note

Why lumbar hernia is common on the left side?

Because presence of liver in the right hypochondrium prevents lumbar hernia formation on the right side.

SPIGELIAN HERNIA (Fig. 10.27)

- *It is a variety of intraparietal hernia with hernial sac dissecting between the internal and external oblique muscles.*
- This hernia protrudes *through the linea semilunaris along the lateral border of the rectus muscle at the level of arcuate line. Arcuate line lies midway between the umbilicus and symphysis pubis.*
- The hernial sac, composed of peritoneum, is covered with skin and subcutaneous tissue only.
- It appears as a small swelling to one side of the abdominal wall along the lateral margin of the rectus muscle just below and lateral to umbilicus. *Expansile impulse* on coughing is present.
- *It has a high incidence of incarceration or strangulation* because of the narrow and rigid neck.

Differential diagnosis

1. Haematoma within the sheath – tender swelling following history of trauma. Cough impulse absent.
2. Pyaemic abscess of the abdominal wall commonly in diabetic patient. Tenderness with high temperature is significant.
- Diagnosis is confirmed by:
    (i) U/S scan – can be performed in the

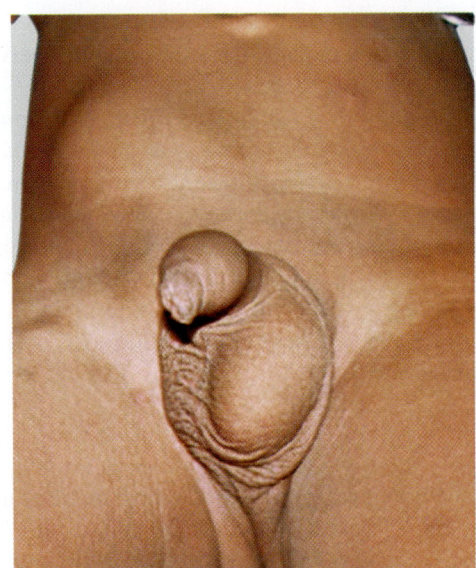

Fig. 10.27: Right spigelian hernia + right-sided undescended testis. Abdominal swelling was reducible and cough impulse was positive—so, a hernia. Same patient had right-sided undescended testis. On exploration, hernial sac was found protruding through the lateral margin of rectus abdominis. The content was found to be right testis—*a surprising content of the hernia at this site.* Testis was mobilised and implanted to the right scrotum. Hernia was repaired. *The picture in this case is that of a child.*

standing position, if no defect is visible in supine position.
    (ii) CT scan.
- Operation is the treatment of choice to avoid the risk of strangulation – open or laparoscopic approach.

Note

Most spigelian herniae develop after 4th decade of life. These are usually associated with obesity. Fig. 10.27 shows spigelian hernia in a young boy.

OBTURATOR HERNIA

This rare hernia protrudes through the obturator foramen and proceeds into the medial side of the thigh in the femoral region under the pectineus and adductor brevis muscles. *Hence, clinically not detectable.*

Patient may complain of referred pain in the knee, the pain radiates from the obturator nerve via its genicular branch.

Irreducibility, intestinal obstruction and strangulation are more common with this hernia. Many a time patient presents with intestinal obstruction *when exploratory laparotomy only can settle the diagnosis of obturator hernia* as the cause of intestinal obstruction.

Recently, *CT scan* is widely used for the purpose which is helpful in the diagnosis of the condition.

Differential diagnosis of a lump in the groin

When a patient presents with a lump in the groin one must think of anatomical structures in and around the area and correlate the pathological lesions arising from the structures.

1. *The hernial orifices*
   - Inguinal hernia
   - Femoral hernia
2. *The lymph nodes*
   - Lymphadenopathy
     - Inflammatory
     - Neoplastic
     - Reticuloses
3. *The vein*
   - Saphena varix
4. *The artery*
   - Femoral aneurysm
5. *The testicular apparatus*
   - Hydrocele of the cord or canal of Nuck
   - Lipoma of the cord
   - Undescended testis
   - Ectopic testis
6. *The psoas sheath*
   - Psoas abscess
7. *The skin and subcutaneous tissues*
   - Lipoma
   - Neurofibroma
   - Sebaceous cyst.

Note
- Most common of all hernias – indirect inguinal hernia.
- Most common hernia in elderly – direct hernia.

- Most common hernia in female – indirect inguinal hernia.
- Indirect inguinal hernia obstructs or strangulates more commonly than direct inguinal hernia.
- All hernias that reach the stage of vascular compromise produce local symptoms and signs of intestinal obstruction except omentocele, Richter's hernia, Littre's hernia.
- Femoral and indirect inguinal hernia are more prone to strangulation.
- In a patient with femoral hernia, femoral vein would be immediately lateral to the sac of the hernia.
- Right-sided femoral hernia is more common than the left-sided one.
- Rule that constipation is present in intestinal obstruction does not apply in cases of Richter's hernia (where only a portion of circumference of intestine is herniated).
- The initial symptoms in a strangulated omentocele are similar to strangulated bowel but vomiting and constipation are rare.
- Truss is contraindicated in infantile hernia and sliding hernia.

Note

Important but rare herniae
- **Sliding hernia:**
  - Common in elderly male.
  - Common on left side.
  - Usually sigmoid colon on the left side (commonest) or caecum on the right side or urinary bladder *on either side slide down along with posterior wall of the sac.*
  - Posterior wall of the sac is formed by a viscus.
  - Chances of injury to these viscera during repair are common.
  - Oesophageal hiatus hernia, cystocele, rectocele in women often with uterine descent are also categorised as sliding hernia.
- **Dual hernia (saddle bag or pantaloon hernia):** This type of hernia *consists of two sacs that straddle the inferior epigastric vessels* – one sac being medial and the other lateral to

this vessel. This condition is not rare and is a cause of recurrence because one of the sacs having been overlooked at the time of operation.

- **Parastomal hernia:** Hernia most commonly associated with end colostomy.
- **Sciatic hernia:** Hernia through greater or lesser sac foramen.
- **Phantom hernia:** Localised muscle bulge following muscular paralysis.

Rare named herniae

- **Richter's hernia:**
  - When *the content of the hernial sac is a portion of the circumference of the intestine.*
  - *Usually complicates femoral hernia.*
  - Commonly associated with gangrene or perforation of the content.
- **Littre's hernia:** Meckel's diverticulum is the content of the sac.
- **Holthouse hernia:** Inguinal hernia with extension of the loop of intestines along the inguinal ligament.
- **Cloquet's hernia:** Hernia through pectineal fascia.

- **Serafini's hernia:** Hernia occurring behind the femoral vessels.
- **Velpeau's hernia:** Hernia in front of femoral vessels.
- **Gibbon's hernia:** Hernia with hydrocele.
- **Amyand's hernia:** Inguinal hernia containing appendix with or without caecum into the right hernial sac (cf. sliding hernia – Fig. 10.8).
- **Ogilvie's hernia:** Hernia through the defect in conjoint tendon just lateral to where it inserts with the rectus sheath.
- **Grynfeltt's hernia:** Primary lumbar hernia – may also occur through the superior lumbar triangle known as Grynfeltt's hernia. Very rare.
- **Petit's hernia:** Primary lumbar hernia through inferior lumbar triangle.
- **Beclard's hernia:** Femoral hernia through the opening of saphenous vein.
- **Petersen hernia:** Hernia under roux-en-Y gastric bypass.
- **Berger's hernia:** Hernia in the pouch of Douglas.
- **Stammer's hernia:** Internal hernia occurring through the window in the transverse mesocolon after retrocolic gastrojejunostomy.

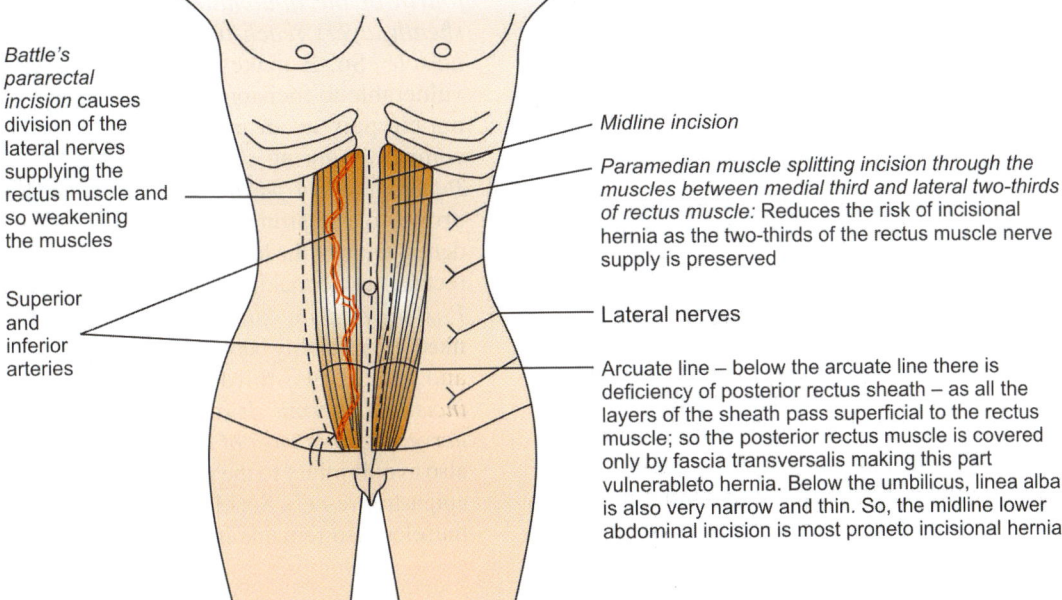

Battle's pararectal incision causes division of the lateral nerves supplying the rectus muscle and so weakening the muscles

Superior and inferior arteries

Midline incision

Paramedian muscle splitting incision through the muscles between medial third and lateral two-thirds of rectus muscle: Reduces the risk of incisional hernia as the two-thirds of the rectus muscle nerve supply is preserved

Lateral nerves

Arcuate line – below the arcuate line there is deficiency of posterior rectus sheath – as all the layers of the sheath pass superficial to the rectus muscle; so the posterior rectus muscle is covered only by fascia transversalis making this part vulnerableto hernia. Below the umbilicus, linea alba is also very narrow and thin. So, the midline lower abdominal incision is most proneto incisional hernia

Fig. 10.28: Different abdominal longitudinal/vertical incisions for exploratory laparotomy

Note

Diverication of recti

Usually a young or middle-aged man may present *with a lump as an epigastric bulge.* This becomes prominent during strenuous jobs or while exercising in a gym. *It is otherwise asymptomatic* except causing worry. Clinically, both erect and supine positions reveal a midline swelling or gutter in the upper abdomen which becomes prominent on Valsalva manoeuvre. No scar mark noted in and around the bulge. *Chances of obstruction are very rare.*

Note

Hiatus hernia

There are four types:

- Type I or sliding hernia: Upward displacement of gastroesophageal (GE) junction into the posterior mediastinum. *The stomach remains in normal position.*
- Type II: Normal position of GE junction with upward herniation of the fundus of the stomach along side it.
- Type III (mixed type): Defined by displacement of the GE junction with a large portion of the stomach cephalad into the posterior mediastinum.
- Type IV: Dilatation of the oesophageal hiatus to such an extent that the hernial sac also contains other contents of the abdomen like spleen, small bowel and colon.

Note

Rectus abdominis muscle is considered as red muscle because it contains more myohaemoglobin, so it is a strong muscle and heals quickly. Both the rectus muscles prevent protrusion of the abdominal viscera during abdominal distension. *It is also a powerful flexor of the thoracic region* specially at the lumbar vertebral column.

Both the rectus muscles also compress the abdominal contents thus keeping the contents in their place. It also opposes the diaphragmatic pressure thus keeping the viscera in its place.

Note

Rectus abdominis muscle is considered as red muscle because it contains more myohaemoglobin, so it is a strong muscle and heals quickly. Both the rectus muscles prevent protrusion of the abdominal viscera during abdominal distension. *It is a powerful flexor of the thoracic region* specially at the lumbar vertebral column.

Note

In TAPP repair, access to peritoneal cavity is required and mesh is placed intra-abdominally between the peritoneum and posterior abdominal wall.

Note

Abdominal longitudinal incisions for laparotomy (Fig. 10.28)

1. *Midline vertical incision specially in the lower abdomen – more prone to incisional hernia because the linea alba is narrow below the umbilicus and there is deficiency of posterior rectus sheath in the lower fourth of the abdominal wall as all the sheath layers reach in front of the rectus muscle.* So, it makes the posterior wall vulnerable to incisional hernia because of poor repair in an emergency operation commonly during cesarean section.
2. *Battle's vertical pararectal incision* is also prone to incisional hernia as it causes denervation of the lateral nerve supply of the rectus muscle making it weak.
3. *Paramedian incision* through the rectus muscle, preferably between medial one-third and lateral two-thirds, is *less prone to incisional hernia. It avoids injury to the nerve supply of most of the rectus muscle.* It also avoids injury to the inferior and superior epigastric vessels. So, blood supply of rectus muscles also remains intact.

Testis, Epididymis and Scrotum

Disorders of the testis and epididymis are commonly encountered in clinical practice. Most of them give rise to solid or cystic scrotal swellings with the exception of imperfect testicular descent.

Classification of disorders

Testis and epididymis

1. Imperfect descent (cryptorchidism)
2. Inflammation
3. Tumours
4. Cysts
   Cysts connected with the epididymis
   (a) Cyst of the epididymis
   (b) Spermatocele

Spermatic cord

1. Torsion
2. Varicocele

Tunica vaginalis

1. Hydrocele
2. Haematocele

▌CRYPTORCHIDISM

Cryptorchidism means a hidden testis. When absent from the scrotum, the testis is hidden from the sight, i.e. the testis cannot be externally appreciated by inspection or palpation.

Before we consider the pathology under this heading we should discuss the development of the testis.

Development of testis

The testes are formed in the abdomen from the mesenchymal cells derived from the yolk sac. The testes develop retroperitoneally in the lumbar region from the genital ridge on the medial aspect of *the mesonephros (Wolffian body)*, and so in early life they lie in the coelomic cavity. *The epididymis and vas deferens develop from Wolfian ducts.*

The primitive testis is attached to the posterior abdominal wall by a fold of peritoneum, the mesorchium, which contains the testicular blood vessels, and nerves derived from the tenth and twelfth dorsal segments respectively (*hence the testicular pain is referred to the umbilicus*). Most of the Wolffian body disappears, but the Wolffian duct persists as the epididymis and vas deferens.

A strand of fibromuscular mesoblastic tissue (*the gubernaculum*) is attached to the lower pole of the testis and bottom of the scrotum. *It acts as a rudder to guide the descent of the testis to its* normal position, i.e. scrotum (Gubernaculum means rudder).

During its descent the testis is preceded by a fold of peritoneum (processus vaginalis) which projects into the foetal scrotum and this obliterates at birth.

Contraction of the gubernaculum, together with increased intra-abdominal pressure, brings about the normal descent of the testis.

Patent processus vaginalis may lead to the formation of a congenital hydrocele or indirect inguinal hernia.

Timetable of testicular descent (Fig. 11.1)

- Third month of foetal life – iliac fossa.
- Seventh month of foetal life – deep inguinal ring.
- Later part of the seventh month of foetal life – travelling down the inguinal canal.
- Eighth month of foetal life – superficial inguinal ring.
- By nine months, i.e. shortly before or at birth – drops into the scrotum, i.e. the final seat of destination.
- Right testis descends little later than the left testis and remains at a slightly higher level.

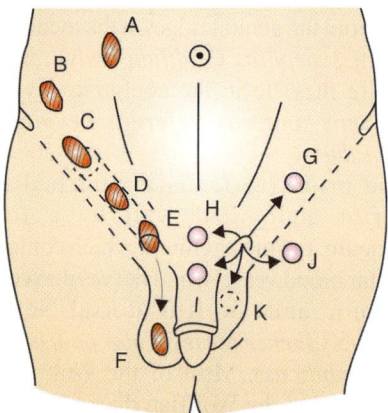

Fig. 11.1: *The time table of testicular descent on the right side (these are also the different positions of undescended testes).* A, lumbar region; B, iliac fossa; C, deep inguinal ring; D, inguinal canal; E, superficial inguinal ring; F, scrotum. *On the left side showing common positions of ectopic testes:* G, superficial inguinal pouch; H, pubic; I, penile; J, femoral triangle; K, perineum.

- *Spontaneous descent of testes occurs in most boys by 3 months of age after birth and uncommonly thereafter.*
- 4% of full term infants and 20% of premature infants have cryptorchidism at birth. The incidence of cryptorchidism in adults is 0.8%.

Factors helping the descent of testis

1. *Shortening of and traction of the gubernaculum testis.*
2. Differential growth of the body wall in relation to a relatively immobile gubernaculum.
3. Raised intra-abdominal pressure due to faecal accumulation and relative growth of the abdominal viscera – pushing the testis through the inguinal canal that is engorged by the swollen gubernaculum.
4. Development and maturation of the epididymis inducing testicular descent.
5. Higher temperature inside the abdomen, which is detrimental to spermatogenesis.
6. *Hormonal factors* supposed to play the major role in promoting testicular descent. The hormones are chorionic gonadotrophin from maternal circulation, testosterone and dihydrotestosterone from the testes, Mullerian inhibiting substance.
7. CGRP, calcitonin gene related peptide released from the sensory branch of the genitofemoral nerve is also responsible for testicular descent.

Factors interfering with the descent of testis

1. Retroperitoneal adhesions.
2. Obstruction, e.g. lateral adhesion at the deep inguinal ring.
3. Short vas deferens.
4. Short testicular vessels.
5. Short pampiniform plexus.
6. Inefficient pull by the gubernaculum testis.
7. Deficiency of maternal human chorionic gonadotrophin and/or testosterone.
8. Imperfectly developed testis (e.g. dysgenesis) which makes the testis insensitive to gonadotrophins.

9. Deficiency of Mullerian inhibiting substance which is secreted by fetal Sertoli cells which is essential for testicular descent.

10. Maternal exposure to exogenous estrogens (oral contraceptives) during the first trimester of pregnancy has been identified as a risk factor.

11. *Prune-Belly syndrome* leading to poorly developed abdominal wall.

Note

There should be two testicles.

• If one testis fails to develop, it is known as monorchism. So, palpate the opposite inguinal canal also for hidden testis.

• If both testes fail to develop, it is known as anorchism. So, palpate both inguinal canals for hidden testes.

• If no testes can be found or palpated in both the scrotums and inguinal canals and both the scrotums are hypoplastic or small – *consider karyotyping the patient before any surgical interference.*

Pathological changes of undescended testis

1. *Growth of the testis:* An undescended testis fails to develop normally. *After the age of 6 years,* growth of the testis is retarded and the testis becomes hypoplastic. *By the time of puberty* the incompletely descended testis is soft and flabby and hardly more than half the size of its intrascrotal counterpart. Testis becomes soft and flabby due to atrophy in view of the fact that scrotum acts as a thermoregulator to the testis maintaining the temperature at least 2 °F lower than that of the inguinal canal, *but the undescended testis is subjected to a higher temperature.*

2. Epididymis is separated from the testis *by a long mesorchium* – a factor for torsion of undescended testis.

3. An incompletely descended testis is *often associated with a hernial sac.*

4. *Histological changes:* Epithelial elements become grossly immature after 6 years of age.

By the age of 16 irreversible, destructive changes occur in the germinal epithelium. Interstitial cells development will however proceed normally.

5. *External secretory function:* The spermatogonia content starts diminishing from the age of 2 years, and spermatogenesis becomes feeble over the months or years and ultimately ceases by about 12 years of age . *Unless the testis is placed in the scrotum by the age of 10 years spermatogenesis will be defective. The placement of testis outside the abdomen is essential for normal spermatogenesis,* as high intra-abdominal temperature is detrimental to this process. When the condition is unilateral, the spermatogenesis is carried out by the normally descended testis but *may develop subfertility* due to defective spermatogenesis in the normally descended testis. *Bilateral cases invariably develop sterility.*

6. *Internal secretory function:* Interstitial cells (Leydig cells) development will, however, proceed normally and *secondary sex characters* appear. In bilateral cryptorchism about half the normal amount of androgen is produced. Nevertheless, the secondary sex character is noticeable in most of the cases and *endocrinologic cause of impotence is rare.*

7. Postnatal growth of testis passes through three stages:
   • The resting stage (0–4 years).
   • The growth stage (4–10 years).
   • The maturation stage (10 years and throughout adolescence).
   At the growth stage (4 to 10 years) spermatogenesis begins to appear and seminiferous tubules become tortuous. It is at this stage that an abnormally placed testis undergoes imperfect but reversible spermatogenesis; *permanent and irreversible changes at the maturation stage will occur if the testis is not in the scrotum by the 10th year.*

8. Cryptorchism may be associated with abnormalities of urinary tract system (13.3%).

Incidence

- Approximately 4% of all full-term newborns have an undescended testis or testes (about 80% cases are unilateral). It may be bilateral (20%).
- The frequency is significantly higher in premature neonates (20%).
- By one year of age, 95% of full terms and 75% of premature cryptorchid testis descend spontaneously into the scrotum.
- Family history is positive for cryptorchidism in roughly 15% cases.
- Undescended testis is *more common in the right side* (50%) than in the left side (30%).
- *Why common in the right side in unilateral cases?* Because the right testis usually descends later than the left testis.

Types of maldescended testis

A. *Undescended testis:* Arrested along the normal line of descent.
B. *Ectopic testis:* Deviated from the normal line of descent.

Undescended testis

An undescended testis is one which fails to reach the scrotum but which is retained at any point along the normal path of its descent (Fig. 11.1). This is better termed incompletely descended testis. *A testis when absent from the scrotum after 3 months of birth is unlikely to descend spontaneously.*

Different types

Based on the location of the testis (can be remembered by the mnemonics 'AIRES')

(AIRE means penis, in Portuguese)

A **Abdominal:** Retroperitoneally in the posterior abdominal wall.
I **Iliac:** Deep to the deep inguinal ring.
  Inguinal: Lies in the inguinal canal: Most common location – about 80%.
  In early life, the testis is soft and lies over the non-resisting floor of the inguinal canal and is covered by the overlying tendinous aponeurosis of the external oblique; so this variety is also clinically difficult to palpate.

R **Retractile testis:** Here, *due to contraction of overactive cremaster muscle,* the normally descended testis is pulled upward either in the inguinal canal or in the superficial inguinal pouch (a space lies superficial to the aponeurosis of external oblique but deep to the fascia of Scarpa. The space lies lateral to the superficial inguinal ring).

  So, in retractile variety the testis can be coaxed down in the scrotum, i.e. its normal position and it remains there after traction is withdrawn for few hours or days. The scrotal sac is also normal. In infancy, 80% of inapparent testes are retractable testes and require no treatment. *The testis is usually of normal size. This variety of testis requires neither endocrine nor operative treatment.* In course of time (may be delayed up to puberty) the testis will take up its normal position permanently.

E **Emergent testis:** Movement of the testis ranges from the inguinal canal to the superficial ring. Emergent testis is transiently palpable outside the superficial inguinal ring, but liable to slip back again into the inguinal canal.

S **Simple undescended or high retractile testis:** Movement of the testis ranges from the superficial inguinal ring to the upper scrotum.

Note

Most common location of undescended testis is the inguinal canal.

Note

Incomplete descended testis is commonest on the right side.

Note

Approximately 70 to 80% of cryptorchid testes will spontaneously descend usually by 3 to 6 months of age.

Ectopic testis

An ectopic testis is one which fails to descend into the scrotum *but has also deviated from its usual path of descent and presents in an ectopic site.*

Ectopic testes are far less common than incompletely descended testis.

An ectopic testis may be found in one of the following positions, in order of frequency (Fig. 11.1).

1. *Superficial inguinal pouch* (i.e. above and lateral to the superficial inguinal ring and superficial to the external oblique aponeurosis but deep to fascia of Scarpa) – commonest site.
2. *Suprapubic* – at the root of the penis.
3. *Perineum* – located at the anterior perianal region.
4. *Femoral triangle* – near the fossa ovalis.
5. *Opposite scrotal compartment* – transverse testicular ectopia is the rarest of all ectopic testes.

Note

Ectopic testis is not found in lumbar region/abdomen.

Explanation regarding ectopic position of testis

According to Lockwood, the gubernacular band has got 4 other additional or accessory tails known as *tails of Lockwood*, in addition to the scrotal tail. These are (Fig. 11.2):

1. Superficial inguinal tail
2. Pubic tail
3. Perineal tail
4. Femoral tail.

Normally all these accessory tails disappear, not the scrotal tail. But in ectopic testis the scrotal tail becomes ruptured. As a consequence, the

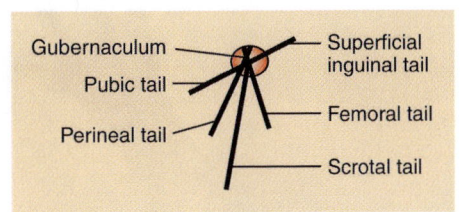

Fig. 11.2: Left 'gubernacular tails' of Lockwood.

testis follows one of the accessory rudders, and takes up the position as mentioned above (Fig. 11.2). *In ectopic testis, the cord structures are not short*; adequate mobilisation will be possible to put back the testis to its normal position.

Note

Complications of ectopic testis

- Atrophy
- Torsion
- Tumour (seminoma)

Diagnostic criteria (cryptorchidism)

Symptoms

1. Parents usually seek advice for the baby because of empty scrotum either one side or both sides due to absence of testis/testes.
2. If the parents fail to notice, the patient may notice it during adolescence or in adult life.
3. A small proportion of patients may present in adult life because of subfertility or infertility.

Local examination (Figs 11.3 to 11.7)

Examination must be done in supine position and when the baby can stand, in upright and cross-legged position also. With the legs adducted the cremaster muscles are relaxed and this facilitates examination.

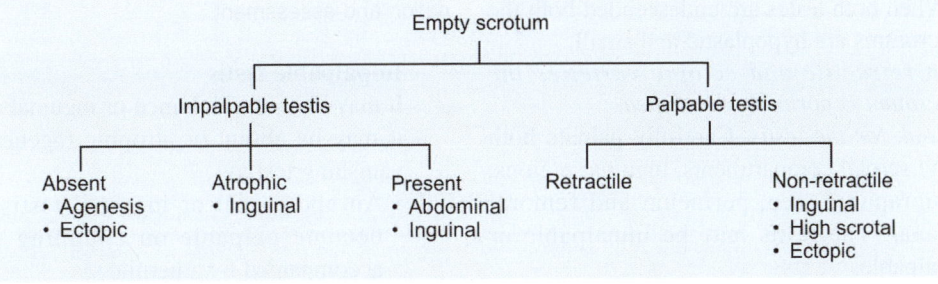

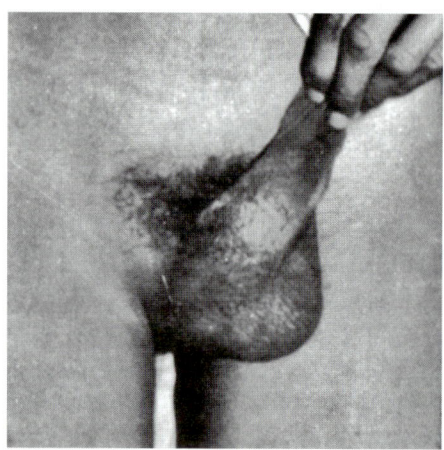

Fig. 11.3: Right-sided undescended testis. Right scrotum was not developed. Right testis was not palpable in the groin. Left testis is in left scrotum.

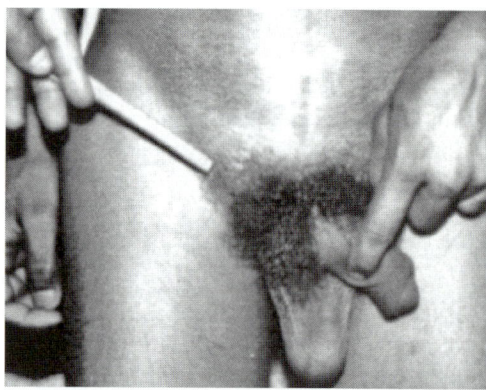

Fig. 11.5: Right-sided undescended testis. Right scrotum was not developed. There was a swelling at the groin—at the medial end of inguinal canal. The swelling imparted testicular sensation and was smaller and softer than the normal counterpart.

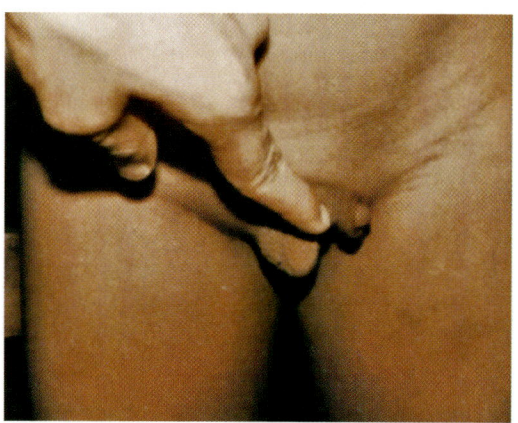

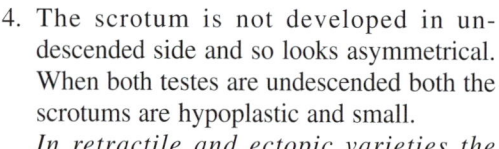

Fig. 11.4: Right-sided undescended testis. Right scrotum was not developed (cf. retractile and ectopic testis). Look for the testis—testis is not palpable anywhere in the groin.

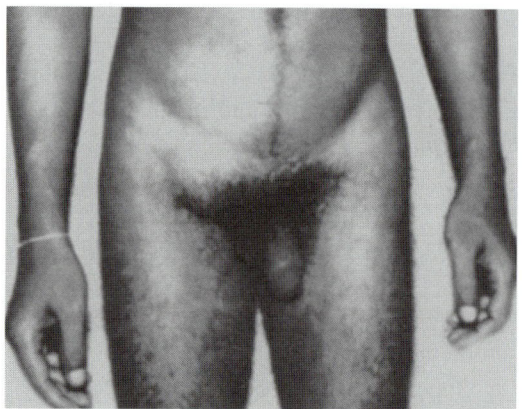

Fig. 11.6: Bilateral undescended testis. Lump noted on the right groin suggestive of testis. Left testis was not palpable in the scrotum and in the groin or perineum. So, intra-abdominal testis. CT/MRI of the abdomen to be done to locate site of the left testis. Once confirmed, the left testis should be removed to prevent future malignancy. *Right testis* should be brought down to right scrotum for regular examination and assessment.

4. The scrotum is not developed in undescended side and so looks asymmetrical. When both testes are undescended both the scrotums are hypoplastic and small.

   In retractile and ectopic varieties the scrotum is normally developed.

5. *Look for the testis.* Carefully palpate both the scrotal compartments, inguinal regions, suprapubic area, perineum and femoral canal. The testis may be impalpable or palpable.

Impalpable testis

It may lie in the abdomen or inguinal canal; it may be absent or atrophic (agenesis or vanishing testis).

- An abdominal or inguinal testis may become palpable on coughing when accompanied by a hernia.

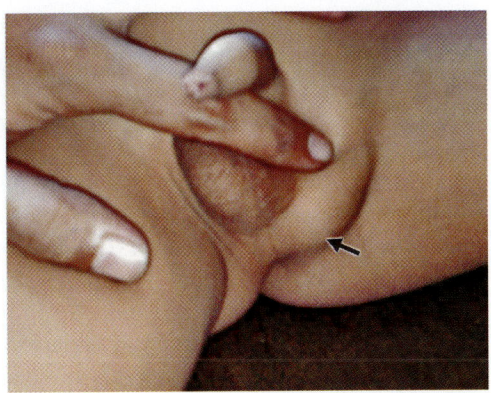

Fig. 11.7: Left ectopic testis in the perineum. Right scrotum developed with right testis. Left scrotum not developed. *Left testis noted in left perineum (marked by arrow).* (*Courtesy:* Professor Sugato Banerjee, MS, MCh)

- The undescended testis in the inguinal canal is very difficult to feel but every attempt should be made to coax it down to the superficial inguinal ring by pushing it medially and downwards so that the external oblique aponeurosis no longer covers it, thus rendering it palpable. *Pressure along the line of the inguinal canal from the lateral to medial end may evoke tenderness or testicular sensation.*

Sometimes examination under anaesthesia can definitely locate the testis in 70 to 80% cases. *Right side is more often involved.*

Bilateral undescended testes are found in about 20% cases.

Palpable testis

It may be either inguinal, high scrotal, retractile, or ectopic.

- *Retractile testis:* The testis can be coaxed down to the scrotum.
- *High retractile testis:* The testis is usually palpable just beyond the superficial inguinal ring but cannot be coaxed down into the scrotum.
- *Non-retractile palpable testis:* The testis is either high scrotal, inguinal or ectopic.

6. The testis is smaller in size and soft in consistence in undescended variety. *So the undescended testis is very difficult to feel.*

In ectopic and retractile variety the testis is normal sized and lying very superficially. A well formed scrotal sac is in favour of retractile testis.

7. *Testicular sensation: Indicates that the swelling is testis.* In case of a child, while the testis is pressed the child will cry. In an adolescent or adult while the testis is pressed, a sickening pain will be felt in the lower abdomen.

8. Range of mobility should be looked for to differentiate the different varieties. It also indicates the planning of operation.

9. Look for the presence of any complication – *particularly hernia.* Undescended testis almost always will have an associated hernial sac. *So, look for a cry/cough impulse in the inguinal region.*

10. Patients with unilateral undescended testis will have a normal puberty and secondary sex character. *Patients with bilateral undescended testes are inclined to be fatty with poorly developed sexual character.*

In cases of bilateral undescended testes, if the penis is very small and/or is associated with epispadius, one should suspect an 'intersex' problem.

(*One should be cautious about the overweight boys* who always appear to have small genitals, as the penis is swallowed up in the abdominal fat and the scrotum appears smaller than what it should be; *parents should be reassured about this and advised to take measures to reduce the body weight.*)

11. Look for the other congenital abnormalities. *Cryptorchid is usually associated with epispadius but not with hypospadius.*

How to differentiate between the undescended testis in the inguinal canal and the ectopic testis in the superficial inguinal pouch?

There are two valuable physical signs:

1. The patient is asked to tense his abdominal muscles (and hence the external oblique aponeurosis) by raising his head and shoulders from the couch – *in case of ectopic variety*

the testis becomes more prominent and easier to feel as it lies on the taut external oblique aponeurosis. Moreover, the mobility of the testis will be unaffected.

In undescended variety the testis becomes less prominent or impalpable with restricted mobility.

2. The ectopic testis, when pushed laterally and upwards, becomes more prominent and goes merely to a higher level, superficial to the aponeurosis.

The undescended testis within the inguinal canal: Testis disappears into the abdomen through the deep inguinal ring.

3. The scrotum on the side of ectopic testis is usually well developed.

Carnett's test: The testis becomes more prominent in ectopic testis on asking the patient to raise legs.

How to differentiate between retractile testis in the superficial inguinal pouch and ectopic testis in the superficial inguinal pouch?

In retractile variety, the testis can be coaxed down into the scrotum but not in case of ectopic variety. The testis can remain there for some period of time even after letting it free. Retractile testis rarely requires active treatment.

Note

Superficial inguinal pouch lies between fascia of Scarpa and external oblique aponeurosis.

Investigations for undescended testis

Though investigation plays a minor role in the diagnosis of an empty scrotum, the following may be helpful in locating the testis particularly the intra-abdominal testis.

- Selective gonadal venography for proving the presence and position of a testis. Demonstration of a pampiniform plexus makes it almost certain that a testis is attached.
- Herniography.
- Radionuclide testicular scan.
- Ultrasound scan: Testis within the inguinal canal or positioned just inside the internal ring can be detected. Intra-abdominal testis is difficult to detect with U/S.

- CT scan: Useful in prepubertal patient when the intra-abdominal testis is sufficiently enlarged to be detected.
- MRI shows high success rate in determining the non-palpable testis.
- **Laparoscopy:** Most useful in identifying the impalpable testis or testes: Anorchism or agenesis. It has become the first choice of investigation recently. Moreover, therapeutic measure, i.e. orchidopexy after mobilisation can be taken at the same sitting. If on laparoscopy, blind ending testicular vessels are seen, do nothing and close the laparoscopic wound.
- Hormone studies: Serum testosterone, LH, FSH, in case of bilateral undescended testis. When basal gonadotropin levels are extremely high in a boy of 7 years and there is no response by testosterone to exogenous hCG, the diagnosis is in favour of bilateral anorchia.
- Karyotyping: If no testicles can be palpated in the scrotum or in the inguinal canal consider karyotyping the patient before any surgical exploration.

Note

Best investigation for retractile testis in inguinal region is inguinal exploration followed by orchidopexy.

Complications of maldescended testis

Can be remembered by the mnemonics 'SATHI'.

S   Sterility – in bilateral undescended testes
A   Atrophy/ambiguous genitalia syndrome in bilateral undescended testes
T   Trauma/Torsion/Tumour
H   Hernia
I   Inflammation
    Infertility

Sterility or infertility

It is the rule in bilateral cryptorchid testes, treated or untreated. The fertility of patients with unilateral cryptorchid is also poor because of the usual defect in spermatogenic activity of the contralateral scrotal testis also. Evidence of decreased fertility exists even in unilateral cryptorchid patients who had undergone prepubertal orchidopexy. *The prospects of fertility (spermatozoa count >20 million/ml and mobility >30%) after unilateral orchidopexy may be as high as 80%.* The placement of testis outside the abdomen is must for normal spermatogenesis as high intra-abdominal temperature is detrimental to the process.

Atrophy of the testis

It occurs if descent does not occur by puberty. It may occur even earlier when the testis is situated in the inguinal canal due to repeated trauma.

Very rarely, atrophy rather than a lump is the first sign of malignancy, and so may be an indication for orchidectomy supplemented with prosthetic implantation.

Occasionally, the patient may present with the complaint that a previously small atrophic testis has enlarged to the size of the normal contralateral testis – *it should arouse suspicion of malignancy in atrophic testis*. Malignancy can develop also in atrophic testis.

Ambiguous genitalia syndrome

* When no testes are visible or palpable in both the scrotums – scrotums appear small and rudimentary. The penis is also small and *is associated with epispadius* – ambiguous genitalia syndrome.
* *Requires urgent karyotyping for sex/gender determination.*
* In bilateral anorchia in a boy of 7 to 8 years there will be no response by testosterone to exogenous hCG.

Trauma

An inguinal testis is liable to oft-repeated trauma, giving rise to pain and atrophy.

Torsion

Because the undescended testis is very often suspended by a narrow mesentery and also because of the abnormal anchorage of the testis to the scrotum, torsion may occur. Torsion of an imperfectly descended testis gives rise to painful tender swelling which is difficult to differentiate from a strangulated hernia or acute epididymo-orchitis. *Deming's sign* – tender lump at superficial inguinal ring (high positioned testis).

Note

* *Prehn's test* in a high positioned testis: *On elevation of the scrotum*, the weight of testis is off and pain is relieved in acute epididymo-orchitis. *But in torsion pain increases.*
* *Detorsion:* The pain decreases when the anterior surface of the testis is rotated outwards towards the thigh.

Note

Any adolescent or adult person presenting with *painful testis if pain is not relieved on elevation of testis* – expect torsion of testis.

In a suspected case urgent colour Doppler study will show decreased blood flow and so, requires immediate surgical exploration and fixation.

Tumour

The risk of malignant change in an undescended testis is 50 times greater than in a fully descended testis. Approximately 10% of all testicular tumours occur in an maldescended testis. *Chances of malignancy are:*

* higher in abdominal type (1 in 20), and
* lower in inguinal type (1 in 80).

In case of unilateral undescended testis, the opposite palpable testis which has normally descended on other side, is also more prone to malignant change than normal individual.

All types of malignant testicular tumour may develop in undescended testis, *but seminoma is commonest followed by embryonal carcinoma.*

Orchidopexy does not reduce the risk of malignancy, but facilitates easy and early detection of changes in size, shape and consistency when it is in the scrotum.

The appearance of a lump in the line of testicular descent, whether within the abdomen or the inguinal canal, and an empty scrotum *should arouse the suspicion of malignant change in the undescended testis.*

Note

Incidence of malignancy is also seen in the opposite normal descended testis of the same patient.

Hernia

Either indirect inguinal hernia or interstitial hernia is often associated with undescended testis due to imperfect obliteration of processus vaginalis (about 90%). *Note that hydrocele is not seen in undescended testis.*

Inflammation

Epididymo-orchitis is rare because the abnormal testis is less likely to become involved by descending infection. *Pain due to torsion is to be excluded.*

Right-sided epididymo-orchitis in an incompletely descended testis may simulate appendicitis. Ultrasound may be helpful.

Infertility

With bilateral undescended testes.

Note

Unilateral undescended testis may also be associated with infertility due to defective spermatogenesis in normally descended testis of the opposite side.

Note

A maldescended testis should be brought down early in the scrotum to prevent torsion, trauma, infertility and to enable early diagnosis of a tumour, torsion. *Orchidopexy does not reduce the chances of malignancy but facilitates early detection and early operation.*

Treatment

I. UNDESCENDED TESTIS

Surgery is the treatment of choice. *Hormonal therapy has no role in this case.*

For a boy under 12 years of age there is no question of orchidectomy; testis should be restored in the scrotum at the earliest.

Procedures available

1. *Orchidopexy*, i.e. fixation of the testis in the scrotum as early as possible, ideally around 2 years of age, in any case not later than 4 years of age.
2. *Orchidectomy*, i.e. removal of the testis. It is advisable to resect an intra-abdominal testis that cannot be brought down into the scrotum

provided there is a normal testis on the other side, because of high risk of malignancy of the undescended testis.

Orchidopexy

Indication of orchidopexy

1. Inguinal or abdominal testis
2. Ectopic testis
3. Undescended testis at the root of the penis

Idea of orchidopexy

1. To allay worries and anxiety of both parents and patients – to improve cosmetic and psychological outcome.
2. To maximise the prospects of fertility.
3. To minimise the risk of tumour development. *Though orchidopexy does not confer immunity against malignancy, it may help screening for malignancy easier and earlier by placing the testis in a readily palpable position and prompt evaluation by U/S.*
4. To reduce the risk of torsion.
5. To repair the associated inguinal hernia.
6. To retain the hormonal function.

Principles of operation: Four essential steps

1. Mobilisation of testis and the spermatic cord to obtain adequate length of the spermatic vessels allowing placement of the testis into the scrotum. But skeletenization of cord structures to gain length should be avoided.
2. Repair of any associated hernia – herniotomy.
3. Eversion of tunica vaginalis to prevent future hydrocele.
4. Fixation of the testis in the scrotum (orchidopexy), preferably without tension.

Ideal time for operation

Because some undescended testes, even in premature infants, *descend by 1 year of age*, the infant is usually observed till that time. *All testicles should be brought into the scrotum by the age of 2 years to improve the spermatogenesis power.* Postponement of operation beyond the age of 4 years results in germ cell atrophy. *Moreover, early orchidopexy also reduces the incidence of malignancy.*

Prior to 2 years of age, the cord structures are so small and thin that operation may endanger the arterial supply to the testis as well as injury to the thread-like vas.

So, *ideally, orchidopexy should be performed at or just after 2 years of age*, i.e. after the child is dry, before he goes to school and before any permanent histological changes have developed.

In bilateral cryptorchidism, one side is operated upon at a time *with an interval of 6 months* between the operations.

Note

Postponement of operation beyond 4 years of age results in germ cell atrophy.

Methods

Three stages of operation:

1. Mobilisation of cord structures.
2. Scrotal fixation of the testis (orchidopexy).
3. Dealing with associated hernia, if any.

Various methods of fixing the testis in the scrotum are available and each merits its advantage according to the length of the cord after mobilisation.

1. Ladd and Gross technique – external anchorage.
2. Denis-Brownes operation – narrowing the neck of the scrotum and external anchorage.
3. Ombredanne's technique – placing the testis to opposite scrotum.
4. Keetley-Torek technique – placing the testis in thigh pocket.
5. Placing the testis in 'Dartos pouch' – *commonly done nowadays.*
6. Fowler-Stephen procedure.

Ladd and Gross technique: External anchorage

In this technique the testis after mobilisation is placed into the scrotal sac followed by narrowing of the neck of the scrotum. The testis is anchored below by passing a non-absorbable stitch through the tunica albuginea at the lower pole of the testis, and the stitch is brought out through the bottom of the scrotum, and anchored to the skin of the thigh by tying it over a piece of rubber tube. This tension apparatus is left in place for 2 to 4 weeks.

Disadvantage: Chance of recurrence after removal of tension stitch.

Ombrédanne's technique (Fig. 11.8)

In this technique the testis is placed in the contralateral scrotal compartment by traversing the median septum of the scrotum. After re-positioning the testis, the hole in the septum is narrowed taking care so as not to make it too narrow to cause obstruction of the structures of the cord.

The method is difficult to perform, and has no special advantage.

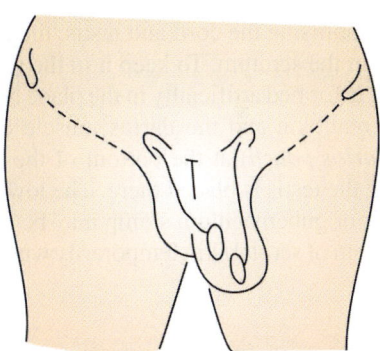

Fig. 11.8: Ombrédanne's technique.

Keetley-Torek technique (Fig. 11.9)

In this technique the testis is placed into a pocket made into the upper and inner aspects of the thigh superficial to the fascia lata, adjacent to the scrotal sac. The testis is brought out through a scrotal incision and either the tunica albuginea covering its lower pole or the stump of the gubernaculum is stitched to the fascia lata of the thigh thus allowing the cord structures to elongate. *Margins of the scrotal incision and thigh incision are then united.* This tension apparatus is maintained for 3 to 6 months.

At a second operation, 3 to 6 months later, the scrotum and the testis are separated from the thigh and thus the testis is replaced into the scrotum.

Disadvantages:

1. The child has to undergo two operations.
2. There is considerable tension on the testis which is likely to interfere with the blood supply hence may lead to atrophy.

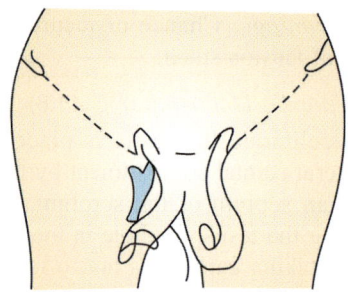

Fig. 11.9: Keetley-Torek technique.

Placing the testis in the dartos pouch
(Fig. 11.10)

After mobilising the cord and testis, the testis is placed in the scrotum. To keep it in the scrotum, a space is formed artificially in the plane between the scrotal skin and the dartos muscle (*sub or extradartos pouch*) at the bottom of the scrotal sac and the testis is placed there. The lower pole of testis or gubernaculum stump may be fixed to the bottom of scrotal skin temporarily with catgut stitch.

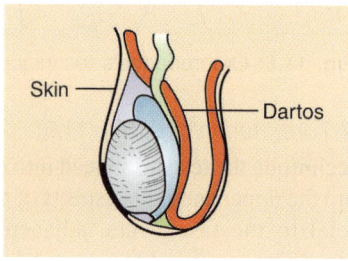

Fig. 11.10: Placing the testis in dartos pouch.

Advantages:

1. Rubber bands and traction are not necessary, if the mobilisation of the cord has been adequate.
2. One stage operation.

Problems during operations

Inability to obtain sufficient length of the cord to bring the testis down. Following methods are available to deal with this problem:

1. During mobilisation, if necessary, the fascia transversalis may be incised medially from the deep ring, and the inferior epigastric vessels are divided between the ligatures, *so* that the cord structures can take a more direct course to the scrotum and thus gain in length.

   This procedure would seem to weaken the posterior wall of the canal, *but tendency to hernia is little.*

2. *Two-stage orchidopexy:* In the first stage, after possible mobilisation the testis is brought outside the superficial inguinal ring and anchored as low down as possible by non-absorbable suture. *At a second stage, after about months to 1 year* a tedious re-exploration and attempt to obtain sufficient length of the cord can be made followed by orchidopexy.

3. *Fowler-Stephens procedure:* The technique relies on the assumption *that the collateral blood supply, primarily from the anastomoses between the artery to the vas and the testicular artery, will prevent infarction of the testis.* The testicular vessels are clamped atraumatically for 5 minutes, and then the tunica albuginea is incised. *If there is brisk bleeding from the testis* it is assumed that the collateral blood supply from the artery to the vas is sufficient to obtain a viable testis. *The testicular vessels are then sacrificed to gain length and the testis is placed into the scrotum.*

4. *Silber procedure of microvascular anastomosis of the testicular vessels:* With the aid of operating microscope the testicular artery is anastomosed to the inferior epigastric artery and the testicular vein to the epigastric vein, but the vas and vasal artery are left undisturbed.

5. *Orchidectomy, in unilateral cases is considered if there is atrophy, torsion, inability to bring down the abdominal testis. It may be followed by either simultaneous or subsequent placement of a testicular prosthesis to avoid emotional trauma.*

Note

Advantages of orchidopexy in cryptorchidism

Orchidopexy can prevent:

• Epididymo-orchitis
• Torsion of testis

- Allays anxiety of patient's parents
- Helps in easy examination and early detection of testicular tumour. *Orchidopexy does not reduce the chances of malignancy.*
- Doubt of sexual ambiguity in bilateral cases

Note

For associated indirect hernia, *simple herniotomy would suffice.* Repair of posterior wall, i.e. herniorrhaphy may be considered on the merit of local anatomy.

Note

Recently, orchidopexy is being performed between 8 and 12 months of age as the microscopic changes in undescended testis start by 1 year of age.

Note

Tumour can occur in ectopic testis also.

Orchidectomy (removal of the testis)

Indication

1. The undescended testis is either hopelessly atrophic or cannot be brought down due to insufficient length of the cord structures, *provided the contralateral testis is normal.*
2. Unilateral undescended testis in adolescent or adult, because of the risk of malignancy.
3. Bilateral undescended testes – when neither testis can be brought down, the smaller testis is removed and the *larger one is preserved for its androgenic function.*

If the testis cannot be found in the inguinal region it is advisable to look for an abdominal testis and remove it because of the high risk of malignancy.

Laparoscopic management of undescended testis/cryptorchidism

- Recently laparoscopic intervention is in favour of the treatment of undescended testis (anorchism) at 2 years of age.
- Laparoscopy has both diagnostic and therapeutic roles to play in the management of undescended testis in the same sitting.

- Laparoscopy helps to detect the location of the undescended testis: *Peeping testis, testis lying at the internal inguinal ring* or *testis lying 2.5 cm proximal to the internal ring or above.*
- *Intra-abdominal testis lying proximal to internal inguinal ring is difficult to be brought down to scrotum by conventional/open inguinal approach.*
- Laparoscopy offers the choices of single stage as well as two-staged orchidopexy.
- Laparoscopy offers to treat bilateral undescended testes in the same sitting.
- Laparoscopy may detect the absent (agenesis) or atrophic testis.
- *Testicular absence (agenesis) can be established only when blind ending testicular vessels are found.* Do nothing and close the wound.
- If the spermatic vessels are seen entering the deep inguinal ring, the next step is inguinal exploration and orchidopexy.
- Atrophic testis should be removed when contralateral testis is in normal position, *because tumour may also develop in atrophic testis.*
- The laparoscopic orchiectomy is a simple procedure in experienced hand to prevent or to detect malignancy early.

Diagnostic laparoscopy and Fowler-Stephens procedure

Fowler-Stephens procedure can be performed laparoscopically also in two-stage procedure or one-stage procedure *for high intra-abdominal testis (>2.5 cm proximal to internal ring).*

- *Two-stage procedure: In the first stage* the testicular vessels are clipped *in situ* with a hulka clip. *In the second stage*, 6 months later, the testicle is brought down after division of the testicular vessels into the dartos pouch of the scrotum *based on the vasal vasculature.*
- *One-stage procedure:* The testicular vessels are clamped atraumatically for 5 minutes, and *then the tunica albuginea is incised.* If there is brisk bleeding from the testis it is assumed that the collateral blood supply is sufficient to obtain a viable testis. The testicular vessels are then sacrificed and the testis is brought down in the dartos pouch of the scrotum.

Problem with impalpable testis or testes – whether cryptorchidism or agenesis

When bilateral:

The diagnosis of *bilateral agenesis or anorchism* should always be considered in the presence of bilateral impalpable testes. *So, consider karyotyping the patient before surgical exploration.*

- First diagnostic laparoscopy is performed before hormonal studies: *The absence of bilateral testicular vessels* or *blind ended testicular vessels suggest that the testes are absent on both sides – agenesis.*
- Then patient is referred to endocrinologist for hormonal studies: Serum testosterone, LH and FSH followed by hormonal stimulation test.
- Serum testosterone level is normal in unilateral undescended testis as the other testis is normal.
- Serum testosterone level is also normal in bilateral undescended testis, provided they are not a case of bilateral agenesis.
- *Hormonal stimulation study is available to distinguish bilateral agenesis from bilateral undescended testes.*

A short course of human chorionic gonadotrophin (hCG 2000 IU daily for 3 days) is given. *In bilateral agenesis* basal serum gonadotrophin (FSH and LH) levels are extremely high with a low serum testosterone level – *the low serum testosterone level does not respond to the challenge with hCG.*

In bilateral cases, if required, surgery is done with an interval of 6 months for each side. *Both sides not to be done in the same sitting.*

When unilateral:

- Unilateral agenesis poses a unique diagnostic problem. Hormonal studies and stimulation test does not help.
- *Testicular venography may be useful:* The absence of pampiniform plexus or a blind ending testicular vein suggests that the testis is absent.
- *Diagnostic laparoscopy is very helpful:* The absence of testicular vessels or presence of blind-ended testicular vessels suggests that the testis is absent on that side (agenesis).

II. ECTOPIC TESTIS

An ectopic testis, like the undescended testis, should be placed in the scrotum as soon as the condition is suspected *as the tumour can develop in ectopic testis also*. Moreover, spermatogenesis is also reduced in ectopic testis.

In these cases orchidopexy is usually a simple procedure *because of the sufficient length of the cord*, the scrotum is usually well developed and the processus vaginalis is usually not patent, so facilitates comfortable orchidopexy.

Hormonal treatment is of no value.

A comparison between undescended and ectopic testes is shown in Table 11.1.

III. RETRACTILE TESTIS

Retractile testis does not require any treatment. Reassurance to the parents that testicular descent will occur normally (may be delayed up to puberty) is all that is necessary.

Hormonal treatment is of little value.

Role of hormone therapy

Much controversy exists regarding the efficacy of hormone therapy in truly cryptorchid patients. Most consider it to be efficacious only in retractile testis. It may be used in patients with bilateral palpable (inguinal) cryptorchid testes with or without hypogenitalism and obesity.

Drugs used

At present two types of hormones are available: hCG and GnRH (LHRH). hCG is given IM in the dose of 1500 IU/m^2 on alternate days for 9 doses.

GnRH is given in the dose of 1.2 mg/day *as a prenasal spray* for 4 weeks.

Drawbacks of hormone therapy

- Injections are painful.
- It may precipitate precocious puberty.
- Mechanical barrier is almost always present in truly cryptorchid testis on which hormone has no effect. Rather it will be a waste of time.
- Inguinal hernia coexists in majority of the cases and if the hernia is not timely treated there is a chance of strangulation.

Table 11.1: Comparison between undescended and ectopic testes

Undescended testis	Ectopic testis
1. Arrested descent of the testis which lies in the normal path of its descent.	The testis deviates from its normal path of descent.
2. Cause: Already mentioned.	Cause: Already mentioned.
3. Undescended testis is poorly developed (cf. retractile testis – the testis is usually of normal size).	Usually well developed.
4. Scrotum is not developed and is empty (cf. retractile testis – the scrotum is usually developed but empty).	Scrotum is usually developed but empty.
5. Undescended testis lies deep in the inguinal canal (cf. retractile testis).	*It lies superficial to inguinal canal.*
6. On pressure – the testis disappears upward, backward and laterally. It may disappear deep into the abdominal cavity.	No effect on pressure.
7. Length of the cord is usually short.	Length of the cord is usually adequate.
8. Power of spermatogenesis becomes poor.	Power of spermatogenesis usually normal.
9. Treatment requires operation and depends on the age and may be satisfactory (cf. retractile testis).	Treatment requires operation.
10. Complications and hazards – so many – remember 'SATHI' (p. 270).	Tumour can also occur/develop. The other hazard is liability to injury (rarely the testis may be associated with an oblique, or interstitial inguinal hernia).

Note

- *Management of undescended testes detected at puberty – orchidopexy (if viable) to preserve the function of hormone production (testosterone) and to provide mental satisfaction and to keep the testes under regular surveillance for early detection of testicular tumour.*
- Orchidopexy does not protect against the risk of development of testicular tumours, but it can prevent epididymo-orchitis, torsion of testes, sexual ambiguity in bilateral cases. *Orchidopexy cannot prevent testicular tumours, but it allows easy and early examination of the testis during checkups, particularly to exclude or rule out tumour suspicion.*

Note

Gynaecomastia may be seen with anorchism but is usually not a feature of cryptorchidism.

CYSTS IN RELATION TO EPIDIDYMIS

A cyst of the epididymis may arise due to cystic degeneration of the vestigial remnants in the epididymis. These may include:

- Remnants of the mesonephric or Wolffian duct system:
  - · The appendix of the epididymis.
  - · The paradidymis.
- Remnants of the paramesonephric or Mullerian duct system
  - · The appendix of the testis (Fig. 11.11A).

CYST OF THE EPIDIDYMIS

It is a *multilocular degeneration cyst* in relation to head of the epididymis.

Diagnostic criteria

1. Though congenital in origin, cysts of the epididymis are usually *found during middle life.*

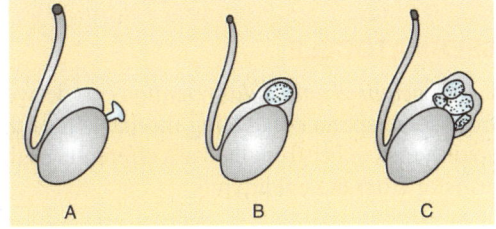

Figs 11.11 A to C: Cysts in relation to epididymis. (A) Cyst of the hydatid of Morgagni; (B) Spermatocele; (C) Cyst of the epididymis.

2. Patient complains of swelling in the scrotum. The swelling enlarges very slowly over many years. *It may be bilateral.*
3. The swelling is situated at the head of the epididymis and hence *above and behind the testis. The testis can be distinctly felt apart from the swelling* (Fig. 11.11C).
4. On careful palpations: *Multilocular cystic swellings*; the swelling feels somewhat lobulated or like a branch of tiny grapes (because it consists of an aggregation of small cysts (Fig. 11.11C). *The testis can be distinctly felt apart from the swelling.*
5. *Fluctuation:* Positive.
6. *Transillumination: Brilliantly positive* but is finely tessellated (due to the presence of numerous septae) giving *Chinese lantern or marble floor appearance.*
7. *U/S scan: Confirms multilocular cysts.*
8. *On aspiration: Crystal clear fluid* without any sperm will be obtained.

Treatment

1. If the swelling is small – it does not require any treatment.
2. If the swelling is large enough to cause persistent pain or discomfort—
   • Excision of the cyst completely via a scrotal incision.
   Disadvantage: Excision will almost certainly cause infertility from blockage and the patient should be informed of it before undertaking the operation.
   • Aspiration of the cysts may be performed but it is useless as the cysts are multilocular and repeated aspirations may introduce infection.

SPERMATOCELE

It is an *acquired unilocular retention cyst* derived from some sperm conducting mechanism of the epididymis, either from the vasa efferentia of the testis or from the epididymis.

Diagnostic criteria of spermatocele

1. A soft, painless cystic swelling situated in the head of the epididymis and hence above

and behind the upper pole of testis (Fig. 11.11B). *The testis can be distinctly felt apart from the swelling.*
2. *Fluctuation:* Positive.
3. *Transillumination:* Poorly positive (cf. cyst of the epididymis).
4. U/S scan: Confirms unilocular cysts.
5. *On aspiration: White, opalescent (barley water-like) fluid* containing dead spermatozoa is obtained (cf. cyst of the epididymis).

Treatment

1. If of a smaller size – it does not require any treatment.
2. If of a larger size causing discomfort—
   • *Aspiration* may be useful as it is a unilocular cyst.
   • *Complete excision* of the cyst is performed via a scrotal incision.

Differential diagnosis

The *cyst of the epididymis* and *spermatocele: Both the types of cysts* are to be differentiated from a vaginal hydrocele by the following points.

• Both these cysts are situated above and behind the testis. *So, they can be distinctly felt apart from the testis. In hydrocele, the testis cannot be felt separately.*
• They are softer in feel but *hydrocele is a tense cystic swelling.*
• *Transillumination test:*
  – Cyst of the epididymis – *positive with Chinese lantern appearance in multilocular cyst.*
  – Spermatocele – *poorly positive in unilocular cyst.*
  – Hydrocele – *brilliantly positive and uniform appearance.*
• Aspiration test: The aspirated fluid:
  – *Cyst of the epididymis* – crystal clear.
  – *Spermatocele* – white opalescent (barley-water like).
  – *Hydrocele* – amber-coloured (urine-like).

Note

Tuberculosis of epididymis:
• Tuberculosis attacks epididymis – affects the globus minor first.

- *The epididymis becomes firm and craggy, and the vas becomes beaded.*
- *Cf. – (1) syphilis* – attacks the body of the testis; *(2) filariasis* attacks both epididymis and testis.

PROCESSUS VAGINALIS

Its source and fate (Fig. 11.12)

Processus vaginalis is a peritoneal diverticulum dragged down by the testis during its descent from the abdomen to the scrotum.

After the testicular descent is completed, the processus vaginalis becomes occluded at two points soon after birth – *first at the deep inguinal ring, and secondly, just above the testis leaving* behind a part of the sac in relation to the testis which is known as the tunica vaginalis of the testis. *The tunica vaginalis surrounding the testis has two layers – the visceral layer and the parietal layer.*

The portion of the processus vaginalis between the two occlusions is known as *funicular process*, which normally becomes obliterated forming a fibrous cord, the rudiment of processus vaginalis.

In some children, this process of occlusion and/or obliteration may not take place and *the persistence of the processus vaginalis is the principal factor* in the development of congenital hernia and hydrocele.

The difference between a congenital hernia and congenital hydrocele in a child is the size

and the contents of the processus vaginalis. A hernia contains an intra-abdominal structure whereas a *hydrocele contains only peritoneal fluid which is brilliantly transilluminate.*

▌HYDROCELE

A hydrocele is an abnormal collection of fluid within some part of the processus vaginalis, commonly in the tunica vaginalis of the testis. It is *a type of exudation cyst* limited to scrotum.

Processus vaginalis is an outpouching of peritoneum that enters into the scrotum when the testis reaches the scrotum. Proximal portion of processus vaginalis obliterates whereas the distal portion persists and forms the tunica vaginalis.

Clinically, two types are encountered according to the presence or absence of a communication with the peritoneal cavity.

1. *Communicating hydrocele:* Generally present in neonates and children, and results from the incomplete obliteration of the processus vaginalis. This patent processus vaginalis contributes to the collection of peritoneal fluid in the tunica vaginalis. *Also called congenital hydrocele* (Fig. 11.12A).
2. *Non-communicating hydrocele:* Typically appears in adult life.

Causes of hydrocele

- Congenital
- Acquired
  - Primary or idiopathic
  - Secondary

Primary or idiopathic hydrocele

The cause is unknown. *There is no associated disease of the testis or epididymis.* It is thought that an imbalance of the secretory and absorptive capacities of the layers of the tunica vaginalis is responsible for the collection of fluid within the sac.

Primary hydrocele usually develops slowly without pain and becomes large and tense.

Secondary

It occurs *due to some pathological condition of the testis or epididymis*, e.g.

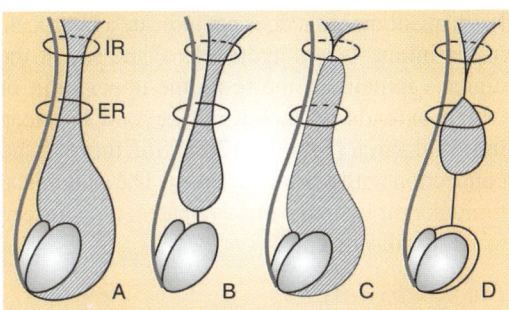

Figs 11.12 A to D: Abnormalities arising in relation to the processus vaginalis. (A) Congenital hydrocele; (B) Funicular hydrocele; (C) Infantile hydrocele; (D) Encysted hydrocele of the cord. ER, external ring; IR, internal ring.

- Inflammation – epididymo-orchitis. Most common. Subsides with resolution of epidi-dymo-orchitis.
- Lymphatic obstruction – filariasis
- Trauma
- Tumour – malignancy

Most secondary hydroceles appear rapidly and remain small and lax. *Exception is hydrocele due to filariasis* which can be large and tense.

Types of primary hydrocele

Seven anatomical varieties are encountered:

1. Congenital hydrocele (Figs 11.12A and 11.13)
2. Funicular hydrocele (Fig. 11.12B)
3. Infantile hydrocele (Fig. 11.14)
4. Encysted hydrocele of the cord – rare (Figs 11.15, 11.16 A and B)
5. Hydrocele of the canal of Nuck
6. Vaginal hydrocele – commonest
7. Hydrocele en-bisac or bilocular hydrocele.

CONGENITAL HYDROCELE (Fig. 11.13)

Here the processus vaginalis remains patent throughout communicating with the abdominal cavity and fluid accumulates in it – communi-cating hydrocele; but the communication at the deep ring is too narrow to admit the bowel or omentum to allow development of hernia; it only admits the escape of normal peritoneal fluid (cf. hernia) while the child is up and playing around.

Diagnostic features

1. *Congenital swelling* present since birth.

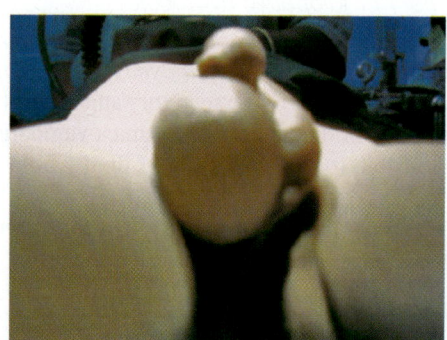

Fig. 11.13: Congenital hydrocele—brilliantly trans-illuminable.

2. It appears as an inguinoscrotal or scrotal swelling which becomes more prominent on standing or walking. It is a type of special form of indirect hernia which allows egress of fluid only.
3. The hydrocele volume fluctuates, with the scrotum being full by evening after a day's activity, *but relatively empty in the morning after the fluid has drained back into the abdominal cavity through the patent processus during night rest – communicating hydrocele.*
4. Testis cannot be felt separately from the swelling.
5. *Cystic swelling:* Fluctuation positive.
6. *Cough impulse: Present.*
7. *Transillumination:* Positive.
8. *Reducibility:* Reducible, partly on lying down and on gentle pressure and this confirms the presence of a patent processus vaginalis; *no gurgling on reduction.*

FUNICULAR HYDROCELE (Fig. 11.12B)

This is also congenital but largely incomplete, i.e. the processus vaginalis is shut off from the tunica vaginalis just above it.

The features are the same as those of congenital hydrocele except that the testis can be felt separately from the swelling.

INFANTILE HYDROCELE
(Figs 11.12C and 11.14)

It is a misnomer as it does not indicate a hydrocele in the infant. It is a hydrocele of the sac of the tunica vaginalis of the testis the upper limit of which extends up to but not beyond the deep inguinal ring (Fig. 11.12C). So, there is no connection with peritoneal cavity. The anatomical funicular process remains as a patent tract instead of being fibrous cord.

Diagnostic features

1. *Inguinoscrotal swelling: Bilocular swelling,* one in the scrotum and one in the inguinal region between superficial and deep inguinal ring communicating with each other.
2. *Testis* cannot be felt separately.
3. *Cystic swelling: Cross fluctuation positive.*

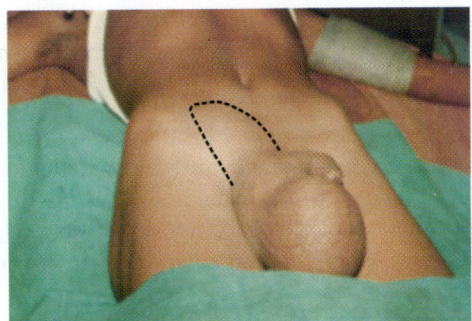

Fig. 11.14: Right-sided infantile hydrocele (also called *bilocular hydrocele*). Scrotal swelling extending above to the inguinal region up to the mid-inguinal region (note the ink marking over the inguinal region). On examination—cystic swelling, cross fluctuation positive and transillumination positive. *Not reducible and cough impulse negative* (cf. complete inguinal hernia) (*Courtesy:* Dr RL Modak, MS)

4. *Cough impulse:* Absent.
5. *Not reducible* (cf. inguinal hernia).
6. *Transillumination:* Positive.

Treatment of hydroceles in infants and childhood

Spontaneous closure and resolution of the patent processus vaginalis usually occur by 12 to 18 months of age. *So, if the hydrocele persists beyond 2 years of age surgical treatment is necessary.*

Congenital hydroceles are treated by hernio-tomy as they do not resolve spontaneously.

Operation is performed through a small inguinal crease incision, as the primary abnormality is at the level of the deep inguinal ring. The operation consists of high ligation of the patent processus vaginalis at the deep ring followed by excision of the part of the distal sac. The remaining part of the opened sac is left intact.

ENCYSTED HYDROCELE OF THE CORD
(Figs 11.12D, 11.15, 11.16 A and B)

This condition develops when a portion of the funicular process fails to shrink into a fibrous cord and persists (Fig. 11.12D), being shut off from the tunica vaginalis below as well as from the peritoneum above, and becomes distended

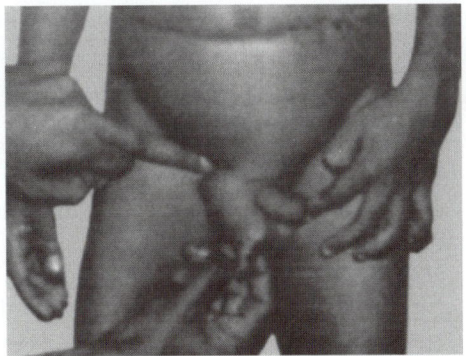

Fig. 11.15: Right-sided encysted hydrocele of the cord—inguinoscrotal swelling. Note that the testis was felt separated from the swelling. The upper margin of the swelling extended to the inguinal canal. Cough impulse negative. Transillumination positive. Traction test positive.

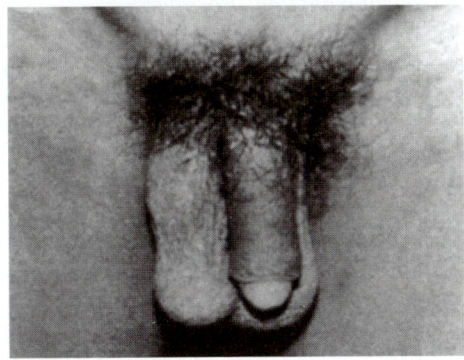

Fig. 11.16A: Right-sided encysted hydrocele of the cord—scrotal swelling. Cough impulse negative. Transillumination positive.

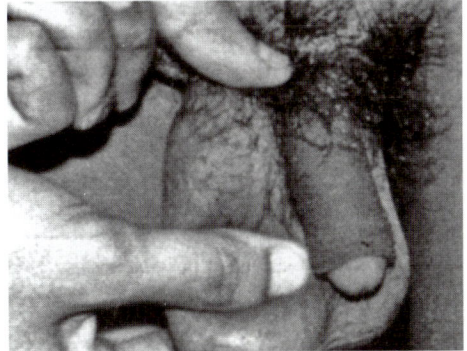

Fig. 11.16B: Same patient. The scrotal swelling was limited both above and below and the testis could be felt apart from it. Traction test positive.

with fluid. *It appears as a localized elongated swelling in relation to the spermatic cord.*

Diagnostic features

1. The swelling may be found in the inguinal, inguinoscrotal or in the scrotal region depending on which part of the funicular process is patent (Figs 11.15 and 11.16 A and B).
2. Elongated cystic swelling in relation to the spermatic cord.
3. The swelling is limited both above and below and the testis can be felt apart from it (Figs 11.12B and 11.16B).
4. Cystic swelling: Fluctuation positive.
5. Cough impulse: Absent.
6. Not reducible.
7. *Transillumination: Positive.*
8. *Traction test: Positive*, i.e. when gentle traction is exerted on the testis, the swelling comes down and becomes fixed or less mobile.

Treatment

Excision of the encysted cyst.

HYDROCELE OF THE CANAL OF NUCK

It occurs in the female rarely, in relation to the round ligament, *always in the inguinal canal.*

    This is female counterpart of encysted hydrocele of the cord in male. Treatment – excision.

HYDROCELE EN-BISAC OR BILOCULAR HYDROCELE

Here the hydrocele has two intercommunicating sacs – one above and one below the neck of the scrotum. The upper sac has no connection with the processus vaginalis. This is, in fact, the herniated tunica vaginalis.

    Treatment – excision.

VAGINAL HYDROCELE

Here the fluid collects between the visceral and parietal layers of the tunica vaginalis of the testis. It gives rise to a scrotal swelling. It is limited to

scrotum *giving rise to scrotal swelling. Vaginal hydrocele is the most common type of hydrocele.*

Composition of hydrocele fluid

Hydrocele fluid is *amber or straw-coloured.* It contains water, inorganic salts, traces of albumin and fibrinogen. In long-standing cases the fluid may contain cholesterol and tyrosine crystals. *The fluid does not clot until it comes in contact with blood.*

Diagnostic criteria of vaginal hydrocele

1. *Age: Primary hydroceles* are most common in the middle-aged or the elderly men, but it is not uncommon in early childhood. Secondary hydroceles are common in young

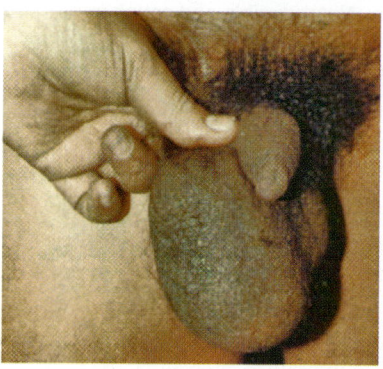

Fig. 11.17: Right-sided vaginal hydrocele. Scrotal swelling. The upper limit of the swelling can be reached—**getting above the swelling** one can feel the cord of the testis above the lump. Fluctuation positive. Transillumination positive.

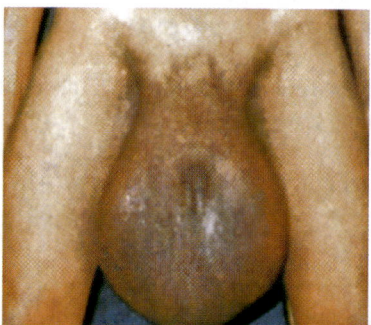

Fig. 11.18: Large bilateral vaginal hydrocele with buried penis. Fluctuation positive. Transillumination positive. After eversion of vaginal sacs the penis regained its shape.

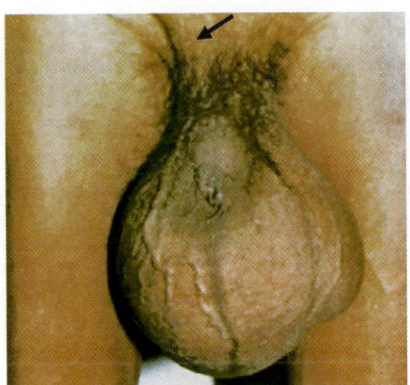

Fig. 11.19: Bilateral vaginal hydrocele right > left. Also note the right inguinal swelling—incomplete inguinal hernia. *So, always examine inguinal region for hernia while examining for hydroceles and vice versa.*

adults because trauma, infection and neoplasm *are most common during this period.*

2. The patient presents with *a scrotal swelling* which may cause social embarrassment. There may be pain or discomfort in secondary hydrocele but idiopathic hydrocele can reach a considerable size without causing pain.

3. The swelling may be unilateral or bilateral.

4. The swelling is confined within the scrotum. The upper limit of the swelling can be reached, i.e. *one can get above the swelling* (Fig. 11.17) (cf. congenital hydrocele, infantile hydrocele, inguinoscrotal hernia).

5. *One can feel the cord of the testis above the lump.*

6. *The testis cannot be felt separately* as it is surrounded by a bag of fluid. (cf. encysted hydrocele of the cord, cyst of epididymis).

7. Uniformly cystic – *fluctuation is positive.*

8. The swelling may be tense or lax depending on the amount of the contained fluid.

9. *The swelling is not reducible* (cf. hernia).

10. *Transillumination: Positive* as the hydrocele fluid is clear. *Transillumination may be negative if the tunica or skin is thick, or the fluid is turbid (filariasis).* (But one must be careful to exclude testicular tumour when transillumination is negative in a scrotal

swelling. *Any scrotal swelling when felt hard do transillumination test; if negative, the testicular tumour is suspected.*)

Differential diagnosis

1. Inguinoscrotal hernia.
2. Cysts in relation to epididymis.
3. Tumour of the testis.
4. Chylocele.
5. Haematocele.
6. Filariasis of the scrotum.
7. Encysted hydrocele of the cord.
8. Hydrocele en-bisac.

Complications

1. Rupture – haemorrhage
2. Haematocele following aspiration or trauma
3. Infection may lead to pyocele
4. Atrophy of the testis
5. Hernia of the hydrocele sac through the dartos muscle.
6. Calcification of the sac.
7. Cosmetically unsightly when very big causing physical disability, embarrassment both to patient and his relatives or friends.
8. Bars entry to army or police service.
9. Masking an underlying testicular disease, e.g. malignancy.

Treatment

Indication

1. When the scrotal mass is cosmetically unsightly.
2. Uncomfortable for the patient and relatives.
3. If any complication arises.
4. Appears to be a bar to entry into the armed or police service.

Methods

Various methods are available including surgery, aspiration, aspiration followed by injections of a sclerosing agent, e.g. tetracycline within the sac, tapping.

Surgery

Surgery offers the best chance of cure and recurrence is unlikely. *It can be performed also under local anaesthesia.* Types of operations are:

1. **Lord's procedure:** A more or less bloodless operation often *practised in small hydroceles* and when the sac is reasonably thin-walled – *plication of the sac.*

   After draining the fluid the testis is delivered through the incision in the hydrocele sac. *The edges of the sac are plicated around the periphery of the testis with several interrupted sutures.* When these sutures are tied, the whole tunica is bunched at the periphery of the testis, thus eliminating the potential space for further collection of fluid. *The scrotal wound is then closed without drain.*

2. **Jaboulay's operation:** *Eversion of sac* mostly practised nowadays *for medium-sized hydroceles.*

   Principle:
   - The vaginal sac is incised anteriorly and the fluid is drained out.
   - *The sac is then everted behind the testis and epididymis* so that the secreting surface of the tunica vaginalis will be lying outside. The everted margin of the sac is stitched with a running suture. Then the testis is placed back inside the fascial pouch of scrotum prepared by dissection of the fascial plane by index fingers of both hands inside the scrotum.
   - Meticulous haemostasis is achieved.
   - The scrotal wound is closed with or without drain.

3. **Excision of the sac**, may be necessary in a very *large hydrocele*, haematocele, chronically inflamed hydrocele (e.g. chylocele), as the *sac wall becomes thickened in these cases.*

   After draining the fluid, most of the vaginal sac is excised *leaving behind a margin of 2 cm by the side of the testis. Bleeding from the cut margin is always considerable and should be controlled* either by continuous mattress suture or with diathermy. *The scrotal wound is closed preferably with a drain.* Excision of the distal part of the scrotal skin may also be required to reduce the size of the scrotum.

Aspiration

Aspiration with or without infusion of a sclerosing agent such as tetracycline, is *often tried as an alternative to surgery, especially in patients who are poor surgical candidates*. But this method is associated with a high rate of recurrence with or without pain in almost half of the patients.

Aspiration is often required in secondary hydroceles, so that the underlying testis can be accurately palpated for any underlying pathology (e.g. tumour of the testis).

Tapping

Tapping may be tried for relief of discomfort as an alternative to surgery in large hydroceles, *especially in patients who are poor surgical candidates*. But it never cures the condition.

Before tapping with trocar and cannula one must perform the transillumination test which will indicate the site of the testis and scrotal vessels which must be avoided during puncture.

Complications after aspiration or tapping are infection, haematocele, injury to the testis, high rate of recurrence. Because of these complications and the ability to perform operation of hydroceles using local anaesthetic, many prefer to avoid aspiration or tapping nowadays.

FILARIAL HYDROCELE (CHYLOCELE)

- Usually occurs *following repeated attack of filarial epididymitis.*
- *Wuchereria bancrofti* is the organism responsible. Adult worms are demonstrated in the epididymis.
- Chylocele develops because of rupture of lymphatic varix with discharge of chyle into the hydrocele sac.
- Commonly occurs in the coastal regions – southern and eastern states of India.
- Filarial hydrocele is usually large in size and the sac is thickened.
- Usually present as tense cystic swelling – fluctuation is positive.
- *But transillumination is negative* because of thick opalescent fluid content.

- *On aspiration or drainage,* thick yellowish opalescent milky fluid is drained – chylocele (cf. pyocele).
- Fluid content is rich in cholesterol and fat.
- *Treatment: Inversion of sac* after draining the thick fluid and a course of antifilarial drugs. *Often requires partial excision of thick-walled sac prior to inversion of sac.*

Note

- *Cystic swellings involving tunica vaginalis:*
  1. *Hydrocele,* contains clear fluid; trans-illumination positive.
  2. *Chylocele,* contains milky lymph; trans-illumination negative.
  3. *Haematocele,* contains blood; trans-illumination negative.

Note

D/D of scrotal lump – hydrocele, inguinoscrotal hernia, lipoma of cord, lymph varix, testicular tumour.

Note

In presence of chylocele, the patient should be advised postoperatively a course of Hetrazan 100 mg tds for 3 weeks.

Note

Surgery for vaginal hydrocele

- Small hydrocele: *Lord's procedure* – plication of the sac.
- Medium hydrocele: *Jaboulay's operation* – eversion of the sac.
- Large hydrocele: *Excision of the sac.*

Note

Causes of secondary hydrocele

1. Filarial hydrocele (chylocele)
2. Chronic epididymo-orchitis
   - Most commonly – tuberculosis
   - Mostly subsides with reduction of epididymo-orchitis following anti-Koch's therapy.
3. *Tumour: How to rule out testicular tumour?*
   - U/S examination to rule out a mass lesion in the testis.
   - By tumour markers – β-hCG and α-feto-protein estimation.

4. Torsion of testes rarely, treated by correction of torsion, plication of tunica vaginalis and then orchidopexy.

Note

Hydrocele of the canal of Nuck

- *Female counterpart of hydrocele of the cord*
- Seen in relation to the round ligament

Spermatocele

- *Unilocular retention cyst derived from some portion of the sperm conducting mechanism of the epididymis.*
- *C/F: Typically lies at the epididymal head and behind the upper pole of the testis.*
- *Transillumination: Poor or negative.*
- Usually painless.
- Most spermatoceles do not need treatment.

VARICOCELE

It is a condition of dilatation, elongation and tortuosity of the veins of the pampiniform venous plexus.

In many cases, it has been found that the testicular veins are normal and the varicosities are present in the cremasteric veins which anastomose freely with the testicular veins.

Surgical anatomy of pampiniform plexus

The pampiniform plexus forms the main bulk of the spermatic cord. It consists of three groups of veins:

1. Veins from the testis and epididymis (testicular veins).
2. Veins accompanying the vas deferens.
3. Veins associated with the cremaster muscle (cremasteric veins).

Veins of testis and epididymis form an anasto-mosing plexus surrounding the vas. From the upper part of the plexus 15 to 20 veins arise and as they ascend the number is reduced to about 12. On reaching the superficial inguinal ring, these unite to form 4 veins and traverse the inguinal canal. On reaching the deep inguinal ring these further join to form 2 veins. The veins thereafter enter the abdomen and unite at various levels to form a single vein called testicular vein. *The right testicular vein drains in the inferior vena cava at an acute angle. The left testicular vein drains in the left renal vein at right angle.* Near the termination, the testicular vein is provided with valve (Fig. 11.20).

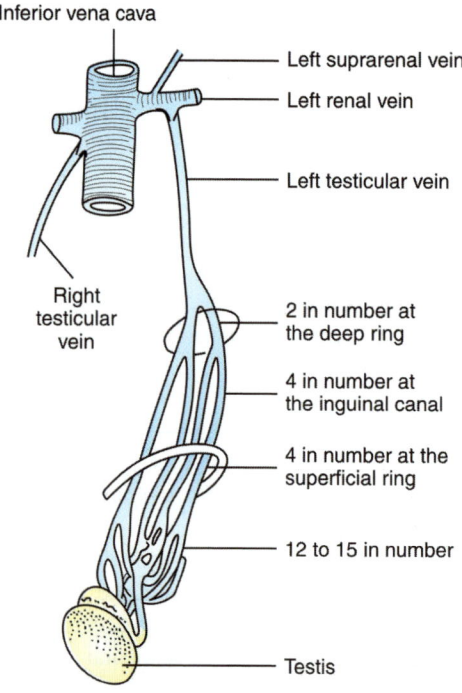

Fig. 11.20: The pampiniform venous plexus and mode of drainage of testicular veins.

The cremasteric veins and the vein accompanying the vas anastomose with the testicular veins. So, they provide an alternative pathway (collateral) of venous return from the testis and epididymis. *The cremasteric veins drain into the inferior epigastric vein.*

Surgical physiology

The pampiniform plexus around the testicular artery is believed *to constitute a countercurrent system which serves as a heat exchanger mechanism to reduce the scrotal temperature about 2–3° lower than the abdominal temperature* to keep the testicle cool and thus, this has some useful role to play in normal spermatogenesis.

Types of varicocele

1. *Primary or idiopathic:* Where no definite cause has been found. One hypothesis is that it occurs principally in young unmarried men and due to chronic venous congestion consequent upon unrelieved sexual stimulation. *Most varicoceles (95%) are idiopathic.*
2. *Secondary: Where there is an obstruction of the testicular vein by some intra-abdominal or retroperitoneal pathology, e.g. a tumour in relation to the left kidney.*

Aetiology of primary varicocele

No definite aetiology has yet been found as the contributing factor in case of primary varicocele.

1. *Age:* Mostly seen in teenaged individuals or in early adult life. Tall, thin, visceroptotic men are frequently affected.
2. *Incidence:* About 10% of males between 15 and 25 years have a varicocele.
3. *More common (95%) in the left side* for the following reasons.
   - *The left testicular vein joins the left renal vein almost at a right angle. The right testicular vein joins the inferior vena cava at an acute angle (Fig. 11.20).*
   - *The left testicular vein is longer than the right* because the left testis lies slightly at a lower level and the left testicular vein ends at a higher level. So, the left vein has to bear a long column of blood, and *thus the venous pressure is higher in the left scrotal veins which results in retrograde reflux of blood into the left pampiniform plexus.*
   - Loaded pelvic colon is likely to compress the left testicular vein as it ascends behind the pelvic colon.
   - Sometimes the left renal vein may be sandwiched between the abdominal aorta and the trunk of superior mesenteric artery, so may be compressed between the two. Eventually, it hinders the venous return of the left renal vein and therefore of the left testicular vein, which may culminate into varicosities of the left pampiniform plexus (Fig. 11.21).

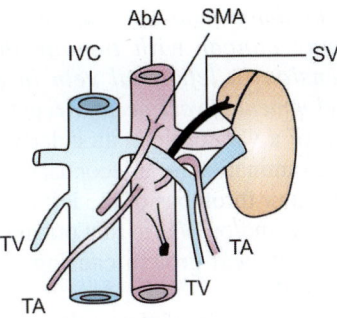

Fig. 11.21: Compression of the left renal vein by superior mesenteric artery (SMA); arching of the left renal vein by left testicular artery (TA); close association between the left suprarenal vein (SV) and left testicular vein (TV). IVC, inferior vena cava; AbA, abdominal aorta.

- Left testicular artery may arch over the left renal vein and thus may cause compression over the vein (found in 16% cases according to Nathan) (Fig. 11.21).
- The close association between the entry of the left suprarenal vein and the left testicular vein in the left renal vein may allow the circulating adrenaline to constrict the testicular vein (Figs 11.20 and 11.21).
4. There may be incompetency or absence of valves near the termination of testicular veins.
5. Rarely the tumour tissue of left-sided renal carcinoma grows along the left renal vein, and thus may cause obstruction to the left testicular vein. *So, renal carcinoma is to be suspected when a recent varicocele appears in a middle-aged individual (secondary varicocele).* U/S of kidney may be helpful.

Power of spermatogenesis in varicocele

Power of spermatogenesis may be seriously depressed (e.g. oligospermia) because the affected testis is subjected to a higher temperature following the stagnation of blood in the varicose veins. It is said that unless the testis is kept at a temperature of 2.5°C lower than the rectal temperature normal spermatogenesis will be hampered. *Varicocele is one of the causes of male subfertility or infertility.* Varicocele raises the temperature in the scrotum which is detrimental

to the spermatogenesis. Both the sperm count and motility are reduced. Operative correction will improve both but mainly the sperm motility.

Surgery can result in improvement in fertility up to 50%.

Diagnostic criteria

1. Mostly seen in the teenaged individuals or in early adult life.

   Gynaecologist many a time refers a male partner with subfertility or infertility to exclude varicocele.
2. More frequent and more troublesome in hot climates.
3. It may give rise to either scrotal swelling (elongated scrotum) or inguinoscrotal swelling. *The left side alone is involved in 90% of cases,* with bilaterality in 5 to 20%.
4. The patient complains of dragging pain in the affected side which may extend into the groin. (The elongated scrotum no longer supports the testis whose full weight is now borne by the cord giving rise to dragging pain).

Examination:

5. *On palpation with the patient standing:* A mass of dilated, tortuous veins lying posterior to, and above the testis is felt which gives the impression of *'a bag of worms'* – *chief characteristic.* The degree of dilatation can be increased by the valsalva maneuver.
6. *On coughing:* The swelling gives an impulse like a fluid thrill (cf. hernia gives an expansile impulse). Fluid thrill may be absent in secondary varicocele.
7. *When the patient lies down and the scrotum is elevated,* the swelling reduces in size and disappears as the veins will be emptied by gravity.

   During this examination, the size of the testis should be compared with that of the opposite testis. Testicular atrophy from impaired circulation may be present. The testis on the affected side is usually somewhat smaller and softer than the opposite testis in long standing cases.

8. *On standing:* The swelling reappears, *the varicocele fills up from the bottom of the scrotum* (cf. hernia).
9. *Fluctuation and transillumination: Negative* (cf. hydrocele).
10. *Bow sign:* The varicocele mass is held between the fingers and the thumb and the patient is asked to bow down – *the tension within the veins becomes appreciably less* (because bowing down will cut off the continuity of the blood inside the varicocele mass with that of the testicular vein).
11. *Always the abdomen should be examined in case of recently developed varicocele particularly in middle-aged individuals* – to note a lump, e.g. renal carcinoma, loaded pelvic colon in chronic constipation.
12. *In renal carcinoma, the varicocele does not decompress in supine position.*

How to differentiate a primary varicocele from a secondary varicocele?

In primary idiopathic varicocele, on elevation of the scrotum in a patient lying down, the varicocele disappears as the veins will be emptied by gravity. But in secondary varicocele, the varicocele will not disappear because either the testicular vein is compressed by a renal lump or the left renal vein is filled up with tumour embolus in case of renal carcinoma, so that it obstructs the drainage of testicular vein. *When suspected IVP, ultrasound, CT scan, selective arteriogram will confirm the renal carcinoma.*

Differential diagnosis

Lymph varix, hydrocele, inguinal hernia, and diffuse lipoma of the spermatic cord.

Investigations

1. *Ultrasound of the scrotum and inguinal region* to confirm varicosities – it may show anechoic multiple tortuous channels along the cord suggestive of varicocele. *Testes may appear smaller.*

   Colour Doppler flow study on standing with or without Valsalva manoeuvre will confirm the presence of varicocele and reflux into the scrotal veins which disappears on compression of the external ring.

2. *U/S of abdomen to detect any SOL, e.g. left kidney cancer with tumour thrombus extension in left renal vein in a recent development of varicocele.* Recent development of a varicocele in an elderly warrants U/S examination for a secondary varicocele by tumour thrombus of the left renal vein.
3. CT scan and/or IVU to rule out any renal or retroperitoneal growth causing secondary varicocele.
4. *Semen analysis of the male patient with subfertility or infertility* – to look for oligospermia or oligoasthenia.

Treatment

A. Conservative

Reassurance and suspensory bandage usually suffice and high Y-front underpants may relieve ache and discomfort if there is mild pain.

B. Operative

Indication:

1. Pain and heaviness are constant sources of discomfort and anxiety to the patient.
2. When gross varicosity is present leading to a big size – causing anxiety not relieved even by any conservative treatment.
3. *Small testis* on clinical examination – varicoceles are associated with testicular atrophy. Varicocele correction can reverse atrophy in adolescents.
4. When the testis hangs at an abnormally low level.
5. *When varicocele appears to be a bar to entry into the armed or police forces* since the condition tends to worsen in hot climates on prolonged standing causing nagging pain in the scrotum; this may be a readymade excuse for malingering.
6. *Subfertility* (a suboptimal semen analysis, e.g. oligospermia, oligoasthenia) or infertility in unilateral or bilateral varicosity.

   Aim of operation: To reduce to a minimum number of veins in the pampiniform plexus.

   Operative procedures: Different methods are available which account for their own merits.
   • Inguinal approach – classical.
   • Scrotal approach.
   • Abdominal extraperitoneal approach.

1. Inguinal approach – classical approach

- *Through inguinal approach*, the canal is opened and the spermatic cord is delivered.
- The coverings are incised. The vas deferens together with its artery and one or two veins are carefully separated from the main mass of dilated vessels.
- Then the clamps are applied both above and below the isolated mass of dilated veins with a gap of about 2 inches and the intervening segment is removed.
- The clamps are then approximated and the individual masses are tied off together with a single ligature of strong silk.

Advantage of this procedure is twofold:
(a) Occlusion of most of the dilated veins, and
(b) Shortening of the cord so that the testis is suspended at a higher level.

Disadvantage: Chance of damage to the testicular artery and/or cremasteric artery.

2. Scrotal approach

- *Through scrotal incision* the varicose veins are exposed right down to the level of the testis.
- Tortuous and varicose veins are divided and ligated individually *keeping behind sufficient veins to maintain venous return.*

Disadvantage of this method: Separation of the veins becomes more difficult near the testis where a free anastomosis exists; bleeding is therefore more troublesome, and a scrotal haematoma is more liable to complicate the convalescence. There is every chance of damage to the testicular artery also.

3. Palomo's operation – suprainguinal approach

- A small oblique incision is made 3 cm above the level of the deep inguinal ring.
- *Splitting of the parietal muscles is done in 'gridiron' manner.*
- Extraperitoneal fat and peritoneum are exposed and they are swept medially, upwards and forward.
- The testicular vessels are exposed *as they lie on the posterior abdominal wall, lateral to the external iliac artery which serves as a useful guide.*

- The testicular vein is identified, separated and divided between the ligatures.

Advantages of Palomo's method:
(a) Simple operation, it can be performed under local anaesthesia.
(b) Less chance of endangering the blood supply to the testis, as the operation is carried out well above the deep inguinal ring.
(c) *Even if the testicular artery is divided and ligated*, the testis will get adequate blood supply via the anastomosis between the cremasteric artery and the artery to the vas which cannot be injured at this higher level (Fig. 11.22) (*cremasteric artery* – a branch of the inferior epigastric artery; *artery to vas* – a branch of the superior vesical artery).

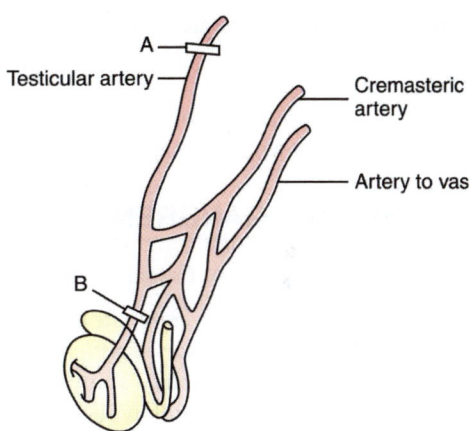

Testicular artery
Cremasteric artery
Artery to vas
A
B

Fig. 11.22: The anastomoses of the testicular artery with cremasteric artery and artery to the vas; ligature of testicular artery at A—still the blood supply to testis is maintained. But ligature at B imperils the blood supply to the testis.

(d) Moreover, *the cremasteric vein*, which anastomoses with the testicular vein and thus provides an alternative pathway (collateral) of venous return from the testis, *is not destroyed by this method*. So, the testis can be drained by this route (cremasteric vein) to the external iliac vein.

Disadvantage: It aggravates the varicocele in about 10% cases.

Laparoscopic ligation

The principle of operation is the same as Palamo's operation. Laparoscopically, the testicular vessels are exposed. The testicular vein is identified and separated. The testicular vein is endoclipped with endoscopic ligaclip applicator. The vein is then divided between the clips with endoscissors.

Note

After division of testicular vein for treatment of varicocele, *venous drainage of testis is maintained by cremasteric veins.*

Note

Most common cause of surgically treatable male infertility is varicocele. Varicocelectomy improves spermatogenesis and sperm function and improves pregnancy rate. The testicular volume may also improve and return to normal.

Note

Treatment of recurrence of varicocele – femoral vein catheterisation with spermatic vein ablation.

▎FOURNIER'S GANGRENE

Syn. Idiopathic gangrene of the scrotum

- It is a variant of *synergistic gangrene* involving the scrotum *due to vascular insufficiency of infective origin* (cf. Meleney's superficial gangrene of the abdominal wall). *It is a vascular gangrene of infective origin following infection with gas forming organisms leading to necrotising soft tissue infection.*
- It may be idiopathic.
- It may follow minor injuries or procedures in the perineum such as bruise, scratch, dilatation of stricture urethra and drainage of perineal abscess.
- It is common in patients of low socioeconomic groups living in an unhygienic condition.
- In recent times, the disease has been observed in chronic alcoholics who develop pressure sores of the scrotum and perineum after sitting in the same position for a long time in a drunken stupor.

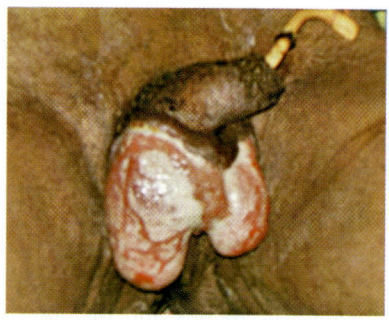

Fig. 11.23: Fournier's gangrene involving both scrotums. (*Courtesy:* Dr Sandip Chakravorty, MS, DGO)

- Diabetic and immunosuppressed patients are also prone to this condition.
- Mortality rate is nearly 100% without surgical debridement.

Causative organisms

Polymicrobial infection with a mixture of gram-positive and gram-negative aerobes and anaerobes. *Multiple organisms are:*

  (i) *Haemolytic streptococci* (sometimes micro-aerophilic): Gram-positive
 (ii) *Staphylococci:* Gram-positive
(iii) *Cl. welchii/perfringens:* Gram-positive, anaerobic, rod-shaped, spore-forming bacterium
 (iv) *E. coli:* Gram-negative
  (v) *Bacteroides fragilis:* Gram-negative and anaerobic

At first these organisms set up a fulminating inflammation of the scrotal subcutaneous tissue *that results in obliterative arteritis of the arterioles supplying the overlying skin* leading to gangrene and necrosis.

The testes covered by tunica and the spermatic cord are usually spared because of thick tunica albuginea.

Diagnostic features

1. Common in *apparently* healthy young men between 25 and 50 years of age.
2. Initially the patient presents with sudden pain of the scrotum with prostration, pallor, and pyrexia. *The scrotum becomes inflamed, red, swollen and tender.*

3. Within one or two days, extensive superficial gangrene develops *resulting in necrosis and sloughing of the scrotal skin*. The sloughing may be partial or total extending to the base of the penis.

4. The cellulitis may spread along the fascial planes (so well known as in superficial extravasation of urine) to the perineum and anterior abdominal wall. *Occasionally penile skin may be involved*.

The testes and spermatic cord are usually spared. The urethra is also not involved.

Treatment

1. *Antibiotic therapy:* Pending the bacteriological report, following antibiotics should be started immediately:
   (i) *Penicillin or ampicillin* for gram-positive organisms
   (ii) *Chloramphenicol or gentamicin* for gram-negative organisms
   (iii) *Metronidazole* for anaerobes
   (iv) Cephalosporin may be added if required particularly after antibiogram.

2. *Surgical debridement of the devitalised scrotal skin and subcutaneous tissue:* As soon as possible to provide early drainage and thus to prevent spread of gangrene. May require repeat exploration within 24 to 36 hours to confirm that no necrotic tissue remains behind.

3. *If the testicles are exposed*, they can be implanted in the thigh.

4. Once the infection and necrosis subside, the wound is covered with split skin graft.

5. If the penile skin is necrotic, it can be debrided down to but not through Buck's fascia followed by secondary non-meshed thick split thickness skin grafting for penile shaft.

CARCINOMA OF SCROTUM

• *Squamous cell carcinoma of scrotum* most commonly due to exposure to environmental carcinogens like chimney soot, tars, paraffin and petroleum products and also due to poor hygiene and chronic inflammation leading to chronic ulcer formation.

• Present with ulcers which refuse to heal.
• Enlarged superficial lymph nodes – first node involved lies medial to saphenofemoral junction – sentinel lymph node (SLN).
• *Typical nature of job should arouse suspicion.*
• Diagnosis confirmed by biopsy of scrotal skin.
• *Treatment: Wide local excision with 2 cm margins beyond the lesion.*
   Prognosis correlates with presence or absence of nodal involvement.
• *Change of job* to avoid spoiling of scrotal skin with exposure to carcinogens as mentioned above.

Differential diagnosis of scrotal swellings

While examining a scrotal swelling one should decide first *whether the lump is in the skin of the scrotum* (e.g. sebaceous cyst, filariasis) or not.

Once a scrotal skin swelling is ruled out, one should next decide *whether the swelling is a true scrotal swelling* or *an inguinoscrotal swelling*. To decide this, one should examine the swelling with the patient standing up and *try to get above the swelling* (Fig. 11.17) to feel the cord of the testis above the swelling.

Getting above the swelling is not possible: Inguinoscrotal swelling (e.g. hernia).

Getting above the swelling is possible: Scrotal swelling.

Once the inguinoscrotal swelling is ruled out one should consider *true scrotal swelling*. True scrotal swelling may be hydrocele, spermatocele, cyst of the epididymis, epididymo-orchitis and testicular mass.

Transillumination test is a must for all scrotal swellings to confirm vaginal hydrocele.

A testicular mass is a tumour until proven otherwise – consider urgent U/S scan and test for tumour markers β-hCG and α-fetoprotein.

A painful enlarged testis may be either torsion testis, epididymo-orchitis, or rarely testicular tumour. *Do urine analysis for pus cells* – if normal consider for torsion or tumour – *do urgent U/S scan. U/S scan also detects tumour.*

Note

Testicular tumour is not discussed as this case is not given both short and long cases in examination.

Table 11.2: Algorithm for examination of scrotal swellings

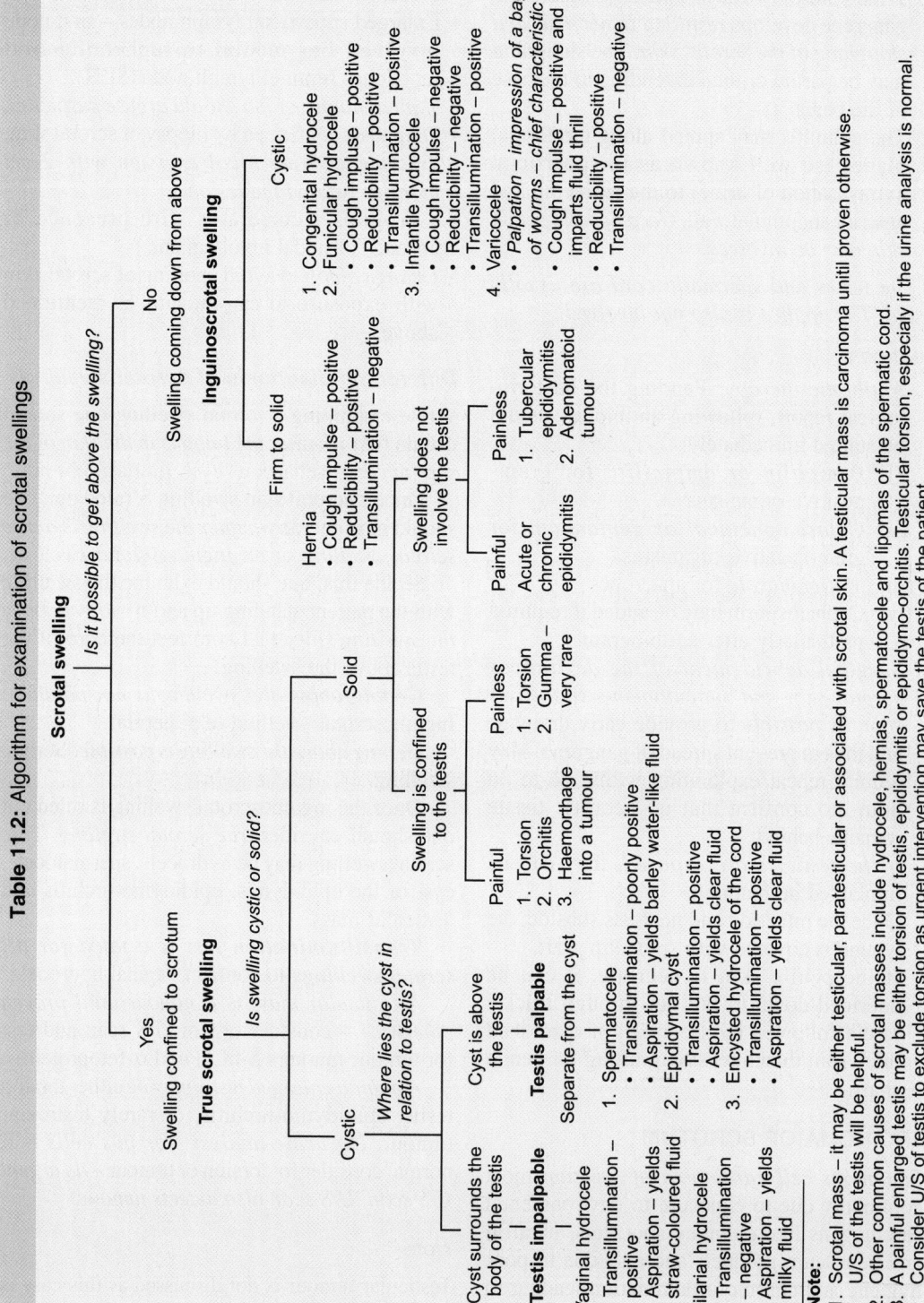

Note:
1. Scrotal mass – it may be either testicular, paratesticular or associated with scrotal skin. A testicular mass is carcinoma until proven otherwise. U/S of the testis will be helpful.
2. Other common causes of scrotal masses include hydrocele, hernias, spermatocele and lipomas of the spermatic cord.
3. A painful enlarged testis may be either torsion of testis, epididymitis or epididymo-orchitis. Testicular torsion, especialy if the urine analysis is normal. Consider U/S of testis to exclude torsion as urgent intervention may save the testis of the patient.

Penis

PHIMOSIS

Phimosis (Fig. 12.1) is the narrowing of the end of the prepuce (foreskin) *so that it cannot be retracted to expose the glans penis.* Because of this, the child may have difficulty in passing urine.

Phimosis should not be confused with redundancy of the prepuce, where the foreskin can be retracted to expose the glans penis.

In neonates and children up to 6 years the prepuce may be normally adherent to glans penis. So it is not possible to expose the glans by retracting the prepuce *but the external meatus can always be clearly seen.* So, that is not a true phimosis.

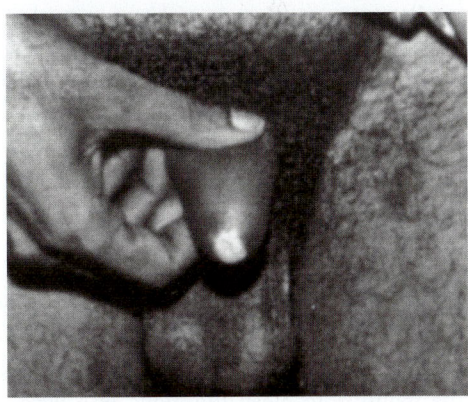

Fig. 12.1: Phimosis. Narrow preputial opening, external meatus not visible. Skin cannot be retracted proximally over the glans.

Causes

Congenital

Not common. The preputial orifice is narrow since birth and there is often a history of ballooning of the prepuce, followed by a thin stream of urine during micturition.

Acquired

1. *Inflammatory:* Due to scarring following long-standing infection from poor local hygiene, e.g. balanoposthitis (inflammation of glans and prepuce), ammoniacal dermatitis. *Most cases occur in uncircumscribed males* especially in diabetics with poor hygiene resulting in narrowing of the preputial orifice.

2. *Traumatic:* The trauma of forcible retraction causes scarring.

3. *Neoplastic:* Underlying carcinoma may lead to narrowing of the preputial orifice.

4. *Chancre:* Painless genital ulcer most commonly found *during primary stage of syphilis* – can cause preputial adhesion over the glans.

Diagnostic criteria

1. Babies may be brought by the parents with the complaints of difficulty with micturition, and inability to retract the prepuce. There may be history of *ballooning of the prepuce during micturition followed by a thin stream of urine – an important criterion of true congenital phimosis.*

   If necessary, the prepuce can be gently separated from the glans by a blunt probe, or dorsal slit under general anaesthesia, enabling retraction of prepuce over the glans.

   Young adults may present with the difficulty of retraction of the prepuce causing interference with masturbation, erection and sexual intercourse.

   Patient may present with recurrent balanitis causing pain and purulent discharge.

2. Difficulty in retracting the preputial skin with narrowing of the preputial orifice.

3. There may be associated pinhole meatus.

Complications

1. Balanitis – inflammation of glans
2. Posthitis – inflammation of prepuce
3. Balanoposthitis – inflammation of both glans and prepuce

   All these may be causes of phimosis. Because of the inability to clean the glans in a case of phimosis the person is prone to develop recurrent balanitis, posthitis or balanoposthitis due to irritation by the smegma and/or infection. The patient may present with local pain, redness and swelling of prepuce and glans and purulent discharge. Bacteria involved are *Staphylococcus*, coliforms and gonococci. In diabetic and immune compromised patients, *Candida* infection is a further risk. So, diabetes should be controlled. Local hygiene and proper antibiotics are necessary. *Also, early circumcision is to be done when infection subsides.*

4. Balanitis xerotica obliterans (BXO) – dyskeratotic skin disorder and affects 30–50 years age group causing thickened white plaques and fissures on the prepuce and glans leading to non-retractile prepuce and/or preputial discharge – requires urgent

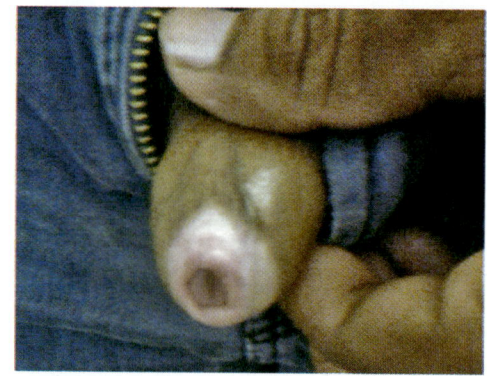

Fig. 12.2: Phimosis with BXO involving the prepuce leading to non-retractile prepuce.

circumcision and dilatation or meatotomy if meatal stricture is present. *BXO is considered precancerous* (Fig. 12.2).

5. *Paraphimosis:* This is a condition in which the tight foreskin or prepuce once forcibly retracted over the glans becomes stuck behind the glans penis and cannot be replaced in its normal position. The everted skin fold acts as a constricting band at the corona glandis and results in venous congestion leading to oedema and swelling of the glans, which leads to more difficulty in reducing back the tight prepuce over the glans. The constricting band of preputial skin also *becomes oedematous and swollen.*

   In neglected cases, arterial occlusion leading to gangrene and necrosis of the glans may occur. *The urethra is usually not involved and micturition is possible.*

   Emergency surgical relief is performed under general anaesthesia when multiple punctures are made over the oedematous preputial skin and then compressed to let out the fluid completely. Once the prepuce becomes supple it will be pulled forward over the glans distal to corona, up to the tip of the glans. *If required, a longitudinal dorsal incision may be made on the dorsal aspect of the thick band also to prevent imminent gangrene of the glans.*

   Following emergency relief, the patient must return back early after a month for elective circumcision.

Note

Paraphimosis may be catheter-induced when long preputial skin is not retracted back to its original position following catheterisation.

6. *Ballooning of the preputial sac:* In extreme cases the preputial sac balloons out with the accumulated urine due to narrowing of the preputial orifice. When the patient micturates, a weak narrow stream of urine flows. Immediate dilatation or a dorsal slit of narrow preputial orifice is required to let the urine out. *Requires circumcision later at an earliest.*

7. *Concretions or calculus:* May form in the preputial sac. Smegma along with urinary salts make such calculus.

8. *Obstruction to the flow of urine* may cause retention of urine, residual urine, hydro-ureter, hydronephrosis from back pressure. These are rarely due to phimosis alone; *more often there is associated pinhole meatus. So, check for **pinhole meatus** in every case of phimosis.*

9. *Recurrent urinary tract infection: Paediatrician many a time refers the children to a surgeon for correction of phimosis.*

10. *Carcinoma:* Phimosis itself is an aetiological factor in the development of carcinoma of the penis. Development of carcinoma has been attributed to the *chronic irritation by the smegma* which is a product of bacterial action on desquamated cells retained within the preputial sac. *Smegma is carcinogenic.*

    Circumcision carried out soon after birth confers total immunity against carcinoma of the penis. Ritual circumcision is a religious practice in Jews and Muslims and so penile carcinoma is very rare in these communities. Jews – circumcision is done soon after birth. *Muslims* – circumcision is done 4 years after birth.

    On the other hand, carcinoma can give rise to phimosis. So, any old man presenting with phimosis should be examined properly to exclude a hidden carcinoma of the prepuce or the glans penis. *Often, a dorsal slit of the prepuce is required to exclude a hidden carcinoma of the glans penis.*

Treatment

Circumcision

Excision of the long preputial skin to expose the glans penis and the corona glandis under general or local anaesthesia. *The frenulum, considered to be the sexually sensitive area, should not be damaged* and if it is found to be too short, it may be lengthened by V-Y frenuloplasty.

When phimosis is associated with narrow external urethral meatus particularly in congenital variety *meatotomy* is performed also.

When it is associated with considerable inflammation of the prepuce a dorsal slit is performed first, followed by circumcision at a later date when infection subsides.

Complications of circumcision

1. Too little or too much skin excision.
2. Local and/or general infection.
3. Haemorrhage – mostly from the frenal artery.
4. Meatal stenosis.
5. Urethral fistula.

Note

Neonatal circumcision is practised in developed countries and by Jews using a Hollister plastibell or a Gomco clamp – the excess foreskin is crushed and excised. No suturing is required.

Note

- Neonatal circumcision confers immunity against carcinoma penis, HIV and STDs.
- Most important carcinogens are smegma and HPV infection.

Note

Rarely, Fournier's gangrene of scrotum may develop following plastibell circumcision.

PEYRONIE'S DISEASE

- It is an acquired connective tissue disorder causing formation of *fibrous scar tissue inside the penis mainly on the dorsal surface.*
- It causes *curved, painful erection with dorsal curvature of penis.*
- It causes difficulty in introducing penis in the vagina during coitus.

- It can impede both ejaculation and micturition also.

Treatment

- Incision or excision of the fibrous plaque on the dorsum of the penis followed by *tissue grafting* derived from the patient's body or synthetic graft – *but associated with worsening erectile function.*
- *Erectile function can be improved* by implantation of semirigid silastic prosthesis which allows the patient to straighten the penis during coitus and bend it down after coitus.
- Collagenase clostridium histolyticum (Xiaflex) is being tried at some centres.

CARCINOMA OF THE PENIS

Carcinoma of the penis (Figs 12.3 to 12.7) commonly occurs in middle-aged and elderly persons. It is uncommon in Europe and USA but relatively frequent in the East, including India.

In 97% of cases, it is squamous cell carcinoma and is relatively prevalent among people of low socioeconomic class who have poor health practices and inadequate hygiene.

Sporadic cases of non-squamous malignancy like melanoma, basal cell carcinoma, lymphoreticular tumours, mesenchymal tumours and metastatic tumours have been reported.

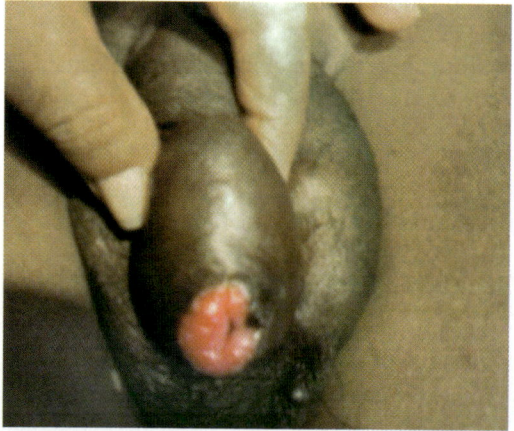

Fig. 12.3: Carcinoma of glans giving rise to phimosis. On retraction of the preputial skin proximally exposed the growth.

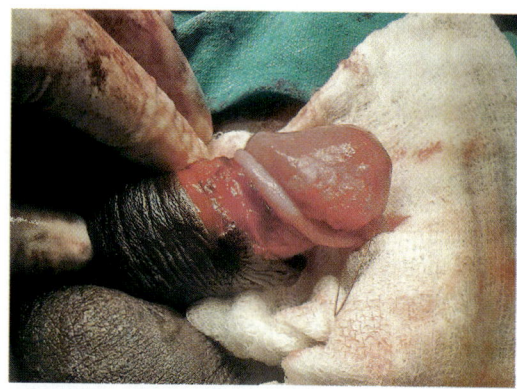

Fig. 12.4: Carcinoma on the base of the glans penis: Right side—exposed only after circumcision.

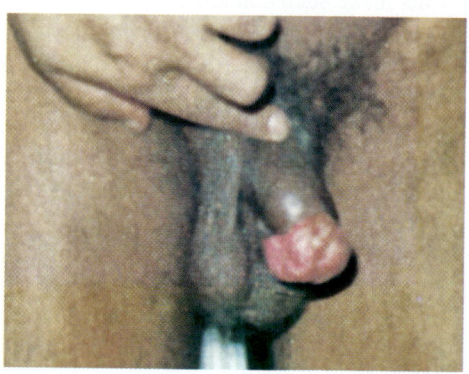

Fig. 12.5: Carcinoma penis involving the glans (proliferative type) with induration extending to the shaft. The external urethral meatus was difficult to see, but the patient did not have any difficulty in passing urine. Inguinal nodes were not palpable in this patient.

Rarely, there may be an adenocarcinoma when it arises from the *Tyson's gland, the smegma secreting gland on either side of the frenum.*

Aetiology

1. Phimosis: *More than 50% of carcinoma of penises are associated with phimosis. It has been attributed to the chronic irritation by the smegma collected in the preputial sac. Smegma is carcinogenic.*

   Circumcision carried out soon after birth confers almost total immunity against carcinoma of penis, but circumcision done after early infancy or in adult life does not provide the same degree of protection. The reason is not known.

It is almost rare in some communities, e.g. Jewish, where ritual circumcision is performed soon after birth. Moslems, in whom the ritual circumcision is done between the ages of 4 and 9 years, may be affected.

2. *Balanoposthitis:* Recurrent attacks due to poor hygiene may predispose to carcinoma.
3. *Viral papilloma:* Condyloma acuminatum or venereal warts of long-standing due to HPV type 16 & 18 infection and HSV type 1 & 2 following sex.
4. *Buschke-Löwenstein tumour* (Fig. 12.9): A giant penile condyloma acuminata. It is cauliflower-like lesion. *Also known as verrucous carcinoma of penis.*
5. *Leukoplakia of the glans.*
6. *Bowen's disease:* Intraepidermal carcinoma of prepuce developing in the apocrine gland bearing areas.
7. *Paget's disease of the penis:* A variant of Bowen's disease.
8. *Erythroplasia of Queyrat* (Fig. 12.10): Persistent rawness of glans penis – a variant of Bowen's disease.
9. *Balanitis xerotica obliterans:* Affects 30–50 years age group; uncommon. Thickened white plaque and fissures on prepuce and glans. *Present with non-retractile prepuce or preputial discharge and meatal stenosis.* Requires urgent circumcision and/or meatotomy.
10. *Keratin horn on the glans penis:* Extreme hyperkeratosis over pre-existing warts often related to HPV16 infection.
11. *Syphilis:* Doubtful.

Pathology

The lesion usually occurs on the glans (48%) and the inner surface of the prepuce (21%) near its reflection from the corona. *The growth starts either commonly as a nodule, a wart or an ulcer.*

Origin from the skin of the shaft is very rare.

Macroscopic appearance

1. *Ulcerative type* with rolled out and everted margin.
2. *Proliferative or cauliflower type* which may be warty or nodular. This type is less malignant than ulcerative type.
3. *Fissure type* looks like a small fissure situated over the glans.
4. *Plaque type* situated over the glans.

Microscopic appearance

The histologic features of penile carcinoma resemble *squamous cell carcinoma* occurring elsewhere in the body and is usually moderate to well-differentiated type.

Spread

Direct spread: Through the prepuce and proximally along the shaft. The growth is slowly growing and remains localised for many months. *Spread to the body of the penis is prevented for a long time by Buck's fascia surrounding the corpora.* Once the neoplasm penetrates the fascia and tunica albuginea of the corporal body, rapid dissemination takes place and vascular dissemination is possible.

Urethra remains uninvolved even in late cases though scrotal skin may be involved by direct contact.

Lymphatic spread is the earliest: It usually occurs by embolisation through the lymphatics first to the superficial and deep inguinal nodes and then to the iliac lymph nodes. *It is to be noted that penile lymphatic drainage is essentially bilateral.*

- N_1: Metastasis in single superficial inguinal LN.
- N_2: Metastases in multiple or bilateral superficial inguinal LN.

Glans penis drains into the *Cloquet's lymph node* which is a deep lymph node in relation to the femoral septum lies at the sphenofemoral junction under the cribriform fascia (SLN).

Blood spread: Distant metastases by blood is very rare and commonly involve the lungs, liver and bones.

Diagnostic criteria

1. *Age:* Common in middle-aged and elderly persons. It may also occur in young males below the age of 40 years (40% cases).
2. *Duration:* Usually short and of a few months only. The progress is slow.

Symptoms:

3. (a) *The patient usually presents with a lump, plaque or an ulcer*, representing the papilliferous or ulcerating varieties of penile carcinoma respectively. *The lesion as such is a painless condition* but may be painful if infected.

(b) Other symptoms may include mild irritation with penile discharge – serosanguineous, purulent or blood stained.

(c) The patient may also present with phimosis which may be the cause of carcinoma or may be caused by carcinoma. In these circumstances the primary lesion is hidden under the preputial skin and eventually produces an offensive discharge. *A dorsal slit is required to expose the lesion.*

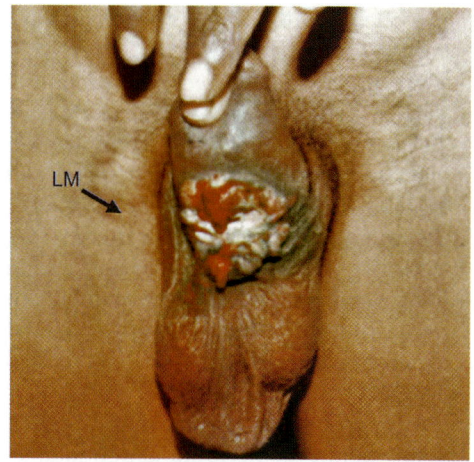

Fig. 12.6: Carcinoma penoscrotal junction ulcerative type—right inguinal nodes were enlarged (stage III).

(d) Unfortunately many patients delay to report to the doctor early because of embarrassment, guilt, denial, fear or ignorance. They present late with a fungating and foul smelling mass destroying a good portion of the body of the penis.

(e) *The patient may present with enlarged inguinal lymph nodes* – which may be secondary to deposits or infections.

(f) Pain, oedema, tenderness, redness develop once infection occurs.

(g) General features of malignancy – anaemia, anorexia, loss of weight, cachexia are rare.

On examination:

4. *Site: The lesion may be anywhere on the glans* or *the inner surface of the foreskin.* The penis may be swollen at the tip due to mass beneath the prepuce. When the tumour is large it may appear through the preputial opening or erode through the preputial skin. *If phimosis is present, doral slit under local anaesthesia may be required for proper inspection.* Note the status of the prepuce and meatus location and calibre – adequate or inadequate.

5. *Shape and consistency:* It may appear as *an ulcer* with a raised, everted edge and necrotic

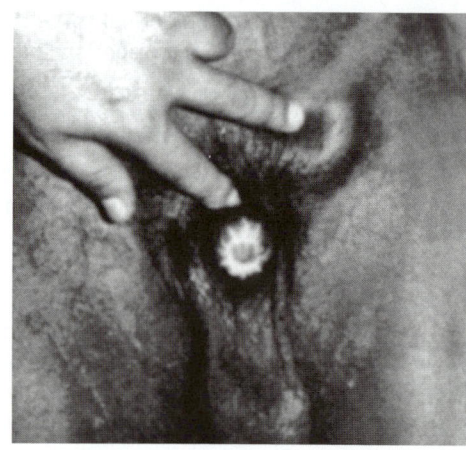

Fig. 12.7: Partial amputation of penis for carcinoma penis. 10 months later patient developed metastatic lymph node at left groin—pointed by the tip of the middle finger. Index finger pointed the penile stump.

indurated base, or as *a sessile papilliferous growth* with indurated base. Occasionally, the lesion may be *fungating with partial or total length of the penile shaft involvement.* The growth is hard in consistency particularly at the base. The surface of the papilliferous variety is soft and friable and bleeds easily. Any part of the penis which is infiltrated also feels hard. *Entire shaft, root of the penis and scrotum have to be examined for evidence of tumour infiltration.*

6. *Lymph nodes: Inguinal lymph nodes are found to be enlarged in about 60% cases,* but a half of these enlargements is due to secondary infection from the primary growth. *Bilateral inguinal LNS should be examined for enlargement.* Metastatic lymph nodes are hard in feel and may be mobile or fixed. *In advanced case,* the lymph nodes may appear as fungating growth through the skin of the groin. In very late case, the fungating growth may erode the underlying femoral vein or artery *to cause torrential haemorrhage.*

7. Urethra is rarely involved in carcinoma penis because it is protected by the Buck's fascia. In a large fungating lesion involving the glans it may be difficult to identify the external urinary meatus. In such situations, patient will point out the site of exit of urinary stream, i.e. the site of external urinary meatus.

8. Rectal and bimanual examination to assess if pelvic spread is present.

Investigations

1. *Biopsy of the lesion and FNAC or FNAB of the bilateral inguinal (SLN) lymph nodes. An edge biopsy of the lesion is mandatory prior to therapy even in frankly malignant tumours on clinical examination.* Biopsy helps in two ways:

   (a) Diagnostic value.
   (b) Therapeutic value – whether radio-resistant or radiosensitive.

   If there is phimosis a dorsal slit has to be made to take a wedge biopsy of the lesion.
   No open biopsy of lymph nodes as it causes metastatic spread to both superficial and deep (pelvic) nodes. SLNB or FNAC is practised nowadays.

2. Blood for WR and Kahn tests.

   Importance:

   (a) Syphilitic ulcer and malignant ulcer may coexist or a malignant ulcer may supervene on a preexisting syphilitic ulcer.
   (b) *Carcinoma supervening on preexisting syphilitic ulcer is mostly radioresistant* and hence should be treated by surgery.

(Radiosensitivity depends on the vascularity of the lesion. Syphilis causes endarteritis obliterans.)

3. Chest X-ray, lymphangiography, U/S abdomen, abdominopelvic CT scan, bone scan may be required to note the nodal involvement and dissemination in presence of enlarged inguinal nodes.

Tumour staging

Stage I Tumour confined to the glans or foreskin or both.

Stage II Tumour involves the shaft of the penis.

Stage III Tumour associated with superficial inguinal lymph nodes involvement but mobile and operable.

Stage IV Disease is disseminated, i.e. the disease is associated with inoperable inguinal lymph nodes or distant metastasis or scrotal involvement.

• Distant metastasis occurs in less than 10% of patients.
• *Most important prognostic factor is the presence and extent of superficial inguinal lymph node involvement which can be confirmed by FNAC/SLNB of the inguinal nodes.*

Termination of the lesion

1. Haemorrhage – following erosion of the femoral artery or external iliac artery by the fungating metastatic lymph nodes. There may be torrential haemorrhage which often causes death of the patient.

2. Malignant cachexia in late stage, due to:

   (a) exhaustion from pain, and
   (b) septic absorption leading to septicaemia.

Treatment

It includes:

1. Treatment of the primary growth.
2. Treatment of the secondary lymph nodes.
3. Treatment of distant metastasis.

TREATMENT OF THE PRIMARY GROWTH

• Surgery
• Radiotherapy

- Chemotherapy
- Cryosurgery
- Laser therapy

The objectives of selecting therapy are to eradicate the primary lesion, prevent local recurrence, and *preserve maximum usable penile length. In most cases surgery is preferred for management of the primary lesion.*

Surgery

Indications

1. Growth larger than 3 cm and invasive.
2. Infiltration of the shaft of the penis.
3. Anaplastic growth.
4. Radiotherapy failed.
5. Carcinoma supervening on leukoplakia or syphilitic ulcer – *usually radioresistant.*
6. Elderly males, who do not mind the mutilation as much as the discomfort or pain apprehended from the extensive reaction to radiotherapy.

Types of surgery

1. *Circumcision alone* can be performed for non-invasive tumours involving only the foreskin/prepuce but the recurrence rate is unacceptably high, up to 50%. *It is curative for carcinoma in situ only.*
2. *Local wide excision of the small tumour confined to the glans should be avoided because recurrence rates are high,* as much as 40% with a worsened prognosis.
3. *Partial amputation,* including 2 cm of benign tissue proximal to the tumour margin is indicated – *for growths involving the glans penis or distal shaft,* provided the remaining penile length is sufficient to allow to direct his urinary stream from the standing position. *This is carried out with the use of long ventral flap, and the urethra is brought out through an opening in it.*
4. *Less aggressive surgical resection such as Moh's micrographic surgery and local excision directed at penile preservation is performed in some centres recently.* This is generally followed by brachytherapy, using isotope mould, to sterilise the base.

5. *Total amputation of penis with perineal urethrostomy.*

Indication of total amputation:
(a) Anaplastic growth – invasive and high grade.
(b) Growth involving the proximal shaft or base of the penis.
(c) Growth in which the extent of disease precludes salvage of sufficient length *to allow upright voiding (at least 2 cm of the dependent stump is required).*

The procedure includes the removal of the corpora cavernosa from the pubic bones followed by division of the corpus spongiosum *leaving at least 1.3 cm of the urethra at the proximal end,* which will be taken out through a separate incision behind the scrotum in the form of perineal urethrostomy.

Problem with urethrostomy

1. Ammoniacal dermatitis of scrotum.
2. Stricture of perineal meatus – requires repeated dilatation by Hegar's dilator or meatal dilator.

Note

Many surgeons believe that once corpora cavernosa is involved technically entire shaft is involved; hence nothing less than total amputation should be performed.

Problem with the scrotum and testes during surgery

There are three views:
1. The scrotum and the testes are preserved to avoid psychoneurotic disturbances.
2. The scrotum and the testes are removed. The advantage is twofold.
   (a) The removal avoids disturbance during passing of urine particularly in total amputation.
   (b) It kills the sexual desire. If the testes are not removed, the patient has got the desire but no way of satisfaction after operation because of total amputation or partial amputation leaving a very small stump.

3. The scrotum and the testes are preserved *but the testes are ablated by radiation to kill sexual desire.*

Radiotherapy

Radiotherapy is appropriate only for limited number of cases. *Circumcision with or without meatotomy are necessary prior to irradiation.*

Indications

1. Small lesion less than 3 cm located on the glans penis, which is superficial and non-invasive.
2. Young patients with small lesions.
3. Patients of any age refusing surgery.
4. Squamous carcinoma *in situ* (Paget's disease, erythroplasia of Queyrat, Bowen's disease) as reported after biopsy of the lesion.

Advantage: Radiotherapy preserves the penile structure and function.

Contraindications

1. Carcinoma supervening on leukoplakia and syphilis.
2. Lesions invasive and larger than 3 cm.

Problems with radiotherapy

1. Meagre facilities of radiotherapy, particularly in our country.
2. Longer course of treatment.
3. Chances of urethral stricture, stenosis, fistula.
4. The penis becomes withered, and shrivelled up.
5. Chance of postradiation sterility due to testicular damage.
6. There may be erythema and oedema, transient severe pain, ulceration and necrosis of penis as an extensive reaction to radiotherapy that may force cessation of therapy.
7. Recurrences are common after radiotherapy.
8. Infection accompanying penile carcinoma decreases efficacy of radiotherapy.

Available methods

1. *Interstitial:* Implantation with flexible radioactive tantalum wires (total dose 6000 rads in 5 to 7 days).

2. *Surface:* Radium mould applicators worn either intermittently or continuously (total dose 6000 rads in 7 to 10 days).
3. *Megavoltage:* Electron beam (total dose 5000 to 5700 rads in 3 to 5 weeks).

Chemotherapy

Topical chemotherapy with 5-fluorouracil cream is only advocated *for the treatment of squamous carcinoma in situ lesions* (Paget's disease, erythroplasia of Queyrat, Bowen's disease).

Systemic chemotherapy has not proved useful even in disseminated disease. Bleomycin, methotrexate, cisplatin, and 5-fluorouracil may be tried in tumours associated with lymph nodes involvement.

Cryosurgery

Recently *cryosurgery for carcinoma in situ lesions* of the penis is tried with encouraging results. Cosmetic results are as good as those achieved with radiotherapy. No recurrence after 5 years has been reported.

Laser surgery

In few sophisticated centres *the Nd:YAG laser (photoirradiation)* are being tried in *carcinoma in situ lesion* with encouraging results and good cosmetic effect.

Note

Recently, small, non-invasive lesion is being treated with chemotherapy, cryosurgery, laser surgery and Moh's micrographic surgery at some centres with good success and results.

TREATMENT OF THE SECONDARY LYMPH NODES

1. **Clinically no palpable nodes:** Bimonthly observation for 3 years. If nodes appear, staged *bilateral* ilioinguinal block dissection preceded by FNAC of the palpable nodes.
2. **Lymph nodes are palpable but mobile:**
   (a) Primary lesion is treated.
   (b) A course of antibiotic is given post-operatively for 6 weeks after resection of primary tumour and the patient be observed:

(i) *if the nodes disappear or diminish in size* – suggestive of reactive lymphadenopathy due to sepsis. So, no block dissection but bimonthly observation is required for 3 years.

(ii) *if the nodes remain unaltered or become more enlarged* – suggestive of malignant involvement. So, *bilateral block dissection* is to be performed preceded by FNAC of the palpable nodes. *Excision biopsy of lymph nodes is unwarranted.*

Block dissection: It includes *removal of the nodes of both the sides: Bilateral ilioinguinal block dissection – the more affected side is*

removed first followed by contralateral block dissection at a later date.

Complication – marked lower limb lymph-oedema, delayed wound healing, wound infection, flap necrosis.

Following block dissections, the sartorius muscle is detached from its origin and then fixed to inguinal ligament over the femoral vessels.

3. **Lymph nodes are palpable and fixed** – so inoperable. Palliative radiotherapy and/or systemic chemotherapy is given which can cause temporary regression.

The wait and watch policy, i.e. removing the inguinal nodes only when they become palpably

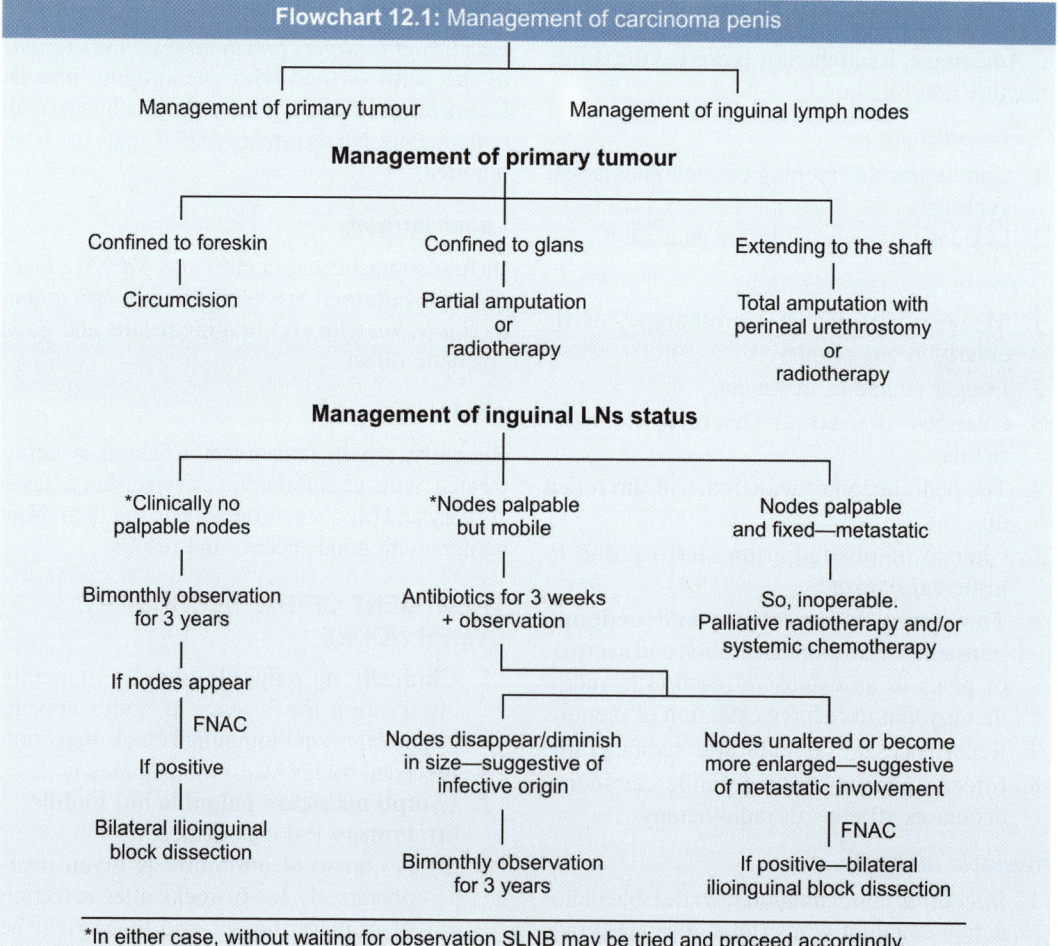

Flowchart 12.1: Management of carcinoma penis

Management of primary tumour — Management of inguinal lymph nodes

Management of primary tumour

- Confined to foreskin
  - Circumcision
- Confined to glans
  - Partial amputation or radiotherapy
- Extending to the shaft
  - Total amputation with perineal urethrostomy or radiotherapy

Management of inguinal LNs status

- *Clinically no palpable nodes
  - Bimonthly observation for 3 years
  - If nodes appear
    - FNAC
    - If positive
    - Bilateral ilioinguinal block dissection
- *Nodes palpable but mobile
  - Antibiotics for 3 weeks + observation
    - Nodes disappear/diminish in size—suggestive of infective origin
      - Bimonthly observation for 3 years
    - Nodes unaltered or become more enlarged—suggestive of metastatic involvement
      - FNAC
      - If positive—bilateral ilioinguinal block dissection
- Nodes palpable and fixed—metastatic
  - So, inoperable. Palliative radiotherapy and/or systemic chemotherapy

*In either case, without waiting for observation SLNB may be tried and proceed accordingly.

suspect, has resulted in greater morbidity and mortality. So, some surgeons advocate *excision biopsy of sentinel lymph node in clinically non-palpable inguinal nodes* – if biopsy is positive *an ipsilateral ilioinguinal lymphadenectomy is performed.*

Importance of sentinel lymph node biopsy (SLNB) in carcinoma penis

The penile lymphatics first drain in *a sentinel lymph node or nodes* (Cabanas). *It is the most medial node of the superficial horizontal group and is located above and medial to the junction of saphenous and femoral veins* (**sapheno-femoral junction**) *in the area of superficial epigastric vein. This sentinel lymph node is the first node to get involved in penile malignancy.* So, this SLN, which is stained blue after isosulphan blue dye injection in the primary lesion, is first identified. FNAB/FNAC of this node is performed. *The involvement of SLN(s) will indicate complete bilateral ilioinguinal block dissection.*

If FNAC is negative – no block dissection of inguinal nodes is performed, but bimonthly checkup is required for 5 years.

Prognosis

This depends on the site and stage of the growth, and lymph nodes involvement.

Stage I   Tumour restricted to the glans penis – 70% 5 years survival.

Stage II Tumours involving the shaft of the penis – 60% 5 years survival.

Stage III Tumours associated with inguinal lymph nodes involvement – 30% 5 years survival.

Secondary carcinoma of the penis

- May occur, but rarely.
- Primary source of the lesion is usually the prostate, bladder or rectum.

   Way of spread from the primary – three ways:

   (a) By direct spread.
   (b) By retrograde spread.
   (c) By retrograde venous embolism via the dorsal vein of the penis.

PREMALIGNANT LESIONS OF THE PENIS

Condyloma acuminatum (Fig. 12.8)

1. Rarely occurs before puberty.
2. Caused by human papillomavirus.
3. Transmitted by sexual contact.
4. These are mostly situated near the coronal sulcus.
5. These appear as sharp pointed red, papillary excrescences, sessile or pedunculated and usually moist with an offensive discharge.
6. HPE shows koilocytosis, irregular size, shape or colour of the nuclei: *Precursor of cancer.*
7. Can involve the urethra in 5% of cases.
8. *Treatment:*
   (a) 20% solution of podophyllin in tinct. benzoin application.
   (b) 0.1% bleomycin application.
   (c) Circumcision and fulguration of the lesion.

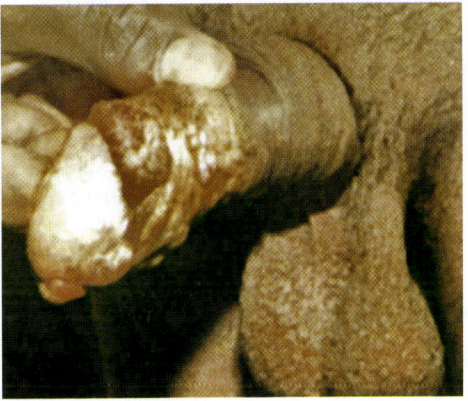

Fig. 12.8. Condyloma acuminata—a precancerous lesion.

Buschke-Löwenstein tumour (Verrucous carcinoma) (Fig. 12.9)

1. A giant variety of condyloma acuminatum.
2. It appears as large exophytic lesion.
3. It penetrates and destroys adjacent tissue.
4. It is a benign lesion with a premalignant potential.
5. Because of its large size it frequently is grossly indistinguishable from squamous cell carcinoma. Excisional biopsy or multiple

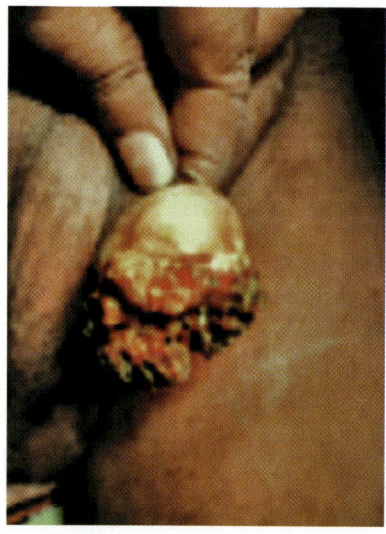

Fig. 12.9: Buschke-Löwenstein tumour. A large exophytic growth on the undersurface of glans nearly obscuring the meatus. Wedge biopsy performed—reported condyloma.

deep biopsies are necessary to exclude true penile carcinoma.
6. *Treatment:*
(a) For small lesions – local excision of the tumour that spares penile anatomic structure, so function is adequate.
(b) Large lesions may require partial amputation of the penis.
(c) Bleomycin topically may be helpful.

Leukoplakia of the glans

1. It is a condition of hyperkeratosis of the epithelial cells (cf. tongue, cheek, vulva and vagina).
2. It appears as greyish white plaque.
3. The condition is painless.
4. Premalignant.
5. *Treatment:* Local excision.

Erythroplasia of Queyrat (Fig. 12.10)

1. *It appears as a dark red, velvety, well-margined, flat or slightly raised indurated patch on the glans penis, or coronal sulcus.* Occasionally it becomes superficially ulcerative when there may be discharge and pain.

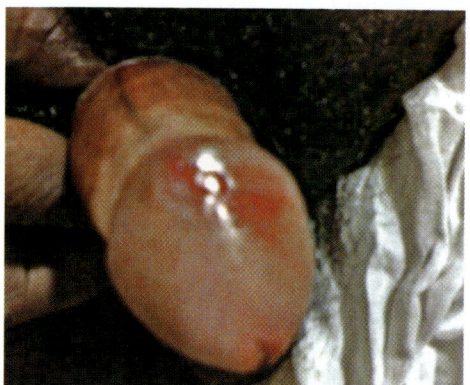

Fig. 12.10: Erythroplasia of Queyrat—a premalignant condition.

2. It is similar to Bowen's disease of penis on histology and represents carcinoma *in situ* changes.
3. Prior to initiating therapy multiple biopsies of adequate depth should be taken.
4. Premalignant.
5. *Treatment:*
(a) Local excision of the lesion is adequate.
(b) If a lesion is preputial, circumcision will suffice.
(c) 5-fluorouracil cream topically is helpful. Cosmetic results are excellent.
(d) Nd:YAG laser fulguration is also adequate.

Bowen's disease

1. It is an intradermal precancerous condition.
2. It is similar to erythroplasia of Queyrat histopathologically and clinically but the lesion is drier in appearance and is often crusted and ulcerated.
3. Premalignant.
4. *Treatment:* Topical application of 5-fluorouracil or bleomycin cream.

Balanitis xerotica

1. It presents as white atrophic lesion with or without oedema involving the glans or prepuce or both.
2. Premalignant.
3. *Treatment:* Local excision and/or topical steroid application.

Note

Sir James Paget, an English surgeon and pathologist

- Diseases named after Paget
  - Paget's disease of penis
  - Paget's disease of breast
  - Paget's disease of bone

Paget's disease of penis

A rare cutaneous slow growing *intraepidermal adenocarcinoma* developing in the apocrine gland bearing areas of the epidermis – *mostly penile skin.*

- This lesion may involve the scrotum and perineum.
- It may also involve the vulva in the female.

Paget's disease of breast

A rare form of *intraepidermal adenocarcinoma* of breast in which cancer cells collected in and around the nipple and areolar surfaces *with the appearance of eczema.*

It can spread to the ducts of the nipple and causes underlying duct carcinoma. Sir James Paget first described this disease.

Paget's disease of bone

Osteitis deformans: There is *interference of replacement of the old bone tissue with new bone tissue and so hinders* new bone formation and remodelling of the bone *leading to osteoporosis and fragile bone.*

- *Mostly occurs in pelvis, skull, spine and legs.*
- Causes bone pain and deformities.
- Fracture is common.
- *Mainstay of treatment: Biphosphonate* orally or by injection. *Calcitonin* injection or nasal spray may also help if biphosphonate cannot be tolerated.

Raynaud's Syndrome and Thoracic Outlet Syndrome

Raynaud's syndrome is defined as recurrent, episodic attack of vasospasm of the digital blood vessels resulting in **triphasic colour changes** of the digits, i.e. pallor → cyanosis → rubor in that particular sequence (*remember mnemonics PCR*): Raynaud's phenomenon.

This phenomenon *affects the fingers and hands most commonly*, though it may occur in the feet, ear, nose and lips.

This syndrome usually develops on exposure to cold or emotional disturbance and is usually paroxysmal and episodic.

Causes

1. Primary or idiopathic variety

This variety is known as Raynaud's disease. In this condition the digital vessels appear to be healthy but very much sensitive to the cold leading to vasospasm. There is no demonstrable structural change in the arterial tree or associated systemic disease. *Raynaud's disease refers to occurrence of Raynaud's phenomenon* **due to vasospasm** *without an underlying disease of the digital vessels:* **Vasospastic** *Raynaud's disease.*

2. Secondary variety

In this condition Raynaud's syndrome occurs *due to obstruction of blood flow in the digital vessels*

complicating a known disease or local trauma: **Obstructive** *Raynaud's disease,* e.g.

(a) *Collagen vascular diseases* – causing vasculitis
   • Scleroderma – commonest
   • Polyarteritis, polymyositis
   • Rheumatic arthritis
   • Systemic lupus erythematosus (SLE)
   • Dermatomyositis

(b) *Obliterative arterial diseases*
   • Thromboangitis obliterans (TAO)
   • Atherosclerosis of subclavian artery

(c) *Occupational and industrial exposure to vibrating tools* such as riveting machines and earth impactors which disturb the neuro-vascular control in the hands and fingers, *particularly the pacinian corpuscles: nerve endings in the skin responsible for sensitivity to vibration and pressure.*

(d) *Irritation of nerves and vessels*
   • Thoracic outlet syndrome such as cervical rib, scalene syndrome
   • Cervical disc protrusion
   • Spinal cord disease – syringomyelia, tumours
   • Old poliomyelitis

(e) *Peripheral embolism arising from*
   • Damaged subclavian artery crossing a cervical rib

- Subclavian aneurysm secondary to cervical rib
- Atherosclerotic stenosis of the subclavian artery

(f) *Blood abnormalities*
- Cold agglutinins
- Cryoglobulins

Both cause vascular damage *due to agglutination of red cells,* e.g. in multiple myeloma.

(g) *Ingestion of drugs*
- Ergotamine preparations
- Methysergide
- β-blockers, e.g. propranolol
- Amphetamine
- Cytotoxic drugs – bleomycin, vinblastine, cisplatin

(h) *Poisoning* by lead and arsenic

(i) *Atrophic changes in the limb* following poliomyelitis, frostbite, etc.

(j) Trauma – vibrating tools injury, hammer hand syndrome, electric shock, cold injury, typing, piano playing

So, basically Raynaud's syndrome may be divided into two distinct pathophysiologic disorders:

(a) **Vasospastic disorder** in primary variety or Raynaud's disease due to cold sensitivity.

(b) **Obstructive disorder** in secondary variety.

Sympathectomy is avoided in secondary variety of Raynaud's syndrome as it produces very poor results.

RAYNAUD'S DISEASE

It is a recurrent paroxysmal vasospastic disorder of the apparently healthy digital blood vessels in response to abnormal hypersensitivity to cold resulting in alternate vasoconstriction and vasodilatation of the digital arterioles.

The disease was first described by Raynaud in 1862.

Pathophysiology

The exact cause of this arteriolar vasoconstriction is not known. It may be due to:

(a) *Hypersensitivity of the arterioles themselves to cold.* The vessels show no evidence of organic disease.

(b) Abnormality of the sympathetic nervous system *α-adrenergic receptors:* Causes constriction of the blood vessels.

The disease is usually precipitated by exposure to cold and/or emotional stress with an abrupt onset.

It passes through three stages and is associated with *cyclical triphasic colour changes in the digits*, and *often disturbances of sensation*. To remember the colour changes remember the mnemonics WBC (White Blood Cell).

W   White or pale (stage of blanching)
B   Blue or cyanosis (stage of dusky anoxia) (Fig. 13.1)
C   Crimson or red (stage of red engorgement)

Three pathological changes are encountered for these triphasic colour changes.

Stage of local syncope: On exposure to cold the digital arterioles go into spasm resulting in diminished blood flow locally *which is evident*

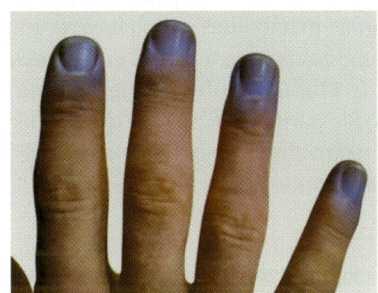
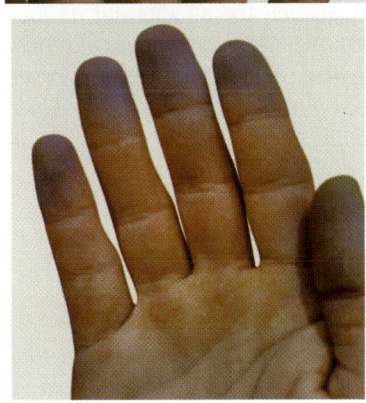

Fig. 13.1: Note the colour changes of the fingers (both the dorsum and palmar surfaces of the fingers)—Raynaud's disease. The digits are cyanosed and blue—*stage of dusky anoxia.*

by pallor or blanching of the fingers (**stage of blanching**). *The fingers become cold and waxy pale white*. These changes start at the tips of fingers and gradually spread to the base of the fingers. There is also associated *tingling and numbness*.

Stage of local asphyxia: As the hand is warmed or the general body temperature is raised the spasm relaxes and the capillaries are slowly dilated and filled up with blood. Then as the red cells reach the anoxic tissue *they become acutely deoxygenated*. The digital vessels gradually become filled up with this deoxygenated blood so that *the digits become cyanosed or blue (**stage of dusky anoxia**)* (Fig. 13.1). *The digits are still cold and numb*.

Stage of recovery: With rewarming or passing of the attack, further relaxation of the spasm occurs and the blood flow is increased and *the digits become crimson or red (**stage of red engorgement**), hot and swollen*. The redness is also due to a reactive hyperaemia set up by the local tissue metabolites which have accumulated during the cold phase. *There is also an **acute pain which is tingling and burning in nature***. The pain is due partly to increased tissue tension and partly to irritation of cutaneous nerves caused by local metabolites.

Late features

In the early stages of the disease the digits are normal between the attacks *but as the disease progresses, obliterative changes may occur in the peripheral vessels – stenosis and/or occlusion* followed by *trophic changes in the skin and nails of the fingers*: atrophic but shiny skin, alopecia, dry scaly or erythematous skin, chronic pigmentary changes, brittle nails.

The patient may eventually **get rest pain and dry gangrene** of the finger tips or ulcer.

Diagnostic criteria

1. *Sex:* Raynaud's disease is *ten times more common in women than in men* (F : M = 10 : 1).
2. *Age:* It *usually occurs in young adult* after puberty and before the menopause (between 20 and 40 years).

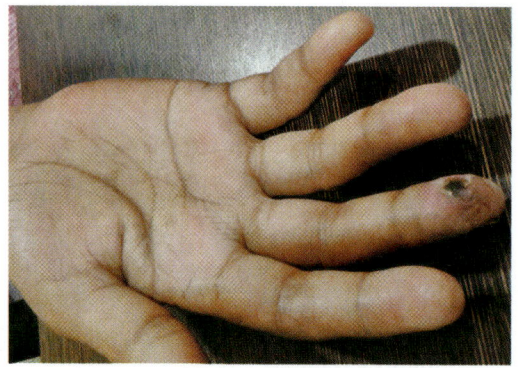

Fig. 13.2: Raynaud's disease involving the fingers (note the cyanotic changes of the fingertips and also ulcer at the tip of right middle finger). (*Courtesy:* Dr A Anand, MS)

3. In about 50% cases there is a family history.
4. *It affects the digits of the upper extremity more commonly* and more severely than of the lower.
5. Initially one or two fingers are affected but gradually all the fingers are involved to include the distal palm. *The thumbs are usually spared*.
6. *Commonly bilateral.*
7. *Usually symmetrical.*
8. *May be paroxysmal* (sudden occurrence) *and episodic* (periodical) *and painful* (cf. acrocyanosis).
9. *On presentation, the fingers and hands may look white, and feel cold*. Or they may look normal between the attacks.

   An attack can be precipitated by asking the patient to dip her hand into ice-cold water, when the fingers and hands become *waxy pale white*. If this white hand is then put into warm water, *it turns blue or cyanosed and finally a dusky red colour due to hyperaemia*. The patient often experiences a *throbbing painful sensation*.
10. In late cases, there may be the *presence of trophic changes* when the diagnosis can be guessed correlating the patient's description of her typical symptoms with the local findings. *The trophic changes* may be one of the following.

    (a) Permanently blue ischaemic fingertips;

(b) Thin and pointed finger tips due to atrophy of the pulp;

(c) Necrosis of small areas of skin followed by small scars;

(d) Small very painful ischaemic ulcers on the finger tips.

(e) Recurrent infections around the nails (paronychia) are common. These are painful and slow to heal.

(f) *The patient may eventually present with gangrene of the finger tips and rest pain.*

(g) *Sclerodactyly:* Thickening and tightening of digital subcutaneous tissues may develop in few patients.

(h) Fewer than 1% of these patients may lose a part of the digit.

11. *Pulses:* At the wrist and above are usually palpable. *Presence of peripheral pulses, yet obvious ischaemic changes of the digits is a typical finding in Raynaud's disease* (cf. Buerger's disease – *peripheral pulses are absent*).

12. The return of capillary circulation after blanching produced by pressure on the pulp or nail bed may be very slow. *Raynaud's disease involves the small arteries, i.e. digital arteries. Radial artery is not involved. So, radial pulse will be palpable.*

13. Exclude the causes of secondary Raynaud's phenomenon, e.g. cervical spondylosis, cervical rib, scleroderma, history of drug ingestion etc.

Note

• Raynaud's syndrome or phenomenon is usually unilateral.
• Raynaud's disease is *usually bilateral.*

Note

• Raynaud's disease: *Peripheral pulses are usually palpable.*
• Buerger's disease: Peripheral pulses of arteria dorsalis pedis and posterior tibial arteries are absent.

Note

• All patients with history of Raynaud's phenomenon should be asked about symptoms

of autoimmune disease such as arthritis, dry eyes or dry mouth, myalgias, fever, skin rash, cardiomyopathy abnormalities.

• *ANA assays* are highly sensitive for connective tissue disorder.

Investigations

Diagnosis of Raynaud's disease is made on the typical history and findings.

Special investigations may be performed *to rule out* any associated systemic disorders leading to secondary Raynaud's syndrome to come to a diagnosis of Raynaud's disease by exclusion.

1. *X-ray of the cervical spine* AP and lateral views – to exclude cervical rib or spondylosis.

2. *Angiography* to establish the diagnosis by:
   (i) demonstrating the presence of spasm of terminal arterioles on exposure to cold.
   (ii) Demonstrating subclavian artery stenosis or dilatation, thrombi or emboli.

3. *Doppler ultrasound:* To detect the presence of peripheral pulses. *It has outdated angiography.*

4. *ESR*

5. *Rheumatoid factor:* Rheumatic arthritis

6. *Antinuclear antibody:* Collagen vascular disease

7. *Cold agglutinins* ⎤ Raised in multiple
8. *Cryoproteins* ⎦ myeloma

Treatment

No cure for Raynaud's disease. The treatment of primary Raynaud's disease remains unsatisfactory. There are currently no specific means for overcoming the local fault and the hypersensitivity of the digital arteries to cold.

Conservative

To palliate symptoms and decrease the severity and perhaps the frequency of the attacks:

1. *Avoid exposure to cold.*
2. *Avoid any emotional stress.*
3. *Stop smoking or tobacco in any other form.*
4. *The patient is advised to keep her hands and body warm – to dress warmly, to wear socks*

and gloves, to keep the house and specially bed warm at night during winter and cold weather. *Warmth of the central body induces peripheral vasodilatation.*

5. *Avoid drugs* such as ergotamine, methysergide, β-blockers, amphetamine.
6. *In presence of nail bed infection:* Oral antibiotics and antifungal drugs like griseofulvin or fluconazole may be advised.
7. *Analgesics and neurotonics to give immediate pain relief.*
8. *Drug therapy to improve vascularity.*
   (i) *Vasospastic antagonistic drugs: Drugs that block sympathetic vasoconstriction:* Reserpine, guanethidine, α-methyldopa, phenoxybenzamine, pentoxifylline and α-blockers like prazosin may be useful.
   (ii) *Vasodilators:* Arlidine, Complamina, nifedipine (*calcium channel blockers*). *Nifedipine 10 mg BD is commonly used nowadays.* Diltiazem is also used.
   (iii) IV prostaglandin E and prostacyclin are potent vasodilators and inhibit platelet aggregation. May be used in acute stage.

   Patients with spasmodic Raynaud's syndrome respond better than obstructive Raynaud's syndrome with drug therapy.

   (iv) *Ketanserin* is a selective serotonin receptor blocker which antagonises serotonin-induced vasoconstriction and inhibits platelet aggregation. *This drug is useful in treating Raynaud's syndrome induced by scleroderma.*
9. *Drugs used during acute severe spasmodic attack:*
   (i) Intravenous low molecular weight dextran may alleviate the attack.
   (ii) Intra-arterial injection of reserpine (1 mg in 10 ml normal saline) injected slowly in brachial artery may alleviate the attack.

Operative
- Sympathectomy
- Amputation

Cervicodorsal sympathectomy

Procedure
In this operation the following are removed.

(i) The portion of sympathetic trunk that includes the *lower one-third of the stellate ganglion (containing T_1 ganglion), T_2 and T_3 ganglion* which contain most of the postganglionic fibres supplying the upper limb.
(ii) All rami communicantes associated with the T_2 and T_3 ganglion.
(iii) The nerve of Kuntz, gray ramus which arises from the T_2 ganglion and goes to the 1st thoracic nerve.

The stellate ganglion is identified as it lies on the neck of the 1st rib. It is dumbbell-shaped with upper larger inferior cervical ganglion and lower smaller T_1 ganglion fused together with a waist between them. The postganglionic fibres supplying the head and neck pass through the inferior cervical ganglion present in the upper larger part of the stellate ganglion.

Removal of the whole of the stellate ganglion will cause Horner's syndrome.

Routes
Cervicodorsal sympathectomy can be done through the supraclavicular route or transthoracic route via an axillary incision at the third intercostal space.

Thoracic route has the advantage of:

(i) Cosmetically better because of hidden scar at axilla, particularly in female.
(ii) Removal of sympathetic chain up to T_5 ganglion is possible.

Endoscopic sympathectomy is being tried at some centres recently.

Result
- The results of cervicodorsal sympathectomy is unpredictable and short lasting.
- *The patient may derive some benefit, if it is done in the early stages.* In the later stages when the vessels are partly or completely occluded by fibrosis or thrombosis *sympathectomy is useless.*

- *The operation will not provide a permanent cure*, as there is no evidence that sympathetic abnormality is only responsible for the disease.
- The maximum result that can be achieved from such operation is *some permanent increase in warmth of the digits due to reduction in tone of the cutaneous arterioles.*
- There is also some increase in thermal insulation around the digital arteries which can provide a protection against local cooling to critical levels.
- *But in over 75% patients the symptoms return with increased vasomotor tone within 5 years of operation.*

Note

The results of lumbar sympathectomy for Buerger's disease in the lower limb are much better and late relapses rarely occur provided patient stops smoking for the rest of life.

Limitations

Sympathectomy should be avoided in secondary causes of Raynaud's syndrome as it produces very poor results.

Complications of cervicodorsal sympathectomy

- Perforation of pleura leading to pneumothorax.
- Haemorrhage leading to retropleural haematoma.
- Lymph fistula following damage to the thoracic duct during left cervical sympathectomy.
- Horner's syndrome – when total stellate ganglion is removed. *Stellate ganglion is a large ganglion formed by the fusion of two lower cervical ganglions with the 1st thoracic ganglion* – hence known as cervicothoracic ganglion.

Features of Horner's syndrome

- Ptosis
- Myosis
- Enophthalmos
- Anhydrosis (loss of sweating) of the ipsilateral face
- Loss of ciliospinal reflex – normally, pinching the skin over the neck produces dilatation of the pupil due to ciliospinal reflex. *This reflex is lost in Horner's syndrome.*

Amputation

Local amputation may be required rarely in cases when there is necrosis of tissues and gangrene of the digits. Since the circulation of proximal vessels of the hand is usually satisfactory, major amputations are seldom required. *Any amputation should be supplemented by prior sympathectomy.*

ACROCYANOSIS

- This is a chronic *persistent vasospastic condition of the cutaneous arteries and arterioles producing* cyanosis or blue discoloration of the hands and feet including digits.
- Common in young females.
- There is **persistent and painless cyanosis and coldness of the hands and feet** (cf. Raynaud's disease – which is *episodic* and *painful*).
- The cyanosis may also be noticed at the tip of the nose and ears. Often legs are involved.
- The involved parts are also cold with excessive perspiration.
- *The peripheral pulses are normal.*
- *The cyanosis may aggravate on exposure to cold.*
- *Though the condition is painless* (cf. Raynaud's disease), *it is susceptible to chilblains. But the digits are not subjected to gangrene.*

Treatment

(a) Conservative: Reassurance and avoidance of undue exposure to cold which can cause chilblains.

(b) Oral vasodilator drugs: α-adrenergic blockers or calcium channel blockers.

(c) Sympathectomy in the presence of severe cyanosis or if the chilblain is particularly troublesome. The effect may be transient.

Note

- Acrocyanosis – *painless* and *persistent cyanosis* of hands and feet.
- Raynaud's disease – *periodic or episodic painful cyanosis* of hands and digits.
- Chilblains – *itchy sores/bumps* of the hands and feet including digits.

Note

Indications of sympathectomy

1. Raynaud's disease – caused by stable arterial occlusion
2. Cervical rib syndrome when associated with vasomotor disturbances.
3. *Thromboangitis obliterans (TAO):* Lumbar sympathectomy is *not effective in claudication* but it may occasionally relieve rest pain and ulceration.
4. Hyperhidrosis – *best respond to sympathectomy.*
5. Causalsia.
6. Acrocyanosis.
7. Frostbite sequelae.
8. Inoperable atherosclerotic arterial occlusion with pain or limited tissue loss. Sympathectomy can be justified only when it is technically not possible to operate or employ balloon angioplasty to relieve distal ischaemia.

THORACIC OUTLET SYNDROME

It is a syndrome complex due to neurovascular bundle compression in the thoracic outlet (Fig. 13.3). The thoracic outlet syndrome has a host of synonyms depending on the variation of normal anatomy or the presence of abnormal structures at the thoracic outlet. The synonyms are:

• Superior thoracic aperture syndrome

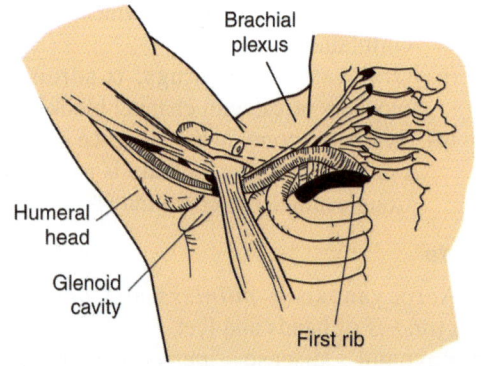

Fig. 13.3: Thoracic outlet: Pectoralis minor syndrome on hyperabduction of the arm leading to compression of the vessels and nerve.

• Cervical rib syndrome (additional rib)
• Scalenus anticus syndrome (scalene triangle)
• First thoracic rib syndrome (wide rib)
• Costoclavicular syndrome (costoclavicular space)
• Pectoralis minor syndrome
• Hyperabduction syndrome

All these syndromes give rise to symptoms arising due to neural or vascular compression of subclavian artery or neurovascular compression.

Surgical anatomy

Boundaries of superior thoracic aperture (*Syn.* Thoracic outlet in the neck)

Thoracic outlet is a limited space *at the root of the neck* bounded by the bony structures all around.

• *Posteriorly* – first thoracic vertebra (protruding or convex posterior boundary)
• *Anteriorly* – by the manubrium sterni
• *Laterally* – by the first pair of ribs and their costal cartilages on either side

Clinicians refer to superior thoracic aperture as the thoracic outlet as they are emphasizing that the subclavian artery and T_1 spinal nerve that emerge from the thorax pass through the aperture to enter the lower neck and the upper limbs.

At the superior thoracic aperture of thorax, the subclavian vessels and brachial plexus traverse the cervicoaxillary canal to reach the upper limb. Cervicoaxillary canal is divided into proximal *costoclavicular space* and *distal axilla* by the first rib.

Costoclavicular space is bounded *superiorly* by the clavicle, *inferiorly* by the first rib, *anteromedially* by the costoclavicular ligament and *posteromedially* by the scalenus medius muscle along with overlying long thoracic nerve.

Scalenus anterior muscle divides the costoclavicular space into two compartments – the *anterior one* contains the subclavian vein and the *posterior one* contains subclavian artery and the brachial plexus. This posterior compartment is called *scalene triangle* as it is bounded *anteriorly* by scalenus anterior, *posteriorly* by scalenus medius and *inferiorly* by the first rib. Then the neurovascular bundle enters the axilla deep to the insertion of pectoralis minor muscle into the coracoid process.

Presence of abnormal cervical rib narrows the scalene triangle and causes compression of C_8T_1 nerve roots and subclavian artery.

So, there are three potential areas of constrictions:

1. *In the neck* – scalene triangle
2. *Costoclavicular space* – between the first rib and the clavicle
3. *Axilla* – behind the insertion of pectoralis minor muscle.

The thoracic outlet syndrome results due to neural or vascular compression or both neuro-vascular compressions at one of these potential areas of constrictions. *The manifestations of the syndrome involve the upper limb.* However, *neural compression is the common presentation* and comprises 90% of the symptoms and signs.

CERVICAL RIB SYNDROME

(*Syn.* Scalene syndrome, superior thoracic aperture syndrome)

This is a condition characterised by pain, par-aesthesia and muscular wasting of the upper extremity due to some abnormality at the scalene triangle, *commonly due to a cervical rib protruding in the scalene triangle.*

Boundaries of scalene triangle (Fig. 13.4)

• *Anteriorly:* Scalenus anterior muscle which is inserted on the scalene tubercle on the first rib. A groove is found on the first rib anterior to scalene tubercle for the subclavian vein.
• *Posteriorly:* Scalenus medius muscle
• *At the base:* First rib.

The trunks of five spinal nerves (C_5–C_8, T_1) forming the brachial plexus and the subclavian artery pass through this triangle behind the scalenus anterior muscle. The subclavian vein passes over the first rib in front of the scalenus anterior muscle. *At the scalene triangle, the neurovascular bundle may be stretched or angulated by one of the following factors:*

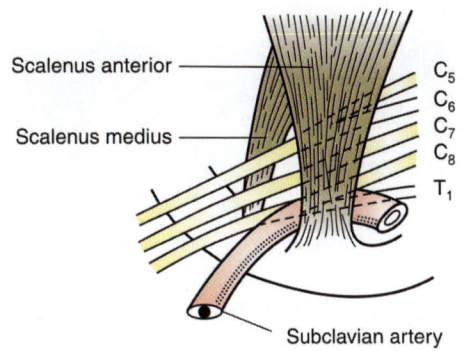

Scalenus anterior

Scalenus medius

C_5
C_6
C_7
C_8
T_1

Subclavian artery

Fig. 13.4: Scalene triangle and brachial plexus with subclavian artery.

1. Abnormalities of the rib (Fig. 13.5)

Usually an extra rib springs from the 7th cervical vertebra – *the cervical rib* (cervical rib syndrome). The rib may be complete or incomplete.

(a) A complete cervical rib – Articulates with the manubrium sterni or first rib (Fig. 13.5A). The scaleni muscles may be attached to such a rib.

(b) An incomplete cervical rib –
    (i) The free end of the rib expands and forms a large bony mass (Fig. 13.5B) often palpable in the supraclavicular region.
    (ii) The rib may end in a tapering point which is connected by a fibrous band to the scalene tubercle of the first rib (Fig. 13.5C).

Cervical rib (supernumerary rib) is seen only in 1% of the populations, and is bilateral in 80% of cases. Only 10% of the cervical ribs give rise to symptoms.

2. *Sometimes, there is no extra rib; only a fibrous band is present* extending from the seventh transverse process to either the first rib or scalenus medius muscle (Fig. 13.5D).

3. *Occasionally, long transverse process of the 7th cervical vertebra* may act as a cervical rib.

4. *In absence of a cervical rib, if the first thoracic rib is too wide*, the similar symptoms may arise (*first thoracic rib syndrome*).

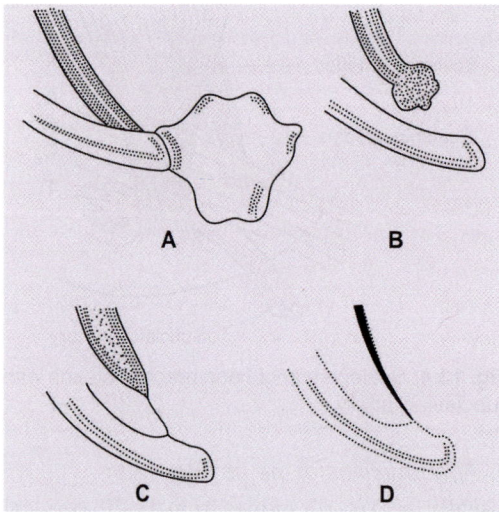

Figs 13.5 A to D: Different types of cervical ribs. (A) Complete rib articulates with the first rib; (B) Incomplete rib ends in a large mass; (C) Incomplete rib ends in a tapering point which is connected by a fibrous band to the first rib; (D) No rib but only a fibrous band.

5. Other factors:
   • Fracture of clavicle or the first rib with callus formation or malunion.
   • Cervicothoracic scoliosis may put the neurovascular bundles on stretch.
   • Apical lung tumour – pancoast tumour.

In all the above mentioned conditions, the neurovascular bundle climbs over the abnormal structure and becomes stretched or angulated.

Abnormality of the muscle

In the absence of a cervical rib, muscle pathology may play a major role.

(a) There may be a close proximation of the insertions of the scalenus anterior and scalenus medius, narrowing the triangle.
(b) Scalenus anterior muscle may be wide and thick.
(c) There may be an additional scalene muscle.

Angulation of the first thoracic nerve

When the brachial plexus is postfixed, the first thoracic nerve becomes stretched or acutely angulated over the first rib.

All the above mentioned abnormalities, congenital or acquired, may not produce any symptoms throughout life; or if produced, *the symptoms are usually rare before the age of 30 years. The probable explanation* is that with the decline of youth there is gradual sagging of the shoulder girdle, perhaps in association with some atrophy of the regional musculature allows the thoracic outlet to narrow and compress the neurovascular structures.

Pathology

There may be angulation or compression of the artery and/or of the first thoracic nerve.

Artery (Fig. 13.6)

(a) The subclavian artery or axillary artery is rarely compressed, rather it is angulated over the rib. Owing to the elevation and angulation, there is constriction or narrowing of the lumen of the artery over the rib – followed by poststenotic dilatation (Figs 13.6 A and B).

(b) Due to traumatic arteritis, there is thrombus formation within the poststenotic dilatation

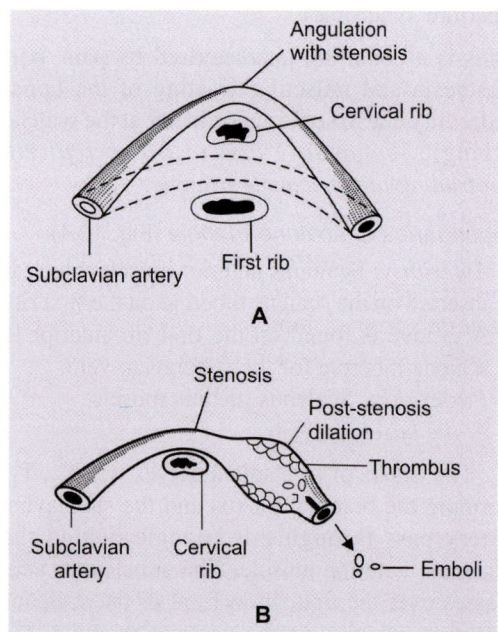

Figs 13.6 A and B: The changes of the subclavian artery in relation to cervical rib.

and/or possibly at the site of constriction. A portion of this thrombus may become dislodged and carried distally giving rise to an embolus or emboli of the digital arteries and ultimately gangrene, particularly, of the tips of the fingers.

Rarely, the thrombus may extend proximally and involve the vertebral artery and thus cerebrovascular embolic episodes may occur.

Nerves

(a) Following stretching or compression of the first thoracic nerve (or the lowest trunk) there will be friction neuritis causing *at the beginning sensory disturbances* and *later also the motor disturbances* along the distribution of C_8 and T_1 fibres identified by weakness and wasting of the muscles of the hand: *hypothenar muscles and muscles of ulnar two fingers of the hand.*

(b) Irritation of the periarterial sympathetic fibres, or paralysis of the sympathetic fibres contained in the lower trunk may be responsible for the vasomotor disturbances.

Predisposing factors of TOS: Cervicothoracic scoliosis, obesity, breast hypertrophy, stress/depression, poor posture, overuse and bad habits *all can lead to forward head tilt and shoulder drop* – allow the thoracic outlet to narrow and compress the neurovascular structures.

Diagnostic criteria

Diagnosis is primarily by clinical examination and *based on reproducibility of symptoms resulting from* compression of neurovascular structures at the thoracic outlet.

Common in women around the age of 30 years. *A thin woman with a long narrow neck is more susceptible.*

Symptoms

• Usually, there are no general or neck symptoms. Rarely, *dull aching pain in the neck* may be caused by expanded bony end of the cervical rib.

• The patient may come with the symptoms depending on the structures compressed.

• *Neural symptoms are the commonest.*
• Arterial symptoms are observed frequently.
• Venous symptoms are rare.

Neural compression symptoms: Initially result in *pain, paraesthesia (pins and needles) principally in the little and ring fingers* innervated by the ulnar nerve (C_8–T_1). Later, it may be felt in the ulnar side of the hand (hypothenar eminence) and forearm. Often the pain becomes worse after carrying a heavy weight, e.g. shopping basket or ironing. Later *numbness* develops.

Arterial compression symptoms: Mainly subclavian artery. *Results in pain, numbness, coldness and weakness.* Pain is the prevailing prominent symptom, usually an aching pain. *The pain is located in the hand and forearm and may radiate to upper arm.* Characteristically the pain is brought on by the excessive use of the arm; *the onset of pain is accelerated when the arm is in a raised position at the time of exercise, e.g. during weightlifting. The pain is relieved by rest.* This pain is ischaemic muscle pain similar to intermittent claudication pain of the leg. In late cases pain is also felt during rest.

Vasomotor symptoms: May be noted as *coldness of the fingers and hand, periodic colour changes from pale to blue (cyanosis), increased sweating, trophic changes* with ulceration and rarely gangrene of the tips of fingers. *These symptoms are akin to typical Raynaud's phenomenon and are uncommon. Moreover, the symptoms are usually unilateral (cf. Raynaud's disease which is bilateral).* The symptoms appear towards the end of the day or at night and are improved by raising the limb.

Venous compression symptoms: Rare and present as heaviness due to oedema, pain, cyanosis in the hand due to compression of the subclavian vein which passes in front of the scalenus anterior muscle.

Signs

• *Neurovascular signs:* Can be grouped under three headings:
  · Signs of neural compression
  · Signs of arterial compression
  · Signs of venous compression
• Signs in the neck

Neurovascular signs

Signs of neural compression

1. Signs of neural compression are less frequent though neural symptoms (*pain and paraesthesia*) are common. Usually features of sensory or motor deficits in the distribution of ulnar nerve may be present:

   (a) *Sensory deficit of* fine touch, vibration, pain and temperature may be present along the medial aspect of the forearm, hypothenar eminence, medial two fingers.

   (b) *Wasting of the small muscles of the hand supplied by the ulnar nerve (C_8–T_1),* i.e. interosseous and hypothenar muscles are affected. Hollows between the metacarpals on the dorsum of the hand indicate atrophy of the interosseous muscles.

   (c) *Loss of tone and muscle power:* Movements of the fingers are clumsy and slow.

   (d) *Rarely, there may be clawing of the ulnar two fingers.*

2. *The following are the tests to confirm ulnar nerve paralysis.*

   (a) *Paralysis of interosseous muscles –*

      (i) Patient is asked to spread out (abduct) and close (adduct) the fingers. Patient will be *unable to do it* [dorsal interossei are abductors (DAB) and palmar interossei are adductors (PAD)] (Figs 13.7 and 13.8).

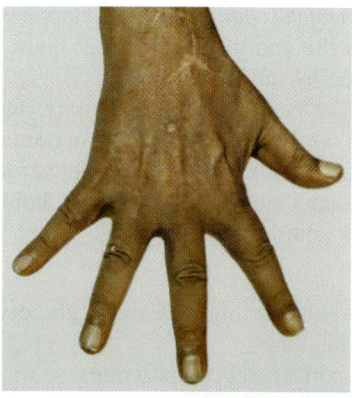

Fig. 13.7: Abduction of fingers—DAB—dorsal interossei: Abductor.

(ii) **Card test:** Patient is asked to hold a thin paper or card in between the fingers: *The patient is unable to hold the card tightly* due to paralysis of palmar interossei (Fig. 13.8).

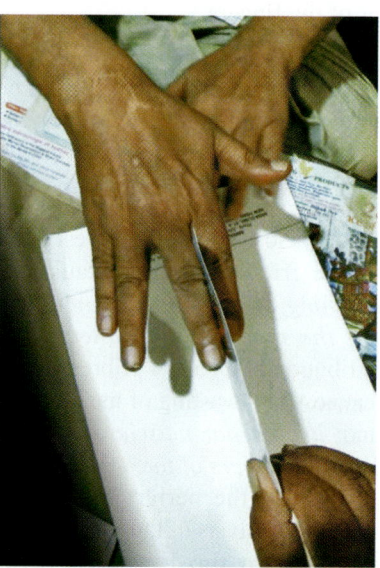

Fig. 13.8: Card test—PAD—palmar interossei: Adductor.

   (b) *Paralysis of the first palmar interossei and adductor pollicis:*

      Book test (Froment's sign): Patient is asked to hold a book firmly between the thumbs and other fingers of both hands tightly. In the normal side the thumb remains straight *whereas in ulnar nerve*

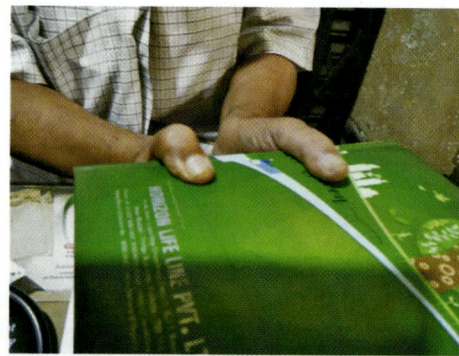

Fig. 13.9: Book test (Froment's sign): Flexion of the right thumb.

paralysis the terminal phalanx of the thumb of the affected side will be immediately flexed (because in presence of paralysis of palmar interossei and adductor pollicis supplied by the ulnar nerve, the flexor pollicis longus (supplied by median nerve) takes upper hand and flexes the terminal phalanx of the thumb in its attempt to hold the book firmly (Fig. 13.9).

(c) *Paralysis of adductor pollicis muscle supplied by the ulnar nerve:* Due to paralysis of this muscle, *the patient is unable to hold a piece of paper or post card between the thumb and palm.*

(d) *Pen test* – for adduction of thumb: *Adductor pollicis causes adduction of thumb* (Fig. 13.10).

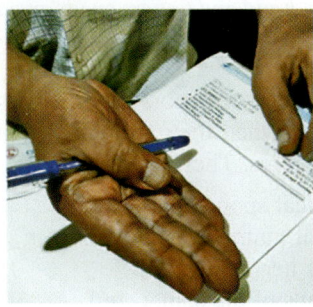

Fig. 13.10: Pen test for adduction of thumb—adductor pollicis causes adduction of thumb.

Signs of arterial compression

1. Coldness of the fingers, pallor, cyanosis, increased sweating – *vasomotor symptoms* may be present.

2. *Rarely, evidence of trophic changes of the fingers is noted* – atrophy of the skin, pulp wasting, brittle nails with or without ulceration.

3. *More rarely, finger tip necrosis or gangrene is noted.* These are due to migration of emboli arising from the thrombus at poststenotic dilatation of subclavian artery (Fig. 13.6). Pallor on elevation of the arm and features of chronic ischaemia such as atrophy of the skin, brittle nails, digital ulceration occurs in late cases.

4. *Feeble radial pulse.*

5. **Adson's test (Scalene test):** This is a test *to determine the presence of subclavian artery compression.*

Feel the radial pulse of the patient sitting on a stool. Now the patient is asked to take a deep breath and hold it, and then the patient is instructed to turn his chin up and to the affected side as much as possible. *If the pulse disappears or becomes feeble on the affected side – indicates the presence of compression of subclavian artery.*

The radial pulse is also feeble or lost during abduction and external rotation of the shoulder.

Signs of venous compression

Very rare:

1. Distended superficial vein mainly evident on the dorsum of the hand and forearm.

2. Oedema of the hand.

Signs in the neck

1. *A palpable lump at the end of the cervical rib in the supraclavicular region:*
   (a) The lump may be mushroom like, finely bosselated, hard and fixed bony mass (due to expanded bulbous free end of the cervical rib) (Fig. 13.5).
   (b) The lump may be pulsatile (the sub-clavian artery being elevated by the abnormal rib).
   (c) On auscultation over the supraclavicular region – a bruit may be heard.

2. Lowering of the shoulders on the affected side with evidence of muscular wasting.

Investigations

1. X-ray of the neck, shoulder and chest: May show presence of
   (i) a cervical rib or long transverse process of the 7th cervical vertebra;
   (ii) anomalies of the first rib – bifid or wide;
   (iii) clavicular deformities, e.g. excessive callus formation following fracture healing;
   (iv) narrowing of intervertebral foramina by disc protrusion or exostosis;
   (v) narrowed intervertebral foramen by cervicodorsal scoliosis.

2. MRI: May be useful:
   (i) to identity the brachial plexus and angulation or compression of the lower trunk of brachial plexus;
   (ii) to delineate aneurysm or poststenotic dilatation of subclavian artery and presence of any thrombus in it;
   (iii) to identify the cervical disc protrusion and narrowing of the intervertebral foramina by disc or tumour.
3. Electromyogram and nerve conduction study: *To show prolongation of conduction in presence of nerve compression.*
4. Arteriogram: Not performed nowadays because of non-invasive colour Doppler ultrasound.
5. Colour Doppler ultrasound study to know:
   (i) the exact location of the arterial compression, aneurysm and presence of any thrombus;
   (ii) the site of venous obstruction.

Note

Provocative tests

For vascular compression

- *Halstead test (Costoclavicular manoeuvre):* This is done by bringing the wrist behind the trunk, to reach the opposite sacroiliac joint, which depresses the clavicle and narrows the space between it and the first rib *causing compression of subclavian artery leading to diminution of radial pulse.*
- *Wright test (Hyperabduction test):* Hyperabduction of the upper limb with or without external rotation causes compression of the subclavian artery by the pectoralis minor muscle *causing diminution of radial pulse.*
- *Adson's test (Scalene test): The radial pulse becomes feeble* when the patient turns his/her head towards the affected side with extended neck and takes deep breath. This puts stretch on the scalenus anticus muscle and causes compression of subclavian artery leading to diminution of radial pulse.
- *Allen test: To know the patency of radial and ulnar arteries.* The surgeon feels the pulses of both radial and ulnar arteries and then occludes

both of them by grasping the forearm tightly just above the wrist. Patient is asked to clinch his fist tightly for one minute. Now the pressure over the radial artery is released and change in colour of the palm is noted. If it appears white the radial artery is blocked. Similar manoeuvre is repeated to check for patency of the ulnar artery.

For neural compression

- *Roos test (5-minute elevated arm test): For neurogenic compression.* The patient abducts his/her arm at 90° with external rotation of the shoulder and maintaining this position, the patient exercises his/her hand by opening and closing the fingers rapidly for 5 minutes. A normal individual can perform this without difficulty. *But in presence of TOS, the patient will complain of fatigue and paraesthesia of the forearm, hand and fingers on ulnar side mainly.*

Differential diagnosis

Many disorders resemble cervical rib syndrome particularly when they are present with neurological features. These are:

1. Cervical spondylosis
2. Carpal tunnel syndrome
3. Ulnar nerve lesions
4. Lesions of the spinal cord
5. Pancoast syndrome
6. Brachial neuritis
7. Raynaud's disease.

Investigations

1. Straight and lateral X-rays of cervical spine.
2. MRI of the cervicothoracic spine.
3. CT angiography to confirm vascular anomalies.

Treatment

Before any treatment is undertaken other causes of pain and paraesthesia in the upper limb should be eliminated (*see* differential diagnosis).

Conservative

Physical and occupational therapy:

1. Avoid heavy weightlifting like shopping basket or iron, etc.

2. Postural exercises of the muscles of the shoulder girdle to strengthen the muscles and to lessen the tendency of the shoulder to drop.
3. Analgesics and neurotonics to give immediate relief of pain.
4. Local heat therapy by ultrasound or short-wave diathermy.

50–90% patients can be improved with the conservative treatment.

Operative

Indication:
1. Failure of conservative treatment
2. Presence of severe pain and paraesthesia
3. Wasting of the muscles of the hand
4. Evidence of vasomotor disturbances: Hot flushes and sweating

Essentials of operation:
1. *Division of scalenus anterior muscle* and/or
2. *Complete excision of the abnormal rib* or *the fibrous band.*
   These procedures may not cause relief of symptoms. So some surgeons advocate to divide all the three sides of the scalene triangle, i.e. *division of scalenus anterior and medius muscles, excision of cervical rib or any fibrous band, excision of a portion of the first rib.* When a cervical rib is excised, it should be removed along with its periosteum; otherwise there will be a chance of regeneration.
3. If vasomotor symptoms like hot flushes, sweating are prominent, the above mentioned operation should better be supplemented with sympathetic denervation of the upper limb, i.e. *cervical sympathectomy where the 2nd and 3rd thoracic ganglions as well as the lower one-third of stellate ganglion containing T_1 ganglion are removed on the involved side.*
   Removal of whole stellate ganglion will cause *Horner's syndrome.*

Costoclavicular syndrome

This syndrome is *due to the compression of the subclavian artery* between the first rib and the clavicle.

This leads to the features of arterial compression, i.e. pain or paraesthesia, coldness of the fingers, periodic changes in skin colour from pale to blue (cyanosis), trophic changes with ulceration, necrosis and gangrene of the tips of the fingers.

Costoclavicular test (Halstead test)

Patient's radial pulse is felt and the patient is asked to brace his shoulders backward and downward as is seen in exaggerated military position – *if the pulse becomes feeble or impalpable the test is positive.*

Treatment

Excision of the middle one-third of clavicle or the portion of the 1st rib below the subclavian vessels.

Pectoralis minor syndrome
(*Syn.* Hyperabduction syndrome)

This syndrome is *due to the compression of the subclavian or axillary artery beneath the pectoralis minor muscle* onto its insertion to the coracoid process. *This leads to features of arterial compression* – coldness of the hands and fingers with ischaemic pain, blanching and poor radial pulse.

Hyperabduction test

Patient's radial pulse is felt and then the arm is passively hyperabducted with or without external rotation, if the pulse becomes feeble or impalpable, the test is positive.

Treatment

Through axillary approach, the pectoralis minor muscle is divided from its insertion onto the coracoid process.

Pancoast syndrome

This syndrome comprises the following components.

- *Pancoast tumour – a peripheral lung carcinoma arising at the apex of the lung.*
- Invasion of the lower roots of brachial plexus (C_8–T_1) resulting in symptoms and signs in the

distribution of ulnar nerve: *Weakness and atrophy of the hand muscles.*

- Invasion of the cervical sympathetic chain leading to Horner's syndrome.
- Compression of the blood vessels with oedema of hand and forearm.
- Erosion of the first rib – as evident on X-ray.
- Common in elderly men who are chronic smokers.

Complications of surgery in thoracic outlet syndrome

1. Brachial plexus injury
2. Injury to long thoracic nerve leading to winging of scapula
3. Horner's syndrome
4. Vascular injury – subclavian artery and vein
5. Air embolism as a result of subclavian vein injury
6. Pneumothorax

Note

Causes of upper limb ischaemia

1. Atherosclerosis – including subclavian artery
2. Acute thromboembolism
3. Raynaud's syndrome
4. Vasculitis:
   (a) Autoimmune vasculitis: SLE, scleroderma, giant cell arteritis, polyarteritis
   (b) Thromboangitis obliterans (Buerger's disease)
5. Thoracic outlet syndrome
6. Occupational disorders:
   (a) Vibration-induced injury following using earth impactor or riveting machines
   (b) Hypothenar hammer syndrome
7. Haematological disorders and dysproteinemias
8. Vascular compression – Volkmann's ischaemic contracture following tight plaster immobilisation for fracture both bones of forearm or supracondylar humeral fracture.

Aneurysm

An aneurysm is defined as a *localised dilated sac filled with blood* in direct communication with the lumen of an artery (Fig. 14.1).

Causes

Every aneurysm is caused *by the weakening of the wall of the artery*. The weakness may be congenital or acquired.

1. Congenital

(a) *Berry aneurysm* which occurs *in the cerebral blood vessels* particularly in the circle of Willis is *due to congenital deficiency of the elastic lamina* at the sites of branching. Berry aneurysm is located commonly in relation to the anterior communicating branch of anterior cerebral artery.

   These aneurysms are usually asymptomatic but may rupture giving rise to life-threatening subarachnoid or intracerebral haemorrhage.

(b) *Congenital arteriovenous fistula* where there is a direct shunt between an artery and a vein without the interposition of capillaries. *Common in the limbs.*

(c) *Cirsoid (racemose) aneurysm:* Tortuous complex of dilated arteries and veins. *Common in the scalp* and presents as a pulsating mass due to AVM *with serpentine arteries and veins around it.*

(d) Aneurysm of the aorta may occur proximally to a coarctation.

(e) *Marfan's syndrome and Ehlers-Danlos syndrome* are *rare inherited connective tissue disorders* (collagen diseases) and may cause *dissecting aneurysm of the aorta.*

   Marfan's syndrome is characterised by excessive height, thin body habitus, *aortic aneurysm*, valvular regurgitation, ocular lesions and skeletal abnormalities like kyphosis/scoliosis.

2. Acquired

(a) *Degenerative:* Atherosclerosis (commonest), arteriosclerosis, arteriomegaly, cystic medial necrosis. *Atherosclerosis* is the commonest cause of aneurysm, commonly thoracic or abdominal aorta *due to significant loss of elastin in tunica intima and media.*

   Cystic medial necrosis is the common cause of *aortic dissection.*

(b) *Traumatic:* The wall of the artery may be damaged by a trauma either single or repeated and the weakened wall may subsequently distend to form aneurysm – *false aneurysm.*

Examples:
- (i) Subclavian aneurysm may be related to a cervical rib.
- (ii) Penetrating wound to the artery may cause an aneurysm – pulsating haematoma common in limb arteries.
- (iii) Arteriovenous fistula may develop after trauma.
- (iv) Radiation injury may cause aneurysm.

(c) *Infective:*
- (i) Specific: *Syphilis* due to endarteritis of vas vasorum; nowadays relatively rare; thoracic aorta most commonly involved and often presenting as a pulsatile swelling eroding the sternum.
  Tuberculosis: Microaneurysms may develop within a tuberculous abscess of the lung which may leak and cause recurrent haemoptysis.
- (ii) Non-specific: Mycotic aneurysm *due to bacterial infection,* e.g. subacute bacterial endocarditis.

(d) *Arteritis:* Particularly polyarteritis nodosa.

(e) *Microaneurysm* associated with hypertension and affects smaller arteries and arterioles especially in the brain.

Risk factors for aneurysm
- Diabetes, atherosclerosis, hypertension, obesity
- Tobacco use, alcoholism, copper deficiency
- Collagen diseases: Marfan's syndrome and Ehlers-Danlos syndrome cause aortic dissection or aneurysm of the ascending aorta or arch of aorta.

Most common cause of abdominal aortic aneurysm – atherosclerosis.

Sites

Aneurysm may involve both large and small arteries:

(a) Aorta: Arch of aorta, descending thoracic, abdominal aorta.

(b) Carotid, subclavian, axillary, femoral and popliteal arteries.

(c) Smaller vessels like cerebral, mesenteric, renal and splenic arteries.

(d) Berry aneurysm occurring in the circle of Willis, may be multiple.

Types

1. True aneurysm
2. False aneurysm
3. Arteriovenous fistula.

True aneurysm contains all the three layers of vessel wall of the artery.

False aneurysm contains single layer of fibrous tissue as wall of the sac and it usually occurs after trauma and/or infection.

TRUE ANEURYSM

A true aneurysm is due to actual localised dilatation of an artery, either symmetrical or eccentric. It may be fusiform, saccular or dissecting in nature. *The sac wall is lined by all the layers of the arterial wall.*

Types

Fusiform, saccular, dissecting (Figs 14.1 and 14.2).

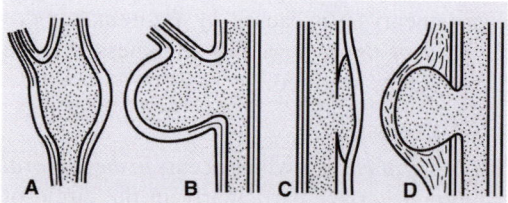

Figs 14.1 A to D: Different types of aneurysms. (A) fusiform; (B) Saccular; (C) Dissecting; (D) False.

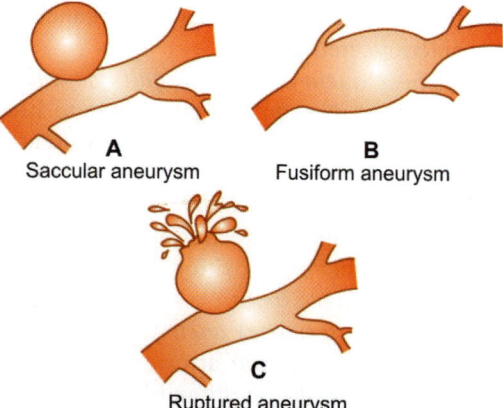

A Saccular aneurysm   **B** Fusiform aneurysm

C Ruptured aneurysm

Figs 14.2 A to C: Different types of aneurysms and common complications.

Fusiform aneurysm

There is a uniform expansion of the entire circumference of the arterial wall in all directions along the long axis of an artery: *spindle-shaped* (Figs 14.1A and 14.2).

Saccular aneurysm

There is an expansion of a part of the circumference of the arterial wall, i.e. on one side of the wall (Figs 14.1B and 14.2).

Dissecting aneurysm

A dissecting aneurysm is *due to intimal injury in which the blood dissects its way along a tunnel* between the intima and part of the medial coat and the adventitia permitting longitudinal propagation of blood-filled space within the aortic wall. It is not true aneurysm, because the vessel is not dilated, but, rather, *a haematoma of the arterial wall* (Fig. 14.1C).

The leakage of blood may occur at the site of an atheromatous ulcer of the intima, or at the site where the intima has been weakened either by mucoid degeneration or by obliteration of the vasa vasorum.

It usually occurs in elderly hypertensive patients and affects commonly the ascending thoracic aorta or near the origin of subclavian artery. *With the onset of leakage the patient experiences a sharp pain and a tearing sensation in the chest and there is a severe shock closely mimicking cardiac infarction. If the lesion is untreated, death occurs within 24 hours in 50% cases because of rupture causing massive haemorrhage in the thorax or abdomen.* Rarely, a false channel tunnels back into the proper lumen of the aorta and spontaneously relieves the pain.

Besides atherosclerosis, other degenerative disease of vessel wall, such as *cystic medial necrosis may also produce dissection.*

FALSE ANEURYSM

A false aneurysm is a sac formed by condensed periarterial fibrous tissue and it communicates with the lumen of the artery through an opening in its wall accidentally formed (Fig. 14.1D). *Commonly due to penetration or rupture of the arterial wall following trauma* (pseudoaneurysm) or *iatrogenic* following traumatic rupture.

The sac wall is lined by periarterial fibrous tissue, not by the layers of arterial wall.

Effects of aneurysm

Remember the mnemonics PTI (Press Trust of India)

P   Pressure
T   Thrombosis
I   Ischaemia

I. Pressure on the neighbouring structures

1. *Pressure on the adjacent veins* can block the vein or cause thrombosis leading to congestion and oedema of the distal part, e.g. popliteal aneurysm pressing over the popliteal vein leading to oedema leg.
2. *Pressure on the adjacent nerves* causing altered sensation like pain, tingling and numbness, paraesthesia or rarely paralysis. An aortic arch aneurysm may give pressure on the recurrent laryngeal nerve causing aphonia.
3. *Pressure on the adjacent bones* causing erosion of the bones, e.g. a vertebral body, sternum, or rib giving rise to backache and local bony tenderness. The intervertebral discs are resilient structures and do not undergo erosion.
4. *Pressure on the adjacent organ*, e.g.
   (i) pressure of an aortic aneurysm on the oesophagus causing *dysphagia*;
   (ii) stomach may be pushed forward by an aneurysm of the abdominal aorta; ultimately the aneurysm may leak or burst into the stomach or third part of duodenum causing severe *haematemesis.*
5. *Pressure on the adjacent skin:* The aneurysm with increased size may bulge under the overlying skin; *the overlying skin becomes stretched, red, oedematous and appears inflamed simulating an abscess. (So, one must be very careful to exclude aneurysm if an abscess lies in the line of a known artery which may be pulsatile. One should aspirate*

first before making an incision, particularly when situated in the chest wall, axilla, groin or popliteal fossa.)

II. Thrombosis

There may be formation of a classical laminated thrombus, consisting of *alternate layers of pale platelet thrombus and red blood clot*. The process is slow, but eventually the sac becomes filled with thrombus. *It may be protective by preventing rupture but it often causes ischaemia in the distal territory. This is a common occurrence in popliteal aneurysm.*

III. Ischaemia

This may be due to one of the following causes.
  (i) due to pressure of the aneurysm on nearby branches of the artery;
 (ii) due to occlusion of the ostia of emerging vessels by the contained thrombus;
(iii) due to embolism from contained thrombus, e.g. formation of multiple small emboli from subclavian aneurysm which block the digital arteries leading to gangrene.
(iv) due to dissection of the vessel wall.

Complications and terminations

Once diagnosed, an arterial aneurysm will produce some complications in about 95% of patients in 5 years.

Remember the mnemonics **P R I E S T**.

P *Pressure* on the adjacent structures as mentioned under 'Effects' (PTI).

R *Rupture → Haemorrhage* – may be fatal. Rupture frequently occurs due to avascularity of the vessel wall; more common at the sides of the sac. The blood extravasates into the surrounding tissues (retroperitoneal or retropleural haemorrhage, subarachnoid or intracerebral haemorrhage), or the sac may rupture in the peritoneal or pleural cavity (haemoperitoneum or haemothorax), in the oesophagus, stomach or duodenum (causing haematemesis). *During rupture the patient may complain of severe pain associated with severe shock.*

The sudden onset of a severe headache in a middle-aged hypertensive patient is suggestive of spontaneous intracranial haemorrhage *due to rupture of Berry aneurysm.*

There may be double vision due to 3rd nerve palsy. This is caused by compression of the 3rd nerve just before entering the cavernous sinus by the expanding aneurysm or the adjacent haematoma following rupture.

I *Insufficiency of circulation* due to *thrombosis* or *embolism* may lead to ischaemia and gangrene of the distal territory.

Infection usually arises from the organisms in the blood stream. Signs of inflammation may supervene, and if untreated, suppuration, abscess and rupture follow. Infection may lead to pyemia, septicaemia.

E *Embolism* by a thrombus from the fragmented intramural laminated clot causes ischemia with ulceration of the toes, foot and leg. Failure to respond immediately leads to gangrene of the distal territory.

S *Spontaneous cure* may be brought about by the formation of clot and fibrosis within the aneurysmal sac leading to consolidation. This sometimes occurs in small peripheral saccular aneurysm.

T *Thrombosis* leading to circulatory insufficiency which leads to ischaemia and gangrene of the distal territory.

Trauma direct or indirect, may cause rupture of the aneurysm leading to haemorrhage.

Diagnostic criteria

They depend largely on the position of the aneurysm and its rate of growth.

Symptoms

Elderly patients are commonly affected.

1. *Asymptomatic:* When the swelling is detected accidentally during routine physical examination.
2. *Symptomatic:* Symptoms due to local cause when a patient may notice a *pulsatile swelling*. This is common with femoral or popliteal aneurysms – not so common with abdominal aorta aneurysm.

The patient may present with *a dull aching pain* with abdominal aneurysm; this dull ache is felt over the *swelling in the centre of abdomen*.

The aching pain is caused by stretching of the arterial wall. It does not radiate. It is not relieved or exacerbated by any natural event.

Acute pain can occur if the sac suddenly stretches or begins to tear.

A severe pain, bursting in nature, is common when the aneurysm suddenly ruptures resulting in a large haematoma.

Referred pain due to pressure on the adjacent nerve is not uncommon leading to pain and paraesthesia.

Patient may present with the symptoms arising due to the pressure effects on the neighbouring structures by the aneurysm – see *effects of aneurysm* (p. 323).

Aortic dissection produces intense pain, often described as tearing or shearing knife like. It is sudden and very severe. *The pain of ascending aorta dissection* is felt in the anterior chest wall and *that of descending aorta dissection* is felt posteriorly between the scapulae. The pain can migrate downwards into the flank or pelvis as the dissection process propagates distally.

Signs

May be intrinsic or extrinsic.

A. Intrinsic:

1. *Pulsatile swelling* in the course of an artery, *both visible and palpable.*
2. Swelling exhibits *expansile pulsation* and this is synchronous with the heartbeat.
3. *On palpation thrill may be palpable.*
4. Swelling is *cystic and compressible,* direct compression may empty the sac or diminish its size.
5. *Pressure proximal to the swelling,* the swelling diminishes in size and also the pulsation diminishes or ceases. On release of pressure there is reappearance of the swelling with expansile impulse.
6. *Pressure distal to the swelling,* the swelling increases in size, so also the expansile impulse.

7. *On auscultation, systolic bruit* may be detected distal to the sac.

B. Extrinsic:

1. *Distal pulsation on the side of aneurysm found to be delayed and diminished,* when compared with the pulse in the corresponding vessel of the opposite side.
2. *Signs due to pressure effects on the adjacent structures:*
   (i) *Pressure on the veins:* Venous congestion with oedema of the leg, e.g. in popliteal aneurysm.
   (ii) *Pressure on the artery:* Gangrene.
   (iii) *Pressure on the nerves:* Referred pain, paraesthesia or even paralysis, e.g. foot drop in popliteal aneurysm, aphonia due to recurrent laryngeal nerve palsy in aneurysm of the arch of the aorta.
   (iv) *Pressure on the neighbouring structures,* e.g.
      (a) Pressure on the oesophagus by aortic aneurysm causing dysphagia;
      (b) Pressure on the bones causing erosion (as evident by radiology) leading to backache and local bony tenderness when vertebra is involved.
3. Evidence of *distal ischaemia due to embolic phenomenon.*

Differential diagnosis

1. *Swelling under an artery:* An artery may be pushed forward by an underlying structure and thus rendered prominent, e.g. *the subclavian artery by a cervical rib.*
2. *Swelling over an artery:* Transmitted pulsation is liable to be mistaken with the expansile pulsation. *Careful examination and postural change will differentiate it from expansile pulsation,* e.g. a pseudopancreatic cyst lying in front of the abdominal aorta will show a pulsatile swelling in the epigastric region. *A pseudopancreatic cyst,* when examined in the genupectoral position, falls away from the aorta, and consequently pulsation is less definite or absent.

3. *Pulsating bone tumours,* e.g. aneurysmal bone cyst, bone sarcoma, osteoclastoma, and a metastasis especially from a hypernephroma. Careful radiological investigation will differentiate these conditions from aneurysm.
4. *An abscess:* Already mentioned under complications.
5. Arteriovenous fistula.
6. A serpentine artery, usually carotid or innominate. May mimic an aneurysm.

Differentiation between expansile pulsation and transmitted pulsation

Expansile pulsation

An aneurysm is characterized by expansile pulsation. When the two fingers are placed over the sides of a pulsatile swelling, in case of *expansile pulsating swelling, the two fingers are not only lifted up but are also separated from each other,* e.g. popliteal aneurysm. *This sign should be demonstrated in both axes – vertical and transverse.*

Transmitted pulsation

When the two fingers are placed over the sides of a pulsatile swelling situated over a vessel, the two fingers are lifted up but are not separated from each other, e.g.
  (i) Cervical rib pushing the subclavian artery up giving rise to pulsatile swelling in the neck;
 (ii) Pseudopancreatic cyst may feel like a pulsatile swelling in supine position, as the swelling is situated in front of abdominal aorta. *On postural change* (knee elbow position), the swelling will be shifted away from the artery and thus will lose pulsation (cf. aortic aneurysm).

Investigations

1. Blood for sugar and lipids – atherosclerosis. Blood for WR and Kahn to exclude syphilis.
2. Radiology:
  (a) Straight X-ray of chest/abdomen may reveal calcification of the arterial wall, soft tissue shadow or bony erosion.
  (b) *Arteriography to see the extent of the lesion and to study the collaterals above and below the lesion.*
      Arteriography may indicate the scope and nature of operation required. But it is not of much value in the diagnosis, because, due to the pressure of laminated mural blood clot, the aneurysmal dilatation is seldom visualised.
3. *CT or MRI shows the 3-dimensional structure of the aorta and accurate size of the lesion: If the diameter is twice that of a native artery, there is a high risk of rupture.*
4. Ultrasound confirms diagnosis and diameter, extent, accurate size of the lesion.
5. *Duplex ultrasound scanning is more precise test:*
  (a) to see the extent of the lesion, state of the peripheral/distal vessels and any evidence of distal embolism;
  (b) for determining the flow patterns and imaging of both venous system and arterial system;
  (c) *for providing accurate localisation of fistula site in an arteriovenous fistula.*
6. Transesophageal echocardiogram (TEE).
7. MRI angiogram.
8. *Ophthalmoscopy* to ascertain the degrees of atherosclerotic changes in the retinal vessels.
9. *Renal function tests:* Blood urea, serum creatinine, IVP and isotopic renogram. *These are necessary before undertaking any major surgery for abdominal aneurysm.*

Treatment

Indications

1. *If the life expectancy of the patient is more than 5 years,* because 95% of them produce some complications within 5 years of diagnosis.
2. *If the diameter of the aneurysm is twice than that of the native artery* or aneurysm more than 5 cm because of high risk of rupture.
3. *To avoid development of complications* (under complications, *see* mnemonics **PRIEST**).

Procedures

There are various operative procedures which can be remembered by the mnemonics 'WEAL'.

W 1. Wiring } *Reinforcing procedures*
    2. Wrapping

E 3. Excision only
    4. Excision and end-to-end anastomosis } *Excision with reconstruction*
    5. Excision and grafting
    6. Exclusion and bypass grafting

A 7. Aneurysmorrhaphy ⟨ *Reconstructive* / *Obliterative*
    8. Amputation

L 9. Ligation of the artery ← *Proximal* / *Distal* / *Both*

Note

WEAL – means a red swollen mark left on the flesh by a blow or pressure.

Aim of operation

1. To prevent the onset of complications.
2. To preserve the blood supply to the distal territory.

Choice of operation

This depends upon –

(i) the site of the aneurysm;
(ii) the size of the artery concerned;
(iii) the state of the collateral circulation.

In most of the larger arteries aneurysm should ideally be treated by *excision combined with some reconstructive procedures designed to maintain the patency of the artery.*

In the cases of peripheral aneurysms, the nutrition to the distal territory is usually maintained by the collateral channels. So, *the aim of operation here is to reduce or abolish the flow of blood through the aneurysm, if necessary by its obliteration or excision.*

The treatment of aneurysms by proximal and/or distal ligation, intrasaccular wiring, wrapping in cellophane or synthetic cloth, and aneurysmorrhaphy is seldom used nowadays *because of the recent advances in the reconstructive vascular surgery technique and the advent of synthetic graft.*

1. Wiring of the aneurysmal sac

It is *indicated in elderly and poor risk patients with a difficult aneurysm so situated that operative excision carries an unduly high mortality.*

A long fine thread of stainless steel wire (No. 3 and 200 to 1000 ft. in length) is introduced inside the aneurysmal sac with the help of a hypodermic needle. *The wire gets coiled inside the sac and causes clotting of blood within the sac except a central channel which remains open.* The cure is expected by clotting followed by fibrosis. Both the wire and the thrombus provide a strengthening framework for the weak aneurysmal sac.

2. Wrapping of the aneurysmal sac

The aneurysmal sac is wrapped by either a strip of fascia lata, or synthetic cloth, or plastic material like polythene, cellophane sheet – *the idea being reinforcement of the wall and thus preventing rupture.*

This method may be of palliative value where surgery is impossible, e.g. intracranial aneurysm.

3. Excision only

Small peripheral aneurysms can be excised without endangering the peripheral circulation, e.g. aneurysm of the radial artery or the arteries which make up the circle of Willis.

4. Excision and end-to-end anastomosis

Small peripheral aneurysm is excised. The artery proximal and distal to aneurysm is mobilised and *end-to-end anastomosis* is performed.

5. Excision and grafting (Figs 14.3 A, B, C)

This is the ideal method and should be performed wherever possible. It consists of any one of the following.

(i) Excision of the sac and 'End-to-End' graft interposition (Fig. 14.3A).
(ii) Excision of the sac and 'End-to-Side' graft interposition (Fig. 14.3B).
(iii) Excision of the sac and 'Side-to-Side' graft interposition (Fig. 14.3C).

6. Exclusion and bypass grafting (Fig. 14.3D)

This method avoids damage to the adjacent vital structures (e.g. the popliteal vein in popliteal

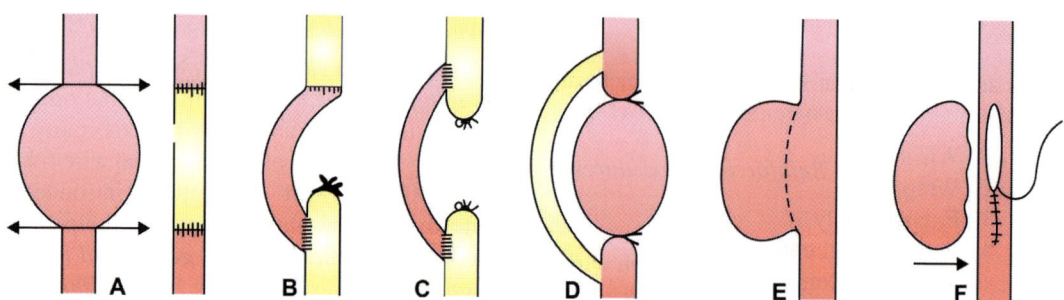

Figs 14.3 A to F: Different methods of operation for aneurysm. (A) Excision and end-to-end graft; (B) Excision and end to side graft; (C) Excision and side-to-side graft; (D) Exclusion and bypass grafting; (E and F) Matas reconstructive endoaneurysmorrhaphy.

aneurysm, the vena cava in aneurysm of abdominal aorta). Here, the sac is ligated both above and below; the blood flow is redirected into the distal segment with the help of a bypass graft (Fig. 14.3D). The excluded aneurysmal sac becomes thrombosed, and rapidly shrinks into a fibrous mass, containing porridge like atheroma and blood clot in the centre. *The bypass graft used is mostly autogenous vein* (e.g. *reversed saphenous vein*). Synthetic grafts may be used but to be avoided in dirty wounds.

7. Aneurysmorrhaphy ⟨ *Reconstructive* / *Obliterative*

Matas reconstructive endoaneurysmorrhaphy is a very useful procedure *for small saccular aneurysm of important arteries, e.g. popliteal or femoral.*

Procedure: The sac is opened. Clots are removed. *A new lumen is reconstructed for the artery from the sac wall* (Figs 14.3 E and F) by suturing of the adjacent healthy sac wall.

Obliterative endoaneurysmorrhaphy can be carried out in traumatic or false aneurysm.

Procedure: The sac is opened. Clots are removed. The mouths of the feeding vessels are closed by ligature from within the sac. The sac is *obliterated* by further sutures of the sac wall.

    Advantages:
  (i) Simple and safe method.
 (ii) *Surrounding structures are safeguarded.*
(iii) Surrounding collaterals are left un-disturbed.
(iv) Effective in preventing recurrence.

8. Amputations

May sometimes be indicated in cases of aneurysm of the limb vessels with threatened or obvious gangrenous changes.

9. Ligation of the artery

This operation is becoming obsolete nowadays. Simple ligature is one of the oldest operations in surgery. John Hunter's name is associated with ligation of the femoral artery in subsartorial (Hunter's) canal for the treatment of popliteal aneurysm.

    The ligature may be applied either proximal or distal to the sac, or both, with or without intervention of the collaterals.

    The idea was to reduce or abolish the blood flow within the aneurysmal sac by diverting the blood into the collaterals and thereby to induce thrombosis within the sac with subsequent fibrosis and shrinking and hence ultimate obliteration of the sac.

    But the result is not always satisfactory, as complete obliteration is rarely achieved due to the return of blood within the sac either through the collaterals entering into it, or by the retrograde flow along the branches of the main vessels. *In addition there is a great risk of gangrene unless there is adequate collateral circulation.*

Site of ligation:

Proximal ligation (Fig. 14.4)
• *Anel's ligation:* The ligature is applied close to the aneurysmal sac.
• *Hunterian ligation:* The ligature is applied at some distance proximally.

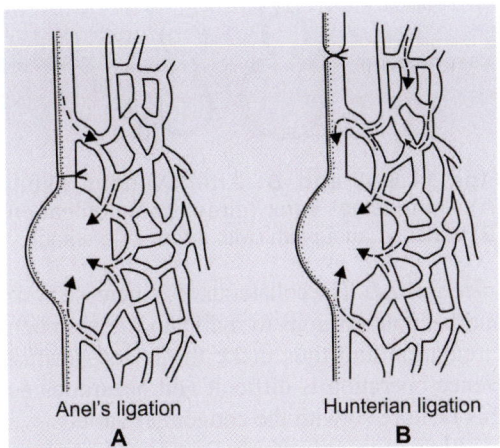

Anel's ligation   Hunterian ligation
A   **B**

Figs 14.4 A and B: Different methods of *proximal* ligation of aneurysmal sac. In either case blood may continue to return to the sac through the collaterals entering into it, or by retrograde flow.

Distal ligation
- *Brasdor's ligation:* The ligature is applied close to the aneurysmal sac.
- *Wardrop's ligation:* The ligature is applied at some distance distally.

Choice of site for ligature:
Aneurysms of the limb vessels may be treated by proximal ligation or by a combination of both proximal and distal ligation, with or without a sympathetic ganglionectomy. *Proximal ligation may also be used in the treatment of intracranial aneurysms.*

   Aneurysms of the great vessels at the root of the neck are usually treated by distal ligation.

Postoperative complications
- Haemorrhage – commonest complication
- Respiratory complications – collapse, consolidation, shock syndrome
- Renal failure
- Spinal cord ischaemia
- Aortoduodenal fistula
- Infection
- Sexual dysfunction

Note

Recently, *percutaneous intraluminal stenting with endovascular prosthesis* is being used successfully for aneurysm of thoracic and abdominal aorta and iliac arteries to exclude the dilated segment from the main bloodstream.

Note

Another novel day care procedure is being used recently *for tiny inaccessible vessels such as berry aneurysm. A catheter with a detachable balloon* is negotiated into the aneurysmal sac under image guidance and then the catheter is withdrawn after deploying the inflated balloon in the sac *to obliterate the sac permanently. This avoids life-threatening rupture in future.*

▌FALSE OR PSEUDOANEURYSM

- A false or pseudoaneurysm is a sac formed by the condensed periarterial fibrous tissues (Fig. 14.5).
- The sac communicates with the lumen of the contained artery through an opening in its wall.
- *Commonly due to penetration or rupture of arterial wall following trauma, or iatrogenic injury.*
- *Iatrogenic pseudoaneurysm occurs most commonly after arterial puncture for vascular access,* e.g. for aortogram or haemodialysis. *The most frequent site is the common femoral artery just below the groin.*

   Iatrogenic pseudoaneurysm *may also occur following mass ligature of vascular pedicles during emergency life-saving operation such* as splenectomy or nephrectomy in a major traumatic case.

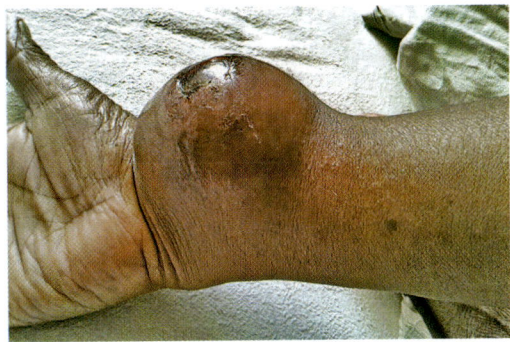

Fig. 14.5: Pseudoaneurysm of right radial artery with overlying inflammatory changes.

- It may also *result from dehiscence of a surgical vascular anastomotic suture line – anastomotic pseudoaneurysm.*
- Pseudoaneurysm is *also common with IV drug abusers* – infected pseudoaneurysm of the radial, brachial or femoral artery commonly.
- *Pseudoaneurysm manifests with pain, a pulsatile mass or effects of compression in the adjacent structures.*
- *Infection* is a common disastrous problem and should be well taken care of.
- *Duplex ultrasonogram may be helpful.*

Treatment of false/pseudoaneurysm

Management includes one of the following.

(i) Pseudoaneurysm less than 2 cm in diameter have a 70% likelihood of spontaneous thrombosis with compression therapy.

(ii) Larger one requires surgical interference.

(iii) Pseudoaneurysm arising in small, nonvital arteries may be treated with ligation, compression or coil embolisation.

(iv) Others require direct surgical repair or exclusion of aneurysm with a stent coil.

(v) Anastomotic pseudoaneurysm requires surgical repair and consists of patching or graft replacement of the disrupted segment.

ARTERIOVENOUS ANEURYSM OR FISTULA

This is a condition in which *an abnormal communication between an artery and a vein is established.* It may be either a *congenital* malformation, or *acquired due to the trauma* of a penetrating wound or a sharp blow.

The communication may be *direct,* when it is known as *aneurysmal varix,* or *by means of an intermediate sac* between artery and vein, when it is called *varicose aneurysm* (Fig. 14.6).

Effect

Structural effect: As the arterial blood directly drains into the adjacent vein, *the vein becomes gradually dilated, tortuous and thick-walled*

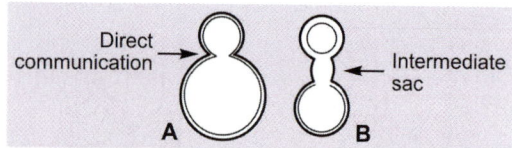

Figs 14.6 A and B: Arteriovenous fistula. (A) Aneurysmal varix (direct communication); (B) Varicose aneurysm (with intermediate sac).

(*arterialised*). The collaterals also increase in size and become tortuous to maintain the peripheral circulation and thus make the lesions diffuse. Hence operation is difficult and hazardous and this is more so with the congenital variety.

Physiological effect: Due to diversion of blood from the normal arterial bed, there is a marked fall of diastolic pressure with a corresponding rise in the *pulse pressure* (systolic pressure – diastolic pressure = pulse pressure).

Increased venous return to the heart will result in an *increase in cardiac output and pulse rate.* Ultimately, left ventricular enlargement and later, cardiac failure will occur. *So operation is indicated before cardiac decompensation has become established.*

Causes

- Congenital
- Acquired
  · Traumatic – most common cause
  · Iatrogenic, e.g. Cimino fistula (temporary AVF for haemodialysis)

Types

1. Localised
2. Diffuse

In the diffuse congenital variety, which is relatively common, the arteriovenous communications are deep (may be in the bone) and clinically indiscernible.

Diagnostic criteria

Majority of the arteriovenous malformations occur in the extremities, pelvis, trunk and shoulder girdle.

Features suggestive of arteriovenous fistula formation vary according to whether it is localised or diffuse, congenital or traumatic.

Local signs

1. When the communication is superficial in situation, the patient may come *with a pulsatile swelling in a limb.*

2. *Presence of distended, tortuous, thick-walled superficial veins* which may be visible even when the patient lies down. *Ultimately, the veins become varicose.*

3. If there is presence of *Portwine discoloration of the skin* in addition – then the combination is highly suggestive of arteriovenous fistula.

4. Presence of *superficial angiomata dilatation* or *neoformation of blood vessels* is suggestive of congenital fistula.

5. The patient may present with *leg ulcer* (which is due to diversion of blood away from the skin). *Often the ulcer is extremely painful. The ulcer is also known as hot ulcer* as the surrounding skin feels warmer than normal.

6. The patient may present with *gigantism of the limb,* i.e. increased growth of the limb supplied by the affected vessel. *This is common in congenital fistula. It may be acquired*, if the fistula occurs before the completion of epiphyseal union of the long bones.

7. *Locally the extremity* is appreciably warmer and usually moister than that of the un-affected side. *Below the fistula* the limb will feel cooler.

8. Muscle wasting below the fistula.

9. *On palpation – a thrill. On auscultation – a buzzing, continuous bruit* (machinery murmur or venous hum) may be present, particularly in the traumatic type.

10. *Pressure on the artery proximal to the fistula causes the swelling to diminish in size and the thrill and bruit to cease.*

Systemic signs

1. *Nicoladoni's or Branham's sign:* When the fistula-shunt is large enough, *digital occlusion of the feeding artery proximal to the fistula causes slowing of the pulse rate (bradycardia) and rising of the blood pressure.*

(Systolic pressure – Diastolic pressure
= Pulse pressure)

(The slowing of the pulse rate is due to vagus reflex effect for the sudden rise of vascular peripheral resistance. The sign becomes negative, if the vagus is blocked by atropine.)

2. Pulse pressure returns to normal.

3. In advanced state, left ventricular enlargement and, later, cardiac failure will be evident.

Complications

- Chronic ulceration
- Compartment syndrome leading to unremitting pain and gangrene
- Bleeding
- Gigantism
- In advanced state, left ventricular enlargement and, later, cardiac failure will be evident.

Investigations

1. *Arteriography:* This is a valuable test to know the site of fistula and also to find out the speed of venous filling.

2. Colour duplex ultrasonography may be helpful.

3. MR angiogram (MRA) or digital subtraction angiogram (DSA) may be helpful.

Treatment

1. *Fistula affecting the smaller vessels: Quadruple ligation* is the method of choice. Both the involved artery and the vein are ligated both above and below. Ligatures are also applied to any other vessels communicating with the sac. Thereafter, the sac may be obliterated with further ligatures. *Every effort is made to avoid damage to important collateral vessels*, on which the circulation of the limb depends.

2. *Fistula affecting the large vessels: Reconstructive operations are indicated*:

    (i) The affected segment of the artery is excised and the gap is replaced by an autogenous vein graft or by a synthetic graft.

    (ii) Occasionally, the artery can be reconstructed at the expense of the vein.

3. *Selective intra-arterial embolisation* is tried in some centres with success.
4. *Stapling of the epiphyses* may be attempted to prevent rapid growth of the limb.
5. *Simple ligature of the feeding artery alone proximal to the fistula, is contraindicated because of a chance of distal gangrene.* (The reason for this is that the collateral circulation lacks the force to drive the blood into the capillary bed distal to the fistula; it takes instead, the course of least resistance through the fistula back to the heart).
6. Amputations may occasionally be required in the following conditions.
   (a) When the giant limb incapacitates the patient.
   (b) In case of intractable pain or gangrene.
   (c) If the associated increased cardiac output leads to cardiac failure.
   (d) If recurrent haemorrhage.

Syndromes associated with AV fistula/AV malformation

1. Klippel-Trenaunay syndrome
2. Kasabach-Merritt syndrome

Klippel-Trenaunay syndrome (Fig. 14.7)

It is characterised by:

- Congenital
- AV malformation
- Cutaneous haemangioma: *Portwine stain*
- *Pulsatile varicose veins* on the outer side of leg
- *Hypertrophy of the involved extremity* due to increased soft tissue and bony growth
- *Absence of deep venous system*

So, *pathological superficial pulsatile varicose vein should not be removed without evidence of an intact deep venous system.* MRI angio will be helpful.

Kasabach-Merritt syndrome

It is characterised by *thrombocytopenia* due to trapping and destruction of platelets within the AV malformations and so *leading to haemorrhagic manifestations:* Haemangioma thrombocytopenia syndrome, commonly affecting the limb.

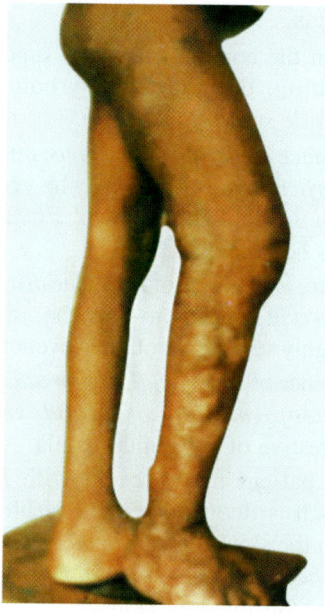

Fig. 14.7: Gigantism of the right lower limb in an 8-year-old child. This was due to arteriovenous fistula. Note the prominent varicosities of the veins and hypertrophy of the limb (*Klippel-Trenaunay syndrome*).

ACQUIRED THERAPEUTIC ARTERIOVENOUS FISTULA OR SHUNT

When surgeons make an arteriovenous shunt for a definite therapeutic purpose *as for haemodialysis – usually a temporary shunt* (Fig. 14.8).

AVF for haemodialysis. Commonly done at the wrist. The diagnosis can be assumed in case of:
   (i) Presence of pulsatile and expansile swelling in the vicinity of an accessible artery and a vein *leading to dilated veins, e.g. at the wrist or ankle.*
   (ii) *Presence of overlying scar mark.*
   (iii) History of operation – *shunt performed for haemodialysis.*
   (iv) *Thrill on palpation.*
   (v) *Bruit on auscultation.*

This type of temporary arteriovenous shunt or fistula is known as *Cimino fistula* and commonly noticed *at the wrist* using the radial artery and the cephalic vein, or *at the ankle* using the posterior tibial artery and a nearby vein.

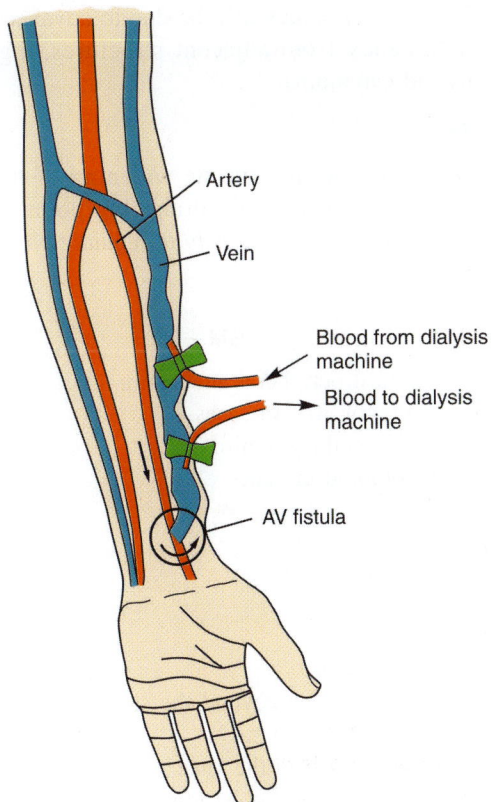

Artery

Vein

Blood from dialysis machine

Blood to dialysis machine

AV fistula

Fig. 14.8: Therapeutic arteriovenous fistula/shunt. Brescia-Cimino fistula.

Scribner shunt – using a silastic tube inter-position between the artery and the vein.

Note

Patient should be asked to exercise the hand and fingers (or foot and toes) to enhance dilatation of veins and to keep the patency of the fistula intact.

Note

Complications of AV fistula

1. Infection
2. Thrombosis
3. High output cardiac failure

Note

Pseudoarterial aneurysm: Common in drug abusers and noted in relation to radial, brachial and femoral arteries.

ANEURYSM OF THE CAROTID ARTERY (EXTRACRANIAL)

Incidence is less than 4% of peripheral aneurysms.

Causes

Due to defective intima and most of the media *because of loss of elastin in the wall of the artery.* Causes are:

- *Atherosclerosis is the most common cause.*
- Hypertension.
- Trauma
- Syphilis
- Marfan's syndrome
- Ehlers-Danlos syndrome
- Congenital
- 10% are bilateral

Types

Fusiform, saccular, false (iatrogenic following trauma).

Clinical features

- *Pulsatile, cystic swelling in the neck* at the level of the thyroid cartilage, *below the angle of the mandible – expansile pulsation.*
- *Smooth, soft, fluctuant, non-tender swelling,* horizontally mobile.
- When tips of two fingers are kept apart over the swelling, *they are not only elevated but they are also separated in both axes – vertical and transverse. Both transmitted and expansile pulsations will be palpable.*
- *Palpable thrill* on palpation and *abnormal bruit* on auscultation.
- Compressibility is present.
- *Proximal compressibility test:* On occlusion of the common carotid artery at the base of neck, swelling diminishes in size.
- On opening the mouth swelling may displace the tonsillar bed towards medially. Can cause dysphagia.
- Neurological features due to embolic episode.
- Hoarseness of voice.
- Horner's syndrome.
- Examine the opposite side also.

Differential diagnosis
- *Carotid body tumour: Solid* swelling, may show transmitted pulsation but not expansile.
- *Neurofibroma arising from vagus:* Solid swelling, non-pulsatile.
- *Abscess in the neck: Soft swelling, non-pulsatile.* Aspiration yields pus.

Complications
- Rupture
- Thrombosis
- Hemiplegia
- Horner's syndrome
- Hoarseness of voice
- Neurological features due to embolic episode.

Investigations
- *Duplex ultrasonography:* Measure the extent of the lesion and determine any mural thrombus.
- Carotid angiogram
- DSA
- CT scan/MRI

Treatment
- Reconstruction of artery using vascular graft.
- Intravascular stenting – endoluminal graft.
- Ligation of the bulb as a life-saving measure.

Note
Horner's syndrome
- Develops due to involvement of inferior cervical ganglion of cervical sympathetic chain either from trauma, persistent pressure or from malignant involvement.
- It consists of unilateral and ipsilateral *ptosis, enophthalmos, miosis, anhydrosis of head and neck* and *loss of spinociliary reflex.*
- *Spinociliary reflex:* Normally pinching of the skin over the nape of the neck produces dilatation of pupil. In Horner's syndrome – *miosis will not dilate.*
- *Surgically induced Horner's syndrome may occur during operation of carotid body tumour or carotid aneurysm. It does not require any urgent treatment as it recovers within a few weeks.*

- This syndrome may also be due to advanced malignancy from adjacent structures, e.g. thyroid carcinoma.

Note
Carotid bulb or sinus is the widening of the carotid artery at its main branching point. *It contains the sensors that help to regulate blood pressure.*

POPLITEAL ANEURYSM
- Commonest peripheral aneurysm.
- Accounts for 70% of cases.
- Often bilateral (two-thirds).
- More common in male.

Types
Saccular or fusiform.

Causes
- Atherosclerosis
- Due to turbulence beyond the stenosis at the adductor magnus hiatus
- Repeated flexion of the knee
- 65% are bilateral. So, examine the other leg also. 25% cases are associated with abdominal aortic aneurysm – so, examine the abdomen also for pulsatile swelling.
- *Iatrogenic following trauma* due to kick on the back of the knee, e.g. during playing games – false aneurysm at the back of knee.

Clinical features
- Presents as *pulsatile cystic mass* behind the knee in the popliteal fossa as a smooth, tense cystic, but *fluctuant and compressible* palpable mass.
- Swelling diminishes in size on extending the knee as the aneurysm is deep in the popliteal fossa.
- *Compressibility is present.*
- *Proximal compression test* – on occluding the femoral artery at the groin the swelling diminishes in size.
- Thrill on palpation and abnormal bruit on auscultation may be present.

- Patient may present with a throbbing pain or claudication pain in the leg, with sores on the toes, numbness of the leg and foot.
- Examine the opposite knee also.

Differential diagnosis

May be distinguished from other masses, e.g. popliteal cyst or lipoma by *palpable pulsation, both transmitted and expansile, with thrill* and abnormal arterial sounds (*bruit*) detected with a stethoscope.

Complications

- 75% cases cause complications in 5 years.
- *Compression of the tibial nerve.* Popliteal artery lies deep to the *tibial nerve.* An aneurysm may stretch or compress its blood supply (vasa vasorum) of the nerve causing referred pain to the skin over the medial aspect of the calf, ankle and foot.
- *Compression of the lateral popliteal nerve* may lead to footdrop due to paralysis of extensor muscles of the foot.
- *Compression of the popliteal vein* may cause pain and oedema of the leg.
- Because of close proximity with the vein, *an injury may result into arteriovenous fistula.* Failure to recognise this occurrence and to act promptly may result in the total loss of leg.
- *Distal embolisation:* Embolisation causes ischaemia, ulceration of the toes, foot and leg.
- *Thrombosis* causes acute ischaemia of the leg (*incidence 40%*): *Potentially requiring a leg amputation.*
- *Rupture* spontaneously or by trauma.
- Because of the close proximity and confinement within the fossa, *a distal femur fracture or dislocation may rupture the aneurysm* resulting in haemorrhage, swelling and pain and tenderness in popliteal fossa.

Differential diagnosis

Popliteal cyst: Firm cystic swelling *but not pulsatile.*

Investigations

- *Duplex ultrasonography: Investigation of choice* which can *measure the extent of the lesion and determine the extent of mural thrombus.*
- Angiography can demonstrate extent of the lesion and *also the patency of the runoff vessels.*
- CT scan/MRI – preferred recently.

Treatment

Indications

- Aneurysm >2 cm^2
- Thrombus in aneurysm
- Angiographic or U/S evidence of distal embolisation

Procedure

- *Exclusion bypass grafting:* Proximal and distal ligation of the aneurysm followed by the *reversed saphenous vein* bypass graft. This method results in total abolition of the sac with revascularisation of the limb – *current gold standard for repair* (Fig. 14.3D).
- *Excision of the sac is better avoided because of chances of adjacent nerve injury.*
  - Lateral popliteal nerve injury causes footdrop.
  - Tibial nerve injury causes wasting of the calf muscles leading to inability to planter flex of the ankle, and clawing of the toes due to paralysis of the intrinsic muscles of the foot.
- *Endoluminal inlay graft using PTFE,* Dacron stenting is also a reasonable option.

ANEURYSMAL BONE CYST

- Aneurysmal bone cyst can occur anywhere in the body, but *commonly in the posterior part of the spine and the long bones.*
- *Presents as expansile pulsatile swelling on the aforesaid areas.*
- *Usually present between first and second decades of life.*
- *Pain and pathological fracture are common,* so confused with neoplasm of the involved bone – *giant cell tumour or osteosarcoma.*
- Radiologically all these lesions may appear similar.
- *Biopsy followed by excision of the cyst and bone grafting are preferred.*
- Simple curettage only leads to high incidence of recurrence.

Note

Most common site of peripheral aneurysm – popliteal aneurysm.

Note

Berry aneurysm which looks like a berry on a narrow stem classically occurs at a point at which a cerebral artery departs from the circle of Willis artery at the base of the brain where the major blood vessels meet. *They make up 90% of all brain aneurysms.*

Rupture of berry aneurysm causes intra-cranial haemorrhage.

Note

Investigation of choice for aneurysm:

* Brain and neck – MRI without dye.

* Abdomen and limb
  · CT with dye, urografin or conray – CECT.
  · MRI with or without dye.

Note

Recently endovascular surgery under radiological control became popular *as minimal invasive method for an aortic aneurysm.*

The aorta is accessed via the common femoral artery which is exposed surgically at the groin. Then, under radiological control, *a delivery system is guided up through a puncture in femoral artery into the aorta*, over which an endovascular prosthesis (made up of Dacron or PTFE) with integral metallic stem for support is introduced to allow firm attachment to the wall of the aorta above and below the sac.

Varicose Veins

Varicose veins may be described as elongated, dilated and tortuous veins: Subcutaneous, mucocutaneous or submucous.

Common sites of varicosity

1. *Superficial venous system* of the lower limb.
   (a) Long saphenous vein ⎤
   (b) Short saphenous vein ⎦ Subcutaneous

   The varicose veins bulge outward under the skin – visible and palpable in standing position – subcutaneous swellings.
2. *Varicosity of the pampiniform venous plexus in the scrotum* (varicocele) – *visible and palpable in standing position* – subcutaneous swellings.
3. *Haemorrhoidal venous plexus* resting on the posterior and lateral wall of the rectum – *visible after parting the anal orifice and/or with anoscope* – mucocutaneous swelling.
4. *Oesophageal varices* – involving the veins at the oesophagogastric junction and bulge inwards under the mucous membrane: *in portal hypertension – visible only with upper GI endoscopy* – submucous swelling.

Only the varicosity of the saphenous venous system will be discussed in this chapter.

VARICOSITY OF THE SAPHENOUS VENOUS SYSTEM

SURGICAL ANATOMY

Venous system of the leg can be considered under three headings:

1. Superficial
2. Deep
3. Perforating

Superficial venous system
(Figs 15.1 and 15.2)

Comprises the long and short saphenous veins and their tributaries. They have the following characteristics.

(i) They lie in the superficial fascia between the skin and the deep fascia, being closer to the skin, *so often are visible when engorged. Saphenous means easily seen.*
(ii) They are low pressure and poorly supported system.
(iii) The middle coat of these vessels is much thicker than that of the other veins and consists mostly of smooth muscles with little fibrous and elastic tissue.
(iv) They are provided with numerous valves.

(v) Normally the blood in the superficial venous system flows into the deep venous system, *except in the sole (and also in the palm) where blood in the deep venous system flows into the superficial venous system.*

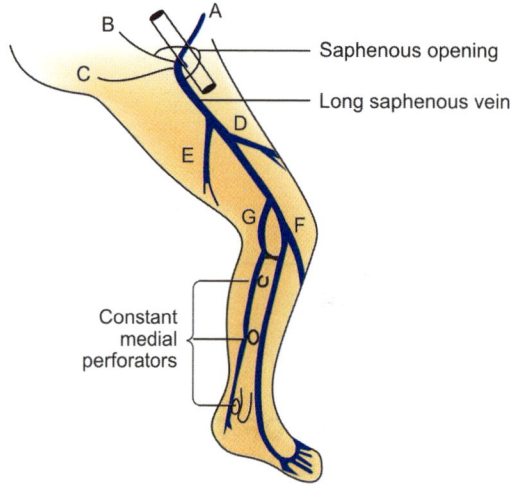

Fig. 15.1: Long saphenous vein and *its tributaries.* (A) Superficial external pudendal vein; (B) Superficial epigastric vein; (C) Superficial circumflex iliac vein; (D) Anterolateral superficial femoral vein; (E) Posteromedial superficial femoral vein; (F) Anterior vein of the leg; (G) Posterior arch vein which lies parallel to and behind the main trunk of long saphenous vein. It anastomoses with the small venous arches connecting the medial perforating veins (H).

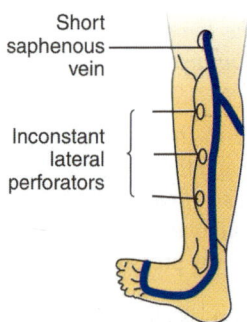

Fig. 15.2: Short saphenous vein and inconstant perforating veins.

The **long saphenous vein** (LSV) is the longest vein of the body. It commences from the medial side of the dorsal venous arch of the foot and *courses in front of the medial malleolus* and *ascends to the posteromedial side of the knee.* Then the vein inclines laterally and forward in the thigh towards the saphenous opening (fossa ovalis) which lies 1½ inches (3.8 cm) below and lateral to the pubic tubercle. It pierces the cribriform fascia and passes deeply to enter the femoral vein. *The saphenous nerve accompanies the vein in the leg, a cutaneous branch of the femoral nerve, supplying the medial part of the dorsum of the foot.*

Tributaries of long saphenous vein are shown in Fig. 15.1.

There are about 20 valves in the long saphenous vein, out of which majority are below the knee.

The usual distribution of varicose veins is below the knee in branches of great saphenous vein.

The **short saphenous vein** commences from the lateral side of the dorsal venous arch and *passes behind the lateral malleolus* and then ascends obliquely backward towards the middle of the popliteal fossa, where it pierces the deep fascia to enter the popliteal vein in most cases. *The sural nerve accompanies this vein in the lower third of the leg.*

Perforator system

The perforating veins are communicating veins between the superficial and deep veins. They perforate through the deep fascia and connect the two venous systems. *They are also provided with the valves near their origin and at their entrance to the deep veins. Under normal conditions they allow blood to flow only from the superficial to the deep veins.* Reversal of blood flow occurs due to incompetence of perforators from deep veins to superficial subcutaneous veins *which will lead to varicose veins.* This system comprises following groups.

1. *Medial perforating veins* (Fig. 15.1): These are *three constant medial leg perforators and situated along the posterior border of the tibia* 2 inches (5 cm), 4 inches (10 cm), and 6 inches (15 cm) successively above the medial malleolus. *The upper two of these perforators enter the posterior tibial vein at*

the precise level where one of the unvalved *'soleal venous sinuses' enters* (Fig. 15.3). So, the clot arising in the soleal veins may extend into the posterior tibial vein and then into these perforating veins, thus destroying the mechanism which obviates reflux.

All these medial perforators again are connected by way of the posterior arch vein to the long saphenous vein (Fig. 15.1G).

2. *Lateral perforating veins* (Fig. 15.2): These are inconstant in their positions and *situated along the posterior border of the fibula* 2 inches (5 cm), 5 inches (12 cm), and 7 inches (17 cm) above the lateral malleolus and are connected with the peroneal veins or venae comitantes.

3. *Central perforating veins:* Usually one or two veins connecting the short saphenous system to unvalved soleal venous sinus in gastrocnemius and soleus muscles. The former enters its muscle on the medial side close to its junction with the tendoachillis while the latter, further up the calf.

Deep venous system (Fig. 15.3)

This is a high pressure system. This accompanies the main arteries and is well supported by powerful leg muscles which compress the veins. It is the powerful muscle contraction that helps in return of the blood to the heart. *The deep vein is also provided with unidirectional valves directing blood upwards to prevent reflux.*

This deep venous system comprises:

(i) Femoral and popliteal vein

(ii) Venae comitantes (paired veins) accompanying the anterior tibial, posterior tibial and peroneal arteries.

(iii) Soleal venous sinuses. Valveless veins draining the calf muscles.

This deep venous system communicates with the low pressure superficial venous system at the following sites:

(i) Saphenofemoral junction – constant.

(ii) Adductor canal by inconstant perforators.

(iii) Short saphenopopliteal junction – constant.

(iv) Posteromedial aspect of the leg by three constant leg perforators.

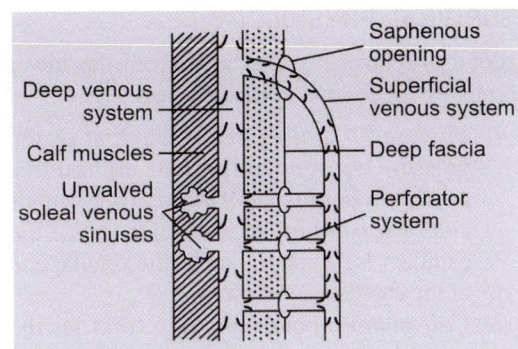

Fig. 15.3: Disposition of superficial and deep venous systems of the lower limb with intercommunication between them.

(v) Posterolateral aspect of the leg by inconstant perforators.

Perforator veins

They perforate the deep fascia of the muscles to connect the superficial veins to deep veins where they drain.

Perforators are of two types:

• *Direct perforators* leave the superficial veins, pierce the fascia and join the deep venous system directly, without any relay channels.

• *Indirect perforators:* Seen mostly in the upper leg; join the intermediary venous channels under the deep fascia, which in turn drain into the deep venous system.

There are perforators in the foot also but allowing the blood flow in reverse direction from the sole to dorsum of the foot (deep to superficial fascia).

Different sites of named perforators

In the leg:

• May or Kuster perforator – inframalleolar perforator

• Bassi's perforator – above the ankle: Supramalleolar

• Cockett's perforator – in the middle of leg

• Boyd perforator – below the knee

In the thigh:

• Dodd perforator – just above the knee

• Hunterian perforator – mid-thigh at the level of Hunterian canal

SURGICAL PHYSIOLOGY

Blood is returned to the heart from the lower limbs by the following mechanisms.

1. *Vis-a-tergo of the circulation*, that is, the pressure transmitted from the arterial tree passes through the capillary bed to the venous side. *Pressure* in the arteriolar end of the capillary is 32 mm Hg and in the venular end of the capillary is 12 mm Hg.

2. *Calf-pump or muscle pump*, that is, the alternate contraction and relaxation of the surrounding muscles of the leg and to a certain extent of the thigh surrounded by their firm fascial sheath act as a pump which increases the return of blood to the heart during walking or running. *A sustained contraction or a continued relaxation will not operate the muscle pump.*

3. *Competent valves in the veins:* Normally the veins of the limbs are provided with *unidirectional competent healthy valves* which allow the flow of blood in one direction, that is, towards the heart. These valves break up the column of blood and thus prevent distension of the veins due to gravity.

4. *Venae comitantes:* These lie by the side of the arteries and may be helped by the arterial pulsation to propel the blood upwards to the heart.

5. Negative intrathoracic pressure during inspiration is transmitted to great veins and causes drop in venous pressure which aids in venous return.

In the resting position, blood returns to the heart mainly by a *vis-a-tergo* imparted by the heart and transmitted through the arteries. The pulsation of the arteries forces the venous blood propelling upwards through the vein.

During walking, the blood returns to heart mainly by the *calf-pumping*.

In addition, the actual pressure in any one vessel is also dependent on the effect of gravity. On standing, therefore, the actual pressure in any vein includes a hydrostatic pressure (up to pressure of 90 mm of Hg) which is equivalent to the weight of the column of blood from the legs to the heart, and this pressure is exerted on the

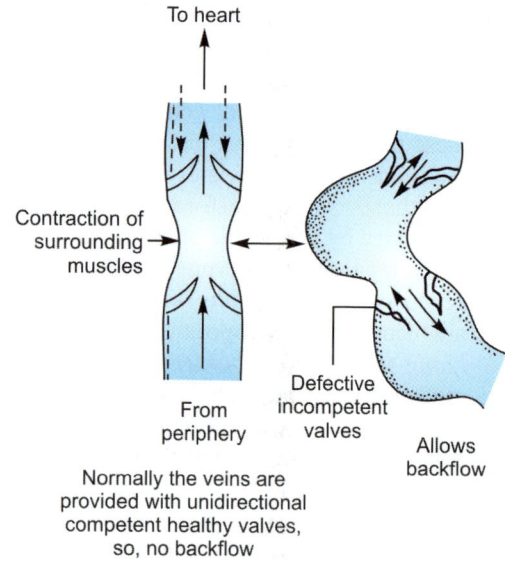

To heart

Contraction of
surrounding
muscles

Defective
incompetent
valves

From
periphery

Allows
backflow

Normally the veins are
provided with unidirectional
competent healthy valves,
so, no backflow

Fig. 15.4

valves, particularly on those guarding the communications between the superficial and deep venous systems of the leg.

The above factors will be effective only if the valves are competent enough to support the column of blood passing each valve 'check point' and the gravitational effects are reduced to a minimum.

Development of varicose veins

Varicose veins develop when the blood leaks continuously from high pressure deep venous system and is allowed to enter the low pressure and poorly supported superficial venous system. Under normal conditions the blood in the superficial venous system flows into the deep veins and the superficial system is protected from reflux of blood from the high pressure deep venous systems *by the unidirectional strategic valves in the deep and perforator venous systems.* But if this mechanism breaks down, *there will be retrograde flow of blood in the superficial veins leading to distension and tortuosity.*

Aetiology

Can be considered under two headings – primary and secondary.

1. Primary or idiopathic

- Exact cause is not known.
- Often familial with onset during young adulthood or pregnancy.
- *Commonly due to weakness of the venous wall* due to defective connective tissue and smooth muscle in the vein wall *that permits valve ring dilatation* or *due to congenital incompetence* or *absence of the valves.*

- **Exciting causes:**
  (a) *Prolonged standing and/or sitting* in one position whereby the gravitational pressure of a long column of blood presses continually upon a weakened valve. It also deprives the veins of the benefits of muscular pump movement during walking, e.g. common in traffic police, military guards, sales girls at the counter or desk – *occupational hazards.*
  (b) *Violent muscular efforts* which are responsible for the frequency of varicose veins *in the legs of athletes.* It is postulated that excessive continuous calf muscle activity may actually force the blood through the perforating system in a reverse direction and *thus causing perforator valve* disruption. This factor is well illustrated by the fact that in our country more commonly *Rickshaw pullers* suffer from varicosity of vein.
  (c) *Obesity:* Soft, virtually fluid, fatty tissue offers poor support to the veins.
  (d) *Aging:* Causes atrophy and weakness of the vein wall.
  (e) *Heredity:* Inherent weakness of the venous valves due to collagen defect or increased lysosomal activity in the venous wall.
  (f) *Pregnancy:*
    (i) Due to increased venous return from gravid uterus leading to high pelvic venous pressure.
    (ii) Due to effect of progesterone from corpus luteum which reduces venous tone and increases venous distensibility with or without telangiectasia – which becomes evident after 20 weeks of pregnancy.

2. Secondary

- *Obstruction to venous outflow* due to following reasons.
  (a) Pregnancy
  (b) Chronic constipation with loaded colon. Sigmoid colon exerts pressure over the pelvic veins on the left side.
  (c) Abdominal or pelvic tumour like uterine fibroid, ovarian tumour or cyst or pelvic cancers.
  (d) Retroperitoneal lymphadenopathy
  (e) Retroperitoneal fibrosis
  (f) Ascites
  (g) Prior deep vein thrombosis (DVT) – leading to destruction of valves.

  Local damage to veins and valves by an inflammatory or traumatic process leading to thrombophlebitis or phlebothrombosis. This causes obstruction of the venous flow. *Also it may destroy the valves.* Following recovery, after an attack of thrombosis, the veins subsequently recanalise but their valves are rendered weak and incompetent.
  (h) *Congenital or traumatic arteriovenous fistula* – the high pressure arterial blood directly drains into the adjacent vein through the abnormal communication thereby causing distension and varicosity of the veins (*see* Fig. 14.6 – Chapter on aneurysm).
  (i) *Extensive cavernous haemangioma.*

  These last two causes [(h) and (i)] should be considered when varicosities are found in persons below the age of 20.

Incidence

- Majority (60–70%) develop as a result of saphenofemoral junction (SFJ) incompetence and long saphenous vein (LSV) reflux. *Usual distribution of varicose veins is below the knee along the branches of great saphenous vein system.*
- 10% develop due to saphenopopliteal junction (SPJ) incompetence and short saphenous vein (SSV) reflux.
- Remainder arise due to both SFJ incompetence and *perforator incompetence.*

Diagnostic criteria

1. *Age:* Varicose veins affect all age groups but common in young and middle-aged.
   A varicose vein in children is invariably due to congenital vascular abnormality.
2. *Sex:* Equally occurs in both sexes. But women are more likely to present early for treatment because of cosmetic reasons.
3. *Occupation:* Many patients with varicose veins have jobs that involve prolonged standing or sitting, e.g. traffic police, guards in military service, bus or tram conductors, shop assistants working in shopping malls. *In our country* rickshaw pullers also suffer from varicose veins (Fig. 15.5).

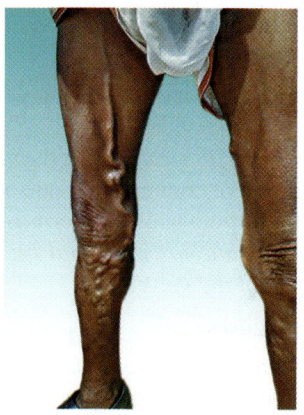

Fig. 15.5: Varicose veins in relation to great/long saphenous vein right leg. (*Courtesy:* Dr Gurusaday Bhattacharya, MS, FRCS)

Symptoms

1. *Swelling of the leg* – always more common towards the end of the day because of upright posture. *The swelling reduces to minimum at the end of night* due to rest in recumbency.
2. *Tiredness, heaviness and dull aching sensation felt in the lower leg or in the calf,* particularly worse at the end of the day resulting after prolonged standing or sitting. *The aching is due to* pooling of blood and venous distension in the limbs. *The aching is relieved by elevation of the limb and exercises.*

   Some patients suffer from *night cramp in the calf* shortly after retiring to bed. This is due to sudden change in the calibre of the communicating veins which stimulate the muscles between which they pass. *The cramp is also relieved by elevation of the limb or exercises.*

   This aching pain or cramps should not be confused with those due to peripheral arterial disease referred to as *intermittent claudicating pain where the pain is made worse by exercise but that of varicosity is improved.*

   The pain may be bursting and severe in nature with deep vein thrombosis, and may be localised at the site of perforating veins when perforator incompetence likely to be present.
3. The patient may present *because of cosmetic disfigurement* with multiple dilated and tortuous visible veins in the leg and/or with its complications (often the presenting features in women) such as:
   (a) Swelling of the foot and leg mostly round about the ankle joint. The swelling is always more towards the end of the day, which reduces to minimum in the early morning due to recumbency.
   (b) Venous stars, blowout or visible varix – a localised dilated segment of vein.
   (c) Blackish pigmentation of the skin.
   (d) Dermatitis and eczema – dry and scaly or moist, itchy and infected.
   (e) Venous ulcers in the lower one-third of the leg.
   (f) Bottleneck deformity of the leg.
4. History of occupation which involves prolonged standing or sitting.
5. Past history: The patient should be asked about any previous episodes of leg swelling, thrombophlebitis or white leg following operation, accident or pregnancy that may have produced damage to the valves of the perforating veins and/or the deep venous system.

Note

Persistent oedema of the leg is the hallmark of deep venous disease.

Signs

- *Examine the patient first in standing position and then in lying down position.*

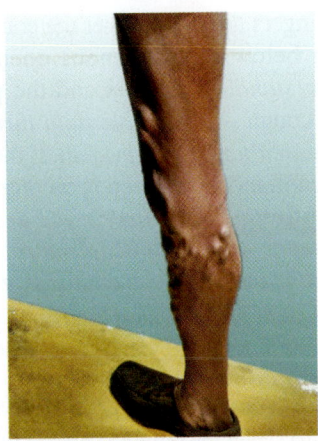

Fig. 15.6: Varicose vein in relation to right leg long saphenous vein. (*Courtesy:* Dr Gurusaday Bhattacharya, MS, FRCS)

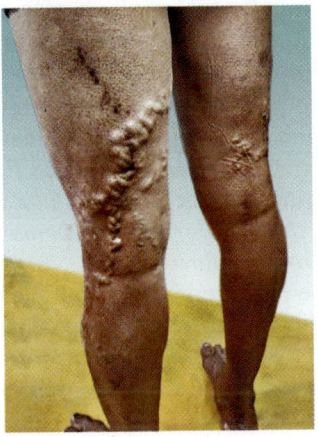

Fig. 15.7: Varicose veins on the posterolateral aspect of the left leg proceeding up to back of thigh. (*Courtesy:* Dr Gurusaday Bhattacharya, MS, FRCS)

• *Expose the patient from umbilicus to toes.*
 1. Presence of dilated, tortuous visible veins in the leg and the thigh. On lying down and elevation of the legs these dilated veins will partially collapse.
 2. *The skin, particularly on medial side of the lower leg (gaiter area),* is inspected for blowout, oedema, brawny induration, pigmentation, ankle flare, eczema, ulceration or healed scars, pale area around the ankle (atrophic blanche).
   • *Blowout* (visible varix): A localised dilated

segment of vein. It signifies underlying perforator.
• *Ankle flare* (corona phlebectatica): Telangiectatic dilated reticular veins caused by the distension of superficial veins giving a reddish hue to the skin. This is seen around the gaiter area of ankle, most apparent over a triangle centred at the medial malleolus (varicular triangle).
• *Healed scar:* Signifies previous ulceration.

Note

Gaiter area of the leg is usually located between the ankle and the calf.

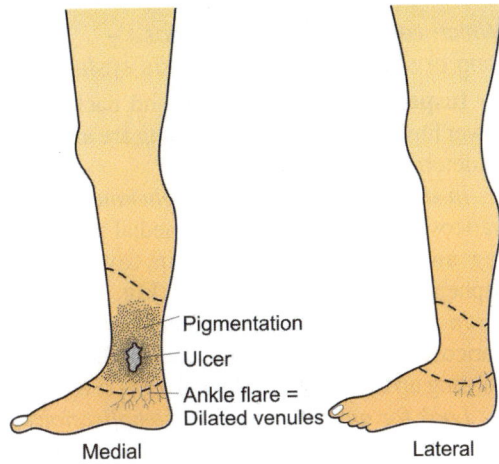

Fig. 15.8: Gaiter area of the leg.

 3. **Saphena varix:** This is a *saccular dilatation* at the upper end of the long saphenous vein at the saphenous opening. The saphenous opening lies medial to the femoral artery below the inguinal ligament about 1½″ below and lateral to be pubic tubercle.
Saphena varix has the following features.
 (a) It is compressible but non-pulsatile (cf. femoral aneurysm).
 (b) It has a positive cough impulse (cf. femoral hernia).
 (c) It disappears when the patient lies down (cf. femoral hernia where spontaneous disappearance is unlikely, and requires manipulation).

(d) The varix has a *fluid thrill* which can be felt over the lump in the groin only when the long saphenous vein lower down the thigh is tapped in standing position.

Clinical tests

There are many clinical tests for examining the varicose veins, which are necessary to diagnose as well as to determine the choice of treatment. For convenience they may be considered in three main groups:

(a) To know which venous system is varicose.
(b) To know which perforator or perforators is/are incompetent.
(c) To know the patency of the deep veins.

*Which venous system is varicose –
long or short saphenous venous system?*

Inspection: Both the front and back of the lower limb *with the patient standing* are inspected to determine the veins affected.

In affection of the long saphenous system, varicose veins are seen on the medial side of the leg and thigh proceeding up towards the saphenous opening at the groin (Fig. 15.1).

In affection of the short saphenous system, varicose veins are seen on the back of the leg proceeding up towards the popliteal fossa (Fig. 15.2).

Look for any local signs of complications of varicose veins (see under symptoms) especially on the medial side of the lower third of the leg.

Schwartz test: With the patient in standing position two fingers of the left hand are placed over or just below the saphenous opening (fossa ovalis) and with the right middle finger the most prominent part of the varicosity lower down the leg and/or thigh is tapped – *a thrill-like impulse will be felt by the fingers at the saphenous opening particularly in presence of saphena varix.* It signifies continuous column of blood due to valvular incompetence.

Which perforator or perforators is/are incompetent – saphenofemoral perforator or leg perforator?

I. Morrissey's sign: *Cough impulse test to determine the saphenofemoral incompetence.*

The fingers are placed over the course of the vein just below the saphenous opening *with patient in standing position* and the patient is asked to cough – *a palpable fluid thrill (and a bruit on auscultation) are evident,* if the valve at the saphenofemoral junction is incompetent.

II. Trendelenburg test: *To detect the incompetence of the saphenofemoral junction (SFJ) and/or the other communicating system.*

The patient lies down on the couch in supine position, the limb is elevated above the level of the heart *to allow the varicose veins to empty* (which can also be helped by stroking the veins proximally). Then the thumb is placed firmly over the saphenous opening or *an elastic rubber tourniquet is applied firmly round the thigh at the saphenous opening.* Now keeping the firm pressure over the saphenous opening, the patient is asked to stand up quickly. *The findings and the remarks are:*

(i) The pressure on SFJ is not released but maintained for about one minute. If there is gradual filling of the veins from below during this time, *it indicates incompetence of the leg perforating veins allowing retrograde flow.*

(ii) The pressure is released. If there is quick filling of the veins by a column of blood from above, *it indicates incompetence of the valves at the saphenofemoral junction.*

Both the above signs (i and ii) are regarded as Trendelenburg test positive and are indications for operation.

If the short saphenous system is involved a similar test can be performed with the thumb or tourniquet pressure over the upper end of the vein at the level of knee crease.

Note

With the tourniquet on, the patient may be asked to walk around to enhance the filling of the veins from below.

III. Pratt's test: *Test for leg perforators.* An elastic compression bandage is applied from toe to upper thigh with the patient in lying down position *with leg elevated* which causes emptying of the varicose veins. A tourniquet is then tied around the upper thigh above the bandage. Now, the patient stands up with tourniquet in position, the bandage is unwinded in downward direction – *a 'blowout'*, i.e. *a visible varix* will appear over the site of constant leg perforators indicating the incompetence of the leg perforators.

Marking these sites with inks or felt pen helps during operation with the patient in supine position to look for the perforator pits and ligate and cut the perforator veins before stripping the main saphenous vein.

IV. Fegan's test: *For seeking the sites of perforator.* First, the varicosities are marked with a skin pencil with the patient standing. The patient lies down. The affected limb is elevated above the heart level and the heel is supported against the examiner's upper chest. Now, the examiner has to palpate along the line of the marked varicosities carefully for any gaps or pits in the deep fascia which transmit the perforators – *they are felt as circular openings with sharp edges* and are marked with these an 'X'. These 'X' marked positions are compared with the anatomical sites of the perforating veins.

This test may also be confirmed by Trendelenburg test to determine whether the superficial varicosities fill from the perforators marked by 'X'.

Leg perforator incompetence may also be evident from the following signs.

(i) *An ankle flare:* Telangiectasia of reticular veins caused by the distension of the superficial veins and is seen around the ankle most apparent over a triangle centred at the medial malleolus (varicular triangle).

(ii) *A 'blowout' or a visible varix*, i.e. a localised dilated segment of the vein – situated over the site of constant medial perforators.

Tests for patency of the deep veins

Perthes' test: *To know whether the deep veins are patent or not.*

This test should be carried out if the patient complains of a bursting or cramp-like pain in the lower leg on standing or walking. A tourniquet is tied tightly round the upper part of the thigh below the saphenous opening while the patient stands with the dilated veins being full, tightly enough to prevent any reflux down the vein. The patient is then asked to walk quickly for about 5 to 10 minutes. *The findings and the remarks are:*

(i) If the varicose vein shrinks or disappears – *it indicates competence of the perforating veins and deep veins.*

(ii) If the varicose vein remains unchanged or becomes more distended – *it indicates that the perforating veins and deep veins are blocked*. There will also be reappearance of pain of which the patient complains.

In the absence of deep veins patency, the superficial venous system is the only vein to drain the blood from the leg, **so, operation is contraindicated**.

Other examinations

(i) In addition to the above tests *the abdomen should be palpated in every case to exclude* pregnancy or pelvic tumour, abdominal lymphadenopathy because sometimes a pregnant uterus or an intrapelvic tumour may be responsible for the development of varicosity (*secondary*).

There may be dilated, tortuous, collateral veins crossing the suprapubic region and abdomen which may indicate inferior vena cava thrombosis, chronic iliac vein occlusion.

(ii) *The peripheral arterial pulses should be palpated* to ensure that there is no accompanying arterial insufficiency. Venous and arterial disease of the lower limb may coexist particularly in elderly men.

(iii) Auscultate the veins to rule out continuous murmur from AV fistula.

(iv) P/R – to exclude pelvic tumour.

Note

Homans' sign

Passive dorsiflexion of the foot will cause pain in the calf – *if positive, suggestive of deep vein thrombosis*. This sign is positive during acute stage of DVT.

Investigations

A careful history and physical examination are usually enough to diagnose the primary or idiopathic varicose veins.

Ascending phlebography may be useful:
(a) to determine the patency of the deep veins;
(b) to localise the sites of perforators.

In the past, phlebography was carried out routinely in some clinics.

Doppler ultrasound may be accurate:
(a) To confirm the presence of incompetence of the saphenofemoral junction, size and status of GSV.
(b) *To determine the patency of the deep veins.*
(c) *To determine the presence of clot in the deep veins. No sound is heard in presence of deep vein thrombosis.* **So, operation is contraindicated**.
(d) To detect the presence of incompetent valves either in deep veins or in the communicating veins.

Duplex ultrasound scanning (Doppler recording and duplex imaging) is *more precise test*:
(a) For determining the flow patterns and imaging of both superficial and deep venous system and *of the arterial system. It demonstrates the retrograde venous flow from deep to superficial venous system (reflux).*
(b) For providing accurate localisation of the sites of perforating veins in the leg and thigh and fistula site in an arteriovenous fistula.
(c) Investigation of choice also for suspected DVT of the lower extremity.

Magnetic resonance venography (MRV) – most sensitive and most specific test to find the causes and sites of anatomic obstruction.

Note

In the absence of deep vein patency, operation for varicose vein is contraindicated. *Why?* Because the superficial varicose veins are the only veins to allow venous return to the heart.

Complications of varicose veins

1. Pigmentation
2. Eczema – itching around the ankle joint
3. Oedema of the leg
4. Brawny induration
5. Ulceration – venous ulcer, Marjolin's ulcer
6. Periostitis
7. Calcification
8. Superficial thrombophlebitis. Deep vein thrombosis – rare.
9. Haemorrhage
10. Deformities of the foot – talipes equinus.
11. Atrophic blanche (white atrophy) – localised often circular whitish and atrophic skin areas surrounded by dilated capillaries and sometimes hyperpigmentation (scars of healed ulceration are excluded from this description).
12. Corona phlebectatica – also called *malleolar or ankle flare*. Fan-shaped pattern of numerous small dilated intradermal veins on the medial and lateral aspects of the swollen ankle and foot.
13. Lipodermatosclerosis.
14. Scars of healed ulceration.

Pigmentation

A brown or dark brown discoloration is usually seen in the medial aspect of the lower one-third of the leg, superior to medial malleolus (**gaiter area**). This is due to deposition of haemosiderin pigment derived from the breakdown of RBC following subcutaneous extravasation of blood which has come out of the thin dilated veins resulting from venous stasis.

Oedema of the leg and ankle

Soft and pitting. Ankle oedema is a feature of persistent venous obstruction. It may not be observed with isolated varicosity. It is usually present in patient with deep vein thrombosis and incompetent perforators.

Brawny induration (lipodermatosclerosis)

It is leg oedema *but hard and indurated* (feel like wood) and *non-pitting*. This is due to increase in the thickened connective tissue due to scarring secondary to fat necrosis, excess protein in tissue fluid, inflammatory changes and hyperaemia leading to thickening of subcutaneous tissue giving *a leathery texture to the skin around the ankle and lower leg*. This is also referred as lipodermatosclerosis (Fig. 15.9).

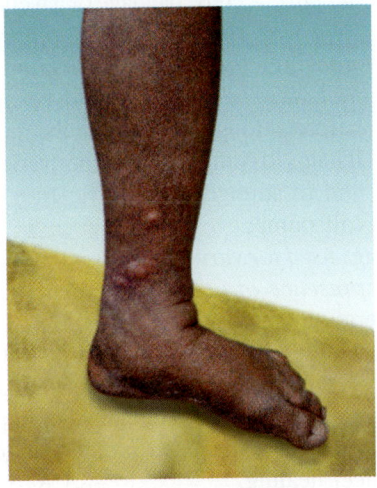

Fig. 15.9: Lipodermatosclerosis of left leg.

Eczema (chronic dermatitis)

Patchy areas of eczema with or without itching may follow minor trauma or self-scratching of the skin, or an allergic manifestation resulting from local application of various ointments or strapping.

Corona phlebectatica (ankle or malleolar flare)

In some patients with chronic ambulant venous hypertension swelling of the ankle with *fan-shaped pattern* of dilation of intradermal venules around the ankle may develop – known as ankle flare.

Ulceration

Venous stasis leading to increased venous pressure is the underlying cause as it results in local tissue anoxia leading to venous ulcers.

- More common in patients with deep vein abnormalities and/or incompetent leg perforators.
- Venous ulcers *commonly develop over the medial aspects of the lower third of the leg, around and above the medial malleoli* because of the presence of large number of perforators

which transmit pressure changes directly into the superficial venous system. This area is called as *gaiter's area*.

- The gaiter's area is the common site for blowouts, ankle flare, induration, pigmentation and ulceration (Fig. 15.8).
- Rarely, carcinomatous change may occur in chronic venous ulcer (*Marjolin's ulcer*).

Periostitis

Occurs in long standing cases if the ulcer is situated over the tibia.

Calcification

Occurs occasionally in the walls of the vein in long-standing varicosity.

Thrombophlebitis of the superficial vein

May occur spontaneously or may be secondary to trauma to the leg. *It may be iatrogenic following injection of sclerosing fluid.* It reveals itself as a reddened tender cord in the subcutaneous tissue. It may be recurrent and may extend in the deep venous system.

Haemorrhage

Usually due to minor trauma to the dilated veins. Such haemorrhage may occur into the subcutaneous tissue causing excessive bruising, or externally causing profuse bleeding due to the high pressure within the incompetent veins. *Bleeding generally stops if the limb is elevated with the patient lying down and first digital pressure and then pressure bandage is applied locally. A tourniquet must not be used.*

Deformities of the foot

Talipes equinus due to the long continued faulty habit of walking on the toes to get relief of pain in the calf resulting in contraction and shortening of tendoachillis. Cases usually respond to remedial exercises.

   Narrow ankle and lower leg with swollen calf above bears the shape of an inverted champagne bottle.

Treatment

Patients with varicose veins seek treatment for one of the following reasons.

1. Severe aching or pain in the legs, particularly after prolonged standing, disturbing sleep at night.
2. Persistent or recurrent complications of varicose veins, e.g. oedema, brawny induration, eczema, ulceration.
3. Because the leg is cosmetically unsightly.
4. *When varicose veins appear to be a bar to join into a particular job,* e.g. nursing, police or the armed forces.

Most patients without symptoms or signs of lipodermosclerosis or ulceration simply require reassurance.

Treatment of varicose veins

Three methods of treatment are available:

(i) Palliative treatment.
(ii) Sclerotherapy.
(iii) Operations.

Palliative treatment

Indications

1. Aged.
2. Pregnancy or puerperium.
3. Patients who refuse operation or who are unfit for operation, or who are waiting for operation.
4. Pelvic tumour.
5. Deep vein thrombosis confirmed by positive Perthes' test, venography or duplex ultrasonography.

Essentials

1. **Bisgaard's regime** $\left\{ \begin{array}{l} \text{Postural drainage} \\ \text{Exercises} \\ \text{Support} \end{array} \right.$

(a) *Postural drainage:*
   (i) Avoidance of prolonged standing, prolonged sitting on chair.
   (ii) Elevation of the limb preferably above the heart level by an angle of 10–15° during rest and at night improves venous drainage and reduces any oedema.

(b) *Exercises:* Exercises of the leg to strengthen the calf muscles which empty the veins are of value. 'Bicycle riding' in the air while lying on the back, walking and cycling are of obvious benefit. Passive and active movements of the ankle are also beneficial.

(c) *Support:* A crepe bandage or a well-fitting *'two way stretch' elastic compression stocking, 'below knee stocking which includes the heel',* should be applied before getting out of bed in the morning. It helps to compress the minor varicosities and to strengthen the efficiency of the calf-pump.

2. *Drugs used for varicose veins particularly in the presence of* oedema, pigmentation and ulceration are:
   • Calcium dobesilate (Dobium) – 500 mg BD. It improves both the venous and lymph flow and reduces oedema. Also improves macrophage-mediated proteolysis to help ulcer healing.
   • Dosmin 450 mg BD or Daflon 500 mg BD may be used in relieving night cramps. But they do not help in ulcer healing.

3. *Ulcer dressing* with hypertonic saline, hydrogen peroxide or EUSOL followed by support with crepe bandage.

4. Patient should reduce heavy body weight.

Conservative treatment with elastic stockings and external compression is an acceptable alternative to surgery, but worsening cutaneous findings and symptoms despite these measures warrant intervention.

Sclerotherapy and compression

Indications

Used to treat varicose veins in the absence of functional incompetence and major perforating veins.

1. Small varicosities and cutaneous spider veins.
2. Recurrent varicosities after operation.
3. *Varicose veins confined below the knee.*
4. Troublesome vulval varicosities.
5. As an alternative to surgery.
6. Cosmetic: But not ideal because of unpredictable staining which may occur.

Principle

Injection of a sclerosant solution into an empty varicose vein. The materials available are:

1. Soap solution such as 5% ethanolamine oleate.
2. 3% sodium tetradecyl sulphate (STD).
3. Polydocanol.
4. Hypertonic solutions of a crystalloid such as sodium chloride or glucose.
5. Organic compounds such as quinine, urethane or sodium salicylate.
6. *Foam sclerotherapy developed by Tessari.*

Idea

- *To induce chemical thrombophlebitis.*
- Sclerosant solution will *damage the intimal lining of the vein* so that an aseptic and firmly adherent thrombus, and later sclerosis develop leading to complete obliteration of the treated vein.

Method

The sclerosant solution should be *injected into an empty varicose vein* and *compression bandage is then applied over the site which is maintained for a few weeks* so that wall adheres to wall with no intervening blood clot. The endothelial lining is destroyed and there will be formation of intravascular granulation tissue which later becomes fibrous and thus obliterates the lumen of the vein permanently. *If the vein is not compressed* it will produce superficial thrombophlebitis which will later get recanalised producing recurrence.

Dose

The maximum dose at one sitting and at any one point is 1 ml. The injection can be repeated at various sites in the leg but the total dose should not exceed 10–12 ml.

When compression sclerosant therapy is used, a latex foam pad is applied over the site of injection and along the length of vein, which is maintained in position by crepe bandage and a full-length two-way stretch elastic stocking *for a period of six weeks* from the last injection or until the pain has gone from the site. *Compression bandage helps to prevent DVT.*

Sites of injections

1. At the maximum point of varicosity.
2. Sites of 'blowout' or perforating veins.
3. At the maximum point of tenderness.

Complications due to injections

1. The injection should always be intravascular. Otherwise, skin ulceration may occur, which is more common with the crystalloids and the organic compounds.
2. Some risk of anaphylactic reactions.
3. Thrombophlebitis.
4. *Chance of deep vein thrombosis because of spread to the deep veins*, if an excess of the sclerosant is injected at one site.
5. There will be local pain, oedema, redness, hyperpigmentation, etc., for a few days which will subside spontaneously.

Patient should be warned of these complications.

Advantage of sclerotherapy

The patient can undergo repeated treatment sessions to ensure that all veins are sclerosed.

Recently, U/S-guided foam sclerotherapy is preferred over 'blind sclerotherapy'.

Operations

Indication

- Saphenofemoral or saphenopopliteal incompetence.
- Persisting symptoms.
- Complications – varicose veins with leg ulcers.
- Deep vein incompetence without DVT.
- Varicosity >3 mm diameter.
- Multiple incompetent perforators.

Contraindication

Presence of DVT along with varicose vein because superficial venous system remains the only channel for proximal venous drainage.

Aim of operation

1. *To stop the retrograde venous flow (and hence high pressure leak)* from the deep venous system, by ligation of the incompetent veins at the:
   (i) Saphenofemoral junction

    (ii) Saphenopopliteal junction and/or
    (iii) At the incompetent perforator sites.
2. To remove the varicosities.

Method

    (i) Ligation alone.
    (ii) Ligation and stripping – the treatment of choice.
    (iii) Multiple stab avulsion or excision of the convoluted veins.
    (iv) Ligation and retrograde injections of sclerosing solutions to the distal segment.
    (v) Cockett and Dodd operation.

Long saphenous vein incompetence

The saphenofemoral junction is dissected out at the groin. All the tributaries of saphenofemoral junction at the groin are divided in between the ligatures. *Then the saphenous vein is ligated flush with the femoral vein proximal to any tributaries, otherwise a recurrence is inevitable. This is known as **Trendelenburg operation**.*

    *The Trendelenburg operation is nearly always supplemented with stripping of the varicose vein with the aid of **Myer's vein stripper** so that the vein is avulsed from the subcutaneous tissue. Stripping of the varicose vein removes the unsightly veins* and also disconnects the other tributaries of the main saphenous system.

    After saphenofemoral flush ligation and disconnection, the long saphenous vein is exposed at the ankle in front of the medial malleolus, and a *flexible wire vein stripper* is introduced into the saphenous vein through a venotomy and pushed upwards towards the groin until it emerges from the proximal end of the vein. The vein is then fixed around the stripper at its lower end by a thread ligature and its distal end is divided and ligated. The ankle wound is closed. *The stripper is then gradually pulled out through the groin incision* with the leg elevated and the leg is firmly bandaged with elastic crepe bandage from foot and ankle up to the groin by an assistant as the stripper advances.

    Just before stripping of the LSV, multiple stab avulsions of the localised dilated segments of the veins (blowouts) using mosquito forceps or avulsion hook can also be made.

Large tributaries may require separate exposure and ligation.

Short saphenous vein incompetence

The short saphenous vein is exposed by a curved transverse incision at the popliteal fossa and *is ligated proximal to any tributaries* close to or flush with the popliteal vein. *Stripping is usually not practised in short saphenous incompetence.*

Perforator vein incompetence

Subfascial ligation of perforators

Incompetent perforator sites are explored subfascially and then ligated and divided. This is known as **Cockett and Dodd operation**.

    In addition to above procedures, smaller varicose tributaries and severely dilated clumps of veins, if present, can be marked out before operation and may then be individually avulsed, ligated or injected by sclerosing solutions.

Complications of varicose vein surgery

   I. Nerve injury – *saphenous nerve* during long saphenous vein surgery radiating along the medial border of the foot. *Sural nerve* during short saphenous vein surgery.
  II. Venous thrombosis in residual varices.
 III. Pain, discomfort and bruising.
 IV. Deep vein thrombosis – prophylactic heparin is used when there is history of previous DVT.

Contraindication of both injections and operative treatment

1. *Women taking contraceptive pills*, because there are chances of deep vein thrombosis and fatal thromboembolism. *Pill alters the viscosity of blood.*
2. *Deep vein thrombosis with oedema of the limb* because here the main axial deep vein has been destroyed and, so, the superficial varicose veins form the major part of the venous drainage of the limb.
3. *Pregnancy.*
4. *Thrombophlebitis.*
5. *Obesity* – reluctant to reduce body weight.

Recent methods of minimally invasive therapy for varicose veins

1. EVLA (Endo venous laser ablation)
2. RFA (Radio frequency ablation)
3. VNUS – under sonographic guidance, vascular endothelium is destroyed by electocautery
4. SEPS (Subfascial endoscopic perforator surgery)
5. TRIVEX – sudden high pressure suction is applied after injecting hypertonic saline into the varicose vein

EVLA, RFA and VNUS

All cause thermal damage of endothelium resulting in endothelial denudation, collagen denaturation and subsequent fibrosis leading to venous occlusion. But they do not provide flush occlusion of the saphenous vein.

Advantages:
- All these minimally invasive methods can be performed at an outpatient department without anaesthesia.
- Patient can return to his/her normal activity early.
- Cosmetically good because of no scars.
- Lower risk of recurrences.

SEPS (Subfascial Endoscopic Perforator Surgery)

- Indicated for leg perforators.
- *Under laparoscopic guidance* subfascial perforators are identified and ligated.
- Procedure is simple and quick.
- Large incisions avoided.
- Morbidity is less.

Advantages:
- This minimally invasive method can be performed at an outpatient department without anaesthesia.
- Patient can return to his/her normal activity early.
- Cosmetically good because of no scars or limited fine scars.

Disadvantage:
- Cost is very high.

Note

Venous diseases of the lower limb are more common on the left side because the venous pressure in the left lower limb is always higher than that of right lower limb due to following anatomical factors.

1. The left common iliac vein joins the IVC at a more acute angle, whereas right common iliac vein joins almost in line with the IVC.
2. The right common iliac artery crosses in front of the left common iliac vein at its entrance into the IVC.
3. Loaded pelvic colon exerts pressure more over the left iliac vein, particularly, in a chronic constipated patient.

Note

Surgical importance of the anatomy of long saphenous vein

1. Varicose veins and their surgical management.
2. Venous cut down as an emergency.
3. Harvesting the vein as a graft in vascular and cardiothoracic surgery.

Note

Role of pregnancy in varicose veins

1. During pregnancy, the gravid uterus, after 20 weeks, exerts pressure on the IVC and common iliac veins.
2. Increased venous return from the gravid uterus.
3. Due to effect of progesterone from corpus luteum, which reduces venous tone and increases venous distensibility.

Note

Gold standard diagnostic test in varicose vein – Duplex imaging.

Note

Best operation for varicose vein – stripping.

Note

Cockett and Dodd's operation – subfascial ligation of perforators.

Note

Most common complication of varicose vein surgery is *ecchymosis*.

Note

Injury to saphenous nerve (branch of femoral nerve), particularly the infrapatellar branch, can cause pain and irritating paraesthesia or anesthesia on the medial side of the leg.

Note

Sural nerve injury

Sural nerve (branch of tibial nerve) during short saphenous vein surgery causing loss of sensation to the skin of lateral foot and lateral lower ankle.

Note

Recently, *foam sclerotherapy* followed by compression dressing are being practised in some centres with good results.

Note

Causes of superficial thrombophlebitis
1. Buerger's disease
2. Varicose veins
3. Polycythemia
4. Occult visceral malignancy
5. Iatrogenic, e.g. IV injection/infusion and catheterisation

Note

Syndromes associated with pulsatile varicose veins of the lower limb
1. Klippel-Trenaunay syndrome
2. Kasabach-Merritt syndrome

Note

Klippel-Trenaunay syndrome characterised by:
1. Congenital AV malformation or fistula.
2. Cutaneous haemangioma.
3. *Pulsatile varicose veins.*
4. Hypertrophy of involved extremity.
5. Absence of deep venous system.

So, pathological superficial distended veins should not be removed without evidence of patent deep venous system.

Note

Kasabach-Merritt syndrome characterised by:
1. Congenital AV malformation or fistula.
2. *Pulsatile varicose veins.*
3. Thrombocytopenia.
4. Haemorrhagic manifestations – due to trapping and destruction of platelets within the varicosities.

Note

Most common cause of superficial thrombophlebitis: Intravenous IV infusion and catheterisation.

Note

Most commonly used donor nerve is the sural nerve.

Note

Varicosity of pampiniform plexus of veins is known as varicocele palpable at the root of the scrotum – commonly on the left side.

Ulcers of the Leg

The lower leg is the common seat of an ulcer and presents a common clinical problem due to disorders of the venous system and also due to a number of other possible causes including the 'Tropical ulcers' occurring in people living in the tropics.

TYPES ACCORDING TO CAUSES

1. Venous
2. Arterial   } Commonest
3. Traumatic
4. Infective
   (a) Specific
      - Tuberculous
      - Bairnsdale
      - Syphilitic
      - Actinomycosis
   (b) Non-specific
      - Pyogenic
5. Neuropathic
6. Neoplastic
7. Cryopathic
8. Diabetic
9. Idiopathic
10. Self-inflicted or artefact
11. Tropical caused by microorganisms including mycobacteria – common in tropical countries.

12. Miscellaneous: Ulcers of the leg may be associated with arteriovenous fistula, sickle cell anaemia, chronic lymphoedema, various collagen disorders, poliomyelitis, ulcerative colitis, etc.

SURGICAL PATHOLOGY OF DIFFERENT VARIETIES OF ULCERS

Venous ulcer

Also called gravitational ulcer. Always associated with incompetent venous systems due to either varicose veins or deep venous thrombosis in which recanalisation of the deep vein has occurred, *but the valves are either destroyed or incompetent due to damage leading to stagnation of blood. The basic defect is* **cutaneous venous stasis** *which results in local tissue anoxia due to stagnation of poorly oxygenated blood.*

As a result of incompetence of the valves of the deep veins and of the communicating veins between the deep and superficial venous systems, there is leakage of blood under high pressure from the deep veins into the superficial veins; *this occurs particularly in the region of a constantly placed perforators over the medial side of the lower leg (the ulcer bearing area or* **gaiter area**). This results in venular dilatation (*ankle flare*) and stagnation of blood. The blood in these varicose veins usually has only two-thirds of the normal oxygen content with a corresponding increase of carbon dioxide. There is also remarkable rise in pressure in varicose veins in the ankle, which may be 30 mm higher than the blood pressure in the arteries particularly when the patient strains during fast walking or running. *Hence, the blood from the superficial capillaries is unable to enter the veins against this pressure, resulting in stagnation of blood and congestion of the skin at the gaiter area. The skin in this area is normally thin, delicate and easily traumatised.* Stagnation of circulation and poor oxygenation combined with effused blood pigment *cause induration and pigmentation of the skin which are the pre-ulceration changes.* If the high pressure leakage is allowed to continue, skin ischaemia can occur and ulceration results, which may be precipitated by a minor trauma.

Venous ulcers usually lie proximal to the medial or lateral malleolus accompanied by lipo-dermatosclerosis and haemosiderosis (pigmentation). If these are not present, then the ulcer is probably not of venous origin.

Arterial ulcer

The basic defect is skin ischaemia following atherosclerotic peripheral vascular disease. It commonly occurs on the toes, dorsum of the foot, or the heel and to start with there is a patch of dry gangrene. *Claudication pain is usually associated with arterial occlusion* commonly in the legs caused by too little blood flow to the leg muscles *usually during exercise or walking.*

Traumatic ulcer

Commonly occurs where the skin is closely applied to bony prominences, e.g. shin of the leg, malleoli and the back of the heel.

Plaster sores and bedsores over the heel are included in this group.

Infective ulcer

(a) *Pyogenic:* Common organism is *Staphylococcus* which may be so potent as to result in multiple abscess formation with subsequent necrosis of the overlying skin resulting in multiple ulcers.

(b) *Syphilitic or Gummatous ulcer:* Occurs in tertiary stage of syphilis, as a result of necrosis of a chronic granuloma of the muscle. The patient complains of deep boring pain in the bone, characteristically worse at night.

(c) *Bairnsdale ulcer:* Starts as a chronic inflammation of the skin caused by the acid-fast bacilli known as *Mycobacterium ulcerans.* First recognised in Australia but common in *Uganda* where it is known as *Buruli ulcer.*

Neuropathic ulcer

The basic defect is sensory loss due to neurological disorder leading to chronic, irregular undermined ulcers. The ulcer occurs due to repeated injury or pressure which is allowed to occur *because anaesthesia leads to loss of appreciation of pain in the area – painless ulcer.* These ulcers are also called *trophic ulcers or penetrating ulcers.*

The ulcer commonly occurs on the sole of the foot: On the heel or over metatarsal heads and it may penetrate the bone or joint.

Common conditions which predispose to neuropathic or trophic ulcers are diabetes or alcoholic neuritis, tabes dorsalis, syringomyelia and paraplegia leading to immobility.

In diabetes mellitus, the ulcer may be precipitated also by atherosclerosis and infection. *The toes and the feet are commonly affected.*

Note

Bedsores are also considered as trophic ulcer.

Neoplastic ulcer

Primary tumour of the skin, e.g. squamous cell carcinoma, basal cell carcinoma, malignant melanoma may present as an ulcer.

Metastasis from a distant primary focus can be lodged in the skin and may undergo necrosis and ulceration.

Marjolin's ulcers: Malignant change (squamous cell carcinoma) may occur in long-standing venous ulcers, or in the scars of old ulcerated burns which refuse to heal, or in keloid, or in chronically discharging osteomyelitic sinuses. *They should be suspected when there is evidence of raised or rolled out edge. They are nothing but squamous cell carcinoma.*

Cryopathic ulcer

The term is used to describe *an ulcer which results from exposure to extremely low temperature.*

(a) *Chilblains (perniosis)*: Intense vaso-constriction of the skin arterioles in areas *exposed to cold of moderate intensity results in tender, red, pruritic swelling followed by blister formation and subsequent ulceration. The lesions commonly affect the feet and toes of individuals particularly susceptible to cold injury.* The lesions are focal and superficial which may heal rapidly when cold exposure is avoided.

Chilblains also involves ear and nose.

(b) *Frostbite:* Exposure of a part of the body in the *wet cold* at or below freezing temperature for a prolonged period results in ischaemic changes of skin and subcutaneous tissue *due to intense arteriolar spasm.* There is also stasis of blood in the damaged capillaries, which aggravates the ischaemia. *Severe freezing injury* may cause freezing of tissues, denaturation of intracellular protein and destruction of enzyme systems to promote ice-crystal formation in the cells. *All these changes may cause gangrene of at least the full thickness of the skin and subsequent ulceration.*

Chilblains and frostbite are *common in soldiers, hikers, homeless people who spend lot of time outside in chilling cold specially when under the influence of alcohol (drunken stupor).*

Idiopathic ulcer

(a) *Tropical ulcer:* Commonly occurs on the legs and feet of the people living in the tropical countries. *Malnutrition* is supposed to be a factor.

(b) *Martorell's ulcer:* Also known as *hypertensive ulcer*, because it occurs in hypertensive patients. But usually there is no

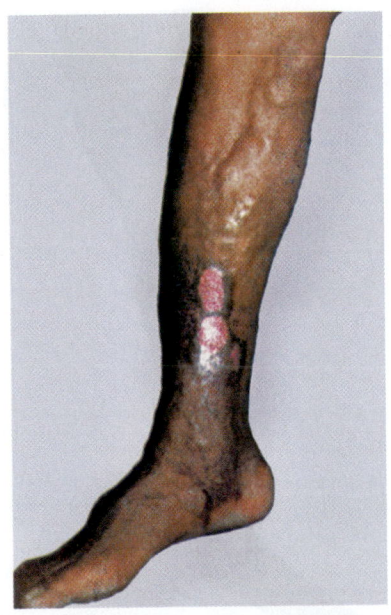

Fig. 16.1: Varicose ulcer on the medial side of lower one-third of the leg. Note the pigmentation, the ankle flare (the spreading of redness or flush due to dilatation of the arterioles), and varicosity at the upper half of the leg with equinus deformity. All these findings led to the diagnosis.

associated atherosclerotic peripheral arterial disease. *The ulcer occurs in the leg over the calf,* and to start with, there are patches of spontaneous skin necrosis. *Often bilateral and painful; takes months to heal; and requires lumbar sympathectomy followed by skin grafting.*

Self-inflicted ulcer

Due to injury to the skin by scratching, cutting or the injection of substances; found most often in those who are psychologically abnormal or who hope for some personal gain.

DIFFERENTIAL DIAGNOSIS OF ULCERS OF THE LEG

A. Varicose ulcer (Figs 16.1 and 16.2)

1. *Site: It occurs typically over the medial aspects of the lower third of the leg around and above the medial malleoli (gaiter area) because of the presence of large number of incompetent perforators in this area.*

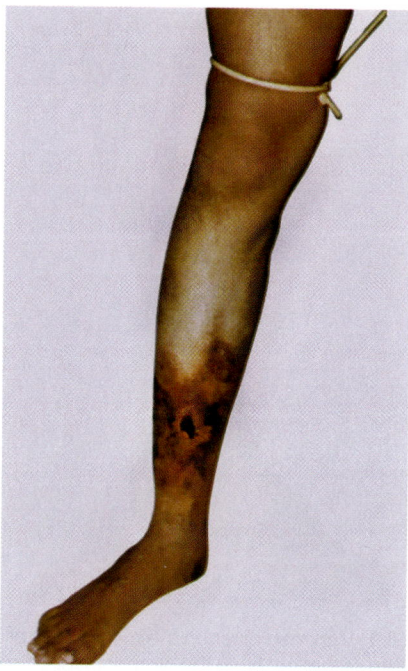

Fig. 16.2: Varicose ulcers. The upper one was healed. The lower one was in healing stage. Note the pigmentation around. No varicosities were noted nearby even after tourniquet test as this patient had Trendelenburg's operation with stripping of the great saphenous vein few years back. *So, ask for the previous operation and look for the scars—at the groin and above the medial malleolus.*

2. Duration – long.
3. Ulcer is ovoid in shape with irregular margin. *Usually single in number.* The ulcer may be fixed to the bone due to associated periostitis. The ulcer may be at the healing stage when it has a slopping edge and a base of healthy granulation tissue. *The ulcer may be painful and tender.*
4. *Presence of associated varicose veins.*
5. *Presence of unhealthy, pigmented skin* (bluish in colour) with or without oedema of the leg.
6. *Presence of deformity (Equinus) and disfigurement* of the leg (bottleneck appearance). Movements of ankle joint may be limited by scarring of the ulcer.
7. Evidence of deep vein thrombosis.
   (a) Pratt's test – positive.

(b) Perthes' test – may be positive.
(c) Homan's sign (passive dorsiflexion of the foot will cause intense pain in the calf) – *if positive*, suggestive of deep vein thrombosis.
8. *Peripheral arterial pulses are normal* (cf. arterial ulcer).
9. *Investigations:* Venography may help, if deep vein thrombosis and perforator incompetence are suspected.
10. Biopsy of the ulcer when doubtful.

Note

Positive Homan's sign and Perthes' test contraindicate varicose vein surgery as the superficial veins are the only veins which allow the venous drainage of the affected limb to maintain or continue.

B. Arterial ulcer (*Syn.* Ischaemic ulcer)

1. *Site: Occurs on the toes, dorsum of the foot, or heel.*
2. *History of intermittent claudication, rest pain* particularly in a person who is a chronic smoker.
3. *Arterial ulcers are very painful.*

On examination:

4. The arterial ulcer varies in size and shape. *The edge is punched out* because healing by the surrounding tissues is poor or absent *as they too are ischaemic.* The skin at the edge may be greyish-blue in colour.

   The base may contain grey-yellow sloughing tissue and is often infected. The ulcer is very often deep penetrating down to the bone or into the underlying joints. Occasionally the bare bone, ligaments or tendons may be exposed at the base of the ischaemic ulcer. *The ulcer and the surrounding tissues are very tender.*
5. *Peripheral arterial pulses: Poor or absent.*
6. *Presence of ischaemic changes in the limb* like dry pale skin, loss of hair, fissuring of nails, etc. *The surrounding tissues are usually cold* because they too are ischaemic.
7. *Arteriography* may help, if peripheral arterial disease is suspected.

C. Neuropathic ulcer

1. *Site: Occurs on the sole or heel of the foot.*
2. *Neuropathic ulcer* is a deep penetrating ulcer like arterial ulcer but it is *painless and non-tender. It occurs over the pressure areas.* The surrounding tissues are healthy and have a normal circulation *but are unable to appreciate pain.*
3. *Evidence of neurological deficits is present,* e.g. loss or diminution of sensation, weakness of the muscles.
4. *Peripheral pulses are usually present* because diabetes affects the smaller vessels like digital vessels mainly.
5. Blood and urine for sugar – to see diabetes mellitus.
6. Blood for WR and Kahn – to exclude tabes dorsalis.

D. Malignant ulcer

See squamous cell carcinoma, basal cell carcinoma and malignant melanoma (Chapter 1).

1. *Squamous cell carcinoma:* The ulcer has a rolled out and everted margin.
2. *Basal cell carcinoma:* The ulcer has raised and beaded edge.
3. *Malignant melanoma:* Pigmented.
4. *Biopsy* must be done, if malignancy is suspected.

E. Marjolin's ulcer

1. *Site:* Malignant change may occur on the long-standing venous ulcer.
2. It is nothing but squamous cell carcinoma developed on a venous ulcer.
3. It should be suspected when there is evidence of raised or rolled out edge in an existing ulcer.

F. Traumatic ulcer

1. *Site: Commonly over the area where the skin is closely applied to bony prominences,* e.g. shin, malleoli, the back of the heel, the back of the sacrum, etc.
2. The ulcer may be due to bedsores or plaster sores.

3. *The ulcer appears as a painful, tender small circular lesion.* In chronic stage the ulcer may be painless.

G. Cryopathic ulcer

1. *Site: Commonly the toes are affected.*
2. *History of exposure to freezing or near freezing temperatures is present causing very poor circulation due to vasospasm and crystallisation of the skin.*
3. To start with there is *blister formation followed by ulceration.*

H. Gummatous ulcer (Syphilitic ulcer)

1. Duration – short.
2. *Site: It occurs classically on the outer side of the leg and more commonly on the upper aspect, i.e. commonly round about the knee.*
3. History of exposure.
4. *The ulcer is typically of punched-out appearance with clear-cut vertical edges and wash-leather slough on the floor.* The ulcer may be round or serpiginous in shape.
5. The ulcer is *painless,* and may be multiple in number.
6. Absence of varicosity.
7. Associated features of neurosyphilis like *ARP* and cardiovascular syphilis like aortic incompetence, aneurysm of the arch of aorta may be present.
8. *Blood for WR and Kahn – highly positive.*
9. *Culture of the ulcer discharge –* may show treponema.

Note

ARP (Argyll Robertson pupils): Bilateral small pupils that reduce in size when looking at a near object, but do not constrict when exposed to bright light.

I. Bairnsdale ulcer (Buruli ulcer) (Fig. 16.3)

1. *Site:* Can occur anywhere, commonly in the limbs.
2. *The ulcer is irregular with thin and under-mined edges* with frequent presence of bluish, pale, watery granulation tissue on the floor.

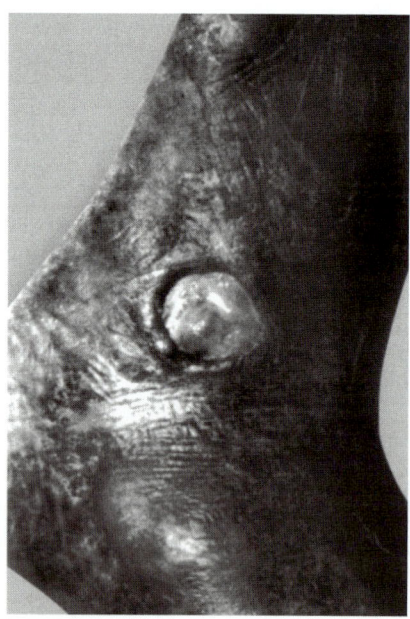

Fig. 16.3: Bairnsdale ulcer over the lateral malleolus of the ankle. Note the undermined edge of the ulcer.

3. Painless ulcer.
4. Smear examination and culture of discharge may show acid-fast bacilli.
5. Absence of varicosity.
6. Treated by rifampicin and streptomycin.

J. Tropical ulcer

1. Also known as *'jungle rot'*.
2. Chronic ulcerative skin lesions thought to be caused by polymicrobial infection with a variety of microbacteria and micro-organisms.
3. Common *over the anterolateral aspect of the lower limbs*. Ulcers may frequently develop on preexisting abrasion or sores developing after minor scratch.
4. Usually painless.
5. May erode the muscles, tendons and sometimes bones.

MANAGEMENT OF LEG ULCERS

1. Careful history taking with particular emphasis on the following.
   (a) Duration

   (b) Painful or painless
   (c) History of claudication
   (d) History of diabetes
   (e) History of DVT
   (f) History of varicosity of long saphenous vein
   (g) History of exposure
   (h) *History of prolonged persistent pressure due to poor nursing care leading to ulcer over the bony prominences – pressure or bedsores.*
2. Local examination of the ulcer regarding the character of the ulcer – site, shape, size, edge, floor, base, any fixity to the bone.

   Note for tenderness and induration of the ulcer margin or base.

   Note for surrounding skin changes and for presence of varicosities and venous ulcers.
3. *Palpation of the peripheral arterial pulses.*
4. Examination of venous system – both superficial and deep venous systems.
5. Examination of the draining lymph nodes.
6. Examination for any evidence of neurological disorders – sensory or motor impairments. Palpation of peripheral nerves, e.g. common peroneal nerve at the fibular neck (leprosy); also palpate ulnar nerve.
7. Investigations:
   (a) Blood for routine, sugar and WR and Kahn.
   (b) Urine for sugar.
   (c) Culture of ulcer discharge for:
       (i) Pyogenic organisms.
       (ii) Mycobacteria.
       (iii) Treponema.
   (d) Arteriography, if peripheral arterial disease is suspected.
   (e) Venography, if deep vein thrombosis and perforator incompetency are suspected.
   (f) Biopsy, whenever a reasonable doubt exists as to the nature of the ulcer, a biopsy should be done.
   (g) Therapeutic test, when self-inflicted ulcer is suspected, plaster immobilisation of the affected part will help in the healing of the ulcer, but amazingly it is found that the patient may deli-

berately create ulcer on some other parts of the body.

8. Treatment of the ulcer – varies according to the nature of the ulcer.

Causes of delayed healing of ulcer

Already mentioned in Chapter 1.

TREATMENT OF VARICOSE ULCER

A. Conservative
B. Operative

Conservative

Indications

1. Severe ulceration of long duration and the ulcer is associated with wide areas of skin involvement with dense fibrosis and brawny induration.
2. Presence of eczema which may be dry and coarse, scaly, moist or infected.
3. Preoperative preparation before any definitive surgical treatment.
4. If operation is refused.

Principle

Principles are laid down according to *Bisgaard's regime* which advocates *elevation* and *proper bandaging of the limb* together with *proper exercises and massage.* By this regime almost any venous ulcer can be healed.

Methods

These depend on whether the ulcer is infected or not.

1. Clean ulcers

1. *Rest in bed with the foot end of the bed elevated* by about 9 inches reduces local oedema.
2. *Application of dressing and compression bandages.*
   (a) Application of zinc cream to the ulcer, olive oil to the dry surrounding skin, and calamine lotion to the eczematous areas that are itchy.
   (b) Dry gauze is then applied over the ulcer.
   (c) A felt pad or sponge rubber piece with bevelled edges, and cut to a size larger than the ulcer is then held over the ulcer by a crepe bandage.
   (d) Over this dressing a firm one-way stretch elastic bandage is applied spirally from the base of the toes to the knee using a good one-half overlap with firm and even pressure, particularly around the foot and ankle. This type of bandaging helps *to reduce oedema, to produce an added pumping and massaging effects of the leg muscle during walking* and *compression of the dilated veins and incompetent perforators.*

   Frequency of application of bandages: The first application of bandage is removed after one week, and thereafter the bandage is renewed at fortnightly intervals until the ulcer is healed.
3. *Massage:* Frequent massage to the whole leg in elevation may help to clear local oedema and to soften the indurated area round the ulcer.
4. *Exercises:* Both passive and active:
   • Passive movements to maintain the mobility of the foot and ankle joint.
   • Active movements of the calf muscles both in elevation and in standing (with bandages on) to improve local blood supply as well.
5. *Walking training:* The patient should be taught proper walking. The heel touches the ground first and then the calf muscles should be used to lift the heel of the back foot. This will give a 'spring' to the walk and thereby improve the venous pump.

Once the ulcer is healed by above procedures, the patient is instructed to wear an efficiently fitted rubberized cotton or nylon stocking, or a crepe bandage, *from the base of the toes to the knee.* The elastic stocking or crepe bandage should be applied before rising from the bed every morning. The bandage may be discarded at night, or during the day for short periods, provided the foot end of the bed is elevated.

The limb should be kept elevated for a while after each walking. *Active toe and foot movements during rest.* Calf muscle massage should be continued particularly in elevation.

Elastic stocking should be worn during walking or prolonged standing at work *for rest of life* particularly in a case of post-thrombotic disease.

2. Infected ulcers

The idea of treatment is to convert an infected ulcer into a clean one which is then treated as above.

a. Swab for culture and sensitivity to antibiotics.
b. *Application of EUSOL and/or hydrogen peroxide to the ulcer to remove the slough and pus* followed by dressing until the ulcer becomes dry with healthy pink granulations tissue at the base.
c. Antibiotics: Local application of antibiotics is unnecessary and may be harmful if a sensitivity reaction or a resistant organism develops.

   Systemic antibiotics may be required in presence of cellulitis, lymphangitis and lymphadenitis.
d. *Rest the patient in bed with the leg elevated when the infective-process shows signs of spreading.*

Once the infection is controlled, the ulcer should be treated along the lines indicated for a clean ulcer.

Operative

Indications

1. Small ulcers with or without localised changes in the surrounding tissues.
2. Extensive ulcer, over 1 inch in diameter, with an induration of the surrounding area over 2 inches in diameter, when the healing is delayed or difficult to achieve or difficult to maintain by conservative methods.
3. When the ulcer is healed – treatment of varicose veins to prevent recurrence.

Contraindications

1. Severe ulceration with wide areas of skin deterioration and/or diffuse brawny oedema, because there is a possibility of skin necrosis in these cases after a perforator dissection.
2. Presence of infected ulcers.
3. Presence of moist or infected eczema.

Methods

1. Subfascial perforator dissection and ligation (*Cockett and Dodd operation*).
2. Excision of associated varicose veins which are the cause of the ulceration or are contributory to ulceration.
3. Excision of the ulcer and also of the nearby unhealthy skin down to healthy fascia or muscle followed by skin grafting. *Pinch graft or mesh graft have shown to provide good result.*
4. Oxerutins are used in the prevention of recurrence of chronic venous ulcers by reducing fluid retention mainly in the legs. *It improves the parietal venous tone and thus microvascular perfusion.*

In order to avoid oedema, pressure bandages must be worn for a few months after operation, including frequent elevation of the legs and active movements. Rest in bed with the leg elevated throughout rest of life will also be helpful to prevent recurrence.

Marjolin's ulcer

- Squamous cell carcinoma developing on a chronic ulcer (e.g. venous ulcer) or on a scar, e.g. post-burn scarring due to chronic infection which ultimately turns malignant.
- The lesion is typically *very slow growing* due to lack of poor blood supply of scar tissue.
- The ulcer is *usually painless* because of impaired sensation following nerve damage around the scar.
- *Lymphatic spread is very rare* because of obliterated lymphatics by the scar fibrosis.
- *Treatment:*

  1. Not radiosensitive because of poor vascularity and extensive fibrosis.
  2. *Surgery is the treatment of choice after four quadrant edge biopsy to confirm the diagnosis:* Excision of the lesion with at least 2.5 cm margin all around is preferred followed by reconstruction of the defect with appropriate skin flaps.

     Lymph node dissection after confirmation of LN involvement with FNAC/FNAB may be considered.

Note

Most important perforator of lower limb – long saphenofemoral junction.

Note

Pulsating varicose vein in a young adult – *arterio-venous fistula*.

Note

Common site for venous ulcer – *lower one-third of leg*.

Note

True about venous ulcer:

1. Always examine deep venous system for DVT.
2. Biopsy should be taken for chronic ulcer to exclude SCC (Marjolin's ulcer).
3. In presence of DVT, superficial venous system should not be removed because it will continue to provide drainage of the limb.

Note

Site of diabetic foot ulcer:

1. Heel
2. Head of metatarsal
3. Head of toes

Swellings of the Leg

Swellings of the lower limb are often encountered in clinical practice. Commonly, they are due to medical conditions such as heart failure, kidney disease or malnutrition. But the surgeons are concerned only with the peripheral causes, the majority of which are venous or lymphatic in origin.

CLASSIFICATION OF CAUSES

Central

Swelling is usually bilateral.

1. *Cardiac*
   - Congestive heart failure
   - Constrictive pericarditis
2. *Renal*
   - Nephrotic syndrome
   - Acute nephritis
3. *Hepatic disorder* – multiple factors are responsible for oedema.
4. *Gastrointestinal*
   - Gastroenteropathies.
5. *Nutritional*
   - Protein deficiency
   - Thiamine deficiency
   - Iron deficiency
6. *Hormonal*
   - Cushing's syndrome
   - Pretibial myxoedema in thyrotoxicosis

- Myxoedema: Fluid retention seen in myxoedema is caused by interstitial accumulation of hydrophilic mucopolysaccharides which leads to lymphoedema.
7. Venous disorder: Inferior vena cava thrombosis.

Peripheral

Swelling is usually unilateral.

1. *Venous disorder*
   - Perforator vein incompetency
   - Calf vein thrombosis
   - Iliofemoral vein thrombosis
2. *Lymphoedema*
   - A. Primary due to developmental anomaly:
     - Lymphoedema congenita present at birth
     - Lymphoedema praecox present at puberty: Meige disease
     - Lymphoedema tarda present in adulthood after 3rd decade
   - B. Secondary – *commonest cause of lymphoedema and is due to obstruction of previously normal lymphatic channels by a known agent such as:*
     - (a) Parasitic infestation of lymph nodes, e.g. filariasis: Most common worldwide

(b) Inflammation:
  - Lymphogranuloma venereum: STD involving inguinal lymph nodes.
  - Tuberculosis
  - Recurrent non-specific infection.
(c) Malignant infiltration of lymph nodes and channels.
(d) Iatrogenic:
  - *Following extensive surgical removal of lymph nodes*, e.g. prophylactic block dissection of lymph nodes in a malignant lesion of lower limb following inguinal block dissection or upper limb following axillary block dissection (e.g. breast cancer).
  - *Postirradiation fibrosis.*
3. *Miscellaneous* (Figs 17.1 to 17.3)
  - Adiposis dolorosa
  - Diffuse neurofibromatosis
  - Arteriovenous fistula
  - Tight plaster or bandage
  - Injuries – fracture, muscle contusion, extensive burn
  - Infection – cellulitis, abscess, gas gangrene.

- Erythrocyanosis frigida
- Angioedema – allergic disorder
- Podoconiosis – cutaneous absorption of mineral particles common in mine workers

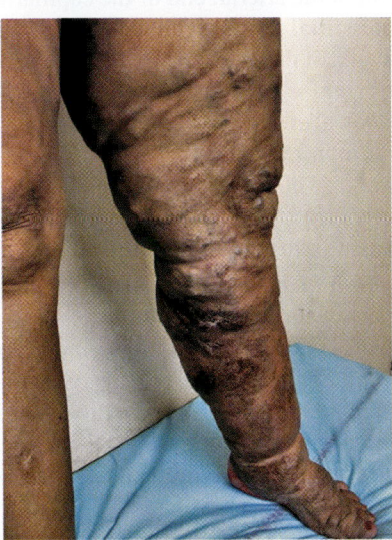

Fig. 17.2: Swelling of the left lower limb: Diffuse neurofibromatosis with multiple nodules.

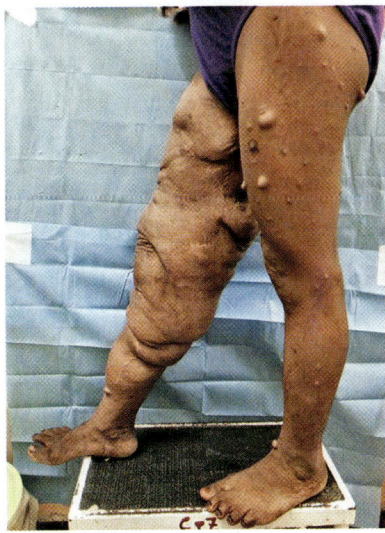

Fig. 17.1: Swelling of right lower limb with plexiform neurofibroma. Also note the multiple nodules over left lower limb. Also note folds on right limb.

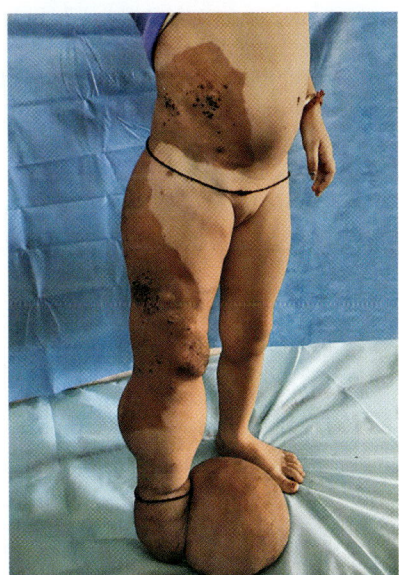

Fig. 17.3: Swelling of the right lower limb with *football size* nodule swelling over the dorsum of the foot. *Also note the pigmentation* right side of abdomen and right thigh and leg: Diffuse neurofibromatosis.

SURGICAL PHYSIOLOGY

Normal tissue fluid circulation

Normally, there is a continuous circulation of fluid out of the arterial end of the capillaries into the interstitial spaces and then back into the venous end of the capillaries. In order to maintain this normal circulation of fluid across the capillary wall *a balance between two main forces, i.e. hydrostatic pressure or capillary blood pressure and plasma osmotic pressure*, operates which controls the rate and direction of fluid movement in the circulation (Fig. 17.4).

Some fluid and most proteins ultrafiltrated at the level of the arterial capillaries enters the lymphatics before eventually returning to the circulation. This may be partly the result of tissue pressure and partly due to osmotic attraction of proteins in the lymphatic system. Normally, about 2–4 litres of lymph is drained into the venous system per day.

Oedema is defined as the swelling of the tissues, caused by an increased interstitial fluid.

- Accumulation of fluid in extracellular and extravascular compartments *mainly occurs in subcutaneous space.*
- *Venous obstruction reduces* the quantity of fluid reabsorbed at the venous end of the capillaries *resulting in oedema containing a large quantity of watery interstitial fluid.*
- *Lymphatic obstruction reduces* the clearance of interstitial protein along with water, and produces the oedema containing interstitial fluid with a high protein concentration.

The main difference between venous and lymphatic oedema is the protein concentration of the interstitial fluid and the rate of increased interstitial fluid formation in the latter.

So, estimation of protein content of oedema fluid gives a useful guide to the nature of the oedema. **In venous oedema** (and also in cardiac and hypoproteinimic oedema), the protein content is usually under 1.0 gm %, *while in* **lymphoedema** (and also in situations of increased capillary permeability following allergy and burns), the protein content is 1.5 gm % or more.

SURGICAL PATHOLOGY

Oedema from venous disorder

Following engorgement of the superficial venous system of the lower limb due to perforator vein incompetence or thrombosis of the deep venous system, the hydrostatic capillary pressure of blood exceeds its plasma osmotic pressure. As a result, the fluid of low protein content accumulates in the interstitial spaces causing *pitting oedema of the limb.*

Extensive oedema of the whole leg is seen after massive thrombosis of whole deep venous system of the leg, the iliofemoral veins (phlegmasia cerulea dolens), or the inferior vena cava. *Thrombosis of the inferior vena cava may*

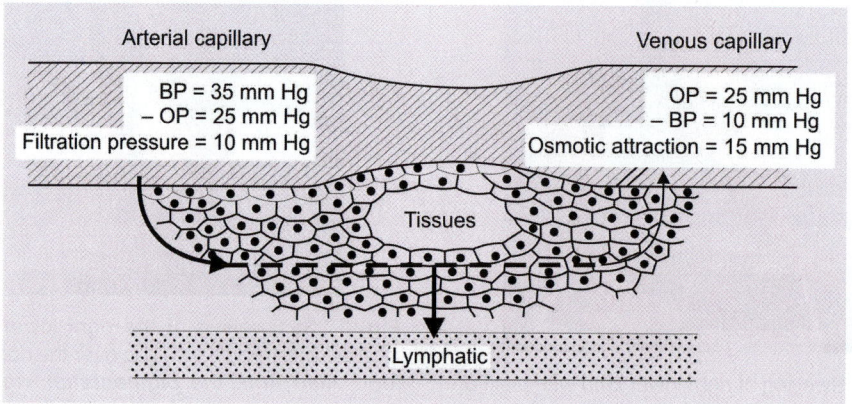

Fig. 17.4: Normal rate and direction of fluid movement.

occur either as an extension from the iliofemoral thrombosis, or in association with abdominal cancer, puerperal sepsis or other infective process. *The oedema then is usually bilateral.*

Oedema of lymphatic disorder (Lymphoedema)

Lymphoedema is interstitial oedema of lymphatic origin resulting in protein-rich fluid accumulation in the interstitial compartment – accumulation of fluid in extracellular and extravascular fluid compartments. *Mainly occurs in subcutaneous space.* It results from the obstruction of lymphatic flow due to fault in the lymphatic system. This fault may be primary or secondary.

Note

- About 2–4 litres of lymph is drained into the venous system per day.
- 40% of the lymph is formed within the skeletal muscles, *but the oedema rarely involves the muscle compartment.*
- *Lymphoedema fluid is classically high in protein content and deposited in the sub-cutaneous tissue.*

Severity of oedema

- *Mild oedema* – one or 2 cm increase in girth measurements between the non-involved and involved limbs.
- *Moderate oedema* >2 to 5 cm increase in girth measurements.
- *Severe oedema* – greater than 5 cm increase in girth measurements.

Causes of lymphoedema

- Congenital – primary lymphoedema
- Acquired – secondary lymphoedema

Primary lymphoedema

It occurs due to developmental defects of the sub-cutaneous lymphatic channels – congenital.

Lymphangiography demonstrates three types of defect in the lymphatic system.

1. *Aplasia:* Where the lymph channels are not formed at all.
2. *Hypoplasia:* Where the lymph channels are too small or too few.
3. *Varicose:* Where the lymph channels are dilated, tortuous and incompetent. When these varicosities extend into the pelvic and para-aortic lymph trunks, retrograde flow of intestinal chyle may occur into the groin and thigh causing chyle-filled vesicles to appear beneath the skin. If ruptures, leakage of milky lymph may occur.

Primary lymphoedema is described in three clinical subgroups according to the age of onset:

Lymphoedema congenita (10%): The swelling is either *present at birth or appears shortly afterwards.* When familial, the condition is known as *Milroy's disease. Patient presents with brawny lymphoedema of both the legs and genitalia*; may involve arms and face.

Lymphoedema praecox (75%): The swelling usually appears in childhood or adolescence. More common in females. It accounts for by far the largest groups.

Lymphoedema tarda (15%): The swelling appears in adult life, after the age of 30 years. Known as Meige's disease. A few are inherited as an autosomal dominant disease. It may involve arms also. *Lymph nodes are replaced by fibrofatty tissues.*

Note

Primary lymphoedema is mostly seen in adolescent girls.

Secondary lymphoedema

It is the most important and commonest cause of acquired lymphoedema and is *due to obstruction of previously normal lymphatic channels by a known agent such as:*

1. *Parasitic infestation*, e.g. *filariasis.* The *Wuchereria bancrofti* infects the lymphatics; a chronic and recurrent inflammatory reaction is set up with consequent lymphatic obstruction leading to gross lymphoedema. *It usually occurs in the lower limbs and genitalia. Common cause of lymphoedema worldwide. Prevalent in India, Africa and South America.*
2. *Malignancy* – commonest cause in developed countries due to:

(a) Advanced neoplastic infiltration of the lymph nodes causes lymphatic blockage, e.g. *brawny arm or carcinoma en cuirasse in breast carcinoma.*
(b) Postirradiation fibrosis.
3. *Trauma or iatrogenic: Following extensive surgical procedures*, e.g. after block dissection of the ilioinguinal, axillary or neck nodes where extensive removal of the lymphatics is performed. This may often be seen in late oedema of the arm after radical mastectomy, or late oedema of the limbs after radical surgery in malignant melanoma.
4. *Inflammation,* e.g.
   • repeated attacks of streptococcal cellulitis may cause fibrosis of lymphatic vessels, common in those who go about barefoot;
   • lymphogranuloma inguinale following sexual/venereal infection;
   • tuberculosis or fungal infection.

Sequence of events in lymphoedema

In the early stage, whatever may be the cause, following obstruction, the lymphatic vessels fail to remove the protein molecules and larger particles adequately from the tissues. As a result, there is an increase in tissue colloidal osmotic pressure which increases filtration of fluid across the capillary membrane and decreases reabsorption so that fluid of higher protein content accumulates in the interstitial space *leading to soft pitting oedema.*

In the second stage, as the process continues and becomes chronic, the skin and subcutaneous tissues become thickened from fibrous tissue replacement and *thus pitting is lost.*

In the third or more advanced stage, as the chronicity persists, there is excessive subcutaneous fibrosis and scarring leading to induration. *The swollen limb becomes firm to hard in consistency with thickened skin with no pitting oedema. Significant pain is unusual at any stage.*

Lymphangitis and cellulitis are common complications of L. praecox but prophylactic antibiotics are not indicated routinely.

Miscellaneous causes

Adiposis dolorosa

There is abnormal and painful accumulation of fat particularly around the thigh, buttocks and ankles.

Arteriovenous fistula (see Chapter 14)

Congenital variety may be localised or diffuse. The diffuse variety is often associated with a giant swollen limb, varicose veins and varicose lymphatics, superficial angiomata in the adolescent (Fig. 14.7).

Traumatic fistula occurs following penetrating injuries. The limb gradually swells and becomes associated with varicose vein formation.

Erythrocyanosis frigida

This condition is *due to hypoplastic microcirculation of the skin arterioles,* but the main blood vessels remain patent. *The condition is almost entirely confined to female adolescents.* Following exposure to cold, the skin of the ankles and legs becomes discoloured with patches of deep cyanosis alternating with reddened areas. *The legs become permanently swollen with thickened subcutaneous tissue, and subcutaneous fat necrosis may result in the formation of hard and tender nodules.* Occasionally the nodules break down, *leaving superficial ulcers which are very painful.*

But the peripheral pulses are palpable.

Diffuse neurofibromatosis

This condition is associated with von Recklinghausen's disease; other areas of the body may be involved. *Pigmented cafe au lait spots* may be noted (Figs 17.1 to 17.3).

Lipedema

A rare condition characterised by *diffuse nonpitting enlargement of subcutaneous tissue of both the extremities seen in patients with obesity and hypothyroidism (myxoedema).*

Chronic venous oedema of the lower limb

Usually resolves within few days of bed rest in elevation and exercises and with oral diuretics.

Lymphangioma

Does not resolve with bed rest. Small lymphatic vesicles may be observed with magnifying glass.

Commonest causes of lymphoedema in developed countries

- Advanced neoplastic infiltration of the lymph nodes and lymphatic vessels causing lymphatic blockage, e.g. brawny arm or cancer-en-cuirasse in breast cancer.
- Postoperative and/or postirradiation fibrosis of lymphatic vessels.

EXAMINATION OF LOWER LIMB OEDEMA

- Whether the leg oedema is *unilateral or bilateral*.
- *Any sign of overlying inflammation over the limb* – thin, red and tender streaks over the skin – suggestive of lymphangitis.
- *Oedema* – pitting or non-pitting after fingertip pressure.

  Stemmer's sign: Try to pinch and lift a skin fold at the base of the second toe in foot (or middle finger in hand) – *if you can pinch or lift the skin, Stemmer's sign is negative*; if you cannot, the sign is positive due to oedema.
- Whether the swelling is *affecting the entire limb* or *localised to the leg, ankle region and/or affecting the toes* (squaring of toes)
  – *Ankle region* is affected in DVT.
  – *Entire limb* is affected in iliac vein thrombosis: Diffuse neurofibromatosis.
  – *Leg, ankle and toes* – filariasis.
- Whether the skin is normal-looking or hyper-keratotic with warty nodules and any vesicular changes – *the hyperkeratotic skin is seen in filarial lymphoedema.*
- Examination of draining lymph nodes:
  – The lymph nodes are enlarged, hard and non-tender along with oedema limb in secondary lymphadenopathy or malignancy.
  – Lymph nodes may be enlarged and tender in presence of distal infection.
  – *Lymph nodes are not enlarged in DVT.*
- Examine the genitalia – scrotum and penis to rule out oedema of either or both and to rule out hydrocele – *both are seen in filariasis.*

- *In female*, mons pubis and labia majora may be involved.
- Examine both breasts in females to rule out lymphatic oedema of the skin. *The glandular tissue of breast itself is not involved.*

DIAGNOSIS

The cause of swelling of the leg can be established by careful history and physical examination. The surgeon is more concerned with the peripheral causes.

Is the swelling central in origin?

Oedema of central origin is usually generalised and *the leg swellings are bilateral and pitting in nature*. Central causes must be excluded by careful history and physical examination: Heart failure, cirrhosis of liver, nephrotic syndrome, venous insufficiency.

Is the swelling unilateral in distribution?

Unilateral swelling of the leg usually indicates a local cause, *which is of venous or lymphatic origin in the majority of cases*; venous pathology is most common.

Is there any history of pain during development of swelling?

- Oedema of central origin or lymphoedema is usually painless.
- Oedema of venous origin is usually painful.

Is the swelling venous or lymphatic in origin?

I. Venous origin

(a) History of deep vein thrombosis with the development of *a painful swollen leg* following operation, prolonged confinement to bed or pregnancy.

(b) History of massive deep vein thrombosis (*phlegmasia cerulea dolens*) with the development of *acute, severe pain over most of the limb in association with marked shock*, rapidly developing extensive oedema, *cyanosis, turgid* (swollen and distended) *subcutaneous veins and superficial skin ulceration.*

(c) Occasionally, deep vein thrombosis may occur without any apparent reason; *the hidden malignancy or the prolonged intake of contraceptive pill* may be considered as possible predisposing factors.

(d) There may be presence of varicose veins, signs of perforator incompetence like blowouts, fascial pits, ankle flare, varicose dermatitis, skin pigmentation, varicose ulcer.

(e) *There may be presence of pitting oedema in the early stage.* The oedema is greatest at the legs and ankle *with sparing of the foot.* The oedema becomes worse after prolonged dependency. *The oedema reduces promptly to overnight elevation of the limbs.*

The oedema may become *non-pitting* when the swelling becomes chronic and associated with skin and subcutaneous tissue thickening.

II. Lymphatic origin

The patient presents with a history of slowly progressive swelling of the limb with or without the affection of genitalia. *The swelling is rarely painful at any stage.*

The skin of a lymphoedematous limb remains remarkably healthy for many years apart from recurrent attacks of cellulitis. *Skin pigmentation, skin ulceration are usually absent.*

Oedema is pitting in the early stage but becomes non-pitting in the chronic stage when skin and subcutaneous tissue thickening is present. Eventually deformity, i.e. *elephantiasis* is developed.

(a) **Primary lymphoedema:** *It is due to developmental anomalies of lymphatics.* It affects commonly female. There may be *family history* in 20% cases (*Milroy's disease*). The swelling is *unilateral in 50% cases.* Usually, the swelling is of gradual onset and *becomes worse in warm weather. In congenital lymphoedema the swelling is either present at birth or appears very shortly afterwards.* Primary lymphoedema is of three types:

• Lymphoedema congenita *present at birth or appears shortly afterwards – Milroy's disease*
• Lymphoedema praecox *presenting at puberty*
• Lymphoedema tarda *presenting in adulthood*

All three types are much *more common in females* – mostly seen in adolescent girls. There may be family history in 20% cases. *Main complaint of the patient is cosmetic appearance.*

When the swelling persists for many years, hyperkeratotic, horny and vesicular changes may occur which may lead to ulceration and discharge of lymph. In the rare cases of lymphoedema, vesicles of milky fluid may appear due to chylous reflux.

The lymph nodes draining the oedematous area will not be enlarged in primary lymphoedema.

(b) **Secondary or acquired lymphoedema:** The swelling is of rapid onset and *unilateral in distribution.* Most often there is an obvious cause for its occurrence, e.g. trauma, infection, inflammation, scar mark due to groin dissection, history of radiotherapy, or malignant infiltration.

Lymphoedema and oedema secondary to iliofemoral thrombosis are very often secondary to malignant disease.

So, a thorough examination of the lymph nodes in the groin and other areas, inspection of the skin of the lower half of the body, a full examination of the abdomen to see any lump or enlarged nodes, inspection and palpation of genitalia, e.g. testes, rectal and vaginal examination are essential to exclude secondary causes.

Lymphoedema secondary to filariasis: The swelling is solid in onset and involves the foot and ankle first and then involves the leg. Very common in South India. Caused by the nematode *Wuchereria bancrofti* (*see* chapter on filariasis).

The lymph nodes draining the oedematous area will not be enlarged in primary lymphoedema, but may be enlarged and hard if they are infiltrated with malignancy.

It must be stressed that one should examine the whole patient, particularly the heart, abdomen, veins of the limb and lymph nodes. *One should exclude central causes of oedema,* e.g. the cardiac and renal causes of oedema before considering the local causes, venous disorder or lymphoedema.

Complications of lymphoedema

Chronically lymphoedematous limb is pre-disposed to:

1. *Thickening of the skin.*
2. *Recurrent soft tissue infection* – most common complication of both primary and secondary lymphoedema is *erysipelas, acute streptococcal bacterial infection of the deep dermis with lymphatic spread.*

   Cellulitis may occur concurrently in lymphoedema because of the pooling rich lymph fluid which makes it easier for the patient to develop infection.
3. Difficulty in movements.
4. Cosmetically ugly.

Is the swelling arteriovenous in origin?

On rare occasions, when central and local causes of oedema are excluded, an arteriovenous fistula may have to be considered. (*See* Chapter on aneurysm).

INVESTIGATIONS

1. Eosinophilia may be seen in filarial infestations.
2. Midnight blood thick smear for microfilaria into the peripheral circulation during the patient's sleep hours is typical diagnostic for filariasis.

When the diagnosis is still dubious some special tests may be helpful.

1. *Venography:* The injection of radio-opaque dye into an ankle vein, femoral vein, or intra-osseous vein at iliac crest will indicate the site and extent of a thrombotic plaque.
2. *Arteriography:* When arteriovenous fistula formation is suspected.
3. *Duplex ultrasound,* a modality that combines Doppler ultrasound and colour flow imaging, is useful for diagnosis of DVT, and arterio-venous fistula.
4. *Lymphangiography:* Dorsal foot lymphatics are visualised following injection of a diffusible dye known as patent Blue V into the interdigital web spaces, 0.2 ml being injected into each space. Then a suitable lymphatic trunk at the dorsum of the foot is exposed under general anaesthesia and injected with radio-opaque solution such as ethiodol and then multiple X-rays are taken over the next 24 hours to outline the nature of the lower limb and abdominal lymphatics and lymph nodes.

   Recently, isotope lymphangiography using radio-labelled (Technitium 99^m) colloid injection in the web space is used for functional assessment of the lymphatic system. Sensitivity and specificity: 92% and 100%, respectively.
5. More recently, high resolution ultrasound scan, CT scan or MRI have replaced lymph-angiography to detect malignant lymph nodes. *MRI is also best for distinguishing between venous and lymphatic causes of a swollen limb.*

TREATMENT

Treatment of venous disorder

Conservative

It should be followed in every case.

1. *Elevation:* Elevation of the limb helps to reduce the swelling. In the beginning it should be prolonged and continuous and when the patient is allowed out of bed he should arrange the intermittent elevation of the leg once during the day, and at bedtime. He should avoid prolonged sitting or standing and should rest his legs upon a chair whenever he sits. While in elevation the patient should perform active movements and exercises of the foot and limb.

   Bed rest with elevated legs helps in simple lymphatic drainage.
2. *Elastic stockings:* Patients should wear *well-fitted elastic stockings* at all times, except when in bed. It helps in reducing the oedema, and counteracts the high venous pressure which develops during exercise. In absence of elastic stockings, crepe bandage may be applied firmly.

3. *Massage:* Massage in a *centripetal direction*, gently and firmly with lanolin or olive oil helps to push the fluid out of the subcutaneous tissue and keeps the skin and subcutaneous tissue soft.
4. *Anticoagulant therapy.*
5. *Fibrinolytic therapy,* if anticoagulants are contraindicated.
6. *Diuretics* may be used intermittently.
7. Compression stockings should provide a pressure between 40 to 60 mm of Hg at the ankle.
8. *MLLB (multilayer lymphoedema bandaging):* Non-elastic MLLB for severe cases and compression type for mild cases.
9. In presence of both streptococcal and staphylococcal infections, flucloxacillin may also be added.

Surgery

When the conservative regimens fail to improve the oedema:

1. *If seen in the early stage (i.e. within 48 hours of onset),* in addition to above measures some advocate thrombectomy in deep vein thrombosis preceded by duplex ultrasound.
2. *If the obstruction is very short*, the obstructed portion can sometimes be resected followed by end-to-end anastomosis.
3. *Palma's operation (Venous bypass on the opposite side):* Localised obstructions in the iliac vein can be bypassed in which the long saphenous vein of the healthy leg is rerouted subcutaneously across the pubis and anastomosed to a vein below the block in iliac vein. Success rate is about 90%.
4. *Trellis procedure:* Deep vein thrombosis may be treated where under catheter guidance the clot is dissolved and patency of the vessel is restored.

Treatment of lymphoedema

Conservative

It should be followed in every case: Both primary and secondary lymphoedema.

- Elevation and exercises
- Elastic stockings
- Massage – manual lymphatic drainage

1. Elevation of the limb at night by raising the foot end of the bed by 12 inches block, above the level of the heart.
2. Exercises of the foot and legs on hourly basis during waking hours.
3. Intermittent pneumatic compression devices are also available to control moderate lymphoedema but it causes sleep disturbance.
4. High quality custom made compression garments or elastic stockings with a pressure gradient of 40 to 60 mm Hg at the ankles should be worn by the patient, preferably at all times except when the limbs are elevated above the heart.
5. *MLD (Manual lymphatic drainage):* Massage with the leg elevated, in centripetal direction, helps to push the protein-rich fluid of the subcutaneous space. It also stimulates lymphangion contraction. This keeps the skin and subcutaneous tissues soft.
6. *MLLB (Multilayered lymphoedema bandage)* helps to reduce oedema. Non-elastic MLLB for severe cases and compression type for mild cases.
7. Exercises during waking hours also help to reduce the swelling by enhancing both lymphatics and venous return. It also helps to maintain joints mobility.
8. Great care of the skin hygiene of the affected part:
   (a) *Regular cleaning* preferably with hexachlorophene soap or Savlon solution.
   (b) Many of these patients have tinea pedis; so, the regular use of *fungicidal ointment* helps to reduce the incidence of cellulitis. In bad cases, oral griseofulvin may be added, if required.
   (c) *Use of antibiotics*, if bacterial infection persists. Mostly the organisms are *Streptococcus*, so, penicillin, or erythromycin in penicillin-sensitive or resistant cases, is preferred.
   (d) *Hyperkeratosis treated by keratolytic agents such as 5% salicylic acid.* Liquid paraffin with mixture of camphor may also be applied over the dry skin.
9. *Diuretics may be used intermittently.*

10. *Diethylcarbamazine (Hetrazen or Benoside)* destroys the filarial parasite but does not reverse the lymph oedema although there may be some regression.
11. *Benzopyrones (e.g. Coumarin)* are being used in USA and Europe. *They are thought to reduce lymphoedema* through stimulation of peristalsis and pumping action of the collecting lymphatics. Benzopyrones have no anticoagulant action.
12. *Oxerutins* improve microcirculatory perfusion and reduce erythrocyte and platelet aggregation. It also stimulates proteolysis to keep the local tissues soft.
13. *Warfarin,* it acts by enhancing macrophage activity and extralymphatic absorption of interstitial fluid and thus helps in reducing lymphoedema.

Surgery

Indication

1. Gross swelling not responding to conservative measures. *Gross swelling incapacitate the individual due to the weight and bulk of the limb causing limitation of movements.*
2. Cosmetic reasons.
3. Chronic, neglected cases with recurrent cellulitis.

Types

- Direct
- Indirect.

Direct surgery

Direct attack to the lymphatic system is rarely performed. Only in a few cases where lymphangiography shows reflux of chyle downwards from the abdominal lymphatics to those of the leg, the reflux can be reduced by ligature and division of the dilated lymphatics *which are usually approached in the inguinal region.*

Indirect surgery

(a) Reducing or excisional operations.
(b) Reconstructive operations to provide new lymphatic pathways.
(c) Amputation.

Reducing operations

There are three types of reducing operations available to reduce limb size.

1. *Partial subcutaneous tissue excision (Homans):* In this operation a long skin flap is reflected along the axis of the limb and *the subcutaneous tissues are excised from one half of the limb.* The skin is closed with simple suture (Fig. 17.5).

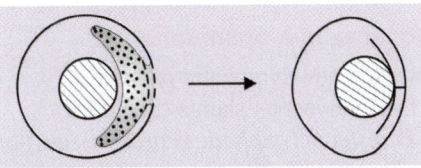

Fig. 17.5: Partial subcutaneous tissue excision (Homans). Reducing operations.

2. *Excision plus buried dermis flap (Thompson):* Also known as Swiss roll operation. This is an extension of the partial excisional procedure in which one of the skin flaps is shaved of its superficial layers of epidermis and then buried deep to the deep fascia. In this way new connections would develop between the dermal lymphatic plexus and the deep lymphatics (Fig. 17.6).

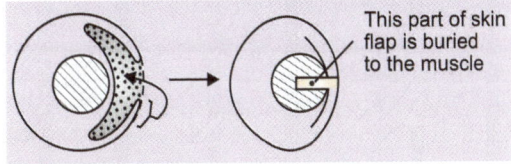

This part of skin flap is buried to the muscle

Fig. 17.6: Excision plus buried dermis flap (Thompson).

No. 1 and 2 procedures can be repeated on the other half of the same limb 3 months later.

3. *Total excision of grossly oedematous tissue (Charles):* This consists of a total excision of the skin and the whole of the oedematous subcutaneous tissue down to the deep fascia *followed by resurfacing of the raw area with split skin grafts.* The skin grafts could be taken either from the healthy part of the body or from the excised skin. This is the most effective operation when there is gross

oedema *but the skin must be healthy and non-infected. The healthy skin is reused for grafting* (Fig. 17.7).

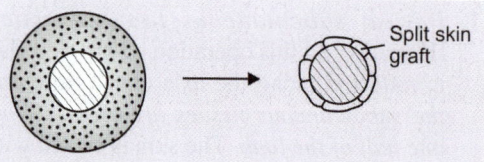

Fig. 17.7: Total excision and skin grafting (Charles).

Reconstructive operations

To provide new lymphatic pathways:
1. Lymphovenous shunts (Fig. 17.8).
2. *Transfer of lymphatic bearing tissue (portion of greater omentum) – omental transposition* – into the effected limb with hypoplastic and fibrotic distal lymphatic vessels in patients with primary lymphoedema.
3. *Alternatively, a segment of ileum is disconnected* from the rest of the bowel and stripped of its mucosa. Then this denuded ileum is mobilised and sutured onto the cut surface of the residual ilioinguinal nodes *in an attempt to bridge the lower extremity with mesenteric lymph nodes.*

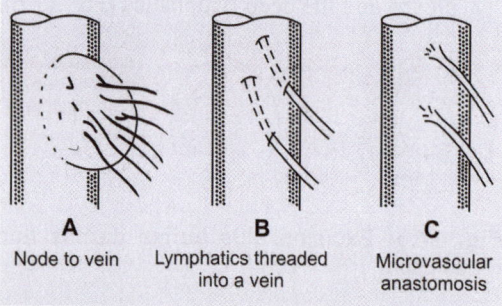

A	B	C
Node to vein	Lymphatics threaded into a vein	Microvascular anastomosis

Figs 17.8 A to C: Methods of lymphovenous shunts.

Lymphovenous shunts

The lymphovenous shunts are *mostly tried for secondary lymphoedema.* The lymphatics can be joined to a vein in three ways:
1. By anastomosing a transected lymph node to a large vein (Fig. 17.8A).
2. By threading lymphatics into a vein (Fig. 17.8B).

3. By microsurgical anastomosis of the dilated lymphatics to a vein (Fig. 17.8C).

But none of these operations are satisfactory.

Amputations

May be required rarely for severe lymphoedema with skin ulceration and leakage of lymph, particularly when it incapacitates the patient and/or leads to a grotesque look of the limb.

The patient becomes movable by using crutch to earn his/her livelihood.

ARTERIOVENOUS FISTULA

See Chapter 14.

Note

Causes of lymphoedema can be remembered by the mnemonics APLASIA.

A   Aplasia or hypoplasia of the nodes/lymph vessels.

P   Parasitic infestation (filarial).

L   Lymphatic obstruction following malignant lymph node involvement.

A   Altered lymph motility.

S   Surgical excision of lymph nodes enlarged due to metastasis from primary lesion.

I   Inflammatory or infective.

A   After radiotherapy of the primary lesion and/or lymph drainage area.

Note

Clinical classification of lymphoedema

Subclinical   No clinical evidence of oedema. Lymphatic changes only on histopathological examination.

Grade I   Pitting oedema which mostly disappears on limb elevation.

Grade II   Non-pitting oedema *with thickening of skin only* which never disappears.

Grade III   Non-pitting oedema *with skin changes* – hyperkeratosis, warty, horny and vesicular changes, e.g. filariasis: *Stage of elephantiasis.* Patient is unable to move around independently due to enormous size of the swelling and heaviness.

Note

Risk factors for oedema leg

- Filariasis.
- Limb surgery, e.g. varicose vein operation.
- Trauma: Bleeding in closed compartment – *compartment syndrome*.
- Deep vein thrombosis (DVT).
- Obesity.
- Family history.
- Air travel for long distance.
- Prolonged operation – more than 2 hours period, particularly in elderly obese patients may lead to DVT.

Note

Malignancies associated with lymphoedema

Carcinoma

- Squamous cell carcinoma
- Malignant melanoma
- Basal cell carcinoma – rare

Sarcoma

- Lymphoma
- Lymphoangiosarcoma
- Kaposi's sarcoma
- Malignant fibrous histiocytoma
- Liposarcoma

Note

Lymphangiosarcoma (dangerous complication of lymphoedema): Very rare but a fatal condition. Originally described for postmastectomy and/or postradiotherapy upper limb oedema following treatment of carcinoma breast – *Stewart-Treves syndrome*. It is suggested that *lymphoedema leads to impairment of immune surveillance* which predisposes to other types of malignancy.

Filariasis and its Surgical Manifestations

Filariasis is a tropical disease *prevalent in the southern and eastern States of India* as well as the other tropical coastal areas of the world.

It is caused by the infestation with the parasite, Wuchereria bancrofti or Brugia malayi. It is a nematode transmitted to human beings by a mosquito bite (*Culex fatigans*).

Wuchereria bancrofti: This parasite passes its life cycle in two hosts – *man and mosquito.* Man is the definitive host; mosquito is the intermediate host for continuation of the life cycle of the parasite. *The stages are:*

1. Adult filariae both male and female are found in the lymphatic system of man (definitive host).
2. After sporulation, the females die and innumerable embryos or microfilariae are produced.
3. These microfilariae enter the peripheral blood particularly at night (*nocturnal periodicity*) where they can live for a considerable time but *do not undergo any metamorphosis* until they pass through the mosquito again.
4. When a female mosquito bites an individual, it sucks in the microfilariae from the peripheral blood through the proboscis sheath.

5. These microfilariae in the mosquito undergo further development and maturation, but they are still sexually immature.
6. These sexually immature microfilariae again enter a human by the bite of the infested mosquito and ultimately reach his lymphatic system where they settle down. Sexual maturity of the worms then occurs and after fertilisation, the microfilariae enter the blood stream. Ultimately microfilariae reach the lymphatic system where they settle down. *The most favourite site for this settling is the inguinoscrotal region.* In the lymphatic system the microfilariae begin to grow into adult forms and again the cycle continues.

Pathological changes

The pathological changes of filariasis are brought about by the adult filariae, living or dead. The microfilariae usually do not produce any pathological changes.

The changes may be classified into two parts – *lymphangitis* and *lymphatic obstruction.*

Causes of lymphangitis

1. Mechanical factor – *irritation and blockage of the lymphatic system* due to the movements of the adult filariae along the

lymphatic system causing spasm leading to obstruction of lymph flow.

2. Allergic factor – *due to helminthic toxins* which are liberated in three ways:
   (a) Liberation of toxins by the fertilised females during parturition.
   (b) Liberation of toxins from the dead worms undergoing degeneration.
   (c) Sometimes in highly reacting individuals, the mild toxins liberated by the microfilariae can produce some allergic reaction.
3. Secondary infection – *due to the associated superadded bacterial infection*, usually streptococci, *often acts as an additional factor*, particularly in presence of lymphatic stasis.

So, the helminthic toxins liberated give rise to foreign body reaction. Clinically this is manifested by *transient attacks of lymphangitis*, which clinically presents with *high grade fever, with chills and rigors* (cf. malaria), and *red streak in the scrotum. Inguinal lymph nodes become swollen and tender.*

Retroperitoneal lymphangitis may produce acute abdominal pain.

Effects of recurrent lymphangitis

1. Proliferation of endothelium of lymphatics and thereby causing occlusion of the lumen – *obliterative endolymphangitis.*
2. *Fibrosis of the lymph vessels* in varying degrees. As a result of fibrosis adult filariae are imprisoned in the lymph nodes and in the lymph vessels causing obstruction: *mainly inguinal lymph nodes are involved.*

Causes of lymphatic obstruction

1. *Mechanical factor:* Imprisonment of the adult filariae, both living and dead, in the lymph nodes and lymph vessels. *This will produce further foreign body reaction leading to further fibrosis and obstruction.*
2. *Sclerosing lymphangitis* leading to fibrosis of the lymph nodes and lymph vessels *resulting in lymphatic obstruction.*

Effects of lymphatic obstruction

I. The lymphatic obstruction will lead to dilatation, elongation and tortuosity of the lymphatic systems giving rise to:

1. *Lymph varix or lymphangiectasis:* Dilatations of the lymph vessels.
2. *Lymphadenovarix.*
3. *Lymph scrotum:* Dilatation and tortuosity of the cutaneous lymphatics of the scrotum.
4. *Hydrocele* due to obstruction of lymphatics there is effusion into the tunica vaginalis.

II. Lymphatic obstruction along with subsequent fibrosis will lead to a condition known as '*elephantiasis*'.

Changes of elephantiasis are brought about in the following way.

Recurrent lymphangitis
↓
Obstruction of lymphatic system
↓
Stagnation of fluid rich in protein in the subcutaneous tissues

This will cause an increase in the tissue colloidal osmotic pressure which increases filtration of fluid across the capillary membrane and decreases reabsorption with the result *that fluid of a high protein content collects in the subcutaneous tissues* – the affected part becomes swollen, oedematous, and *initially pits on pressure.* When the attack subsides the swelling is reduced to some extent with proper treatment – drugs, bed rest and exercises in elevation, *but the normality is seldom attained.*

The presence of deep fascia prevents involvement of the deep muscles of the limb underneath.

With subsequent attacks, the swelling further increases in size and becomes more firm due to excessive growth of connective tissue as a result of stimulation by the protein in fluid. *The lymph stasis provides the suitable nourishment for the luxurious growth of the fibroblasts.* The subcutaneous tissue is replaced by fibrous tissue and lymph-logged gelatinous tissue known as *blubbery tissue* (blubber means jellyfish). *Ultimately, firm, non-yielding and non-pitting swelling is produced.*

The skin becomes enormously thickened, tough and stiff with abundant fibrosis under it. The surface of the *skin becomes uneven and rugose with hyperkeratotic, horny or warty growth.* Chronic eczema, fungal infections of the skin (dermatophytosis) and nail (onycho-mycosis), *fissuring*, *verrucae* and *papillae* (warts) are frequently seen in advanced disease *leading to grotesque appearance and looks like the skin of an elephant* (hence the name, **elephantiasis**). *The dorsum of the foot is characteristically swollen like buffalo hump. The toes become thick and square in shape.*

In between there may be vesicular changes – when vesicles rupture, milky lymph exudes. There is also loss of skin appendages, e.g. *scanty hairs*.

Eventually necrosis and ulceration develop over the swelling due to strangulation of blood supply. These ulcers refuse to heal and provide favourite site for breeding of maggots.

Common sites of involvement of filariasis:
1. Scrotum
2. Penis – may lead to ramhorn penis
3. Lower limb – usually unilateral; *commonly leg, foot and toes*
4. Vulva
5. Arms.
6. Breast – *but the glandular tissue of breast remains unaffected*

Vulva, arms and breast are rarely involved.

The scrotum and the lower limb are the common sites for filariasis probably because of the following reasons:
(a) Great laxity of the subcutaneous tissue and the dependent position of the scrotum.
(b) Dependent position of the lower limb.
(c) *The microfilariae and adult filariae have special predilection for their settlement to the lymphatics of the inguinoscrotal region.*

III. Obstruction and rupture of lymph vessels: Lymphatic obstruction leads to dilatation of the lymph vessels and when the tension is high, they rupture. *Either chyle or lymph escapes* depending on whether the obstruction is situated above or below the cisterna chyle. The results are:

1. Chyle may come out with urine – *chyluria*.
2. Chyle may come out with faeces – *chylous diarrhoea*.
3. Chyle may collect in different serous cavities of the body such as:
   (i) tunica vaginalis – *chylocele*
   (ii) peritoneal cavity – *chylous ascites*
   (iii) pleural cavity – *chylothorax*.

Note

Chyle is milky body fluid consisting of lymph and emulsified fats formed in the small intestine during digestion of foods and taken up by lymph vessels.

Note

Filarial fever: Chills and rigors mostly at night associated with signs of inflammation and tenderness of target organs such as spermatic cord, epididymis and scrotal skin.

Complications of filariasis

1. Chronic lymphadenitis
2. Chronic epididymo-orchitis
3. Hydrocele – 40% hydroceles are of filarial origin
4. Filarial scrotum
5. Elephantiasis
6. Chyluria ⎤
7. Chylous diarrhoea ⎪ Due to rupture of
8. Chylous ascites ⎪ dilated lymphatic
9. Chylothorax ⎦ vessels

▌ FILARIASIS OF THE SCROTUM

Diagnostic criteria

More common in South India and Odisha (coastal zone).

1. In the early stage, the patient may come with scrotal swelling with pitting oedema, and in advanced case present with solid oedema.
2. *The skin is thickened, rough, rugose (wrinkled and corrugated), fissured and hyperkeratotic. There is loss of hairs.* The thickening commences at the most dependent part of the scrotum and extends upwards. In an established case the thickening is maximum

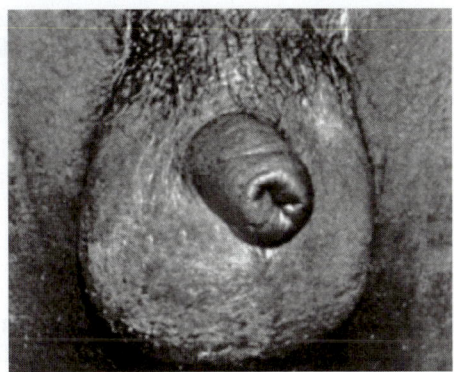

Fig. 18.1: Early stage filarial scrotum and penis with hypertrophied prepuce.

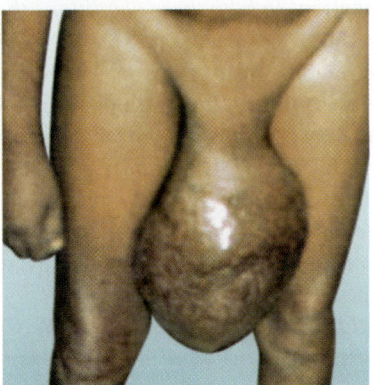

Fig. 18.2: Filarial scrotum with buried penis. (*Courtesy:* Dr Yogesh Salphale, D Ortho)

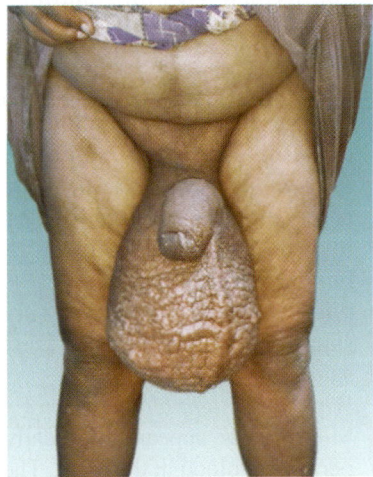

Fig. 18.3: Filarial scrotum with thickened corrugated scrotal skin and also thickened penile skin.

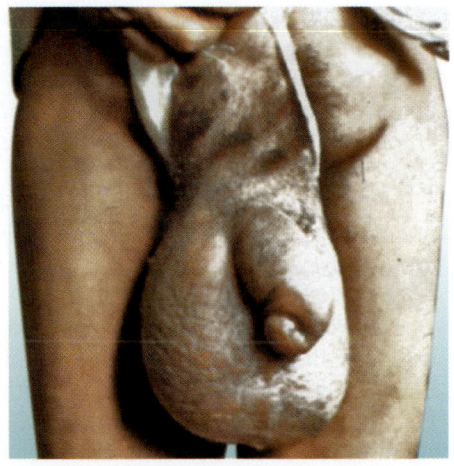

Fig. 18.4: Filarial scrotum with ramhorn penis.

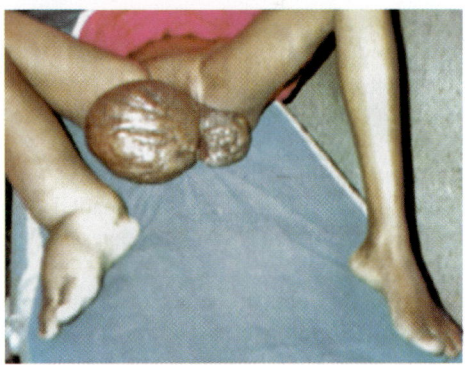

Fig. 18.5: Filariasis involving the labia majora right side. Also note the lymphoedema right leg. This patient had the excision of the filarial swelling of the left labia majora 5 years ago. (*Courtesy:* Dr Subrata Biswas, MD)

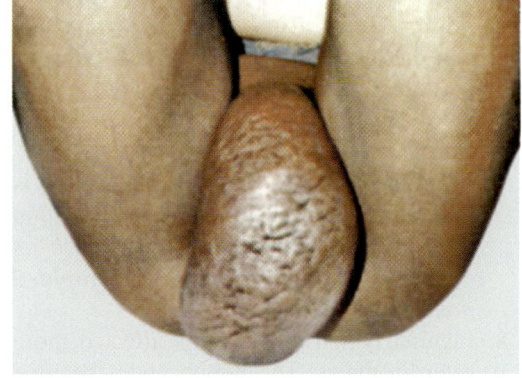

Fig. 18.6: Filariasis involving the right labia majora.

at the bottom (dependent position) and minimum at the root of the scrotum.

3. Over the surface of the skin there may be appearance of lymph filled *vesicular eruptions* which may ulcerate and discharge clear lymph or *milky lymph*.

Between the hypertrophied skin and testis, often with a hydrocele, *remains a thick layer of vascularised adipose tissue (fat) under the skin which feels as blubber*.

4. Due to excessive thickening with unyielding nature of the scrotal wall it is sometimes impossible to palpate the contents within, viz., testis, epididymis, spermatic cord, etc.

5. At the root of the scrotum and over the inguinal canal – *The spermatic cord is thickened* on palpation and may be tender – funiculitis.

Funiculitis can progress to involve the globus major of the epididymis *leading to epididymitis and obliteration of the sulcus between the testis and the epididymis – it is typical of filariasis* (cf. *tuberculosis*, where the epididymis is craggy and beaded with a sinus or cold abscess on the posterior aspect of scrotum).

6. A hydrocele is usually associated, *but fluctuation and transillumination are difficult to elicit* through the thickened skin and milky fluid in the tunica vaginalis sac.

7. The penis may sometimes be involved and associated with filariasis of the scrotum. *The skin and subcutaneous tissue of the penis become hypertrophied.*

Sometimes *the penis is enormously thickened and distorted* owing to unequal contraction of the hypertrophied fibrous tissue and fascia around the penis. Such a swollen and distorted penis is called '**Ramhorn penis**' (Fig. 18.4).

At other times, the penis, being healthy, is buried either completely or partially within the hypertrophied scrotal mass, *when its orifice is indicated by the hypertrophied prepuce* (Figs 18.1 and 18.2).

8. Inguinal lymph nodes may be affected, more often in males. The lymph nodes become enlarged and tender.

9. *The epididymo-orchitis, funiculitis or acute inguinal lymphadenitis* with pain and tenderness often precedes the development of elephantiasis.

10. There may be associated involvement of the lower limb and vulva or breast in female (Figs 18.5 and 18.6).

11. *History of filarial fever is present.*

Characteristics of filarial fever

(a) *Periodic in nature,* i.e. filarial inflammation occurring on full and new moon (not every full and new moon).

(b) *Onset:* Sudden with chill and rigor: *More at night* (cf. malarial fever, fever of urinary tract infection: *In both these conditions there will be absence of swelling and tenderness* of the spermatic cord).

(c) *Temperature:* Often high (103°F to 104°F) and may continue for several days (usually 3 to 5 days). *The temperature comes down by crisis with profuse sweating.*

(d) *Presence of toxic features:* Tachycardia, flushed face, dry coated tongue, severe headache and loss of appetite.

(e) *Simultaneously there may be associated pain, swelling and tenderness of the spermatic cord and scrotum* (these features also help in differentiation from malarial fever and urinary tract infection). There is also an *associated inflammation of the inguinoscrotal lymph nodes.*

Investigations

1. (a) Routine blood examination reveals a transient leucocytosis *with an increase of eosinophils. Eosinophilia (5 to 15%)* is very often noticed in early cases. There may be no eosinophilia in cases of lymphatic obstruction.

   (b) *Midnight blood for microfilariae:* Thick smear of peripheral blood in Leishman's stain.

   Why is midnight blood drawn?
   Microfilariae appear periodically in the peripheral blood in the night. The cause is not known definitely. The probable explanations are:

(i) It is due to night-biting habit of the vector (*Culex fatigans*).

(ii) It is the periodic and cyclical emptying of the gravid uterus of matured adult worm at night.

(iii) It is the habit of the person concerned who sleeps at night when mosquito bite cannot be felt.

(iv) Sunlight repels the microfilariae (not accepted by all).

2. Detection of microfilariae in the hydrocele fluid or in the exudate of lymph varix.

3. Biopsy of the lymph nodes may reveal adult filaria within them – not done routinely.

4. Immunological test with *D. immitis* antigen and complement fixation test – little value.

Treatment

The treatment of choice is surgery. The patient should, however, be prepared preoperatively.

Preoperative treatment

General:

(a) A course of specific antifilarial drug – diethylcarbamazine citrate (DEC) – *hetrazan* or *benocide forte*.

Dose: 6 mg per kg of body weight in three equal doses.

(i) Hetrazen – 2 tablets thrice daily for 3 weeks.

(ii) Benocide forte – 1 tablet thrice daily for 3 weeks.

During the carbamazine therapy *an anti-allergic drug should be given* to combat any allergic reaction caused by the dead micro-filariae.

(b) Antibiotics (benzathine penicillin): If necessary (when routine blood shows poly-morph nuclear leucocytosis also) for combating concurrent streptococcal infection.

(c) Non-specific protein therapy to increase the immunity: Sterodin or milk injection.

(d) Antipyretic, anti-inflammatory and anti-histaminics.

(e) Benzopyrines (e.g. coumarin). Oxerutins, suramin and warfarin may also be used in persistent cases. Suramin is nephrotoxic.

Local:

Treatment of the skin condition, e.g. if lymphoria is present: *Local dressing with lotio Goulard or lotio Acriflavin* (1 in 4,000).

Surgery

Principles of surgery

1. Excision of the hypertrophied and oedematous scrotal and/or penile skin in a ramhorn penis and all the subcutaneous blubbery tissue.

2. Resurfacing of the decorticated penis with skin grafting.

3. Management of the exteriorised testes.

Problems of surgery

1. *Increase in size with increase in vascularity: blood transfusion should be arranged to combat blood loss during operation.*

2. *Injury to urethra* can be avoided by passing Foley's catheter per urethra during operation.

3. *Shortage of skin to house the testes:* When the testes are placed in the subcutaneous pockets made into the upper thigh.

Essence of operation

1. *Dealing with the decorticated penis:* The raw shaft of the penis is covered with either the free skin graft taken from the thigh or the preserved inner layer of prepuce or both. *Advantage of using the inner layer of the prepuce* is that it preserves the all important cutaneous sensations of the organ.

2. *Dealing with the exteriorised testes:* The problem can be dealt with in two ways –

(a) The testes can be covered either by the remnant of posterior scrotal skin which is rarely involved, and/or by approxi-mating the skin from the two sides of the perineum. The mobilised skin flaps are sutured either in 'X' or inverted 'Y' (mercedes) pattern.

(b) If there is lack of scrotal or perineal skin, *pockets in the subcutaneous pouch are made in the medial side of upper part of the thigh superficial to fascia lata*, and the testes are then placed in the pockets of the respective sides.

3. The wound is closed with a drain at its lowest angle which should be kept for 48 hours.
4. A catheter (Foley's catheter) should be passed and kept in position for three weeks in order to prevent contamination of the wound with urine.

Why are the testes placed superficial to fascia lata of thigh?

In order to avoid pressure imparted by the deep fascia particularly during walking or running which may cause pain and pressure atrophy of the testes.

Why are the testes not placed in the inguinal subcutaneous pouch?

Scrotal temperature is 89°F. The temperature in the subcutaneous pouch in the thigh is also 89°F as compared with 98°F in the abdomen or inguinal subcutaneous pouch. So, to avoid atrophy, testes are placed in the thighs.

Note

The involvement of the upper pole of the epididymis is typical of filariasis *causing obliteration of sulcus between the testis and epididymis.*

Note

In tuberculosis, the epididymis is craggy and beaded, with or without a sinus or cold abscess on the posterior aspect of the scrotum, associated with seminal vesiculitis. *There will be suprapubic pain during ejaculation.*

FILARIAL INVOLVEMENT OF THE LEG

Elephantiasis of the leg (Figs 18.7 and 18.8)

Diagnostic criteria

1. Most common in South India and Odisha (coastal areas).
2. More common in male. Mostly common with outdoor workers. Mostly common with people who do not use mosquito nets during sleeping.
3. The lower limb below the knee is almost commonly affected due to the same process as occurs in filariasis of the scrotum and penis.

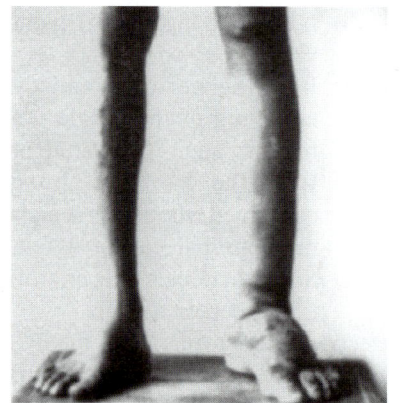

Fig. 18.7: Unilateral left leg swelling due to filariasis.

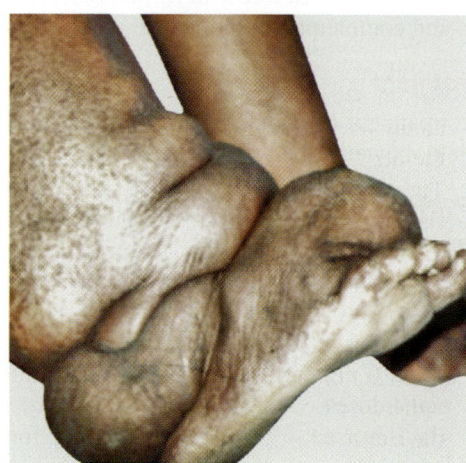

Fig. 18.8: Filarial lymphoedema—elephantiasis of the foot and leg. Grotesque appearance. (*Courtesy:* Dr Yogesh Salphale, D Ortho)

4. *Usually unilateral. The swelling involves the leg, dorsum of the foot and toes – below knee swelling.*
5. *Initially oedema is pitting and reversible –* leg elevation and exercises of toes, foot and legs, use of mosquito nets at bedtime for rest of life along with oral antifilarial drugs.
6. But due to lack of treatment and proper hygienic care, the extravasated tissue fluids excite more inflammation *making it hard, non-pitting and fixed.*
7. So, ultimately patient presents with *solid oedema of the leg with thickened skin.*

Stemmer sign is positive: The overlying skin cannot be pinched at the base of the toes.

8. The *dorsum of the foot is characteristically swollen like buffalo hump* and *the toes become thick and squared*.

9. Eventually, the surface of the skin becomes uneven and rugose (*wrinkled and corrugated*). Later still the skin becomes *hyperkeratotic with horny or warty growth* like the skin of an elephant, hence the name *elephantiasis*.

10. Ultimately, *vesicular eruptions appear* which ulcerate and discharge clear or milky lymph (chylosis).

   These changes are accentuated earlier when recurrent cellulitis occurs due to secondary infection.

   Superadded cutaneous fungal infection (often with epidermophyton floccosum along with bacterial infection) compounds the oedematous process of the limb.

11. There will be decreased range of motion, flexibility and function leading to difficulty in walking and restricted movements.

12. The condition becomes worse after prolonged dependency.

13. *No relief on elevation and exercises*.

14. *Examine the scrotum and penis in male and vulva in female* as they may be involved by the same process at the same time.

Grades of filarial lymphoedema of the leg

Sub-clinical	No clinical evidence of oedema. Lymphatic changes only on histopathological examination.
Grade I	**Pitting oedema:** Completely relieved on rest and limb elevation.
Grade II	**Pitting oedema:** Partially relieved on rest and elevation.
Grade III	**Non-pitting oedema:** *Not relieved on rest and elevation*; skin involvement and subcutaneous thickening is present.
Grade IV	**Non-pitting oedema:** *Not relieved on rest and elevation*; *thickened skin, warty projections over the skin – elephantiasis. Vesicular eruption* may

appear which ulcerates and discharges milky (chylous) lymph – *lymphorrhoea*.

The dorsum of the foot is characteristically swollen like buffalo hump and the toes become thick and squared.

Treatment

Conservative

- General treatment as mentioned under filarial scrotum (*see also* Chapter 17).
- Elevation, exercises, massage and elastic stockings.
- Drugs – *see* page 370.

Surgical options

1. *Excisional surgery or reducing operations:*
   (a) Homans operation
   (b) Thompson operation
   (c) Charles operation
2. *Reconstructive surgery*, e.g. lymphovenous shunt: *See* Chapter 17)
3. *Amputations* for severe lymphoedema with skin ulcerations and leakage of lymph from the involved leg incapacitating the person – above knee amputation may be considered when conservative management and/or surgery fail. At least, the patient can be mobile with a crutch or above knee prosthesis, if affordable. Patient will be able to earn to sustain his/her livelihood.

Note

Elephantiasis of vulva and breast may be encountered also. Causes are:

- Filariasis in endemic areas
- Lymphogranuloma venereum
- Irradiation of groin or axilla due to postoperative radiotherapy to the secondary malignant lymph nodes.

Note

Please *also see* Chapter 17.

- Swellings of the leg – for sequence of events of lymphoedema.
- Surgical options of treatment of filariasis leg: Reducing or excisional operations.

Congenital Anomalies

CONGENITAL ANOMALIES OF THE VERTEBRAL COLUMN AND THE SPINAL CORD

Development of the spinal cord

Spinal cord develops from the neural tube.

1. In the early first week of intrauterine life, a dorsal groove appears on the surface ectoderm of the embryo – *the neural groove.*
2. The neural grove gradually deepens and ultimately becomes closed off forming the *neural tube with a lumen inside. From the walls of this neural tube the entire central nervous system (including spinal cord) is developed. Its lumen persists as the central canal.*
3. *The neural tube becomes separated from the surface ectoderm* by the dorsal ingrowth of the surrounding mesoderm.

Development of the vertebral column

1. Anterior to the neural tube there is appearance of a solid rod of cells, *the notochord, in the mesoderm.* Round the neural tube, *the vertebral bodies develop segmentally from the notochord.*

2. From each side of the vertebral body two projections, one on each side, appear and they are known as neural arches.
3. The neural arches grow posteriorly to encircle the neural tube and ultimately fuse in the midline behind the neural tube to form the spine. The pedicles, laminae are developed from the neural arch. The transverse process is also developed from the neural arch as a lateral extension at the junction of pedicle and lamina.
4. *The fusion of the neural arches occurs first in the midthoracic region.* From there fusion extends up and down.

Developmental anomalies

Failure of the fusion of the neural arches gives rise to spina bifida and its variants.

1. Spina bifida (Fig. 19.1A).
2. Meningocele (Fig. 19.1B).
3. Meningomyelocele (Fig. 19.1C).
4. Syringomyelocele (Fig. 19.1D).
5. Myelocele (Fig. 19.1E).
6. Meningoencephalocele – protrusion of meninges as well as brain – sometimes noted at the root of the nose, anterior fontanelle or occipital region.

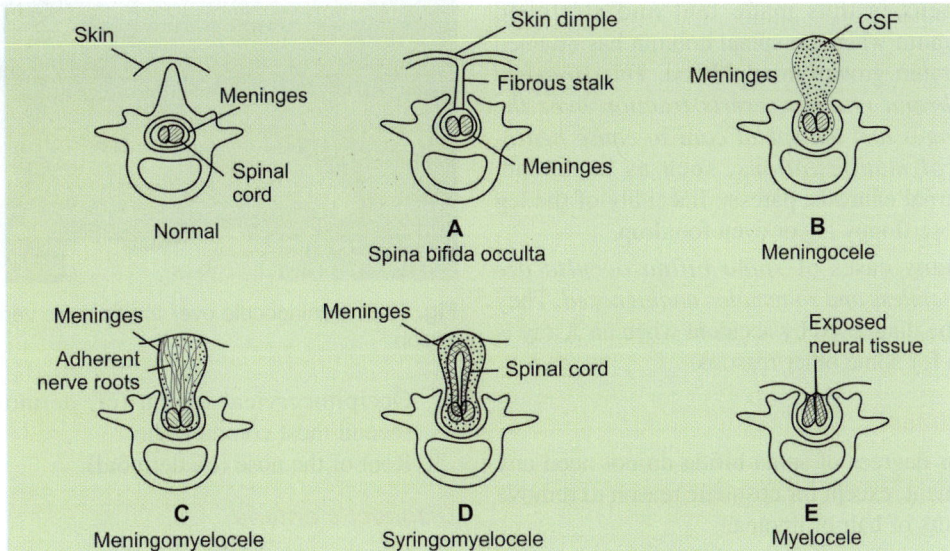

Fig. 19.1: Different anomalies of vertebral column and the spinal cord. (A) Spina bifida occulta; (B) Meningocele; (C) Meningomyelocele; (D) Syringomyelocele; (E) Myelocele.

The above mentioned defects can occur anywhere in the dorsal midline along the neuroaxis but are most common at its extremes, namely the lumbosacral and occipital regions.

Note

Insufficient intake of folic acid (vitamin B) by the mother during pregnancy may lead to spina bifida and/or other birth defects of the child.

SPINA BIFIDA (Fig. 19.1A)

There is a failure of fusion between the neural arches only. So the spinous process will be divided into two, leaving a bony gap giving rise to *spina bifida*. Meninges and nervous tissue develop normally. *The overlying skin usually remains intact*, hence the deformity cannot be seen from the outside and then it is better called *spina bifida occulta*. The deformity is *usually common in the lumbar or sacral region*. Commonest defect usually occurs at L_5 level and is mostly asymptomatic.

Diagnostic criteria

1. *Present since birth.*
2. A depression in the skin (*skin dimple*) at the site of the defect, dermal sinus.

3. Presence of a *tuft of hairs* over the defect at the base of the spine, *it is a sign of spina bifida.*
4. Sometimes there may be presence of *lipoma* or cutaneous haemangioma over the defect.
5. *On palpation,* a bony gap or bony indentation can be felt. *Note the site of the defect in relation to bony landmarks.*
6. Other congenital anomalies may be present, e.g. cleft lip, phimosis, talipes, etc.
7. Neurological manifestations, usually not present; *if any, usually do not appear before adolescence. There will be lower motor neuron signs in the leg.*
8. *X-ray will show the bony defect.*

Explanation of the neurological manifestations

During birth the lower end of the spinal cord and its meninges are connected by a fibrous strand to the skin of the back, known as *membrana reuniens*. At birth the lower end of the spinal cord extends up to the coccyx. As the child grows the vertebral column grows more quickly than the spinal cord as a result of which the lower end of the spinal cord is apparently raised up and lies at the level of first lumbar vertebra. The membrana reuniens is thus made taut and stretched maximum when the spinal column has attained maximum growth in adulthood. *This stretched membrana reuniens exerts traction over the meninges and the spinal cord to cause neuro-logical manifestations*, such as backache, nocturnal enuresis, paresis: flaccidity of the leg or loose floppy leg or even footdrop.

Many cases of *spina bifida occulta are symptomless and so remains undiagnosed*. They may be diagnosed by accident when an X-ray is taken for some other reasons.

Treatment

Minor degrees of spina bifida do not need any treatment, except for cosmetic reason to remove the tufts of hair or lipoma.

MENINGOCELE (Figs 19.1B, 19.2 and 19.3)

There is protrusion of the meninges through the gap in the neural arch posteriorly giving rise to a cystic swelling containing cerebrospinal fluid – *spina bifida cystica*. The spinal cord and its nerve trunks lie in a normal position.

Usually the pia and arachnoid protrude but the dura stops at the margin of the defect. The overlying skin remains intact (Fig. 19.1B).

Commonest defect and usually harmless.

Common sites of meningocele

1. Lumbosacral region – commonest.

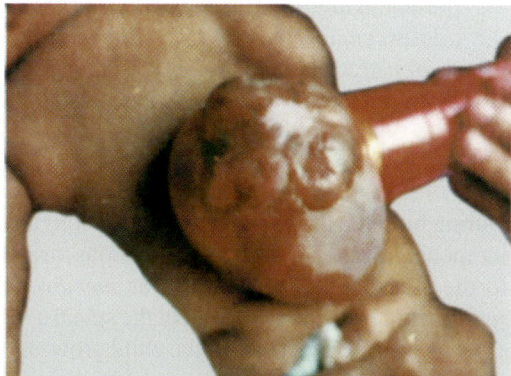

Fig. 19.2: Meningocele thoracolumbar region— cystic compressible swelling at the midline of the back. Transillumination positive.

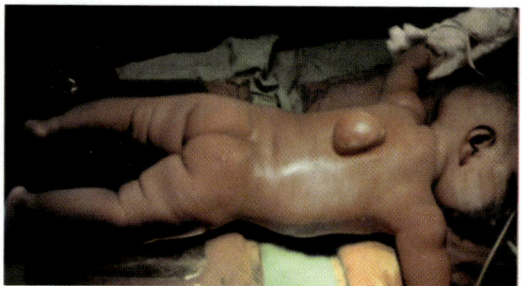

Fig. 19.3: Meningocele over the thoracic vertebral region.

2. Occipitocervical region (cf. dermoid) – second most common site.
3. Root of the nose (cf. dermoid).

Diagnostic criteria

1. Present since birth.
2. *Cystic swelling present at the typical site.*
3. *Fluctuation – positive.*
4. *Transillumination – highly positive* (cf. dermoid).
5. *Swelling is compressible.*
6. *Presence of expansile impulse when the child cries or coughs.*
7. Overlying skin is free and may be thin.
8. *There may be cutaneous stigmata* – a tuft of hair, a lipoma, a haemangioma, or a tail over the defect causing cosmetic problem, and anxiety to parents.
9. The edge of the bony defect or *bony indentation at the margin of swelling is palp-able* (cf. dermoid cyst). *Note the exact bony landmark: Commonly at the lumbosacral region.*
10. May be associated with other congenital anomalies, but *neurological manifestations are usually absent.*

Complications

1. Rupture
2. Infection
3. Ulceration
4. May be associated with hydrocephalus when the condition is known as *Arnold-Chiari syndrome*. Along with this syndrome, there may be severe bilateral limb deformity, bulging perineum and extensive paralysis.

If hydrocephalus is present it requires treatment first before excision of meningocele.

Investigation

1. X-ray will show the bony defect.
2. CT scan of the brain to exclude hydrocephalus.
3. MRI when the swelling is at the lumbosacral region or the craniovertebral junction to note
   - Clear delineation of the swelling.
   - Midline bony spur.
   - Malformed lamina or vertebral bodies.
   - Abnormal curvature of spine.
   - Relation of the swelling to the neural structures.
   - Cord tethering.
   - Position of the lower end of conus medullaris.
   - Associated Arnold-Chiari malformation in craniovertebral lesion.

Treatment

Excision of the sac and the redundant skin and closure of the meninges preferably by plication or sutured together in the midline.

The bony gap is overlapped by the apposition of adjacent erector spinae muscles and the overlying fascia with the help of lateral release incisions. The skin is then closed. Often *myocutaneous flaps* may be necessary to close the defect following excision of a meningocele.

Prognosis is good, the child is expected to lead a normal life.

If associated with hydrocephalus, excision of meningocele or meningomyelocele will aggravate the hydrocephalus. *So, a ventriculoperitoneal shunt is to be performed before undertaking the repair of meningocele.*

Note

Meningoceles may occur in the occipital region of the skull and at the root of the nose when they are categorised under cranium bifida.

MENINGOMYELOCELE
(Figs 19.1C and 19.4)

There is protrusion of the spinal cord or nerve fibres of cauda equina along with the meninges.

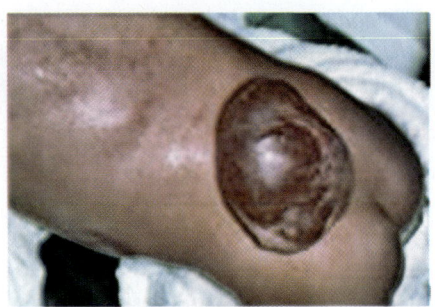

Fig. 19.4: Meningomyelocele over the lumbosacral region—note the parchment-like skin covering the neural placode.

Features

(a) *This is the most common variety.*
(b) *It most commonly occurs in the lumbosacral region.*
(c) *The bony defect is felt at the margin of the swelling* and usually extends over three or more segments. *Note the exact bony landmark.*
(d) The nervous tissue may be adherent to the undersurface of the sac.
(e) *Neurological deficits are almost always present in the form of both sensory and motor deficits.* The motor deficit commonly affects the bladder and bowel sphincters, and the muscles of the lower limb which are flaccid in nature with absent reflexes. Sensation of lower limb is also impaired.
(f) It may be associated with hydrocephalus.
(g) It may be associated with other congenital anomalies particularly of the central nervous system and urinary tract system.

Diagnostic criteria

1. Presence of all the features of meningocele.
2. *Transillumination test – will show opaque bands amidst the red glow. These opaque bands are due to* the presence of nerve fibres.
3. *Neurological deficit usually present*, e.g. bladder or bowel incontinence, flaccid paraparesis, clubfoot, etc.
4. *X-ray will show the bony defect.* It may show other deformities of the vertebrae like hemivertebrae, scoliosis, kyphosis, etc.

5. *CT head to exclude hydrocephalus.*
6. *MRI spine* to note the extent of defect and any adherence of nervous tissue with the sac.

Complications

1. Rupture
2. Infection
3. Ulceration
4. Urinary dysfunction, e.g. infection, incontinence, hydronephrosis.
5. Musculoskeletal abnormalities including scoliosis, kyphosis, dislocation of hip, bilateral talipes equinus – due to muscular hypotonicity and imbalance.
6. May be associated with hydrocephalus, or may develop hydrocephalus after operation.
7. May be associated with Arnold-Chiari malformation.
8. Evidence of intraventricular haemorrhage – which makes it obvious that the baby is likely to die within a few days.

Treatment

The treatment of patients with meningomyelocele includes treatment of the local condition and treatment of the associated problems like hydrocephalus, musculoskeletal abnormalities, and the bladder and bowel dysfunction.

In some 30% patients there is good movement in the legs particularly below the knee and in these children urgent closure of the back lesion is indicated in order to preserve the leg movements.

Time of operation

It is advisable that *the operation should be done within the first 24 hours of birth.* The points in favour of doing early operation are:

1. The sac is smaller in size.
2. The skin is more pliable.
3. There are fewer adhesions between the nervous tissue and the sac.
4. *The chance of infection is minimum* as the skin flora have not yet been established.
5. *The neurological deficit can be reduced to a minimum* (as 24 hours afterwards the spinal cord becomes more prone to infection or

drying or infarction. *The infarction is due to kinking of the blood supply to the spinal cord* as the sac is liable to grow out of proportion to the growth of the child due to distension by the cerebrospinal fluid).

6. As the sac enlarges, the overlying skin will become atrophic and ulcerate.

Principles and steps of operation

1. Operation is performed under local anaesthesia.
2. The child is tied on a splint with the face downwards and head-side is kept at a lower level to minimise the escape of cerebrospinal fluid. The child is given a feeding-bottle during operation.
3. The sac is opened and the redundant membrane is excised.
4. If the neural elements are adherent to the sac, they are either freed by meticulous dissection or separated with a strip of attached membrane. Then the neural elements are replaced, within the spinal canal.
5. The membranes are sutured over the cord preferably by plication.
6. *Adjacent spinal muscles are approximated in the midline over the bony defect.*
7. *The wound may be reinforced with flaps of deep fascia from the erector spinae muscle.*
8. *The skin is closed without any tension.* If necessary, rotation flaps may be fashioned to make an adequate skin cover.

Postoperative management

1. *Regular skull measurements for evidence of development of hydrocephalus.* (Some cases may subsequently develop hydrocephalus from the effect of associated congenital abnormalities at a higher level. Occasionally the hydrocephalus gets arrested spontaneously. *Otherwise, cerebrospinal fluid shunting procedure is to be carried out, e.g. ventriculoatrial shunt).*
2. X-rays of the skull, entire spine and hips, urine analysis, urine culture, intravenous pyelogram are to be carried out routinely at regular intervals. As well as consultation of urologist, orthopaedic surgeon, neuro-

surgeon and a physiotherapist must be necessary for long-term care.

Prognosis: Poor, as the residual neurological defects are always present.

SYRINGOMYELOCELE (Fig. 19.1D)

There is protrusion of the spinal cord and the central canal of the cord is dilated to form a cavity filled with fluid.

Some neurological deficits are always present.

Clinically, very difficult to distinguish from meningomyelocele except that *transillumination test is negative in syringomyelocele.*

MYELOCELE (Figs 19.1E and 19.5)

There is failure of development of the dorsal wall of the neural tube *resulting in exposure of the spinal cord and its central canal to the exterior on the surface of the body.*

There is a *constant dribbling of cerebrospinal fluid through the defect.*

The defect may be complete throughout the length of the cord or it may be partial. *The partial variety is called myelocele.*

Fortunately, the baby with this defect is still born. If the baby is born alive, death ensues within a few days from infection of the cord and meninges.

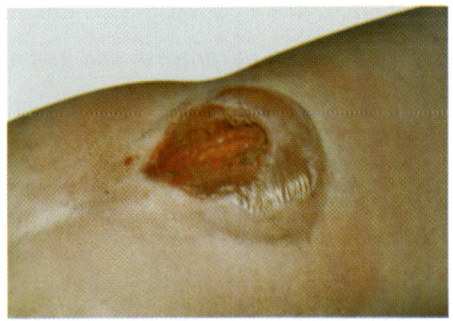

Fig. 19.5: Myelocele on the lumbosacral region—note the absence of parchment-like skin over the neural placode.

Note

Deficient intake of folic acid during pregnancy may lead to spina bifida in the baby.

Note

In every case of spinal defect – neurological examination should be done routinely to detect any distal sensory or motor deficits.

Note

Arnold-Chiari malformation in craniovertebral lesion – when the cerebellum with or without brainstem protrudes or herniates through the foramen magnum leading to severe neurological deficits and hydrocephalus.

Most of these children are stillborn – *thanks God.*

Note

MRI of the spine may detect the different types of spina bifida and any involvement of the spinal cord and/or nerve fibres of cauda equina.

Note

Surgery for meningomyelocele, syringomyelocele, or meningoencephalocele is more complex and often unsatisfactory.

CONGENITAL ANOMALIES OF THE LIP AND THE PALATE

Development of the face, lip and palate

About the 6th week of intrauterine life, five processes appear around the *stomodeum or primitive mouth* at the anterior end of the embryo. These are:

1. Frontonasal process – single.
2. Maxillary processes – two, one on each side.
3. Mandibular processes – two, one on each side.

The frontonasal process arises from the capsule of the forebrain vesicle and descends like a curtain.

The frontonasal process divides into two lateral nasal processes and one median nasal process by the two olfactory pits. The median nasal process becomes bluntly bifurcated, forming two globular processes. The two globular processes ultimately unite to form the central depressed part of the upper lip or philtrum.

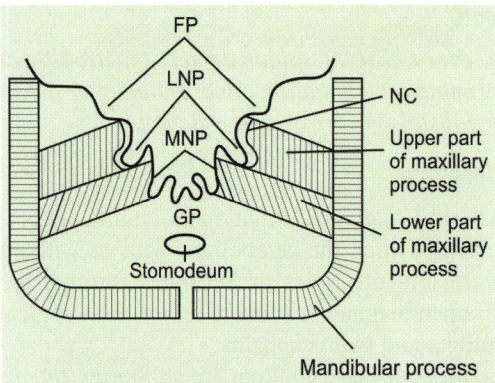

Fig. 19.6: Different processes taking part in the formation of face and hard palate. FP, frontonasal process; LNP, lateral nasal process; MNP, median nasal process; GP, globular process; NC, future site of nasolacrimal duct.

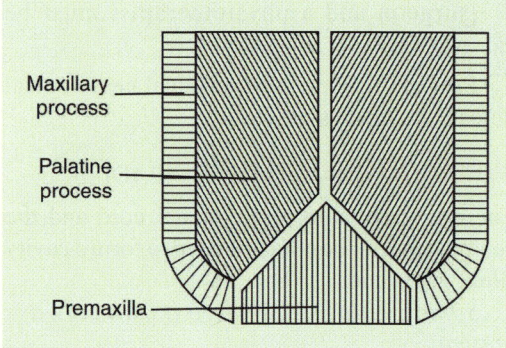

Fig. 19.7: Different parts taking part in the formation of hard palate.

The two maxillary processes, one on either side appear from the dorsal ends of the mandibular processes of the first arches, and grow ventromedially.

The upper part of the maxillary process unites with the lateral nasal process to form the cheek, and the junction of these two processes indicates the position of the nasolacrimal duct. If there is a failure of fusion of these two processes, there will be *a facial cleft.*

The lower part of the maxillary process grows medially beneath the olfactory pits, and unites with the median nasal process to complete the lateral parts of the upper lip.

So, the upper lip develops from two sources:

1. Philtrum – by the fusion of the two globular processes.
2. Lateral part of the upper lip – by the fusion of the median nasal process with the maxillary process.

Two palatine processes appear, one from each maxillary process. They grow downwards and medially beneath the olfactory pits (i.e. between the oral cavity and the nasal cavity) and ultimately fuse to form a part of the hard palate, i.e. the primary palate.

On the anterior aspect of the palatine processes, there is a triangular gap which is filled up by a portion of the median nasal process known as premaxilla, with which the palatine processes fuse to complete the hard palate.

So, the hard palate develops from two sources:

1. From the primary palate which is developed by fusion of the two palatine processes – *one on either side,* derived from the maxillary processes.
2. From the secondary palate, i.e. the premaxilla which is a part of the median nasal process.

These three segments of the palate unite around the incisive foramen. The fusion starts in front and proceeds backwards.

From median nasal process and globular process develop:

• The philtrum of the upper lip.
• The premaxilla.
• The septum of the nose.

From maxillary process develop:

• The cheek.
• The whole of the upper lip except the philtrum.
• The palate.
• Most of the upper jaw.

From mandibular process develops:

• Lower jaw including the lower lip.

These processes unite around the stomodeum to form the face.

CONGENITAL ANOMALIES OF THE FACE

The anomalies can be classified in two groups—

I. Anomalies due to imperfect fusion:
1. Cleft lip:
    (a) Upper lip:
        (i) Central
        (ii) Lateral
    (b) Lower lip – Central.
2. Macrostoma and microstoma.
3. Cleft palate.
4. Facial cleft.

II. Anomalies due to inclusions of surface epithelium along the fusion lines:
1. Sequestration dermoids.
2. Fibrochondromata.

CLEFT LIP (Figs 19.8 to 19.12)

It is a gap in the lip, *mostly congenital* due to non-fusion of maxillary process with medial nasal process.

It may be acquired due to trauma (iatrogenic).

Congenital cleft lip

Commonly affects the upper lip.

Classification

1. *Central cleft:* It is *exactly central and very rare*. It is due to a failure of fusion of two globular processes derived from the median nasal process (Fig. 19.8A).
2. *Lateral cleft: Common type.* The cleft is between the philtrum and the lateral part of the upper lip. It is due to failure of fusion between the median nasal process and the maxillary process. Lateral cleft lip again is classified as follows (Fig. 19.8).
    (a) Unilateral (Figs 19.8B and C) or bilateral (Fig. 19.8D).
        • *Unilateral – cleft on one side of the philtrum:* More common on the left side.
        • *Bilateral – clefts on both sides of the philtrum.* There may be forward protrusion of alveolus along with philtrum in bilateral complete cleft lip. In

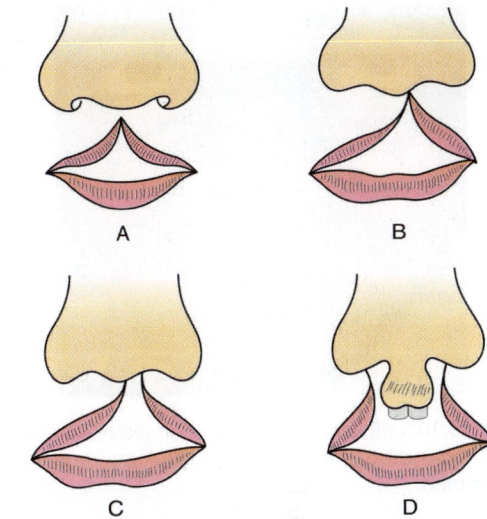

Fig. 19.8: Different types of cleft lip. (A) Central cleft lip; (B) Lateral cleft lip (incomplete); (C) Lateral cleft lip (complete); (D) Bilateral cleft lip. Prolabium is seen in bilateral cleft lips.

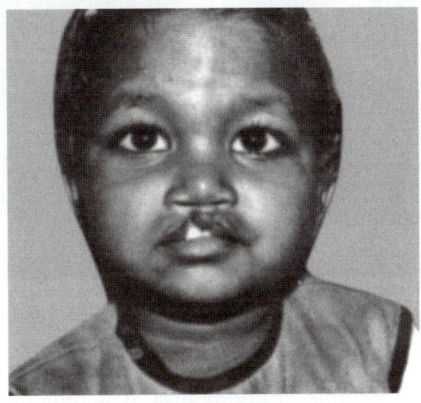

Fig. 19.9: Right lateral cleft lip—incomplete. The cleft not extending into the nostrils. Alae nasi not deformed. The bridge of tissue connecting the central and lateral lip elements is known as Simon's band.

bilateral cleft lips, the muscle origins on both the sides are disrupted leading to forward protrusion of alveolus along with philtrum and prolabium *leading to flattening of the nose.*

(b) Complete or incomplete (partial). It is regarded as complete when the cleft extends into the nostrils or nasal floor (Figs 19.8C and D).

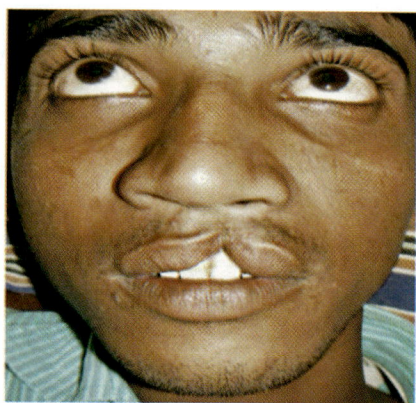

Fig. 19.10: Left lateral cleft lip—incomplete. The cleft not extending into the nostrils. Alae nasi not deformed.

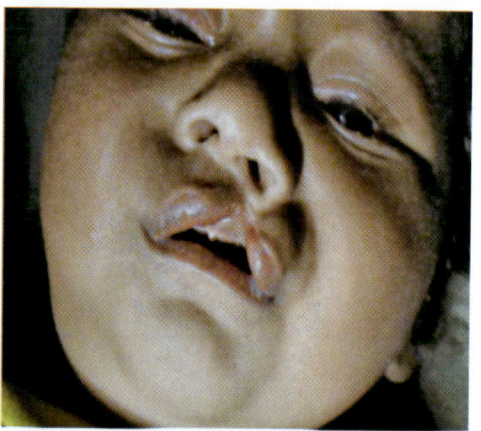

Fig. 19.11: Left incomplete cleft lip. Alveolus intact. But there is deformity of the left alae nasi.

(c) Simple or compound. It is regarded as compound when the cleft lip is associated with a cleft in the alveolus (Fig. 19.12).

(d) Complicated or uncomplicated. It is regarded as complicated when the cleft lip is associated with a cleft in the palate (Fig. 19.14C). The commonest type.

Upper cleft lip may rarely be associated with the presence of two small blind tubes in the lower lip. These tubes are called inferior labial sinuses or mandibular recesses (Sutton). The tubes are lined with squamous epithelium. The cause is unknown, but there is a hereditary tendency.

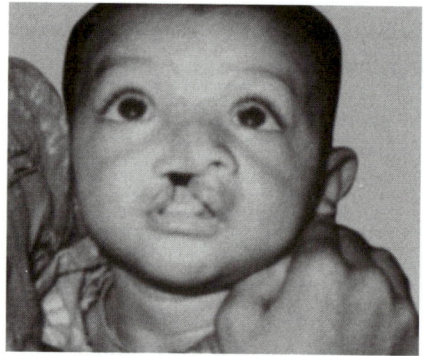

Fig. 19.12: Right lateral cleft lip—complete and compound. The cleft extended into the nostril (complete). The cleft was associated with a cleft in the alveolus (compound). Look inside the mouth cavity to exclude cleft palate. *Note the flattening of the right alae nasi.* Note: Look for congenital defects in other parts of the body.

CLEFT PALATE (Figs 19.13 to 19.19)

It is a gap in the palate at the roof of the mouth, *mostly congenital.*

Classification

Congenital cleft palate may be classified as follows.

Incomplete

1. *Bifida uvula:* Cleft of the uvula only (Fig. 19.13A).
2. Cleft of the soft palate along its entire length (Fig. 19.13B).
3. Cleft of the whole length of the soft palate and the posterior part of the hard palate. This is also known as intramaxillary cleft palate and is due to a failure of fusion of the palatine processes (Fig. 19.13C). In an incomplete cleft palate, the palate remains attached to nasal septum and vomer.

Complete

Cleft on the soft palate and whole length of the hard palate, so that nose and mouth are one cavity.

It is due to failure of fusion between the palatine processes and the premaxilla.

In front the gap may extend on one side of the premaxilla when it is known as bipartite cleft palate (Figs 19.13D and 19.14A).

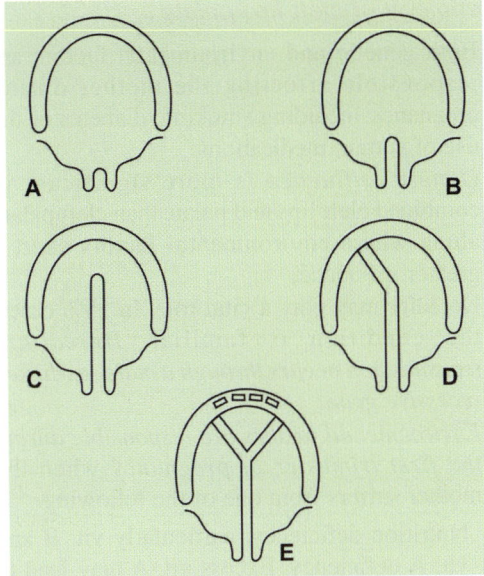

Fig. 19.13: Different types of cleft palate. (A) Bifida uvula; (B) Cleft soft palate; (C) Intramaxillary cleft; (D) Bipartite cleft; (E) Tripartite cleft. A, B and C—incomplete; D and E—complete.

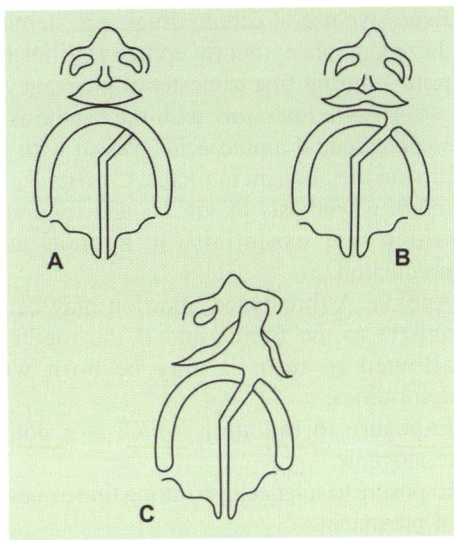

Fig. 19.14: (A) Only cleft palate; (B) Cleft palate and cleft alveolus; (C) Cleft palate, cleft alveolus and cleft lip.

When the gap extends on both sides of the premaxilla, it is known as tripartite cleft palate (Fig. 19.13E).

In both these conditions the cleft may also extend to involve the alveolus without or with the cleft lip (Figs 19.14 B and C).

Incidence

- The incidence varies in different countries and in different races. *Incidence is high in Oriental population* and *low in Negro population.*
- Cleft lip/palate occurs relatively frequently (1 in 800 live births).
- Cleft lip alone: 25%.
  Cleft lip and cleft palate combined: 45%.
  Cleft palate alone: 40%.
- *Cleft lip alone or cleft lip and palate combined predominates in males.*
- *Cleft palate alone appears more in females.*

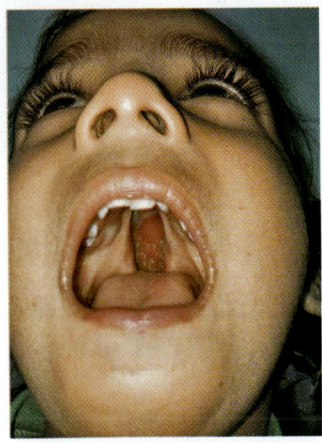

Fig. 19.15: Cleft palate—intermaxillary.

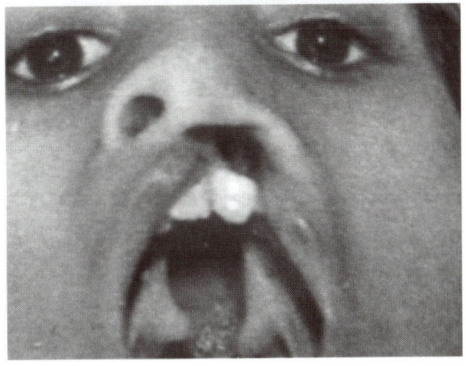

Fig. 19.16: Cleft lip + cleft alveolus (left side) + cleft palate. Note the flattening of alae nasi on the cleft side—on the left side: deformed alae nasi.

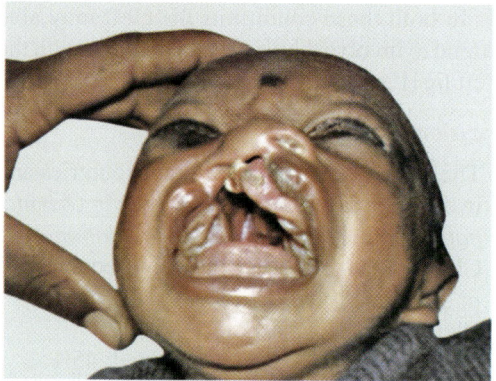

Fig. 19.17: Cleft lip + cleft alveolus (right side) + cleft palate. Note deformed alae nasi.

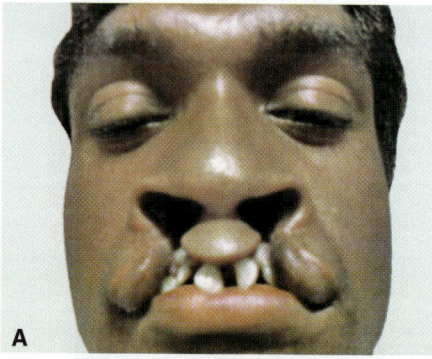

A

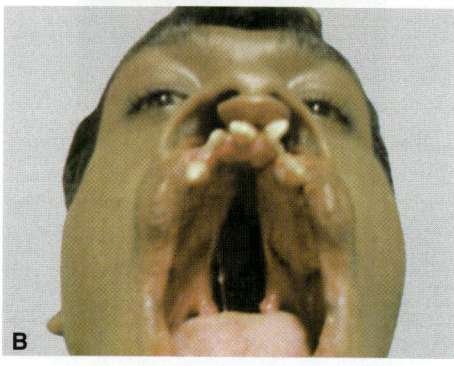

B

Figs 19.18 A and B: Bilateral cleft lips + cleft alveoli + cleft palate. Note the symmetrical deformed alae nasi + protruding premaxilla (prolabium): Seen in bilateral cleft palate.

- Unilateral cleft lip is more common (75%).
- *Left-sided cleft lip is the commonest variety.*
- Incidence of bilateral cleft lip, incomplete or complete, is about 20%.

Aetiology of cleft lip / palate

- Both genetic and environmental factors are responsible affecting the mother during pregnancy including smoking, diabetes or the use of certain medications.
- *Genetic influence* is more significant in combined cleft lips and palate than cleft palate alone where environmental factors exert a greater influence.
- Heredity may play a vital role. In 15% cases, the condition is familial. *Hereditary transmission occurs through a male sex-linked recessive gene.*
- *Environmental factors are responsible during the first trimester of pregnancy* when the mother suffers from one of the following.
  - Nutrition deficiency, particularly vit. B and vit. A deficiency. Excess vit. A may lead to congenital deformities also. *Antenatal folic acid supplement* helps to prevent cleft lip/palate.
  - Endocrine disorders.
  - Certain viral infections, e.g. rubella.
  - Excessive use of certain drugs, e.g. steroids, diazepam, phenytoin (in epilepsy), trimethoprim – during first trimester of pregnancy.
    Cortisone interferes with the synthesis of some essential amino acids and so with the protein metabolism in foetus. *Cortisone also inhibits* synthesis of vit. B_6 and folic acid which are essential for nucleic acid production.
  - Anoxia: A threatened abortion may cause anoxia to the foetus and if the foetus is allowed to term it may be born with deformities.
  - Exposure to radiation which is a potent teratogenic.
  - Exposure to solar eclipse during first trimester of pregnancy.
  - Stress: Excess of endogenous steroid secretion consequent upon stress.
- *Maternal age:* Children born at the late age of the mother are prone to suffer from congenital anomalies.
- *Diabetes:* Diabetic mothers are prone to give birth to deformed children.

- *Consanguineous marriage:* Also are believed to give birth to deformed children.
- Although most cleft lip/palate occur as an isolated deformity, *other syndromes may also be associated with it*, e.g. Down's, Apert's, Treacher Collins, Stickler and Sprintzen syndromes. *Pierre Robin's syndrome* is characterised by cleft palate, retrognathia and a posteriorly displaced tongue.

Diagnostic criteria

The patient is presented before the doctor by the parents mainly because of the deformity.

During examination of a case of cleft lip and/or cleft palate the following points should always be noted.

1. *What is the nature of deformity?* Cleft lip, cleft palate or both. So, *during examination of a cleft lip, the palate should always be inspected* (complicated or uncomplicated). Note the nature of the cleft in the palate (*see* classification).
2. *Site and side of the deformity* (*see* classification).
3. *Presence of any scar tissue* at the mucocutaneous junction of the lip – *scar is absent in congenital cleft lip.* Scar may be due to previous imperfect operation.
4. *Whether the cleft in the lip extends into the nostrils* (complete or incomplete).
5. *Whether there is any cleft in the alveolus* (compound or simple).
6. *Whether the alae nasi are flattened or not –* alae are usually found flattened on the side of the cleft.
7. *Position of the nasal septum.* Whether the nasal septum lies freely (complete cleft palate) or the nasal septum is attached to one side of the palate (incomplete cleft palate).
8. *Age of presentation:* If presented at a later age, the following points should be noted.
   (i) The alignment of the teeth, whether regular or irregular.
   (ii) Forward protrusion of the alveolus.
   (iii) Any speech defect and nasal intonation.
   (iv) Any difficulty in swallowing or drinking.
   (v) Any evidence of chronic ear infection.

9. In addition, examination of the patient from foot to head has to be done for any other associated congenital deformities, e.g. undescended testis, hypospadias or epispadias, supernumerary digits, talipes equinovarus, defects in the spine, neurologic or cardiac anomalies.

Note: Cleft lip may be diagnosed in antenatal period by USG scan after 18 weeks of gestation; but cleft palate cannot be diagnosed antenatally.

Problems with cleft lip

1. *Cosmetically it looks ugly.*
2. *Defective suction:* Effective suction of breast is also helped by effective closure of the lips caused by the tight grip of the orbicularis oris muscle to create a vacuum (or negative pressure) inside the mouth. As there is a gap in the cleft lip, it results in an ineffective grip by the lip, which interferes with effective suction to some extent. So, nutrition of the newborn baby is, to some extent, hampered. So, dropper, spoon feeding may be added.
3. *Defective dentition:* Teeth tend to protrude through the gap along with the alveolus resulting in dental irregularity. Upper lateral incisors may be absent. The maxilla is smaller, causing a relative mandibular prognathism.
4. *Defective speech* particularly with the labial letters B, F, M, P, V, W (ওষ্ঠ্যবর্ণ – প ফ ব ভ ম – ওষ্ঠ্যবর্ণ প্ ফ্ ব্ ভ্ ম্), which need proper apposition of the lips.
5. Unilateral cleft lip is associated with posterior displacement of alar cartilage on the same side.

Problems with cleft palate

1. *Defective suction:* For effective suction a vacuum (or negative pressure) is necessary inside the mouth, which cannot be established in cleft palate due to presence of an abnormal gap between mouth cavity and nasal cavity. Therefore, a baby suffers from malnutrition. *So, in these cases feeding may be assisted by employing spoon feeding or dropper feeding.* In some cases an obturator may be applied to facilitate sucking.

2. *Defective speech:* Particularly with the palatal consonants C, D, E, G, H, J, K, L, N, Q, S, T, W, X, Z (তালব্য বর্ণ / तालव्य वर्ण) which need apposition of the tip of the tongue to anterior part of the palate.

   There will be nasal intonation. To utter these letters there must be a proper closure of the nasopharyngeal isthmus also so that air must not escape into the nose via the nasopharyngeal isthmus leading to nasal intonation.
3. *Defective smell:* Sensation becomes dulled due to constant irritation of the nasal mucous membrane by the regurgitated food.
4. *Defective hearing:* Due to oedema of the orifice of the auditory tube resulting in a blockage consequent upon pharyngeal inflammation from the regurgitated food.
5. Repeated respiratory tract infection.
6. Chance of aspiration bronchopneumonia and lung abscess.
7. Defective dentition because of irregular development of alveolus.
8. Cosmetically ugly look particularly when associated with cleft lip.

Surgical anatomy of nasopharyngeal isthmus

It is the site of communication between oral and nasal parts of the pharynx. It presents the following boundaries.

- *In front:* Posterior surface of the soft palate.
- *Behind:* Passavant's ridge which is a slightly curved transverse ridge close to the arch of atlas and contains palatopharyngeus sphincter muscle.
- *On each side:* Palatopharyngeal arch.

Isthmus is closed during deglutition or blowing of air through the mouth and in expression of some elements of speech (except M and N) by the following muscles.

(i) Levator palati which elevate the soft palate,
(ii) Tensor palati which stretch the soft palate, and
(iii) Contraction of palatopharyngeal sphincter which approximates the Passavant's ridge with the soft palate.

Treatment of cleft lip

Operation

Aim of operation: Mainly for cosmetic reason and also *for functional recovery before speech is developed.* Surgery attaches and reconnects the lip muscles around the oral structures.

Optimum time for operation: The operation on cleft lip should be performed *between 3 and 6 months from birth,* i.e. *before the primary dentition.* Otherwise, the defective dentition is difficult to correct. Moreover, protruded teeth may cause pressure on the suture line and prevent wound healing.

A *'Rule of 10' (Millard)* is usually advocated which indicates that the baby should fulfil the following criteria.

1. The age of the baby should be ≥10 weeks.
2. The weight of the baby should be ≥10 lbs.
3. The haemoglobin content should be ≥10 gm.

So, the operation is better performed when the baby is 10 weeks to 12 weeks old.

Reasons for this timing:
(a) Nutrition of the baby is acceptable for general anaesthesia and operation.
(b) As the lip elements are larger, the repair is technically more precise and easier.
(c) *Dropper feeding in postoperative period is easier,* thereby facilitating healing of the lip wound by reducing the need for sucking with the freshly wounded tissues.
(d) Better cosmesis is expected.

Some authorities advise operation within 48 hours of birth, if the baby is otherwise healthy. They offer the following arguments.
(a) There is no undue risk in doing such early operation because the child is prepared for birth trauma as the child is provided with maternal antibody.
(b) Such early operation facilitates sucking which provides great comfort to the mother and better nutrition to the baby.

But arguments against such early operations are:
(i) The lip is very thin and tiny; so, repair is often inaccurate, necessitating a second operation later on.

(ii) Since this is not an emergency condition and since the deformity will not increase significantly by waiting for 10 weeks, no harm is done.

Advantages of early operation:

1. Better final results are likely: Better cosmesis.
2. It facilitates effective sucking of mother's nipples.
3. It helps in moulding of the alveolus. When cleft lip is associated with cleft alveolus, early operation of cleft lip induces reduction or even closure of the alveolar gap.
4. It avoids defective speech.
5. It allays worries of the parents.
6. When cleft lip is associated with cleft palate, early reconstruction of the lip reduces the gap in the alveolus and palate to some extent.

Principles of operation:

1. The cleft lip should be so repaired that the normal shape and symmetry of the lip is maintained. *For this, adequate mobilisation of the flaps from the underlying maxillae on both the sides of the cleft is necessary.* It also avoids tension on the suture line.
2. To gain adequate vertical length from the nostril floor to the vermilion border to match precisely with the contralateral side of the lip. *To achieve this* various methods (Millard, Mirault-Blair, Le Mesurier, Tennison, etc.) have been proposed which are variations of a Z-plasty.
   Millard's technique is popular and its principle is 'rotation down and advancement closure' of the lip elements.
3. Paring of the edges so that there may be precise union.
4. Accurate apposition of the margins: To achieve this suture should be done in three separate layers.
   (i) Mucous membrane-to-mucous membrane – by catgut.
   (ii) Muscle-to-muscle – by catgut or vicryl.
   (iii) Skin-to-skin – by silk or vicryl.

Essentials of operation:

1. Pouting of the lip: The upper lip must be placed well ahead of the lower.
2. The vermilion border of lip (i.e. the mucocutaneous junction) should be intact; no portion of the mucosa should be everted over the skin.
3. Cupid's bow should be intact and normal looking.
4. Integrity of the orbicularis oris should be maintained by proper suturing of muscle layers to provide good oral sphincter to facilitate sucking of the nipples.
5. Associated nostril deformity should be corrected. Minor deformity can be corrected at primary operation but a major one necessitates a second operation at a later age while the nasal growth is stopped.

Preoperative measures:

1. Mouth cavity should be free of infection. For this throat swab may be necessary for culture and antibiogram.
2. Antibiotic spray in the mouth to eradicate any infection.
3. The baby should be habituated with spoon feeding or dropper feeding starting before operation.

Postoperative measures:

1. *Application of Logan's bow at the conclusion of operation* as an immediate postoperative measure may help. Advantage is two fold:
   (i) It may relieve tension over the suture line.
   (ii) The child cannot scratch over the suture line;
2. The arms and hands should be tied on some suitable splint.
3. Maintenance of nutrition by liquid diet – spoon feeding or dropper feeding. Oral feeding is started as soon as possible.
4. *Antibiotic:* Both systemic and local spray in the mouth.
5. The stitches are removed on the 5th or 6th day after operation.

When will the child be allowed to suck the mother's breast?

The normal tensile strength of a scar is regained in 14 days. Hence, though the stitches are removed on the fifth or sixth day, *the baby should not be allowed to suck the mother's breast before the third week. In the mean time dropper feeding to be continued.*

Note

Different methods of repair of cleft lip
- Millard's method
- Mirault-Blair's method
- Le Mesurier's method
- Tennison's method

Treatment of cleft palate

Operation: Palatoplasty

Aim of operation: To achieve mainly adequate speech without nasal intonations. For these, both length and mobility of the soft palate are necessary to prevent escape of air through the nasopharyngeal isthmus.

So, bring together the mucosa and muscles with minimal scarring to allow: (i) anatomical closure for development and production of normal speech; (ii) to minimise the maxillary growth disturbances and dentoalveolar deformities.

Optimum time for operation: Between 9 months and 12 months, i.e. before the child speaks with nasal intonation which is very difficult to correct. Moreover, the child is reasonably stable to tolerate blood loss during operation.

Reason for this timing: The early repair before 9 months may cause maldevelopment of maxillae leading to facial deformity and dental irregularities which will be evident in later life. So, closure of the hard palate defect should be postponed until facial development is well advanced, i.e. *till the time of primary dentition around the age of 8 months.* Till that time, the defect in the hard palate can be closed either with an obturator or dental prosthesis to facilitate sucking and spoon feeding.

Some prefer only closure of the soft palate before the child begins to speak to allow its development as an essential organ of speech.

Between 9 months and 12 months of age, a child makes efforts to produce understandable sounds as early as that. Once the child has learnt to speak, it is very difficult to control nasal intonation.

Moreover, before the age of 9 months the tissues are delicate and friable and so, difficult to handle. There is a chance of failure of operation.

The child is reasonably safe and stable at this age to tolerate blood loss during operation. *Arrangement for blood transfusion is must during cleft palate operation.*

The cleft palate baby suffers from malnutrition which should be corrected before operation.

Note

There is *a chance of spontaneous reduction of the gap in hard palate up to the age of 1 year.* But spontaneous reduction occurs by dropping or even collapse of palatine vault in limited cases, *which may result in maxillary deformity in later age.* For this reason, waiting for spontaneous reduction is not preferred by some groups of surgeons.

Principles of operation:
1. To repair the cleft in both the soft and hard palates.
2. To create a mobile soft palate of sufficient length to allow closure of the nasopharyngeal isthmus *which is necessary to achieve adequate speech without any nasal intonation* and *also to prevent regurgitation of food in the nasopharynx.*

Essentials of operation:
1. Cleft should be repaired in two layers:
   (i) Mucoperiosteal flaps on the nasal side in the first layer, and then,
   (ii) Mucoperiosteal flaps on the oral side.
2. For mobilisation of the flaps on the oral side, lateral longitudinal release incisions should be made on either side at the junction of palate and alveolus (Fig. 19.19).
3. For adequate mobilisation of the posterior part of the flaps, the pterygoid hamulus is to be broken off on many occasions to release the tensor palati muscles.

4. Greater palatine vessels should be preserved. Otherwise there will be flap necrosis.
5. For adequate closure of the nasopharyngeal isthmus some form of pharyngoplasty may be necessary.

Method of operation: Various methods have been proposed to achieve complete closure of the cleft in the hard palate. Most of these are based on the original Langenbeck procedure.

Fig. 19.19 illustrates Wardill's 'four-flaps' method of repair which combines the repair of the cleft with elongation of the soft palate.

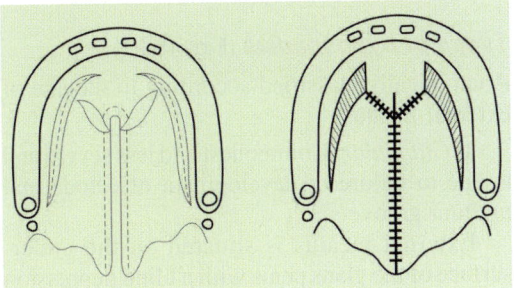

Fig. 19.19: Wardill's method of operation.

Cleft palate closure can be achieved by one- or two-stage palatoplasty also. In the first stage – the soft palate cleft is closed followed by closure of hard palate at the second stage. The philosophy of two-stage closure encourages a physiological narrowing of the hard palate cleft to minimise surgical dissection at the time of the second procedure.

Preoperative measures:
1. *Criteria for suitability of operation:*
   (i) The child must weigh about 20 lbs.
   (ii) Haemoglobin content should be 12 gm %.
2. Normal BT and CT.
3. Mouth cavity should be free of infection.
4. The child should be made habituated with spoon feeding or dropper feeding.
5. 150–175 cc of blood should be kept ready for transfusion during operation, if necessary.
Postoperative measures:
1. Maintenance of nutrition by liquid diet – spoon feeding or dropper feeding.

2. Antibiotic – both systemic and local spray in the mouth.
3. Intensive speech training.

Pharyngoplasty

Pharyngoplasty is used to improve child's speech: most important factor. It is the reconstruction of the pharynx *where the nasopharyngeal isthmus is made narrowed by plastic surgical procedures.* This will prevent nasal escape of air during speech and *thus avoid nasal intonation.* There are several techniques.

1. *Wardill's pharyngoplasty:* Transverse incision is made on the posterior pharyngeal wall at the level of Passavant's ridge – followed by vertical suture.
2. *Denis-Browne pharyngoplication:* Purse-string suture of the mucosa is applied over the posterior pharyngeal wall at the level of Passavant's ridge.
3. *Hynes pharyngoplasty: Pharyngeal flap technique* – either:
   (i) inferiorly based posterior pharyngeal flap – to bridge a smaller gap, or
   (ii) superiorly based posterior pharyngeal flap – to bridge a larger gap.

Note

Baby born with cleft lip and cleft palate – immediate repair of cleft lip first to *facilitate sucking of the nipples of the mother's breasts* which allows baby's nutrition to be maintained.

Note

Many children with cleft lip and palate may require orthodontic treatment to correct the dental problems.

Note

(a) Combination of cleft lip and cleft palate:
   • More common in boys
   • More common on left side
(b) Cleft palate alone:
   • More common in girls
(c) Cleft lip alone:
   • More common in boys

(d) Majority of cleft palates and/or lips are unilateral.

(e) Congenital deformities of lip and palate are common on the left side.

(f) Baby born with cleft lip and cleft palate:
  • *Repair of cleft lip is preferred at 3 months (12 to 18 weeks) of age for better cosmesis and to facilitate sucking of the mother's nipples which maintains baby's nutrition.*
  • Repair of cleft palate better be done between 14 and 18 months of age.

Note

First feed after cleft lip operation should preferably be warm water.

Note

Pierre Robin syndrome

A congenital anomaly present at birth with following features.

(a) Micrognathia – mandibular hypoplasia leading to small lower jaw

(b) Glossoptosis – a tongue that falls back in the throat leading to difficulty in breathing

(c) Cleft palate – an opening in the roof of the mouth

(d) Heart anomaly

Note

Klippel-Feil syndrome is characterised by:

1. Short neck
2. Deformities of cervical vertebrae
3. Cleft palate

Note

Treacher Collins syndrome is characterised by:

(a) Outward slanting of the eyes
(b) Notching of the lower eyelids
(c) High arched or cleft palate

Note

Following congenital anomalies may be associated with cleft palate and lip:

(a) Hydrocephalus
(b) Mental retardation
(c) Congenital blindness

CONGENITAL ANOMALIES OF URETHRA

HYPOSPADIAS

Hypospadias is the most common congenital anomaly of the urethra *where the external urinary meatus is situated on the undersurface (ventral surface) of penis or perineum, instead of its normal position at the tip of the glans.*

In most cases, there would be a ventral bending of penis known as *chordee.*

Incidence

It occurs about 1 in 350 births.

Types of hypospadias (Fig. 19.21)

Anatomically classified according to the site of external meatus.

  1. *Glandular:* Commonest and less severe and is due to failure of development of ectodermal urethral groove.

External meatus is situated on the under-surface of the glans penis with a blind depression at the normal site. *There is no chordee.* Glans is flattened and the penis is straight and rarely bent. This variety does not require any treatment *except a meatotomy if the ectopic orifice is too small.*

  2. *Coronal:* The external meatus is situated at the junction of the undersurface of the glans with the body of the penis (i.e. at the corona glandis). *The chordee is minimum.*

  3. *Penile:* The external meatus is situated at some part of the undersurface of the body of the penis and is *due to failure of fusion of the anterior part of the two medial labial folds.* So, urethra and corpus spongiosum distal to ectopic opening are absent. Instead, a fibrous cord is present known as chordae. *Chordee is a prominent feature and the penis becomes curved ventrally.*

  4. *Penoscrotal:* The meatus opens at the junction of the penis with the scrotum.

  5. *Scrotal:* The meatus is situated anywhere along the median raphe of the scrotum. The scrotum may not be bifid completely but is very often diminutive. *Sex differentiation is usually not a problem.*

  6. *Perineal:* The scrotum is completely bifid and the urethra opens either between its two

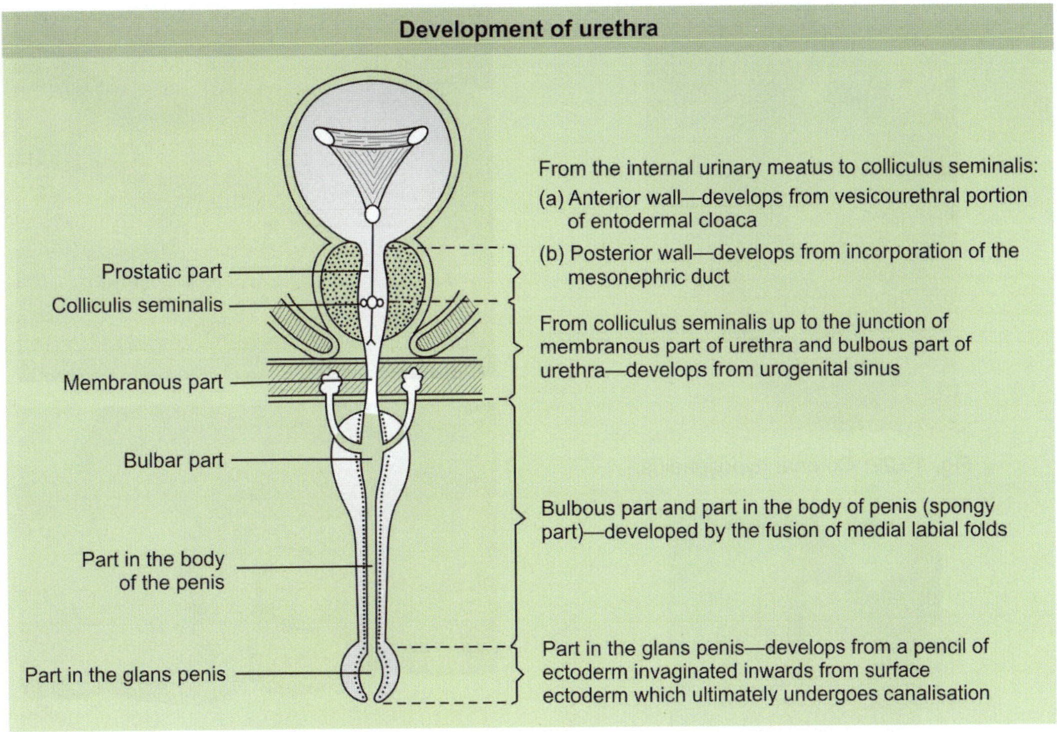

Development of urethra

From the internal urinary meatus to colliculus seminalis:
(a) Anterior wall—develops from vesicourethral portion of entodermal cloaca
(b) Posterior wall—develops from incorporation of the mesonephric duct

From colliculus seminalis up to the junction of membranous part of urethra and bulbous part of urethra—develops from urogenital sinus

Prostatic part

Colliculis seminalis

Membranous part

Bulbar part

Part in the body of the penis

Part in the glans penis

Bulbous part and part in the body of penis (spongy part)—developed by the fusion of medial labial folds

Part in the glans penis—develops from a pencil of ectoderm invaginated inwards from surface ectoderm which ultimately undergoes canalisation

Fig. 19.20: Different parts of the urethra and their development.

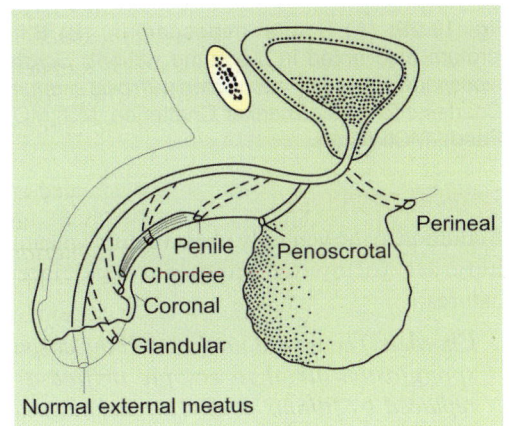

Penile
Chordee
Coronal
Glandular

Penoscrotal

Perineal

Normal external meatus

Fig. 19.21: Different types of hypospadias.

Site		Type	%
Glans penis	Anterior	Glandular	
Corona		Coronal	
	Distal penile		80%
Shaft of the penis ←	Mid shaft	Penile	
	Proximal		
Junction of penis and scrotum		Penoscrotal	
Median raphe of scrotum		Scrotal	20%
Perineum		Perineal	

halves or anywhere along the perineal raphe. The penis is usually quite small with marked chordee.

This type is very often associated with bilateral undescended testes in which event the sex differentiation may be difficult. **Karyotyping should be done.**

- *Both the scrotal and perineal types are due to complete failure of fusion of genital folds after the rupture of urogenital membrane.*
- Anterior groups of hypospadius (i.e. glandular, coronal, penile) are more common than the posterior groups (i.e. scrotal, perineal); *why?* – because the fusion of the medial labial folds begins in the posterior aspect and then proceeds anteriorly. *Hence, deficiency of fusion is more common towards the anterior aspect.*

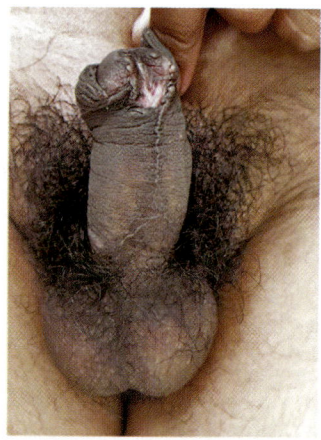

Fig. 19.22: Coronal hypospadius.

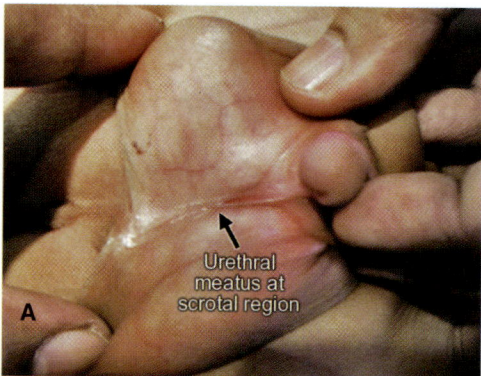

Urethral meatus at scrotal region

A

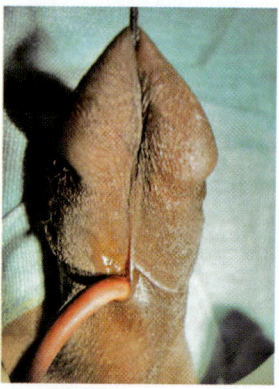

Fig. 19.23: Distal penile hypospadias. [*Courtesy:* Dr Uday Shankar Chatterjee, MS, MCh (Paed), MCh (Uro)]

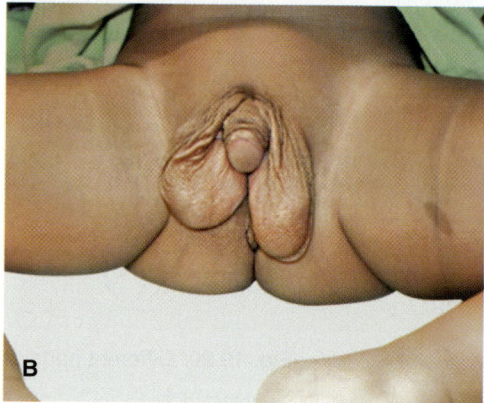

B

Fig. 19.25: (A) Scrotal hypospadias. (B) Bifid scrotum also noted in the same patient. *Scrotal hypospadias is usually associated with bifid scrotum.* [*Courtesy:* Dr Uday Shankar Chatterjee, MS, MCh (Paed), MCh (Uro)]

Surgical pathology

In addition to the ventrally placed ectopic meatus there are following important associated features.

1. *Chordee: The absent urethra and the corpus spongiosum distal to ectopic orifice are replaced by fibrous cord. This is known as chordee. Contracture of this fibrous cord leads to downward (ventral) curvature of the penis.* The more proximal is the ectopic meatus, the more pronounced is the chordee. Whenever there is erection of penis, the chordee becomes more prominent causing ventrally curved penis. This curved penis causes problem in micturition as well as problem during intercourse in adult life.

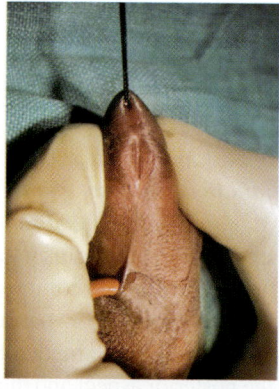

Fig. 19.24: Penoscrotal hypospadias. [*Courtesy:* Dr. Uday Shankar Chatterjee, MS, MCh (Paed), MCh (Uro)]

2. *An incomplete ventral prepuce:* The prepuce is deficient on the ventral aspect and excess on the dorsal aspect of the glans, giving rise to *hooding of the prepuce*. The absence of the prepuce over the ventral aspect of the glans is due to failure of fusion of the genital folds.

   Any child born with hypospadias deformity should not have a circumcision during infancy, since the redundant skin (prepuce) over the dorsal aspect will prove useful later during the reconstruction of urethra.

3. There may be *stenosis of the ectopic external urethral orifice* causing difficulty in passing urine. This is more common with glandular and coronal types. *This needs meatotomy for correction.*

4. There may be a small blind pit on the tip of the glans penis. The glans may be flat.

5. The child with hypospadias usually does not suffer from urinary incontinence.

6. *The perineal or scrotal type is* very often associated with bilateral undescended testes. *Bifid scrotum* may be seen in penoscrotal, scrotal and perineal hypospadias.

7. Multiple urethral orifices may be present, but only one communicates with the urethra per se.

Problem with hypospadias

1. Hypospadias results in an abnormal urinary stream due to difficulty in directing the urinary stream forwards. The stream of the urine is deflected backwards due to downward deformity of the glans penis resulting in spoiling of the undergarments.

2. Chordee is exaggerated during erection and may cause painful erection.

3. Due to chordee, the intercourse may be impossible or uncomfortable.

4. Infertility is frequently associated with a proximal penile, scrotal, perineal and penoscrotal meatus.

5. Hypospadias with ectopic orifice in the scrotal or in the perineal area is *very often accompanied by bilateral maldescended testes with quite a small penis* in which event one should suspect *'intersex' problem* and investigate accordingly. They must be differentiated from adrenogenital syndrome and pseudohermaphroditism. *Before performing urethroplasty, determination of the genetic sex by karyotyping* and *adrenal function test* by determination of 17 oxy-steroids and 17 ketosteroids should be performed. *Laparotomy or laparoscopy and gonadal biopsy may be required.*

6. *Penile torsion and corporal disproportion:* Cosmetically unaccepted by female partner.

7. Some children with hypospadius may have associated upper urinary tract anomalies which need to be investigated.

8. *Infertility* can occur – usually associated with posterior type as it hampers erection, ejaculation and insemination.

Treatment

Objectives of treatment

1. To produce a straight penis on erection.

2. To provide a terminal orifice at or near the tip of the glans, from which to void urine in the long axis of the penis in standing position.

3. To make possible insemination well into the vagina.

4. To achieve a good cosmetic or aesthetic appearance.

5. To achieve a urethra free of meatal stenosis, stricture, fistula, sacculation.

Glandular and coronal hypospadias usually does not require any treatment, but may require meatotomy and dilatation of the orifice, if it is small or stenosed.

All other types are treated by some plastic reconstructive procedures (urethroplasty). A plastic operation is performed to bring the external meatus in its normal position and to remove the chordee to straighten the penis for satisfactory intercourse in adult life. *Several plastic operations are available including two-stage procedures* like Denis-Browne's, Byars, Cecil-Culp, MAGPI and Mathieu operations. Multiplicity of the procedures signifies that no single operation is universally satisfactory or free from complications.

In recent years the trend has been towards one-stage rather than two-stage procedures and

Different other plastic repairs of hypospadius now available according to the site of meatus	
Site of meatus	**Recommended methods**
• Glandular	Usually does not require any plastic repair, except meatotomy if the meatus is stenosed.
• Coronal or subcoronal	MAGPI (meatal advancement and glanuloplasty integrated).
• Distal penile (when the meatus is on the distal shaft approximately 1 cm from the corona)	Mathieu procedure (perimeatal-based flap) – one-stage procedure.
• Proximal penile (with a proximal meatus with or without chordee)	Vascularised preputial island flap mobilised to the ventrum either by Asopa or Duckett technique — one-stage procedure.

towards repairs that give a good cosmetic as well as functional results.

Timing of operation

The operation should preferably be completed before the age of 5 years, i.e. *before the school-going age*.

DENIS-BROWNE'S TECHNIQUE (Fig. 19.26)

It is a two-stage operation for proximal hypo-spadius and is described here because of its simplicity.

Stage I: *Chordee correction* (orthoplasty) to cause straightening of the penis. It is performed preferably between 2 and 3 years of age.

Stage II: *Construction of neourethra:* It is performed preferably between 4 and 5 years of age.

Stage I: Chordee correction

1. The child is placed in supine position.
2. A probe is passed into the ectopic orifice.
3. Incision: A transverse incision is made on the ventral surface of the penis 1.25 cm distal to the ectopic orifice.
4. The skin on either side of the urethra is undermined and mobilised.
5. The fibrous cord distal to the ectopic orifice is exposed which is then dissected from before backwards and excised. As a result, the ectopic meatus recedes proximally towards the perineum, i.e. a coronal hypospadias becomes a penile one or a distal penile hypo-spadias becomes a proximal penile one.
6. The skin flaps are closed longitudinally, and if necessary, to relieve tension a release

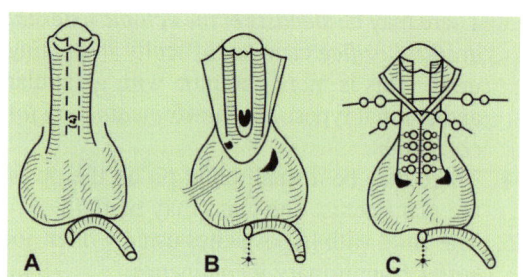

Figs 19.26 A to C: Steps of Denis-Browne's operation.

incision may be given in the midline on the skin of the dorsum of the penis.

Stage II: Construction of the urethra

Principle of reconstruction

The urethral tube is made by burying a strip of skin along the line of urinary meatus which then grows out at its edge and rolls itself into a tube within 8 to 10 days. *This reconstructive procedure is always combined with urinary diversion from the seat of operation* either by:

(a) perineal urethrostomy, or by
(b) suprapubic cystostomy particularly in case of penoscrotal type.

The idea of urinary diversion is to avoid urinary leakage and soiling of the reconstructed urethra.

Technique

Step I: Perineal urethrostomy or suprapubic cystostomy.

Step II:

1. A 'U' shaped incision is made on the under surface of the penis. The incision embraces the ectopic orifice proximally.

2. The skin flaps are undermined and mobilised both in lateral directions and in the direction of perineum beyond the old urethral opening. When the posterior undermining involves the scrotum, two stab wounds are made on either side of the scrotum to prevent haematoma (Fig. 19.26B).
3. A triangular area of skin is raised from the glans on either side of the proposed new meatus.
4. The mobilised skin flaps are apposed and sutured in the midline preferably with 'double stop' sutures of monofilament nylon. The first stop is the sterilised glass beads and the second stop is the sterilised small sections of soft aluminium tubing, which are crushed and thus hold the sutures in place (Fig. 19.26C).
5. A release incision is made on the skin along the whole length of the dorsum of the penis to relieve tension. The release incision prevents necrosis of the flaps and thus urethral fistula.

Nowadays one-stage repair is more popular. Presence of chordee is not an indication of two-stage operation.

Two-stage operation is indicated in scrotal or perineal variety.

Note

• Circumcision is not done in patients with hypospadias as the prepuce can later be used in surgical repair.

Note

• *Bilateral cryptorchidism is not associated with hypospadias. But it may be associated with epispadias.*

Note

Repair of hypospadias:

Two-stage repair:

1. Denis-Browne's technique
2. Bayer technique
3. Cecil-Culp technique
4. Bracka's technique

Stages of operation:

Stage I Involves correction of chordee to straighten the penis – done at 1½ to 2 years of age.

Stage II Involves reconstruction of urethra – done between >2 and 5 years of age.

One-stage repair:

1. Duckett technique – for proximal hypospadius
2. Mathieu technique – for distal hypospadius with preputial islands flap
3. Snogard technique – for distal hypospadius
4. Asopa technique – for mid and proximal hypospadius

Note

MAGPI (Meatal Advancement and Glanuloplasty) – for glandular hypospadias

It consists of the advancement of the meatal pit and closure of a sleeve of glandular tissue over the new pit.

Note

Mathieu flap – for coronal hypospadias

A flap is created based on the ectopic meatus; this flap is folded over and the lateral flap margins are closed over the new urethra.

Note

According to Campbell's urology best time of repair for hypospadias is between 6 to 12 months of age.

Note

Horton's test

Artificial erection of penis is induced to see the presence and extent of the chordee before making incisions for *correction of chordee* – normal saline is injected in the penis to distend the penile tissues, so that any curvature of the penis becomes evident.

Note

Hypospadias may be associated with congenital renal anomalies, undescended or small, firm testis and small penis, Klinefelter's syndrome or inguinal hernia.

EPISPADIAS

It is the congenital anomaly where the external urethral opening is situated on the dorsal aspect of the penis instead of its normal situation at the tip of the glans. There may be dorsal or upward curvature of penis – dorsal chordee.

Incidence

It is a rare condition occurring about 1 in 30,000 births.

Types

Three types (Fig. 19.27)
  1. *Glandular.*
  2. *Penile.*
  3. *Totalis or penopubic* – where the urethra is deficient throughout its whole dorsal extent (Figs 19.28 and 19.29). This variety is very often associated with the ectopia vesicae, termed as *epispadias exstrophy of the bladder when it causes incontinence of urine.*

Incontinence due to maldevelopment of urinary sphincters is commonly associated with most epispadias.

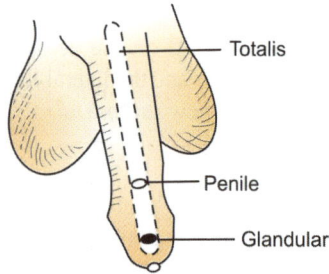

Fig. 19.27: Types of epispadias.

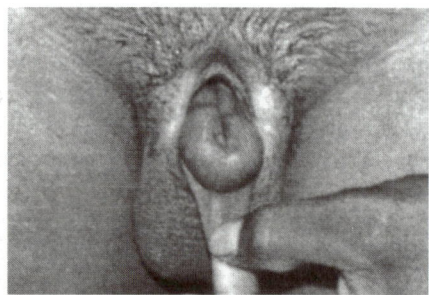

Fig. 19.28: Epispadias totalis. Note the hooded skin (pulled down) on the ventral aspect of the glans penis.

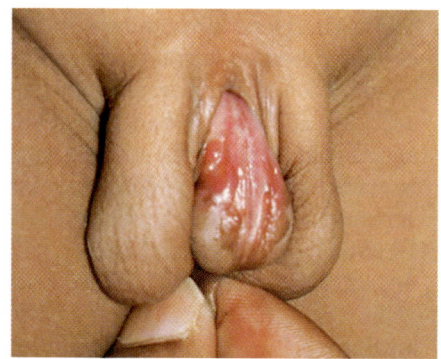

Fig. 19.29: Epispadias totalis.

Treatment

Glandular type usually does not require any treatment.

For penile and penopubic varieties operation are required. A urethroplasty, similar in principle of Denis-Browne's technique, is undertaken usually at the age of 3 years.

ECTOPIA VESICAE (Figs 19.30 and 19.31)

(*Syn.* Exstrophy of the bladder)

It is a congenital anomaly characterised by the absence of the infraumbilical part of the anterior abdominal wall and the anterior wall of the urinary bladder.

Developmental background

The defect is due to failure of migration of mesodermal cells along the genital folds from the

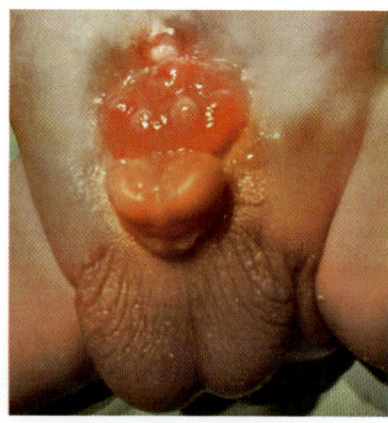

Fig. 19.30: Ectopia vesicae in male. Note the glans penis and the scrotum.

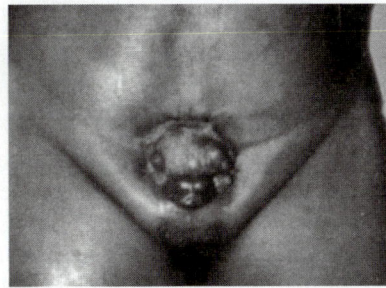

Fig. 19.31: Ectopia vesicae in female. Umbilicus was absent.

primitive streak to the infraumbilical part of the anterior abdominal wall. At the same time the phallus grows from the caudal end of the urogenital membrane. Therefore, when the elongated urogenital membrane ruptures, the interior of the bladder and part of the urethra are exposed to the surface.

Incidence

It is a rare condition occurring about 1 in 50,000 live births.

Diagnostic criteria

1. This condition is two to three times more common in boys.
2. Since the anterior abdominal wall is absent, red congested mucosa covering the posterior wall of the bladder is exposed in the lower part of the anterior abdominal wall. This deep red posterior bladder wall may protrude out through the defect due to the pressure of viscera behind it.
3. When the exposed mucous membrane is drawn upwards, the wet trigone is visible and also effluxes of urine from the ureteric orifices can be seen.
4. The exposed mucous membrane bleeds readily on touch.
5. A well-defined line of demarcation between the protruding mucous membrane and the adjacent abdominal skin (i.e. the muco-cutaneous junction) can be delineated.
6. If the protruding bladder wall is reduced deep to the mucocutaneous junction, the firm edge of the defect in the abdominal wall can be felt.

7. Constant dribbling of urine with excoriation of the surrounding skin and continuous smells of urine.
8. There may be the following associated abnormalities.
   (a) Wide separation of the symphysis pubis, and due to this defect, *the child usually walks with waddling gait. X-ray will confirm the gap.*
   (b) Absence of the umbilicus.
   (c) Umbilical hernia.
   (d) Bilateral inguinal herniae with un-descended testes (when sex differen-tiation is difficult).
   (e) Epispadias totalis: The penis is broader and shorter than the normal. There may be dorsal curvature of penis. The penis is often in two separate portions.
   (f) Bifid clitoris in girls: There may be a wide separation of the labia minora exposing the vaginal orifice.
   (g) Anterior placement of the anal orifice with or without rectal prolapse.
   (h) Rarely ureteric dilatation: *IVU assess-ment of upper urinary tract is must prior to surgery.*
   (i) Occasionally extraurogenital anomalies, e.g. atresia of oesophagus or duodenum.

Complications

1. Painful ulceration of the exposed urothelium.
2. Recurrent attacks of ascending pyelo-nephritis.
3. 50% of the patients die because of renal failure before the age of 30.
4. Continuous bad odour of urine which makes the patient a nuisance to his relatives.
5. Cosmetically unsightly.
6. Squamous metaplasia of the exposed urothelium which may become polypoid in later years.
7. Neoplastic change of the exposed urothelium due to long continued irritation: Adeno-carcinoma which is locally malignant and only rarely metastasizes.

Treatment

Parental distress and inevitable complication demands some form of management policy in these patients. *Surgical treatment is either re-constructive or diversionary.*

Prognosis appears to be better in girls.

A. Bladder reconstruction

To be performed within first 3 years of life.

1. Reconstruction of the bladder wall after mobilisation.
2. *Preliminary iliac osteotomy to allow approximation of symphysis pubis.*
3. Closure of the anterior abdominal wall.
4. In the male, repair of epispadias to be performed at the age of 6 years.
5. *Sphincter control is difficult to achieve* because of absent sphincter muscles and nerve supply; thus the reconstructed bladder becomes an incontinent reservoir.

    Recently, electronically controlled continent device is implanted in bladder neck musculature to achieve continence.

Advantages:

The operation

  (i) removes the unsightly exstrophied bladder and gives a satisfactory external appearance.
 (ii) keeps the patient reasonably dry. The girls may need intermittent self-catheterisation whereas boys may require condom drainage.
(iii) may preserve the genital function in males.

But very soon the operation becomes complicated with ascending pyelonephritis due to the persistence of vesicoureteric reflux. Moreover, there is a chance of stone formation and there may be overflow incontinence. *So, in future a urinary diversion will be necessary.*

B. Urinary diversion

Excision of the urinary bladder is combined with urinary diversion either into the colon (ureterosigmoidostomy) or into an ileal or sigmoid loop conduit.

Ureterosigmoidostomy is contraindicated in presence of anal prolapse with defective anal musculature. Moreover, it carries a high risk of development of chronic renal failure due to ascending infection within 20 years of operation. *So, ileal or sigmoid loop conduit becomes the operation of choice.*

Hazards of urinary diversion:

1. Fistula at the site of anastomosis.
2. Stenosis at the site of anastomosis resulting in bilateral hydronephroses.
3. Recurrent ascending pyelonephritis.
4. Hyperchloraemic acidosis with hypo-potassemia – more in case of ureterocolic anastomosis.
5. Renal failure.

Note

Congenital anomalies associated with increased risk of bladder cancer are:

• Patent urachus
• Exstrophy of bladder

    Both increase the risk of adenocarcinoma.

• Congenital abdominal defects
  – Exomphalos and gastroschisis

Soft Tissue Sarcoma

Soft tissue sarcomas are uncommon malignant neoplasms arising from the soft tissues of connective tissue origin, i.e. *mesodermal in origin.*

In Greek, '*sar*' means flesh; and '*oma*' means tumour. *Sarcoma involves mesodermal and/or ectodermal tissues.*

- **Mesodermal:** Connective tissue origin: sarcoma
  - Soft tissue sarcoma – commonest liposarcoma
  - Bone sarcoma – osteosarcoma
- **Ectodermal origin:** A neuroectodermal contribution corresponding to the peripheral nerves are also included in soft tissue sarcoma.

Note

Endodermal: Epithelial tissue origin: carcinoma.

▌ SOFT TISSUE SARCOMA

Age

- Accounts for less than 1% of all malignancies diagnosed in adults.
- Relatively common in younger population (cf. carcinoma common in elderly population).
- Accounts for 15% of all malignancies diagnosed in children under the age of 15 years.

- Ranked fifth in cancer related malignancy incidence and death in children under the age of 15 years.
- Common varieties noted in different age groups:
  - *Children* – embryonal rhabdomyosarcoma – most commonly in head and neck region
  - *Young adult* – synovial cell sarcoma
  - *Older adult* – liposarcoma or malignant fibrous histiocytoma (MFH), leiomyosarcoma
- Some of the paediatric lesions are congenital.
- *Interestingly it is noted that congenital soft tissue sarcomas rarely behave malignantly though they show an aggressive behaviour in their microscopic appearance.*

Sites

May develop in any anatomic sites:

- 50% in lower extremity, at or above the knee.
- 30% in trunk
- 20% in upper limb and head and neck.
- 10% in retroperitoneum/viscera.

Common histopathology according to anatomic site

- *Extremity:* Liposarcoma, malignant fibrous histiocytoma

- *Retroperitoneal:* Liposarcoma, leiomyo-sarcoma
- *Abdominal wall:* Desmoid tumour
- *Visceral* – GIST (gastrointestinal stromal tumour)

Note

Sarcoma may arise in bone also – osteosarcoma.

Note

Lipoma is the most common soft tissue tumour affecting the adults.

Aetiology

- Little is known about aetiopathogenesis.
- Most of them arise *de novo*.

Table 20.1: Pathological classification (according to histogenic concept) of soft tissue sarcoma

Cells of origin	Benign lesions	Malignant lesions: Sites	Locally malignant lesions
Adipose tissue (fat cell origin)	Lipoma – most common	Liposarcoma – sites commonly involved – arms, legs, trunk	
Fibrous tissue (fibroblast origin)	Fibroma	Fibrosarcoma (low grade malignancy) Malignant fibrous histiocytoma (high grade malignancy) – legs; dermatofibrosarcoma – trunk	Extra-abdominal desmoid
Nerve tissue (Schwann cells origin)	Neurilemoma Neurofibroma	Neurofibrosarcoma; malignant nerve sheath tumour – arms, legs and trunk	
Striated muscle	Rhabdomyoma	Rhabdomyosarcoma – arms, legs and trunk (most common soft tissue tumour in children)	
Smooth muscle	Leiomyoma	Leiomyosarcoma – digestive tract	
Lymph vessels	Lymphangioma	Lymphangiosarcoma – arms	
Blood vessels	Haemangioma	Haemangiosarcoma – arms, legs, trunk; Kaposi's sarcoma – legs, trunk	
Synovial membrane, lining of joint cavities and tendon sheaths	Ganglion Synovioma (giant cell tumour)	Synovial sarcoma – legs	
Mesothelium	Mesothelioma	Malignant mesothelioma	
Histiocytes	Dermatofibroma	MFH – most common soft tissue tumour in adults	Dermatofibrosarcoma protuberans – a cutaneous soft tissue sarcoma: locally aggressive with high recurrence rate
Cartilage and bone	Chondroma Osteoma	Chondrosarcoma, Osteosarcoma	

Note
- *According to age:* Most common soft tissue sarcomas: *In adults* – malignant histiocytoma (MFH), liposarcoma, and leiomyosarcoma. *In children* – rhabdomyosarcoma
- *By site of origin:* Leiomyosarcoma is the most common sarcoma of the organs while liposarcoma and MFH are the most common sarcomas of the extremities.
- *Commonest extremity STS:* Malignant fibrous histiocytoma
- *About 30% of skeletal cancers are chondrosarcoma* – pelvis, hips and base of the skull commonly involved: Cells produce cartilage.
- *Kaposi's sarcoma, clear cell sarcoma of tendon sheaths and aponeurosis, malignant granular cell tumour of the extremities are of uncertain etiology.*

- *Genetic predisposition* – genetic mutations/gene rearrangements: *Two genes are most relevant to soft tissue sarcomas.* These are retinoblastoma Rb tumour suppressor gene and P53 tumour suppressor gene.
  - (i) von Recklinghausen's disease – neurofibrosarcoma
  - (ii) Li-Fraumeni syndrome – consisting of STS, melanoma, breast carcinoma
  - (iii) Retinoblastoma
  - (iv) Gardner's syndrome (familial adenosis polyposis) – may develop desmoid tumour or fibrosarcomas within the abdominal wall or cavity.

- Lymphoedema
  - (a) Postsurgical, e.g. lymphangiosarcoma may develop from postmastectomy lymphoedema of upper limb following axillary dissection for breast cancer with pre- and/or postoperative radiotherapy – *Stewart-Treves syndrome.*
  - (b) Postirradiation – sarcoma affecting radiation fields, e.g. following irradiation for breast carcinoma and Hodgkin's lymphoma – most commonly fibrosarcoma and osteosarcoma.
  - (c) Parasitic infestation (filariasis) – rarely.

- Trauma
  - (i) Postparturition – may give rise to abdominal wall tumour, e.g. desmoid tumour – specially following caesarian section.
  - (ii) Extremity sarcoma – it is uncertain whether trauma induces malignant change or trauma draws attention to already existing lesion.

- Chemical:
  - (i) Polyvinyl chloride. Thorostat used earlier for angiograms
  - (ii) Thorium dioxide
  - (iii) Arsenic
  - (iv) Haemochromatosis.

  } Implicated in hepatic angiosarcomas

- Immunosuppression – Kaposi's sarcoma occurring in HIV/AIDS patients.

It is to be noted that:

- With the ubiquitous presence of connective tissue, soft tissue sarcoma may develop anywhere in the body; *somatic site is more common than visceral site. Extremity tumours are predominant.*
- *Cell of origin is of minimal value for prognostication and treatment schedule.*
- Dermatofibrosarcoma protuberans is a low grade neoplasm.
- Alveolar rhabdomyosarcomas are high grade neoplasms.
- Sarcomatous cells may reproduce tissue similar to that from which it arises, e.g. liposarcoma, fibrosarcoma, osteosarcoma or chondrosarcoma.
- As in other field of oncology, attempts are being made to classify soft tissue tumours on the basis of their gene expression profile.
- Role of trauma – *no etiological role*; probably it helps to draw attention of the patient to the swelling.

Origin

- *De novo:* Large majority of soft tissue sarcomas arise *de novo.*
- *Secondary:*
  - (i) Malignant change may occur in preexisting benign tumours, e.g. lipoma, fibroma, neurofibroma.
  - (ii) May arise as a complication of radiotherapy, e.g. MFH.

Common histological types

1. Malignant fibrous histiocytoma (MFH) and fibrosarcoma – 65%
2. Liposarcoma – 20%
3. Rhabdomyosarcoma – 10%
4. Leiomyosarcoma, synovial sarcoma, angiosarcoma, malignant schwannoma – 5%

Spread

- *Blood spread most common* – pulmonary, skeletal.
- Local spread – by contiguity occurs.
- Lymphatic spread – very rare.

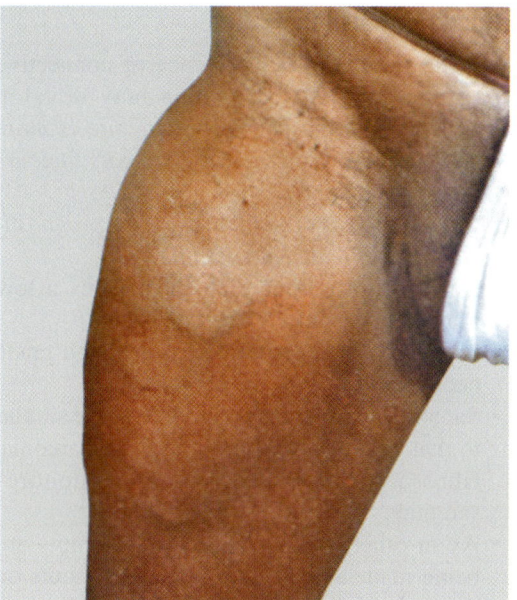

Fig. 20.1: Liposarcoma right thigh. History of soft tissue swelling in the upper part of right thigh for many years. The swelling suddenly started to increase in size during last 6 months with appearance of pain and stiffness more during walking. The lump was firm with ill-defined margin but became hard and less mobile on contraction of quadriceps muscles—the diagnosis was (?) sarcoma. Total excision biopsy of the lump *including 2 cm of surrounding tissue around the lump in continuity was performed.* Histopathology confirmed liposarcoma. Patient was referred to oncologist for radiotherapy.

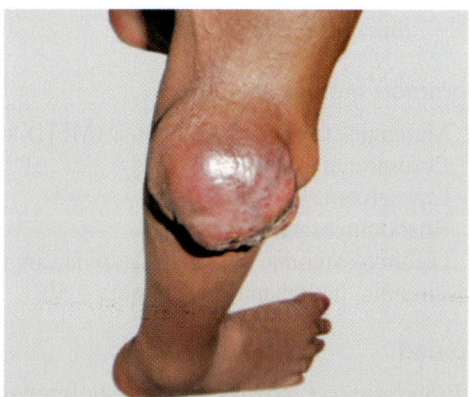

Fig. 20.2: Fibrosarcoma outer side of middle of the right leg. (*Courtesy:* Professor Diptendra Sarkar, MS, DNB, FRCS)

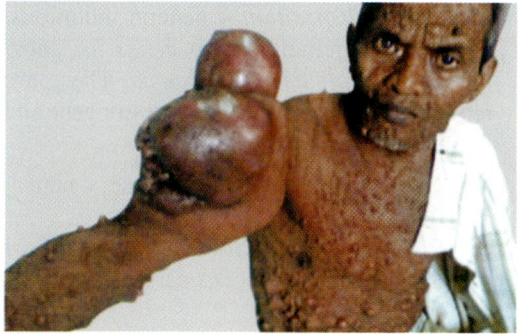

Fig. 20.3: Neurofibrosarcoma of the right upper arm—note multiple subcutaneous nodules over the face, trunk, and right upper limb which were present since childhood. Sarcomatous changes developed on the right arm nodules which were rapidly growing during last 8 months. (*Courtesy:* Professor Bansari Goswami, MS)

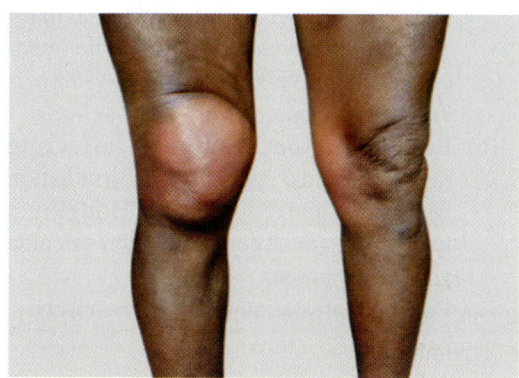

Fig. 20.4: Synovial sarcoma right knee. (*Courtesy:* Professor Sudeb Saha, MS, FAMS)

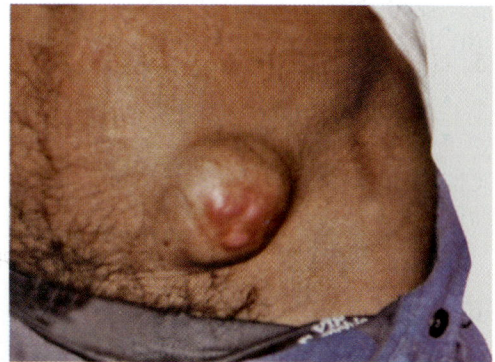

Fig. 20.5: Dermatofibroma left groin—note the cystic degenerative nodules on the surface. (*Courtesy:* Professor Sudeb Saha, MS, FAMS)

Prognosis

Based on following criteria:

1. *Cell of origin:* It is of little value for prognostication and treatment schedule.
2. *Histological type: One of the most important predictors of sarcoma specific death.*
   - Guides therapeutic approach.
   - *Malignant peripheral nerve sheath tumour has the highest risk of mortality.*
3. *Size:*
   - *Less than 5 cm in size* – usually located in distal extremity, is associated with good prognosis regardless of histological grade. Chances of metastasis is low if appropriately excised at the time of initial treatment.
   - *Large size* – usually located in the proximal extremity and retroperitoneum, is associated with poor grading and poor prognosis. Large size is associated with dedifferentiation, so poor grading.
   - Large size is associated with late appearance.
   - Retroperitoneal tumour almost always present as asymptomatic mass.
4. *Depth of lesion:* Superficial lesions do better than the deep lesions. With deep lesions chances of local invasion along the fascial planes, vessels and nerves are more common. *Local spread occurs by continuity.*
   - Spread through musculoaponeurotic plane may occur.
   - Pseudoencapsulation may be noted.
5. *Grade:*
   - *Most important prognostic factor.*
   - Based on several factors as follows:
     (i) Cellularity – hypocellular or hypercellular.
     (ii) Differentiation – well-differentiated or poorly differentiated.
     (iii) Degree of mitoses – less than 10 mitoses or more than 10 mitoses per high power field.
     (iv) Stromal content – very little stroma or abundant stroma.
     (v) Necrosis – absent or present.

- Based on number of mitotic figures:
  - Low grade tumour – low risk of subsequent metastasis (15%).
  - High grade tumour – high risk of subsequent metastasis (50%).
  In soft tissue sarcoma the prognosis depends best upon grading of the tumour and size of the tumour. **Histological grade of tumour is most important prognostic factor.**
6. *Presence or absence of metastasis:*
   (a) *Metastasis by blood spread is common.*
       - Sarcomas often grows rapidly, and dissemination occurs early by blood stream.
       - *Pulmonary metastasis are common with extremity lesion.*
       - Extrapulmonary metastasis is rare, and usually found only with advanced and disseminated disease.
       - Liver is frequent site of metastasis with retroperitoneal or visceral sarcomas.
   (b) Nodal metastases: Rare. *Only occasional, tumour metastases by lymphatics are* (Remember mnemonics – ESR):

       E Epithelioid sarcoma – rarely
       S Synovial sarcoma
       R Rhabdomyosarcoma – commonly

7. Local spread or invasion by contiguity rarely occurs. *Sarcomas of soft tissue origin do not involve the bone.*
8. Some tumours of soft tissues *appear histologically benign but exhibit aggressive biological behaviour* to locally invasive metastasis. Examples are:
   - Desmoid tumour
   - Dermatofibrosarcoma protuberance (DFP)
   - Well-differentiated liposarcomas
9. *Surgical excision:*
   The most important prognostic factors for survival being completeness of resection and grade of the tumour (see treatment).

Diagnosis

A. *Extremity lesion:*
- *Usually presents as asymptomatic, slowly growing soft tissue lump.*

- *Generally painless lump* which is smooth, firm to hard and warm. Many are very vascular.
- Suspicious lesions are:
  - (i) Enlarging lump
  - (ii) Appearance of pain in a painless lump
  - (iii) *Lump greater than 5 cm in size*
  - (iv) Any new lump that persists beyond 4 weeks.

B. *Intra-abdominal or retroperitoneal lesion:*

- Non-specific abdominal pain or discomfort or gastrointestinal symptoms.
- Abdominal palpation detects the lump.

Investigation

A. To establish the diagnosis

For tissue diagnosis and grading – **biopsy**

1. Tissue biopsy of the soft tissue lump is must, *specially to know the grade of the tumour.*
2. *Types of biopsy in extremity lump:*
   - (a) FNAC – grading is not possible
   - (b) With wide bore (Tru-cut) needle *core biopsy:* With CT guidance, *core biopsy* can be taken from deeper structures also – grading may be difficult
   - (c) Incisional biopsy – done when size of the tumour is more than 5 cm and if core cut biopsy is not diagnostic.
     - (i) Provides adequate sample, so grading is possible. At least 1 cc block of tissue should be obtained.
     - (ii) *Advocated for large extremity lump.*
     - (iii) The incision should be longitudinal and be centred over the lump in its most superficial location so that the entire biopsy tract can be included in subsequent radical treatment whether surgical or irradiation.
     - (iv) For truncal lesions – the incision should be placed parallel to the underlying muscle fibres.
   - (d) Excisional biopsy
     - (i) Recommended for small cutaneous or subcutaneous lump between 3 and 5 cm in size.
     - (ii) Grading is possible.
   - (e) Punch biopsy – for small superficial ulceroproliferative lesion under LA.

3. *Types of biopsy in retroperitoneal lump or intra-abdominal lump.*
   - (a) FNAC or CT guided core biopsy has a limited role.
   - (b) May be indicated if abdominal lymphoma is strongly suspected.
   - (c) To confirm or rule out local recurrence or metastatic focus.
   - (d) In most patients, exploratory laparotomy and resection of the tumour settle the diagnosis.

4. *Tumour markers by immunohistochemistry.* Some of these markers may be useful in arriving at a specific diagnosis:
   - S-100 protein – for cartilage and soft tissue tumour
   - Myoglobin – for striated muscle
   - Desmin – for muscle
   - Neurofilaments for nerve – vimentin for mesoderm
   - Glial fibrils for glial stroma

B. To know the extent of the disease

1. Chest X-ray for lung metastases.
2. *Abdominal CT, chest CT to note the site and size and relationship to adjacent structures.* CT chest is preferred over X-ray chest because *sarcoma metastasizes to the periphery of the lung* which may be missed in X-ray chest.
3. *MRI – procedure of choice:* MRI enhances the contrast between the lesion and the adjacent structures. *It is more specific to recognise the tumour and to determine the relationship of the lesion to nearby muscles, blood vessels and nerves. So, helps during dissection.*
4. *Liver* should be imaged as a part of abdominal CT or MRI for metastases.
5. *Angiography:* To find out the tumour vascularity. May be of value in delineating tumour-vessel relationship and hence the treatment.
6. *Lymphangiography: Only when rhabdomyosarcoma or synovial sarcoma is suspected as these sarcomas may metastasize by lymphatics.*
7. Recently, PET-CT scan and MR spectroscopy are being used in some centres for

target biopsy to help in grading, prognostication and determining response to pre-operative chemotherapy.

Staging of soft tissue sarcoma

Based on GTNM

G	**G**rading
T	**T**umour size
N	**N**odal metastases
M	Extranodal **M**etastases, e.g. lung and liver or distal nodal metastases

Grade (G): Major prognostic determinant. The most important diagnostic criterion is high rate of mitotic figures – *over 10 mitoses per 10 high power fields* with or without cellular atypism indicates malignancy.

G0	Benign lesion
G1	Well-differentiated – low grade malignant lesion
G2	Moderately differentiated
G3	Poorly differentiated
G4	Undifferentiated

Tumour (T)

T1	Tumour less than 5 cm in size
T2	Tumour more than 5 cm in size.

Histological grade and size of the primary tumour are the most important prognostic factors.

Nodal metastases (N)

N0	No regional nodal metastases
N1	Regional lymph node metastasis is present.

Lymph node metastasis is uncommon except in those with rhabdomyosarcoma and synovial sarcoma. Moreover, nodal involvement has very poor prognosis. Outcome of the N1 is similar to the M1 disease.

Metastases (M)

M0	No distant metastasis
M1	Distant metastasis present.

- *Lung metastasis is common with extremity lesions.*
- *Liver metastasis is common with retroperitoneal lesions.*

GTNM staging system

Stage I	G1	T1–T2	NOMO
Stage II	G2	T1–T2	NOMO
Stage III	G3	T1–T2	NOMO

NO: No lymph node metastasis.
MO: No distant metastasis.

Stage IV	G1–G3	T1–T2	NIMO
	G1–G3	T1–T2	NIMI

Lymph node metastasis (N1) ± Distant metastasis (M1)

Prognostic factors for STS

1. *Grade:* Most important prognostic factor
2. *Size:* <5 cm, better prognosis
3. *Site:* Superficial STS, better prognosis
4. *Histological type:* Low grade tumours, better prognosis
5. *Margin of resection:* Negative margin, better prognosis

TREATMENT

Surgery

Extremity lesion

Aim is
  (i) to achieve local control, and
  (ii) to treat metastases

Surgical treatment
  (i) *Wide local excision is the first line of treatment for all soft tissue sarcoma.*
  (ii) *The surgical objective should be* complete removal of tumour with negative margins and maximal preservation of function.

Types of surgery
1. *Excisional biopsy:*
   (i) All gross tumour is excised *but tumour may remain behind because of pseudo-encapsulation.*
   (ii) *Recurrence rate is 90%.*
2. **Wide local excision with 2 cm to 4 cm of surrounding normal tissue in continuity** is advocated to prevent local spread but at the same time to provide maximal preservation of function: *2 cm for low grade and 4 cm for high grade tumour.*

Deliberate sacrifice of the major neuro-vascular structures should be avoided.
  (i) *Recurrence after wide excision is 50%.*
  (ii) **So requires adjuvant radiotherapy and/or chemotherapy.**
  (iii) *Wide excision followed by adjuvant irradiation of tumour bed has resulted in the achievement of limb sparing surgery without compromise of survival.*
3. **Radical resection** *implies compartmental excision including the origin and insertion of the entire group of muscles:*
  (i) *Recurrence rate is 20%.*
  (ii) Requires adjuvant radiotherapy and/or chemotherapy for low recurrence rates.
  (iii) Excellent result similar to that seen with amputation may be achieved by this approach.
4. **Amputation** *at suitable level, i.e. one joint above the lesion or disarticulation.*
  (i) Most radical surgery.
  (ii) Recurrence rate is 5%.
  (iii) Little advantage over limb-sparing surgery.
  (iv) May be advocated in below knee lesions or below elbow lesions after reasoning to both patient and patient party.
5. *Prophylactic lymph node resection is not indicated in soft tissue sarcoma.*

Role of radiotherapy

Soft tissue sarcoma is relatively radioresistant.

Aim is to reduce local recurrence.
  Radiotherapy can be given as
  (i) curative
  (ii) postoperative adjuvant
  (iii) preoperative neoadjuvant
  (iv) intraoperative radiotherapy (IORT).

Curative radiotherapy

Radiotherapy has little effect on either the primary growth or on the secondary growth. *Radiotherapy will delay the progression of the disease but does not improve the survival.*
  (a) *Indication:*
    • Poor surgical risk patients
    • Patient refusing surgery

    • Surgery not feasible because of anatomical location, e.g. retroperitoneal tumour.
    • Tumour >5 cm in size.
  (b) *Type of radiation:*
    (i) Sophisticated radiation like mega-voltage or linear accelerator.
    (ii) High dose radiation (7000 to 8000 rads).
  (c) *Results of curative radiotherapy versus combined modality treatment, i.e. surgery + radiotherapy.*
    • Recurrence rate is higher with only radiotherapy.
    • Moreover delayed fibrosis is common with only radiotherapy

Postoperative adjuvant radiotherapy
  (a) *Indication:*
    • Extremity lesion who have undergone surgery less than amputation.
    • Truncal sarcoma who have undergone removal of gross tumour only.
    • Retroperitoneal tumour where total removal of tumour is not possible.
    • Lesions less than 5 cm do not benefit much from radiotherapy due to excellent general prognosis following surgery.
  (b) *Type of radiation:*
    • Brachytherapy for high grade lesions only.
    • External beam radiation therapy for high grade or low grade lesion.

Preoperative neoadjuvant radiotherapy
    • Used in locally advanced disease.
    • Little value.

Note
Sarcoma of bone is sensitive to radiotherapy and so can be used as an alternative to amputation.

Role of chemotherapy
  • As an adjuvant therapy its role is not established.
  • May be used as a part of definitive treatment of metastatic disease.
  • May benefit in large and high grade lesions.
  • May benefit for recurrent lesions.
  • *Combination chemotherapy is used.*

- Leomyosarcoma shows greater resistance to chemotherapeutic drugs.
- *Synovial sarcoma shows good response to ifosfamide based chemotherapeutic drugs.*
- Doxirubicin (adriamycin), ifosfamide, dacarbizine, cyclophosphamide, DTIC and mensa have been used alone or in combination.
  - (i) VAC – vincristine, adriamycin, cyclophosphamide.
  - (ii) DVC – doxirubicin, vincristine, cyclophosphamide.
  - (iii) CYVADTIC – cyclophosphamide, vincristine, adriamycin, DTIC.

  Doxyrubicin (adriamycin) is the single most effective drug but best used with various other drug combinations.

Result of chemotherapy
  - (i) Length of survival may be improved up to 5 years (median survival >1 year).
  - (ii) Rhabdomyosarcoma in young children is more responsive to chemotherapy.

Neoadjuvant chemotherapy with or without radiation therapy
  - (i) May cause downstaging of the tumour.
  - (ii) So, may be used in large primary lesions.
  - (iii) May be used for limb sparing procedures in difficult cases.

SPECIFIC TYPES OF STS

LIPOSARCOMA (Fig. 20.1)

- Commonest type of soft tissue sarcoma arising from fat cells (of primitive mesenchymal cells).
- Can occur *de novo* or from a preexisting lesion.
- Constitutes 90% of all soft tissue sarcomas.
- Common sites: Thigh > Retroperitoneum > Back > Shoulder.
- Different varieties:
  - Well-differentiated
  - Myxoid
  - Round cell
  - Pleomorphic 5% – poor prognosis
- Microscopically, the lesion contains lipoblasts with signet ring malignant cells. It is low grade type.
- Spread to lungs.

- Treatment: Wide local excision of the tumour. Surgical debulking followed by radiotherapy is advocated where complete removal of the tumour is not possible, like in retroperitoneal liposarcoma.

FIBROSARCOMA (Fig. 20.2)

- Origin from mesenchymal cells of fibroblasts and composed of spindle cells.
- May occur wherever there is fibrous tissue.
- Common sites are the trunk and the limbs, particularly the inner and intramuscular fibrous septae of adductors, scapulohumeral and pectoral muscles.
- May occur at any age.
- It may arise as a localised, firm, mobile tumour which eventually gets fixed.
- Usually slowly growing but eventually pulmonary metastases appear.
- Tumour is radioresistant.
- Treatment is by wide local excision or amputation depending on the site of the lesion, supported by radiotherapy.

SYNOVIAL SARCOMA (Fig. 20.4)

- Can originate from the synovial tissue in joints, tendon sheaths or bursae.
- Common in thigh, leg, shoulder, hand and foot. *More common in and around the knee.*
- Synovial sarcoma is highly malignant.
- Predominant cells are spindle shaped.
- Spreads widely, infiltrating its surroundings including bone.
- *Metastasize both by lymphatics and blood.*
- Tumour is usually radioresistant.
- Treatment is by wide local excision or amputation depending on the site of the lesion, supported by radiotherapy.
- *Shows good response to ifosfamide-based combination chemotherapy.*
- *A characteristic feature when present is calcified concretions that can sometimes be detected on X-ray.*
- *Immune histochemistry is helpful* in identifying this tumour, since the tumour cells yield positive reactions for keratin and epithelial membrane antigen differentiating synovial sarcoma from most other tumours.

MALIGNANT FIBROUS HISTIOCYTOMA (MFH)

- Origin from histiocytes and primitive mesen-chymal cells have been proposed.
- Aggressive soft tissue sarcoma
- *Occurs principally as a mass at the extremities (70%); more on the lower limbs.*
- May occur in the abdominal cavity, retro-peritoneum, head and neck, trunk and in other parts of the body.
- Situated in the deep tissues of the extremities and trunk. It involves deep fascia or skeletal muscles. Rarely confines to subcutis without fascial involvement.
- *Occurring principally in middle-aged individuals.* Peak incidence is in the fifth decade.
- Rare symptoms and signs include *episodic hypoglycemia and rapid tumour enlargement during pregnancy.*
- *Diagnosis:* FNAB
- *Treatment:* Wide margin of excision of tumour is advocated.

  Pre- or postoperative radiotherapy is also given to the lesion larger than 5 cm in diameter.

DERMATOFIBROSARCOMA PROTUBERANS (DFSP)

(Figs 20.6 and 20.7)

- *Intradermal sarcoma of low grade malignancy.*
- Rarely metastasizing *but with tendency for local recurrence.* It forms about 2–5% of STS.
- Involving mainly the trunk and extremities in early or mid adult life.
- Rarely turns into a frank sarcoma with a propensity to distant spread (2–5%).
- It is *slowly growing, painless, protruding hard nodular cutaneous mass freely moving* over the subcutaneous tissue.
- There may be surface ulceration more due to stretching of epidermis rather than tumour infiltration (Fig. 20.6).
- Not very radio- or chemosensitive.
- Wide surgical excision is the best option but recurrences are common.
- Mohs microsurgery has been preferred in some cases, which show deeper infiltration.

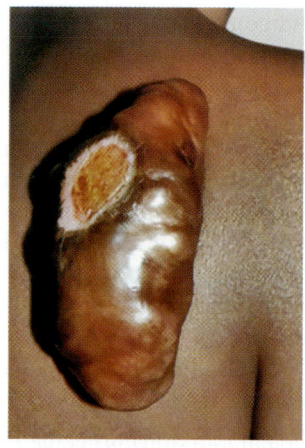

Fig. 20.6: Dermatofibrosarcoma over the upper left back (shoulder)—firm to hard irregular lump. Note the ulcer on the surface with pale granulation tissue. It begins in the middle layer of skin, the dermis. DFSP tends to grow slowly. It seldom spreads to other parts of the body. (*Courtesy:* Prof. Sudeb Saha, MS, FAMS)

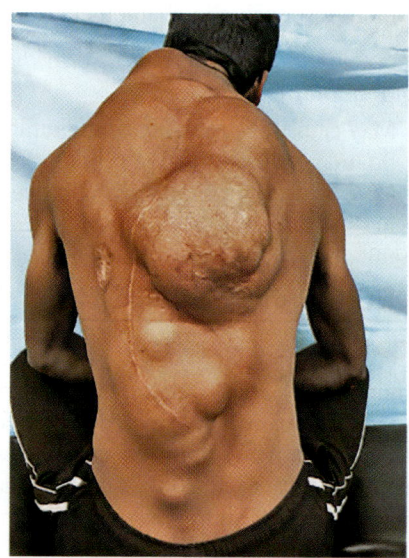

Fig. 20.7: Recurrent dermatofibrosarcoma with multiple swellings—note the scar mark from previous operation.

- *Imatinib mesylate – a chemotherapeutic agent* has shown some promising results in recurrent or non-resectable tumours and appears to be more specific if the tumour is positive for gene translocation.

RHABDOMYOSARCOMA (RMS)

- *Common soft tissue sarcoma in infants and children.*
- Three types are encountered:
    1. Embryonal RMS – arising in orbit or genitourinary tract – *highly chemosensitive with good prognosis*
    2. Alveolar RMS – extremity sarcoma and cytologically resembles lymphomas
    3. Pleomorphic RMS – more common form and has *poor prognosis*

RETROPERITONEAL NEOPLASM

Boundaries of retroperitoneal space

It is a potential space between the peritoneal cavity and the posterior abdominal wall. *It is bounded:*

- *Above* – by diaphragm and the 12th rib
- *Below* – by the pelvic levator ani muscles and coccygeus
- *Anteriorly* – by the posterior peritoneal peritoneum
- *Posteriorly* – by the vertebral column with posterior abdominal muscles on either side – psoas, quadratus lumborum and transversus abdominis muscles.

Contents

1. Structures of mesodermal and endodermal origin with their embryonic remnants. These consist of loose connective tissue, fat, nerves, lymphatics and lymph nodes.
2. Retroperitoneal organs like kidneys and ureters, adrenals and pancreas. *But these are not included in retroperitoneal tumours. These are organ-specific tumours.*

Pathology

Common benign tumours

1. Lipoma, neurofibroma, neurilemmoma, leiomyoma, dermoid cysts
2. Lymphatic or chylous cyst
3. Cysts of urogenital origin
4. Enterogenous cysts
5. Paragangliomas – tumours of embryonal origin from neural crest

Common malignant tumours

A. Primary neoplasms of soft tissues of retroperitoneum of mesodermal origin
    1. Liposarcoma – most common
    2. Leiomyosarcoma
    3. Malignant fibrous histiocytoma (MFH)
    4. Lymphoma
    5. Lymphosarcoma
    6. Fibrosarcoma
    7. Rhabdomyosarcoma
    8. Neuroblastoma
    9. Extra-adrenal chromaffinomas

B. Secondary – *metastatic into the retroperitoneal lymph nodes:*
    - Adenosarcoma – primary from endometrium, prostate, pancreas, kidney, adrenal.
    - Squamous cell carcinoma – primary from squamous cell carcinoma of cervix, vagina, lung.
    - Primary germ cell neoplasm arising from embryonic nest cells.

The most common primary malignancy of the retroperitoneum is sarcoma.

Note

Primary neoplasm in the retroperitoneal organ such as kidney, adrenal, pancreas and colon. These are excluded from the domain of retroperitoneal tumour. *These are organ-specific tumours.*

Note

In children most common sarcoma is rhabdomyosarcoma.

RETROPERITONEAL CYSTIC LESIONS

Causes:

1. Cystic lesions arising from remnants of the Wolffian duct of urogenital tract.
2. Teratomas or dermoid cyst.
3. Cystic lymphangioma or cystic hygroma.
4. Parasitic cysts.

Clinical features of abdominal cystic lymphangioma

- Usually seen in infants and children (3 months to 5 years).
- Most common presentation is abdominal pain or sense of heaviness – *as manifested by frequent crying, off and on.*
- *30% of children present with abdominal mass – felt on palpation.*
- Rarely children may present with intestinal obstruction.
- *Investigations – CT/MRI* – non-invasive and very much informative to confirm diagnosis.
- Treatment – surgical excision.

Clinical features of retroperitoneal tumour

- Swelling – intra-abdominal.
- On palpation – a relatively tense or hard mass is palpable.
- The mass is *usually not crossing the midline.*
- *Relatively fixed mass* – not mobile in either direction.
- *The mass is intra-abdominal* as confirmed by head rising tests (*Carnot's test*).
- *The mass is not falling downwards in knee-elbow position* – suggesting the mass is retroperitoneal.
- *Mobility is restricted.* There will be no movements of the mass with respiration.
- *On percussion, the mass may be resonant* because of the dilated intestinal loops lying in front of the mass.

Retroperitoneal malignancies

Malignant tumours in the retroperitoneal space may result from:

- Primary neoplasm in retroperitoneal organs such as kidney, adrenal, pancreas and colon. *These are excluded from the domain of retroperitoneal tumours. These are organ-specific tumours.*
- Primary neoplasm of the soft tissues of the retroperitoneum of mesodermal origin such as adipose tissue, fibrous tissue, smooth and striated muscles, blood vessels, lymphatic tissues and nerve tissues.

- Primary neoplasm of the retroperitoneal lymphatic system, e.g. lymphoma.
- Primary germ cell neoplasm arising from embryonic rest cells.
- Metastases from a remote primary malignancy into retroperitoneal lymph nodes.

The most common primary malignancy of retroperitoneum is sarcoma.

RETROPERITONEAL SARCOMA

Primary malignant tumours of retroperitoneum arising from the soft tissues of mesenchymal or mesodermal origin occupying the potential retroperitoneal space such as adipose tissue, connective tissue, smooth and striated muscles, blood vessels, lymphatic tissue and nerve tissue – *known as retroperitoneal sarcoma.*

- Incidence is 0.3 to 3%.
- *Sarcomas are solid*, hard and usually fixed mass and deep-seated (cf. *cystic tumours are predominantly benign*).
- Grow slowly and silently and present as asymptomatic abdominal lump when they become quite large.
- Sarcomas may present with following symptoms.
  (i) Vague abdominal pain or heaviness, anorexia, weight loss.
  (ii) Obstructive gut symptoms – vomiting, altered bowel habits, intestinal obstruction.
  (iii) Urinary tract symptoms – haematuria, dysuria and compression of the kidney and ureter leading to renal failure – oliguria/anuria.
  (iv) Neural compression symptoms leading to radicular pain, paraesthesia.
  (v) Vascular and/or lymphatic compression leading to limb swelling and heaviness.
  (vi) With or without any of these symptoms, abdominal palpation may detect the large intra-abdominal mass accidentally.
- They are locally aggressive but rarely metastasize.
- Local recurrence after complete resection is common.

- Patients with high grade sarcoma have a higher risk of systemic disease and death.
- *Associated with a poor long term survival rate, main reason being* the extreme difficulty encountered in performing a complete surgical excision with a rim of normal tissue around the tumour *because of tumour adherence to adjacent major vascular structures and nerves.*
- 5 years survival rate is 25% even after radio- and chemotherapy.

Investigation

1. CT/MRI
   (a) Non-invasive
   (b) Most effective means of delineating abnormalities of retroperitoneum.
   (c) Provide information—
      (i) Regarding exact site, location, size and *extent of the tumour*, physical characteristics – *solid or cystic. Cystic lesions are predominantly benign.*
      (ii) *Tumour relationship to major vascular structures* – more delineated with MRI.
      (iii) *Presence or absence of metastasis.*
      MRI – *Greater accuracy than CT* (100% vs 80%).
2. Chest X-ray.
3. CT chest – preferred over X-ray chest *because sarcoma metastasizes to the periphery of the lung which may be missed in X-ray chest.*
4. Biopsy
   (a) U/S or CT guided FNAC or core biopsy has limited role.
   (b) *Helps to detect the tissue of origin. Grading of tumour is not possible.*
   (c) *Usually reserved for those lesions* with strong suspicion of lymphoma, or germ cell tumour.
   (d) In most patients, exploratory laparotomy and resection of the tumour settle the diagnosis.

Treatment

Multidisciplinary approach is recommended.

1. Surgery
2. Radiotherapy
3. Chemotherapy

Surgery

(a) Complete en bloc resection of the tumour with tumour free margin is the best form of treatment.
(b) Any adjacent involved organ should also be resected, e.g. intestine, kidney.
(c) Parietal fixation does not contraindicate resection
(d) *Only contraindications are:*
   (i) Wide spread metastases
   (ii) Lymphoma.

Lymphoma is chemosensitive and radiosensitive tumour and can be diagnosed preoperatively by U/S or CT guided core biopsy and so surgery is avoided.

Radiotherapy

Indications of radiotherapy:

1. Radiosensitive tumours, e.g. lymphomas
2. All inoperable tumours
3. Residual tumour following incomplete resection
4. As an adjunct to surgery for some tumours
   (a) Neuroblastoma
   (b) Liposarcoma
   (c) Rhabdomyosarcoma
5. Tumour recurrence – RT has a definite role in lowering the incidence of local recurrence. *Radiotherapy will delay the progression of the disease but does not improve survival.*

Chemotherapy

Indications of chemotherapy:

1. Lymphomas
2. Leomyosarcoma showed greater resistance to radiotherapy.
3. In other sarcomas with metastases—may be used as a part of definitive treatment.
4. Chemotherapeutic agents of choice for retroperitoneal sarcoma
   - Adriamycin as a single agent
   - AIM – adriamycin, iposfamide, mensa
   - AD – adriamycin, dacarbazine
   - MAID – mensa, adriamycin, iposphamide, dacarbazine

Prognosis

- Important prognostic factors of RP sarcoma:
  - Histological grade
  - Completeness of surgical excision (RO)
- Prognosis of RP sarcoma: A 5-year survival of 62–92% for well-differentiated tumour after radical excision; 16–48% in undifferentiated tumours.
- Local recurrence rate: About 40–82% with median time of 15 months to 44 months.

Note

- Most common soft tissue tumour affecting adults is lipoma.
- Most of the sarcomas arise *de novo*.
- Most common in the extremities.

Note

Histological type of STS is site-dependent.

- *Extremity* – MFH > liposarcoma
- *Retroperitoneum* – liposarcoma
- *Viscera* – gist, leiomyosarcoma

Note

By age:

- *Most common sarcoma in a child* – rhabdomyosarcoma – commonly embryonal variety
  - More common in lower extremity
  - Most common site of metastasis – lung
- Most common STS in adult is MFH.

Note

Spread:

Soft tissue sarcomas generally metastasize by the haematogenous route.

Most common site of metastasis from soft tissue sarcoma is lung. Exception to this are:

1. Gist and retroperitoneal sarcoma – liver
2. Myxoid liposarcomas – fatty tissues
3. Clear cell sarcomas – bones
4. Rhabdomyosarcomas – lymph nodes

Haematogenous spread is typical of sarcoma and *lymphatic spread is typical of carcinoma.*

Note

Lymph node metastasis is unusual in soft tissue sarcoma and occurs in less than 5% cases.

Soft tissue sarcoma with lymph node metastasis can be remembered by mnemonics **SCREAM.**

S	Synovial sarcoma
C	Clear cell sarcoma – more commonly
R	Rhabdomyosarcoma
E	Epithelial sarcoma – more commonly
A	Angiosarcoma
M	Malignant fibrous histiocytoma (MFH)

Note

Most common site of metastasis from sarcoma is lung.

Note

Kaposi's sarcoma usually presents as multiple lesions on the extremities, *commonly associated with immunocompromised individuals.*

Note

Lymphangiosarcoma (angiosarcoma)

- *A rare tumour develops as a result of complication of long-standing lymphoedema (>10 years).*
- *Stewart-Treves syndrome* – lymphangiosarcoma of the upper extremity in women with ipsilateral lymphoedema after radical mastectomy and postoperative radiotherapy.
- Appear as acute worsening oedema with subcutaneous nodules which are prone to haemorrhage and ulceration.
- Treated by chemo- and radiotherapy followed by surgical excision – radical amputation.
- Associated with poor prognosis.

Note

Embryonal rhabdomyosarcoma

- Common in children – most commonly in head and neck region.
- *Mostly present with proptosis.*

Note

High grade sarcoma

1. Classic osteosarcoma

2. Ewing's sarcoma
3. Angiosarcoma
4. Chondrosarcoma
5. Epithelioid sarcoma ⎤ May cause LN
6. Synovial sarcoma   ⎥ metastases also
7. Rhabdomyosarcoma ⎦

Note

Role of radiotherapy in soft tissue sarcoma:

1. *Internal beam radiotherapy:* Brachytherapy is given in high grade tumour.

2. *External beam radiotherapy:* Teletherapy is given in low grade tumour.
3. All sarcomas more than 5 cm. Need *adjuvant RT* (external beam).
4. Preop RT is also beneficial.
5. Deep-seated tumour, high grade tumour, size more than 5 cm need chemoradiation.

Note

Chemotherapy – imatinib mesylate has shown promising results in recurrent or non-resectable sarcomas.

Intestinal Stomas

A stoma (from Greek 'mouth') is an opening into a hollow viscus either natural or surgically created (artificial) which connects a portion of the body cavity to the external environment. *Natural stomas in the body* are a mouth, a nose, an anus, an urethral meatus.

Any hollow organ can be manipulated into an artificial stoma as required. This includes oeso-phagus, stomach, bowel (small or large), ureters, urinary bladder, kidney, renal pelvis, trachea.

The surgical procedures in which a stoma is created is known as *ostomy* which is prefixed denoting the viscus being exteriorised, e.g. *ileo-*stomy, *colo*stomy, *uretero*stomy, *vesico*stomy, *nephro*stomy, *tracheo*stomy.

Uses of stoma

- Feeding
- Lavage
- Exteriorisation
- Decompression, diversion, drainage

Different types of stoma

- Temporary or permanent
- End or loop

Stoma are based on anatomical location and the organ involved.

Intestinal stoma

It is an artificial opening of the intestine, small or large, surgically created, onto the abdominal wall to divert the faeces and flatus to the exterior, where they may be collected in a changeable bag. *Common intestinal stomas are colostomy and ileostomy.*

Site selection of intestinal stoma

1. Depends on the pathology of the lesion, its location and the organ involved.
2. *Stoma site should be marked properly before elective surgery.*
3. Preferably it should be discussed with the patient and his/her near relative – wife or husband prior to elective surgery.
4. *Stoma should be placed where the patient can see it and easily manipulate the collecting bag by himself/herself.*
5. The selected stoma site *should be away from the potential surgical incision, umbilicus and bony points.*
6. The surrounding abdominal soft tissues should be as flat as possible to ensure tight seal to prevent leakage during movements.
7. A stoma should *preferably be passed within the rectus muscle* to minimise the risk of a postoperative parastomal hernia.

8. Near relatives should also be trained about the method of application of ostomy bag to help the patient at home.

COLOSTOMY

A colostomy is a surgical procedure where an artificial opening is constructed between a part of the colon and the anterior abdominal wall to allow the discharge of faeces.

- A colostomy is designed to be either *temporary* or *permanent*.
- *Colostomy has no sphincteric control.*
- Colostomy appears flush with the abdominal wall or just raised from the surface.
- Most common indication for fashioning colostomy is rectal cancer.

Types of colostomy

1. According to anatomic location
2. According to function
3. According to appearance
4. According to duration

According to anatomic location

- End sigmoid colostomy – *left iliac fossa*
- End descending colon colostomy – *left iliac fossa*
- Transverse colostomy – *above and right to the umbilicus:* Loop or double-barrelled colostomy
- Caecostomy – *right iliac fossa*

The appropriate stoma site must be selected preoperatively for all the elective procedures and for most emergent operations.

According to function that the colostomy is intended for

- Diverting colostomy or defunctioning colostomy.
- Decompression colostomy

Types of colostomy according to function and duration are shown in Flowchart 21.1.

A. Diverting colostomy

Any colostomy may be regarded as 'Diverting' if it is so constructed *that faeces are prevented from entering the diseased bowel distal to it. There are two types: temporary and permanent.*

(a) *Temporary diverting colostomy: Usually loop colostomy – the purpose is to provide temporary diversion of faeces for:*
   (i) Protection of the complicated and threatened distal anastomosis, e.g. following anterior resection for rectal cancer.
   (ii) Grossly infected diverticulitis with or without perforation.
   (iii) Traumatic injuries of the colon or rectum
   (iv) Multiple, complicated and high perianal fistulae.
(b) *Temporary diverting end colostomy:* Hartmann's procedure.
   Once the distal lesions are under control, the temporary colostomy is closed.
(c) *Permanent diverting colostomy:* An end colostomy – *the purpose is to provide permanent diversion of faeces for:*
   (i) Perforated unresectable rectal cancer.
   (ii) Late and unresectable rectal or anal cancer.
   (iii) Unrepairable lesion of rectum or anal canal following trauma, Crohn's disease, hidradenitis suppurativa.

B. Decompression colostomy – temporary

- *The purpose is to provide decompression of hugely dilated large bowel proximal to obstructing growth of the rectum or sigmoid colon.*
- Frequently done on emergency basis to prevent impending rupture of the dilated colon proximal to obstruction.
- Useful and life-saving.
- *Provides opportunity for a subsequent definitive cancer surgery without compromise of the principles of cancer surgery.*

Types of decompression colostomy:
- A loop transverse colostomy
- 'Blow hole' stoma constructed in the caecum or transverse colon.
- Tube type caecostomy

According to appearance of colostomy
   (i) End colostomy
   (ii) Loop colostomy
   (iii) Double-barrelled colostomy
   (iv) 'Blow hole' transverse colostomy
   (v) 'Blow hole' caecostomy
   (vi) 'Tube' caecostomy

According to duration (Flowchart 21.1)

Temporary colostomy – with an intention to reverse it in future

  (i) Loop colostomy
  (ii) Double-barrelled colostomy
  (iii) End colostomy

Permanent colostomy

- *End colostomy* at left iliac fossa, e.g. following APR (abdominoperineal resection) for cancer rectum.

TEMPORARY COLOSTOMY

- **Loop colostomy:** Commonly done with the transverse colon or sigmoid colon.
- **Double-barrelled colostomy:** Commonly done with sigmoid colon or transverse colon.

  Idea: To divert the faecal stream temporarily *to defunct the distal colon:* Diverting colostomy.

Indications

1. To relieve a distal obstruction of the sigmoid colon due to any cause, commonly carcinoma or diverticulitis *for actual or prevention of potential perforation.*
   - *Usually performed as an emergency procedure to relieve obstruction as it is quick and easy to make.*
   - The resection of the diseased part is carried out later on in a completely defunctioned segment of the colon which is empty, inactive and relatively sterile.
2. To defunction the distal colon temporarily and thus *to protect a distal anastomosis after a low colorectal anastomosis.*
3. To prevent faecal peritonitis after perforation of the colon following obstructive cancer, diverticulitis colon, traumatic injuries of colon or rectum.

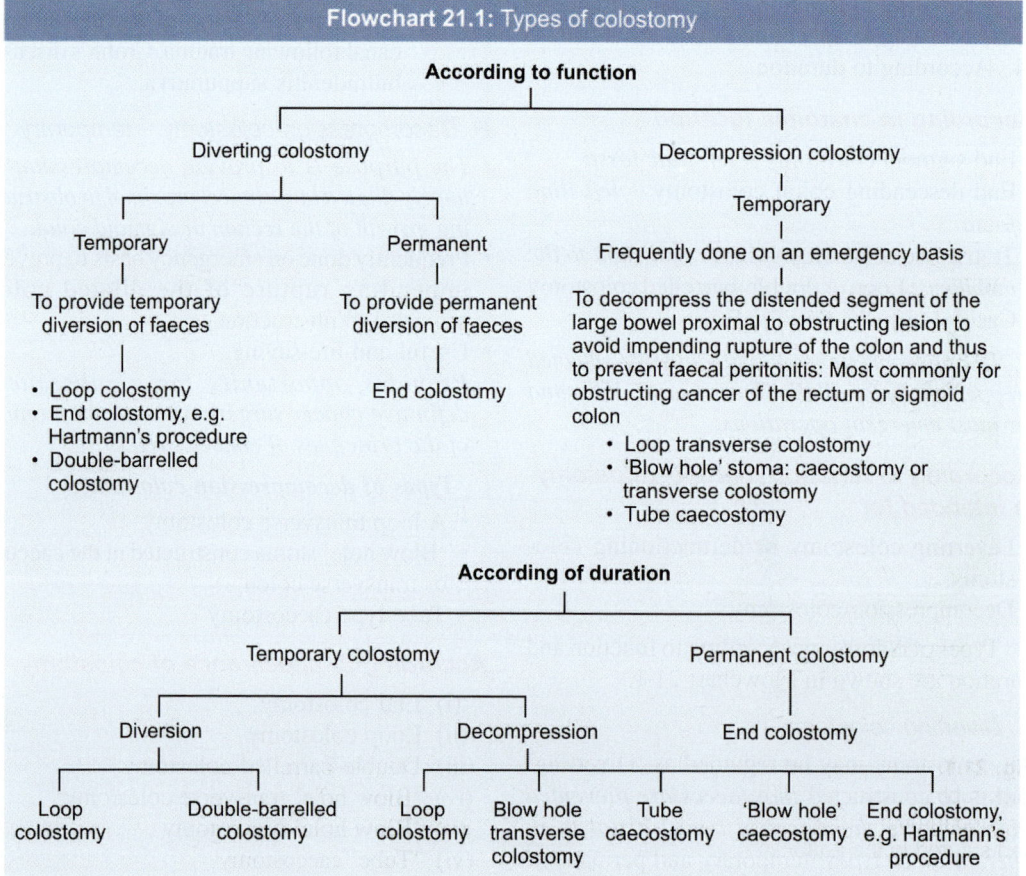

Flowchart 21.1: Types of colostomy

4. To facilitate the operative repair of high fistula in ano.
5. To prevent spoiling of the urinary bladder in vesicocolic fistula or vagina in vaginocolic fistula.
6. Congenital megacolon
7. Anorectal malformation
8. Sigmoid volvulus

Types

A. Temporary loop colostomy
  (Figs 21.1 to 21.3)

Method:
  1. A temporary loop colostomy is made by bringing a loop of bowel to the surface of abdomen.
  2. *The loop is held in place by a glass or plastic rod or a rubber tube passed through the mesentery/mesocolon.*
     • When a glass or plastic rod is used, a piece of rubber tubing is attached to both ends to prevent the rod from slipping out or the ends of the rod sutured to the skin.

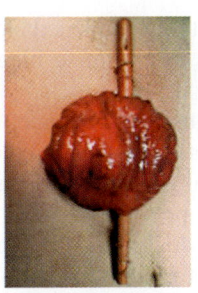

Fig. 21.2: Temporary transverse loop colostomy held in place by a rubber tube. Ends of the rubber tube are sutured to the abdominal wall to prevent retraction.

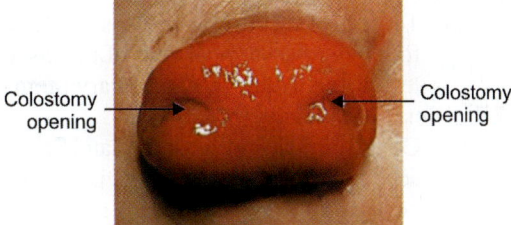

Colostomy opening ← → Colostomy opening

Fig. 21.3: Mature transverse colostomy with healthy moist pink stomas.

     • If a rubber tube is used, it is stitched to skin beyond the stoma.
  3. *So, loop colostomy is made by using the large bowel that has long mesentery,* e.g. transverse colon, sigmoid colon.
  4. Most loop colostomies are made in the transverse colon in diseases involving the left side of the colon.
  5. *Site of election:*
     (a) *Transverse colostomy is usually brought out above and to the right side of the umbilicus,* i.e. right hypochondrium.
     (b) *Sigmoid colostomy is usually brought out in the left iliac fossa.*
  6. *Proximal half of the transverse colon to the right of the middle colic artery is the preferred site,* so that the entire left colon being left available for the subsequent formal operations in the future.
  7. The colonic loop so brought out and the margins of the ostomy are sutured to the layers of the abdominal wall to prevent retraction and/or faecal soiling of the ostomy margin and/or the peritoneal cavity.

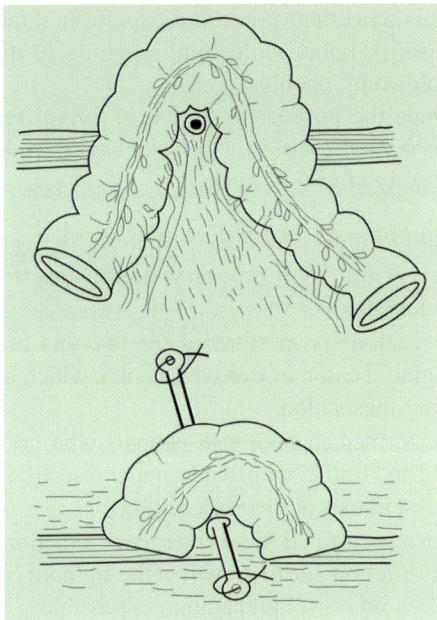

Fig. 21.1: Loop colostomy. Glass or plastic rod or thick rubber tube cut from the malecot catheter is inserted through the mesocolon to support the loop and sutured to the abdominal wall.

8. The colostomy is opened along its exposed tenia coli to minimise bleeding from gut wall.
9. The opening may be made:
   (a) *Immediately* – when colostomy is done specially for distal obstruction, i.e. for decompression
   (b) *After 48 hours* – when colostomy is made for other indications.
10. The glass or plastic rod is removed on the tenth postoperative day and replaced by the rubber tubing, which is finally removed in 2 to 3 weeks.
11. *Closure of colostomy:*
   (a) Temporary colostomy is closed following the surgical cure of the distal lesion for which the temporary stoma has been made.
   (b) Colostomy closure is safely and easily accomplished once the stoma is mature, i.e. *usually 10 weeks after the colostomy has been established.*
   (c) *Intraperitoneal closure of colostomy is preferred over extraperitoneal closure* to avoid closure breakdown resulting in fresh faecal fistula.

B. Double-barrelled colostomy
(Devine or Paul-Mikulicz procedure)

A type of defunctioning temporary colostomy
• A variant of temporary diverting proximal colostomy with mucous fistula (cf. proximal ileostomy with mucous fistula).
• Can be performed with the lesion of sigmoid or transverse colon which has a long meso-colon.
• Rarely used nowadays in poor risk patients, e.g. after resection of a gangrenous sigmoid volvulus, grossly infected diverticulitis or malignant growth of the sigmoid colon with or without perforation.
• *Two types: Devine* procedure and *Paul-Mikulicz* procedure.

Devine procedure (Fig. 21.4)
• A variant of temporary double-barrelled colostomy.
• Occasionally performed with the transverse or sigmoid colon *which has a long mesocolon.*

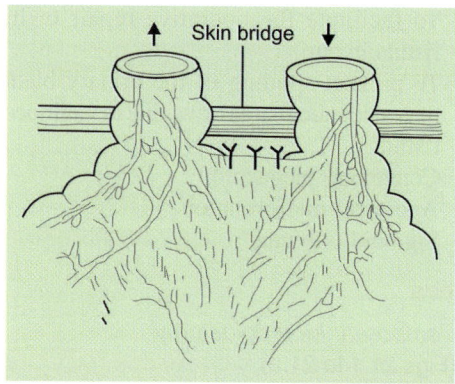

Fig. 21.4: Devine procedure. Skin bridge between the stomas will prevent spillover of faeces from proximal stoma to distal stoma. Requires intra-peritoneal closure of colostomy openings when the purpose is served.

• After resection of the intervening diseased part of the colon intraperitoneally, both the proximal and distal colon ends are brought out to the exterior **through two separate incisions** (openings) on the abdominal surface *thereby fashioning a skin bridge between the stomas.* This skin bridge prevents the spillover of faeces from proximal colostomy opening to distal colostomy opening.
• Once the purpose is served, *a formal intra-peritoneal closure of colostomies is required* usually after 6–8 weeks.

Paul-Mikulicz procedure (Fig. 21.5)
• A variant of temporary double-barrelled colostomy.
• Occasionally, performed for tumours of the sigmoid colon or transverse colon which has a long mesocolon.
• Performed in poor risk patients who are too old and frail to withstand a major resection and anastomosis at the same sitting.
• Also performed in an emergency situation for obstruction due to growth of the sigmoid colon when no bowel preparation is possible.
• The tumour is mobilised and exteriorised through *a separate but same muscle cutting incision* in the abdominal wall, e.g. left iliac fossa for sigmoid growth.

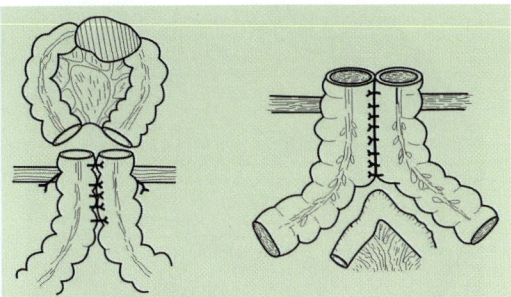

Fig. 21.5: Paul-Mikulicz procedure: *Spur colostomy.* After the purpose is served, the intervening spur between colon ends are crushed by the crushing enterotome and the colostomy openings are closed extraperitoneally.

- The tumour is then resected extraperitoneally.
- The adjacent walls of the two limbs of the colon below the colostomy openings are sewn together at the antimesenteric borders to form a spur keeping the ends of the adjacent guts in contact (*spur colostomy*).
- Once the purpose is served, the colostomy openings are closed *extraperitoneally after crushing the intervening spur by an enterotome* to restore the bowel continuity without laparotomy.

Note

For tumours of the sigmoid colon in a poor risk patient, Hartmann's procedure may also be performed (Fig. 21.9).

PERMANENT COLOSTOMY (END COLOSTOMY) (Figs 21.6 to 21.11)

Types

- **End sigmoid colostomy:** Most common type.
- **End descending colon colostomy:** When the inferior mesenteric artery is transected during an operation of rectal cancer.

   Idea: To provide a permanent opening to allow excretion of faeces for the rest of life in absence of anus.

Indications

Usually performed after abdominoperineal resection (APR) for lower one-third, middle one-

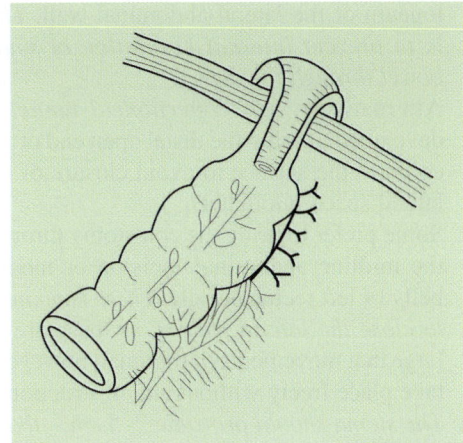

Fig. 21.6: End colostomy. Colostomy opening everted and attached to skin margin of the hole at left iliac fossa. Sutures closing the lateral peritoneal space to prevent small intestine's herniation.

third, and upper one-third of rectal cancer or anal cancer: *APR + left iliac colostomy is commonly done.*

1. *Method:* It is formed by bringing the distal open end of the proximal colon after excision of the distal colon along with rectum and anal canal.
2. *Site of election:*
   (a) Commonly left iliac fossa
   (b) *The stoma location should be flat and away from the skin creases and the bony prominences of costal or iliac margins.* It should be in an area of normal healthy-appearing skin that is visible to the patient. This avoids the faecal spillage from the bag onto the abdominal surface. *In general, the stoma is placed just above the spinoumbilical line at the lateral border of the rectus abdominis muscle or at the middle of the spinoumbilical line.*
      In obese individuals, the stoma may be placed higher, *so patient can see it.*
3. While fashioning the colostomy, after bringing the distal open end of the colon to the abdominal surface, *special care is taken to close the lateral space* between the intra-peritoneal segment of the colon and the peri-

toneum of the lateral abdominal wall. *This is to prevent internal herniation of small bowel through the defect.*

4. Alternatively, a *retroperitoneal tunnel* is developed to bring the distal open end of the colon to the surface to avoid closure of the lateral space (Goligher).

5. Some prefer to bring the colostomy through the midline abdominal incision or medial belly of left rectus muscle. *There is no need to close the lateral spaces,* as these are so large that movements of the small bowel can take place freely without any obstruction.

6. *The stoma should protrude 2–5 cm – like a nipple – above the skin surface. This is to avoid faecal spillage under the bag.*

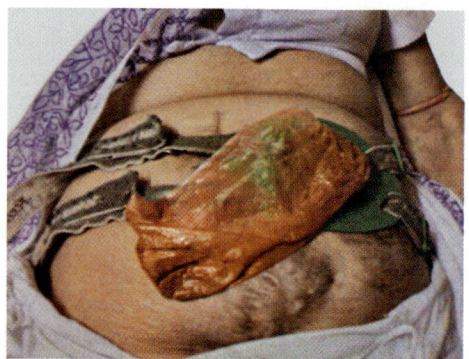

Fig. 21.8A: Permanent left iliac colostomy covered with colostomy bag (following APR for lower third rectal cancer). *Always examine the perineum for scar and absence of anus.* (cf. Hartmann's procedure)

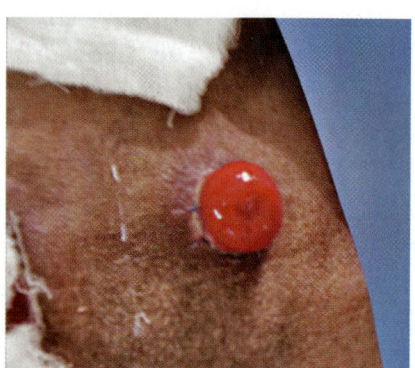

Fig. 21.7: Left iliac permanent end colostomy in an elderly patient after abdominoperineal resection for lower one-third of rectal carcinoma. Note the healthy moist pink stoma projecting well above the abdominal surface like a nipple. *Examine the patient's perineum for presence of scar and absence of anus* (cf. Hartmann's procedure). (*Courtesy:* Dr Sudeb Saha, MS, FAMS)

Note

When possible, the appropriate stoma site must be selected preoperatively for all the elective procedures and for most emergency procedures.

Note

In upper one-third rectal cancer, anterior resection can be performed in selected cases by experienced surgeon which should be protected temporarily by proximal colostomy, caecostomy or ileostomy.

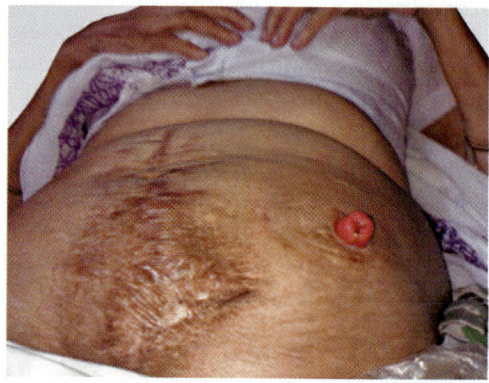

Fig. 21.8B: Same patient after removal of bag. Note that the colostomy was healthy and projecting well from the skin surface but appeared narrow—so, developed stenosis of the stoma. However, patient was managing well with the stenosed stoma with frequent self finger dilatation as advised by surgeon. Note also the hypertrophy of the lower half of the midline scar; but no evidence of incisional hernia on straining or coughing.

Hartmann's procedure (Fig. 21.9)

- It is a form of temporary *end* diverting descending colon colostomy and mucous fistula of distal sigmoid or upper rectum.
- It involves segmental excision of the diseased segment (either from diverticulitis, cancer or gangrene) + closure of the distal stump + temporary end colostomy of the proximal colon – *an emergency procedure.*

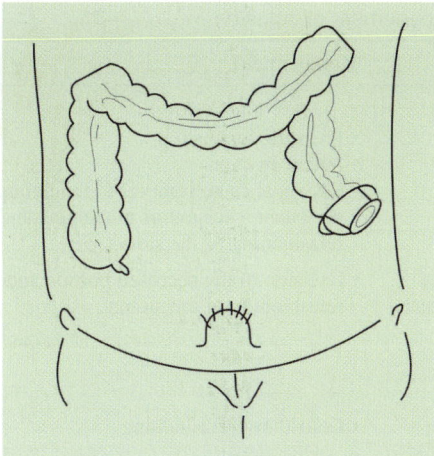

Fig. 21.9: Hartmann's procedure (*see* text) with left iliac end colostomy + sutured intrapelvic rectal stump acting as mucous fistula (cf. left iliac end colostomy following APR). *Examine the perineum* for the presence of anus and digital examination for presence of closed rectal stump. In APR there will be presence of scar in the perineum and absence of anus.

• *This procedure requires a second major laparotomy for reanastomosis of the divided ends of the bowels at a later date*, if necessary, when the patient's emergency condition will settle down, the reanastomosis of proximal colon with the stump of mucous fistula can be performed *to provide normal passage for bowel evacuation. There should be at least 8 weeks interval between the two procedures.*

Indications

1. Grossly infected diverticulitis with or without perforation of the sigmoid colon.
2. Obstructing lesion from cancer of the sigmoid colon or upper one-third of rectum.

Colostomy care

1. Colostomy usually starts functioning during the first 5–7 days following operation. If colostomy fails to function by the seventh postoperative day, straight X-ray abdomen must be done to rule out small bowel obstruction.
2. Look that collecting bag with or without flange or stoma adhesive disc is fitting

properly around the stoma. *Patient and his/ her relative should be trained to learn and manage to apply the bag properly.* Patient may require nurse's assistance during early postoperative period.
3. Patient should take proper care to keep parastomal area clean and dry. Patient and relatives should ensure good local hygiene and *apply properly fitting collecting bag* to avoid parastomal cellulitis.
4. In the presence of parastomal cellulitis, patient requires repeated local application of antiseptic solution and spirit around the stoma and the bag.

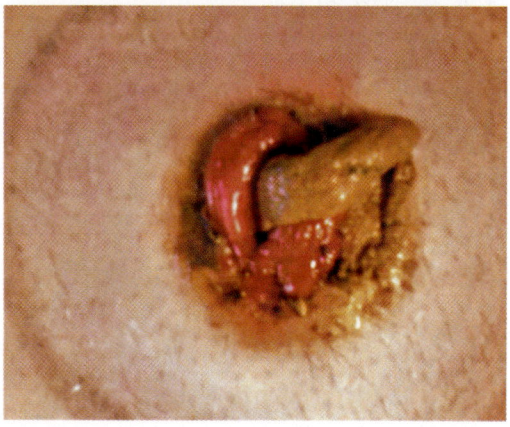

Fig. 21.10: Retraction of colostomy stoma causing spillage of stool onto the abdominal surface. Requires colostomy refashioning.

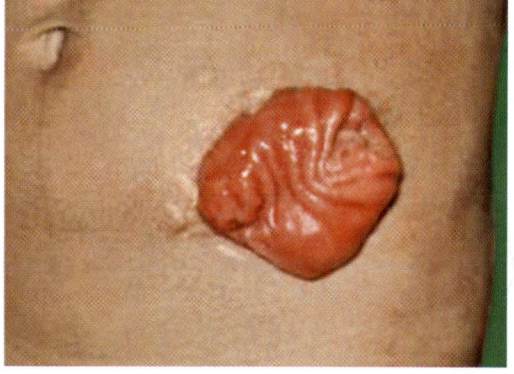

Fig. 21.11: Prolapse of the mucosa through the left iliac end colostomy stoma: Requires colostomy re-fashioning.

Table 21.1: Complications and management of colostomy

Complications of colostomy	Management
Immediate	
1. Bleeding from edges	• Pressure application.
– *Immediate after operation*	• Suture ligation.
– *Delayed*, usually from granuloma around the margin of colostomy	• Chemical cauterisation of granuloma. If persistent, excision of granuloma and refashioning of the stoma.
2. Ischaemic necrosis and sloughing of the distal end of the stoma due to vascular compromise following tight suturing of the sheath and skin around the stoma compromising blood supply of the stoma	• Excision of the necrosed portion and refashioning of the stoma.
Intermediate	
1. Retraction (Fig. 21.10) – partial/total, caused by increased thickness of the abdominal wall due to weight gain	• Colostomy refashioning.
2. Prolapse (Fig. 21.11)	• The protruded bowel should be covered with hypertonic saline packs and then gradually and gently pushed back. If recurrent, colostomy refashioning.
• Common with loop colostomy	
· Leakage of stool may become associated with incarceration with obstructive symptoms, interference with stoma appliance	
• Common with loop transverse colostomy	
· *Ischaemia* – due to inadequate perfusion because of *excessive tension* following inadequate mobilisation or *external pressure* as the bowel passes through the narrow opening of the abdominal wall.	• Urgent attention and exploration – refashioning of stoma.
· Psychological and sexual problems.	• Can be solved by discussion and counselling with nurses and/or members of the 'stoma' club (in European countries many such clubs are present where patient-to-patient communication helps).
3. Stenosis (Figs 21.8 A and B)	• Finger dilatation. If failed, refashioning of the stoma by splitting the constricting abdominal wall layers.
4. Fistula ⎫ 5. Abscess ⎬ Common with 6. Stricture ⎭ Crohn's disease	• Colostomy refashioning.
7. *Parastomal cellulitis* – skin excoriation Poor construction or location of the stoma leads to maceration and inflammation of the skin, pseudoepitheliomatous hyperplasia at the mucocutaneous junction of the stoma. May be due to inadequate adhesive sheet and improper application.	• Avoid loose stool. • Ensure good local hygiene. • Apply proper fitting bag. • Zinc oxide cream application. • Refashioning of stoma in extreme cases.
8. Intraperitoneal abscess	• Drainage with or without antibiotics.
Late	
1. Colostomy hernia – peristomal lateral space ventral hernia with or without prolapse of the stoma – more common in cases of end colostomy	• Closure of the lateral space and refashioning of colostomy.
2. Colostomy diarrhoea	• Avoid constipation.
• Spurious diarrhoea	• Avoid food which causes constipation and/or diarrhoea.
• Infective enterocolitis	• Responds to oral neomycin or metronidazole.

(Contd.)

Complications of colostomy	Management
3. Recurrence of malignancy at the colostomy margin.	• Poor prognosis. Excision of distal bowel segment including stoma and re-establishment of colostomy at a fresh site.
4. High output, foul-smelling affluent.	• Correction of electrolyte imbalance.
5. Cutaneous manifestations of the disease: • Damaged peristomal skin as in psoriasis • Pyoderma gangrenosum in IBD • Parastomal varices in portal hypertension	

5. Patient should avoid diet which produces loose stool. Patient should take high fibre diet and plenty of drinks to avoid consti-pation.
6. Patient should learn self-finger dilatation of the stoma to prevent stomal stenosis.
7. Patient may require frequent colostomy irrigation with 1 litre of plain water through an enema tube *for the purpose of dilating the proximal colon sufficiently to produce a reflex peristaltic contraction of the proximal gut that evacuates the entire distal colon.*

Patient and nurse should take extreme caution while passing the enema tube to avoid perforation of the colon proximal to the stoma which will cause severe abdominal pain during irrigation. This complication represents a surgical emergency and requires urgent laparotomy and reconstruction of colostomy.

CAECOSTOMY

Indications

Severely ill patient with massive distension of large bowel with impending rupture of caecum. The massive distension may be due to:

(i) Growth distal to caecum particularly when ileocaecal valve is competent leading to closed loop obstruction.
(ii) Pseudo-obstructive syndrome, e.g. ileus in elderly patient.

It provides immediate and very effective drainage both of the colon and of the lower ileum.

Purpose

• Caecostomy is performed to prevent faecal peritonitis from rupture of caecum.
• *Colonoscopic decompression is a better alternative for cases of pseudo-obstruction.*
• Caecostomy is performed only when the other methods of decompression fail.

Types

Two types:

1. Skin sutured caecostomy or '*Blow hole*' caeco-stomy.
2. Simple tube caecostomy.

• *A caecostomy is only a temporary measure* to allow a few days to improve the general condition of the patient following decom-pression of large bowel.
• *Definitive surgery is carried out after 5 to 7 days of establishing the caecostomy.*
• *The tube caecostomy requires repeated irrigation with normal saline* to prevent it from being blocked by the faecal matter.
• In tube caecostomy, *the tube may be removed after the 10th postoperative day if it is no longer required.*

ILEOSTOMY

Ileostomy is a surgical procedure where an opening is constructed between the distal ileum and the abdominal wall (for ileostomy, *see* Figs 21.12 to 21.15).

• *Ileostomy has no sphincteric control.* Intestinal waste passes out of the ileostomy and is collected in an external pouching system stuck to the skin continuously.

- Ileostomy is designed to be either temporary or permanent. *Temporary stoma is often constructed as a loop ileostomy. Permanent ileostomy is end ileostomy.*
- Ileostomy is usually sited in the right iliac fossa.
- *An end ileostomy appears to sprout with a nipple* (while the colostomy usually appears flush).
- Care must be taken to leave a 1 cm strip of mesentery with the distal end of the ileum because it carries a vessel supplying the ileal stoma wall and prevent stomal ischaemia.

Indications of ileostomy

Ileostomy is necessary when disease or injury has rendered the large bowel incapable of safely processing the intestinal waste typically because the colon has been partially or totally removed.

Diseases of large bowel which may require surgical removal of the colon include:

- Inflammatory bowel disease—ulcerative colitis, Crohn's disease.
- Familial adenomatous polyposis.
- Total colonic Hirschsprung's disease.
- Occasionally, in the treatment of colorectal cancer where the tumour is causing blockage.

Types

Two types:

- Permanent ileostomy or end ileostomy – an end ileostomy is the preferred configuration for a permanent ileostomy.
- Temporary ileostomy
  (i) End ileostomy
  (ii) Loop ileostomy

Indications

(a) **Permanent end ileostomy:** It is performed in conjunction with a total proctocolectomy in inflammatory bowel diseases like Crohn's disease, ulcerative colitis or polyposis coli: Eversion of the functioning end of the ileostomy *to create a 2.5 cm spigot (nipple) configuration* to eliminate the serositis reaction of the adjacent abdominal wall,

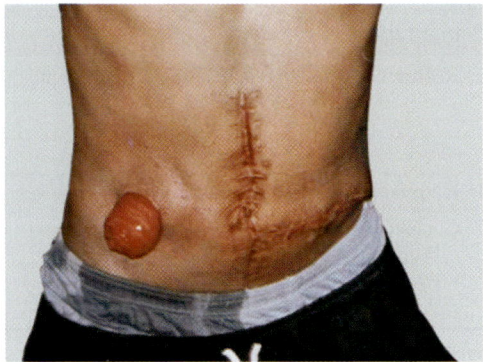

Fig. 21.12: Right iliac permanent end ileostomy— note the stoma was healthy, moist and pink and projecting well above the abdominal surface like a nipple to minimise contact between alkaline effluent (with active enzyme) and skin—Brooke's classic non-conduit ileostomy.

commonly observed from the proteolytic caustic ileal effluent (Fig. 21.12).

(b) **Temporary loop ileostomy:**
- It is performed when temporary diversion of ileal contents is required.
- Commonly performed to divert the ileal contents temporarily *to protect* a tenuous ileorectal, ileoanal, coloanal anastomosis following total colectomy or procto-colectomy, e.g. adenomatous polyposis coli (Fig. 21.13) or carcinoma of lower end of rectum (sphincter preserving operation).

Advantage: To allow healing of the distal anastomosis well and thus allow safe passage of faeces through the anal orifice in future after closure of ileostomy.

(c) **Temporary end ileostomy with mucous fistula:** Occasionally, a temporary end ileostomy (Fig. 21.14) of the proximal end of the ileum and mucous fistula of the distal end of the ileum are constructed, after resection of a gangrenous segment of bowel or a perforated caecal lesion, when primary anastomosis is contraindicated.

Methods

1. *Site of election: Both the types, permanent or temporary, are usually sited on the right*

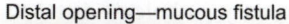
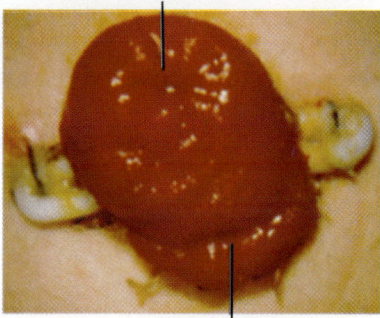

Distal opening—mucous fistula

Proximal opening

Fig. 21.13: Right iliac temporary loop ileostomy held in place by a plastic rod.

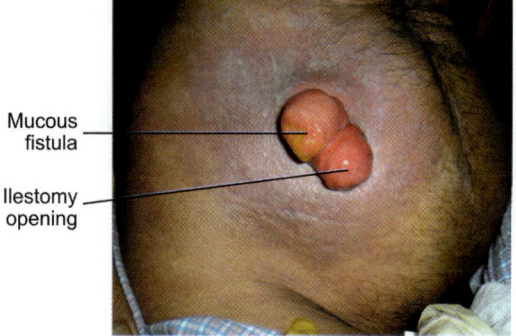

Mucous fistula

Ileostomy opening

Fig. 21.14: Right iliac temporary end ileostomy with mucous fistula—note the maceration and inflammation of the skin around the ileostomy.

iliac fossa, near the outer margin of the right rectus muscle about 5 cm lateral to the midline and 4 cm below the umbilicus.

2. *The ileal stoma should protrude as a nipple for at least 3–5 cm above the skin surface.* The end of the ileum is pulled out through a separate opening in the abdominal wall at right iliac fossa and turned inside out so that the outer margin of everted bowel is sutured to the skin margin of the opening – *Brooke's classic non-conduit ileostomy.* This facilitates the fluid effluent to pass directly into the collecting bag and thus with less chance of seepage between the wafer of the collecting bag and the peristomal skin. *It prevents peristomal skin irritation and break down.*

3. The edge of the ileal mesentery should be sutured to the peritoneum of lateral abdominal wall. *This prevents herniation of small bowel loops through the paraileal stomal space.*
4. *A stoma adhesive disc is applied to the ileostomy stoma in the operation theatre.* An ileostomy bag or pouch is placed over the disc. People with ileostomies *either use a 'closed end' pouch* which must be thrown away when full, *or a 'drainable pouch'* that is secured at the lower end with a leak-proof clip.
5. Ostomy pouches fit close to the body surface and are usually not visible under the regular clothing unless the patient allows the pouch to become full.
6. The ileostomy starts to work within 48 hours.
7. *It produces a daily output of 500 to 700 ml liquid or semi-liquid contents, so, chances of dehydration if more output.*
8. *Ordinarily, the pouch must be emptied several times a day and changed every 2–5 days.*
9. Kock's continent ileostomy with continent intra-abdominal pouch is also being practised by some surgeons.

Complications of ileostomy

Early problems:

1. Ileostomy diarrhoea – treated by diet and fluid control and bowel binding agents.
2. Occasional ischaemic necrosis of the distal ileum due to devascularization.
3. Parastomal infection/irritation.
4. Allergic dermatitis and skin excoriation around the ileostomy – liberal application of zinc oxide cream may help to protect skin excoriation.
5. Parastomal skin ulceration.

Late problems:

1. Fistula
2. Protrusion or prolapse of stoma (Fig. 21.15)
3. Retraction – causing leakage beyond the flange of the bag
4. Stricture/stenosis
5. Obstruction of ileostomy with food fibres, e.g. potato skin, raw vegetables.

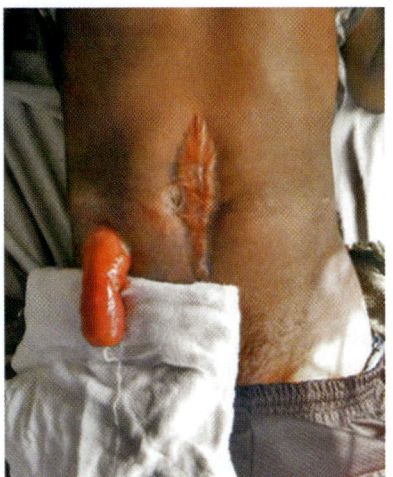

Fig. 21.15: Prolapse of ileotomy: Requires re-fashioning. (*Courtesy:* Dr. Arun Anand, MS)

6. *Ileostomy diarrhoea* – effluent amount larger than 1000 ml/day can cause fluid and electrolyte imbalance. This requires urgent attention and correction of fluid and electrolyte imbalance. Use of drugs like loperamide or lomotil, use of bulk laxatives like isabgol husk may help.
7. Kidney stones formation.
8. Gallstones formation.

   In case of above two points (7 and 8), these are due to loss of absorptive surfaces of ileum and failure of absorption of bile salts.
9. Ileostomy revisions – most commonly performed in patients suffering from Crohn's disease.
10. Parastomal hernia – can interfere with application of bag.

Note

In polyposis coli – ileorectal or ileoanal anastomosis is the preferred choice.

Note

See complications under colostomy also in Table 21.1.

Closure of temporary stoma

Timing of closure

By convention, closure is performed after 6 weeks after ensuring that

(a) The primary pathology distal to the stoma has settled, e.g. pelvic sepsis, peritonitis, multiple fistula-in-ano, rectovaginal fistula, or healing of distal coloanal anastomosis, e.g. anterior resection for lower rectal cancer.
(b) *The defunctional anastomosis has healed and patency confirmed by a contrast study to confirm normal patency of the anastomosis*, e.g. if a low anterior resection had been done.

Closure technique

(a) A loop colostomy is closed *by a simple interrupted anastomosis of the projected margins of the two lumens of the colostomy* keeping the intact posterior wall untouched.
(b) A loop ileostomy is closed by *total resection and anastomosis taking care* that there will be no stenosis after closure.

Examination of a patient presenting with intestinal stomas

Examine:

1. The site of intestinal stoma:
   (a) Left iliac fossa – sigmoid colostomy
   (b) Right hypochondrium – transverse colostomy
   (c) Right iliac fossa – ileostomy, caecostomy

   The ideal stoma site: It should be placed at a site where a patient can see it and easily manipulate the appliance, i.e. the collecting bag.
2. Number of openings:
   (a) *One opening* – end ostomy

      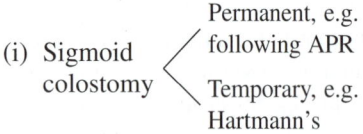

      (i) Sigmoid colostomy — Permanent, e.g. following APR / Temporary, e.g. Hartmann's

      (ii) Ileostomy – permanent (Fig. 21.12)
   (b) *Two openings* – usually temporary
      (a) Loop ostomy
         (i) Transverse colostomy
         (ii) Sigmoid colostomy
         (iii) Ileostomy
      (b) Double-barrelled colostomy
         (i) Devine procedure
         (ii) Paul-Mikulicz procedure

(c) End-descending colostomy and mucous fistula of distal sigmoid – following resection of perforated diverticulitis.

(d) Right iliac temporary end ileostomy of proximal ileum and mucous fistula of distal ileum (Fig. 21.14).

3. Protrusion or projection of the ostomy opening from the skin surface
   (a) Colostomy – at least 2.5 cm above the skin surface
   (b) Ileostomy – at least 3–5 cm above the skin surface
   - Adequate mesenteric mobilisation is necessary for stoma protrusion.
   - Adequate protrusion prevents bowel contents from seeping between the wafer appliance and the peristomal skin.

4. Colour of the stoma – usually pink red.

5. Skin condition around the ostomy opening:
   (a) Smooth, healthy and relatively dry appearance in comparison with the rest of the abdominal surface: Expected.
   (b) Excoriated, macerated and wet surface with or without faecal smell – *mostly due to seepage of effluent. Zinc oxide cream application* over the excoriated surface may help.
   (c) Irregular scar, skin folds or corrugation around the ostomy – allows seepage of the effluent onto the abdominal surface under the flange of the collecting bag which can cause maceration of the skin around the ostomy. *Requires re-fashioning of the stoma.*

6. Whether the ostomy allows introduction of the patient's or examiner's index finger easily – *to exclude stenosis of ostomy.*

7. Examine the patient's perineum in the presence of left iliac end colostomy for linear midline scar and absence of anus. *In the presence of anus do digital examination for rectum:*
   (a) Left iliac end colostomy in APR – anus will be absent.
   (b) Left iliac end colostomy in Hartmann's procedure – anus will be present and will allow digital examination.

8. Enquire what is the *consistency of the effluent:*
   (a) Colostomy – usually solid or semisolid. *If history of constipation or spurious diarrhoea – exclude impaction of stool by digital examination.* This may require enema through colostomy or digital removal of impacted stool. Patient should be advised plenty of drinks, plenty of high fibre diet and frequent purgatives like duphalac.
   (b) Ileostomy – usually liquid or semi-liquid. Enquire the quantity of the daily output – *usually produces a daily output of about 500–700 ml.* Amounts more than 1000 ml/day cause fluid and electrolyte imbalance and increase the likelihood of stone formation.

9. Look for any complication of the ostomy.

10. Enquire for the *type of collecting bags used by the patient* and any problems faced by the patient. *Collecting bags may be*
    - Reusable colostomy bags
    - Disposable colostomy bags with or without flange
    - *Ileostomy bags placed over the stoma adhesive disc.*

11. Ideal stoma appliance should be:
    - Leak-proof.
    - Should not damage the stoma and surrounding skin.
    - Should prevent odour.
    - Easier to use.
    - Easily available.

12. General care and advice to the patients with stoma:
    - Patient *can have normal diet*, which helps to regulate normal bowel action. Liquid intake should be ≤1000 ml/day for patients with ileostomy; and between 1000 and 1500 ml/day for patients with colostomy.
    - *Antidepressants and anticholinergics might cause constipation.* Avoid these drugs.
    - *Patient should have extra stomal bags in his/her possession in case of emergency.*

Note

Types of decompressing colostomy:

- Blow hole caecostomy
- Tube caecostomy
- Blow hole transverse colostomy
- Loop transverse colostomy

Types of diverting colostomy:

- Loop transverse colostomy
- Loop sigmoid colostomy
- Temporary diverting end colostomy – Hartmann's procedure

Note

In polyposis coli – ileorectal or ileoanal anastomosis is the preferred choice.

Note

A *urinary stoma* may also be created surgically to divert urine.

- Suprapubic cystostomy
- Vesicostomy
- Ileal urinary conduit
- Cutaneous ureterostomy

Orthopaedic Disorders

CONGENITAL DEFORMITIES

CONGENITAL TALIPES EQUINOVARUS (CTEV): CLUBFOOT

A congenital deformity involving one foot or both. This deformity is made up of three elements:

1. *Equinus:* The heel is drawn up by tight tendoachillis;
2. *Inversion:* The sole is pointing medially;
3. *Varus:* The forefoot is adducted relative to the hindfoot.

Talipes is a term for foot deformity that centres around the talus and involves the subtalar joint.

Talipes = *Tali* – Talus + *Pes* – Foot

Aetiology

Idiopathic: Common birth defects – about 1 in every 1000 live births. Cause is unknown.

Most cases are due to a defect in the foetal development with imbalance *between the plantarflexor-invertor and dorsiflexor-evertor groups of muscles.*

Milder forms may be due to prolonged malposition of foetal foot in the uterus, but this cannot be accepted for the severe cases. An additional neuromuscular defect is possibly relevant.

Identical deformity *can be seen in babies with neurological lesions* such as spina bifida or polio-myelitis, myelodysplasia, sacral agenesis, Ehlers Danlos syndrome and some other connective tissue disorder or with arthrogryposis multiplex congenita where the muscles are abnormal leading to contracture and curving of the joints.

May be syndromic, e.g. trisomy 15.

Pathological anatomy

The actual defect is subluxation of the talonavicular joint, so that the talus points down-wards (*equinus*) and slightly outwards in relation to the calcaneum, while the navicular along with the entire forefoot is displaced medially upon the head of the talus and rotated into supination (*the forefoot becomes adducted and inverted – the composite **varus** deformity*). There may be internal rotation of the tibia as well in severe cases. Bones of the foot are smaller than normal. The heel is small in size and elevated.

The soft tissues (muscles and ligaments) at the medial side of the foot are also under-developed and contracted *leading to deep creases on the medial side of the foot.* In most cases calf and peroneal muscles (evertors of foot) are underdeveloped and thin as well.

In the absence of early effective treatment secondary growth changes occur in the bones perpetuating the deformity. Untreated TEV *leads to weight bearing on the outer border of foot* which leads to callus formation and significant disability in later life.

Diagnostic criteria

1. *Boys are more affected.*
2. Condition may be bilateral (Fig. 22.1).
3. In mildest form – the forefoot alone found to be adducted relative to the hindfoot.
4. In well-formed cases – *the typical deformity consisting of three abnormal elements are noted:*
   - *Equinus* – plantar flexion at the ankle joint
   - *Varus* – adduction of the forefoot at the talonavicular joint
   - *Inversion* of the foot – at the subtalar joint
   The outer border of the foot is convex and the inner border is concave. The sole is directed medially. *The heel is small and elevated.* There may be *deep furrow at the leg above the heel.*
   The skin of the foot is usually stretched over the dorsum of the foot but thrown into creases along the inner border and the sole (*the skin creases are absent in varieties other than in congenital one*).
   The head of the talus may be seen and felt to protrude on the dorsolateral surface of the foot.
   The leg may be underdeveloped and thinner than that of the healthy side. *There may be some internal rotation of the tibia on its long axis and in a few cases genu valgum.*
5. *Passive movements of the foot are difficult and painful.* As the heel is rotated internally it is not possible to touch anterior surface of the tibia by dorsum of the foot passively.
6. *Different clinical tests for talipes equino-varus:*
   (a) *Dorsiflexion test: In a normal infant*, it is possible to dorsiflex and evert the foot far enough till the little toe touches the front of the leg. This is not possible in CTEV. *This is known as **dorsiflexion test** and **can be used as screening test**.*

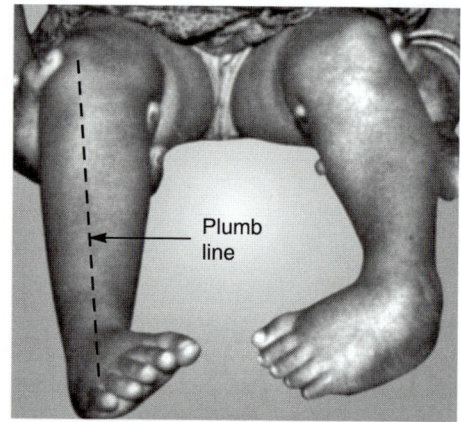

Fig. 22.1: Bilateral congenital talipes equinovarus. Note that the forefoot is adducted and inverted (the sole pointing medially). Equinus (plantar flexion) deformity is not evident from the front in this picture.

   (b) *Plumbline test:* This test helps to detect the tibial torsion. The child is made to sit on the edge of the table with both the lower limbs hanging from the edge of the table. A line is drawn from the centre of the patella down to the tibial tubercle, which when extended down, should cross the foot at the first or second intermeta-tarsal space normally. This is called *Plumbline.* In CTEV, the plumbline cuts the 4th metatarsal space.
   (c) *Scratch test:* This test is performed to detect the muscle imbalance in an infant who cannot obey commands.
   - *Medial scratch test:* In a normal infant when the medial side of the foot is scratched, the foot everts. *This test verifies* the evertor muscles of the foot (peroneus muscles).
   - *Lateral scratch test:* When the lateral side of the foot is scratched, the foot inverts. *This test verifies the invertor muscles of the foot* (tibialis posterior).

X-rays show the shape and positions of the tarsal ossific centres or bones. *In AP view of a* normal foot, the line projecting the long axis of the talus forwards, passes medial to the first meta-tarsal or coincides with it. *In uncorrected club-foot, the line passes lateral to the first metatarsal.*

In lateral view of a normal foot with full dorsi-flexion the long axis of calcaneum should form an acute angle with that of the talus and the *talocalcaneal angle* (kite angle) should be at least 20°. But in CTEV the angle is reduced ≤15°. Normal range of kite angle is 25° to 40°.

Treatment

Depends on the age of presentation.

Primary conservative treatment

Objectives of treatment

1. To correct the deformity early and fully by repeated manual pressure; and
2. To hold the corrected positions until the foot stops growing.

Timing

Ideally the treatment should start within one week of birth.

Correction of deformity:
Ponseti method *(non-operative manoeuvre)*
Each component of the deformity *is corrected in turn* by manipulation and always in the following order.

- *First*, the forefoot adduction;
- *Then*, inversion; and
- *Finally*, the equinus.

It may require three to six manipulations with or without anaesthesia.

Maintenance of correction

The corrected position of the foot is held there preferably by a plaster of pairs cast after each manipulation. The plaster cast must extend to the upper thigh with the knee flexed to 90°, otherwise the infant is able to draw the foot up inside the plaster cast. Repeated manipulation followed by serial plaster casting is known as *Ponseti method.*

Many patients may require a small surgery at the end of plaster casting – *tenotomy of Achilles* tendon to allow correction of equinus deformity.

There are two groups of clubfoot: *Easy and resistant. Easy groups* respond readily to stretching and splinting (Ponseti method). *Resistant groups* respond poorly, and relapse quickly even after repeated manipulations and

plaster immobilisation, and so these groups require early operative corrections.

Complication of CTEV correction

Rocker bottom foot – due to over-enthusiastic overcorrection of equinus deformity before correcting adduction and inversion of foot.

Rocker bottom foot is corrected by Dwyer osteotomy of calcaneum to correct the calcaneus varus deformity.

Operative treatment

The resistant case is best operated upon by 6 weeks. *The operation is soft tissue release at the medial side of the foot and ankle which are tethering the deformity and lengthening of the tendoachillis.* Through a medial incision all the tight ligaments and fascia at the medial side of the foot and ankle are divided and the tight tendons (*the invertors*) are divided. *This is followed by elongation of the tendoachillis usually by tenotomy.* Finally, the foot must be corrected fully and *the corrected position held in plaster for 2 to 3 months.*

Treatment after correction

Whether or not operation was needed, *splintage should be continued with the Denis-Browne splint until the child starts walking*; *thereafter correction can be maintained* by Denis-Browne splint at night and Denis-Browne *shoe during day* which permits walking in eversion during the day. *Splintage may need to be continued until puberty.*

Treatment in neglected or relapsed cases

Several types of operations are available to restore a plantigrade foot.

Between 2 and 5 years of age: Operations involve:

- TURCO operation: Division of contracted soft tissues at the medial side of the foot including the medial talocalcaneal ligament and the posterior capsule of the ankle – *posteromedial soft tissue release*: This may be followed by *lengthening of a short tendoachillis by tenotomy or Z-plasty.*
- *Transfer of the tibialis anterior tendon* to the outer side of the foot, from the first ray (toe) to the third ray (toe) in order to release inward traction of the foot.

- *Transfer of the tibialis posterior tendon* through interosseous membrane to the outer side of the foot, *to supplement the action of the evertor muscles.*

  After the age of 5 years: Some form of bone reshaping is also required. This involves:
- *Dorsolateral wedge excision of calcaneocuboid joint* followed by arthrodesis to shorten the lateral border of the foot (Evans, 1961).
- *Osteotomy of the calcaneum* to correct varus with insertion of a bone wedge in the medial osteotomy site to correct the inversion of the foot (Dwyer, 1963).

  Over the age of 12 years: The best operation is *a dorsolateral wedge tarsectomy,* so that when the gap is closed the foot becomes plantigrade.

  When the patient reaches puberty: A triple arthrodesis could be considered. *It involves fusion of three joints:* TN, talonavicular; TC, talocalcanean; CC, calcaneocuboid.

Note

Three different causes of clubfoot depend on:

- Structural TEV, caused by genetic factors such as Edwards syndrome, a genetic defect with three copies of chromosome 18.
- Breech presentation.
- Ehlers-Danlos syndrome and some other connective tissue disorders.

Note

TEV may be associated with other birth defects such as spina bifida cystica.

SOFT TISSUE LESIONS

A. DISEASES OF FASCIAE

DUPUYTREN'S CONTRACTURE

This lesion consists of *nodular hypertrophy followed by progressive fibrosis in the palmar aponeurosis* that lie deep to the subcutaneous tissues of the hand and superficial to the flexor tendons. This process ultimately leads to shortening and thickening of the fascia leading to flexion contracture of one or more of the

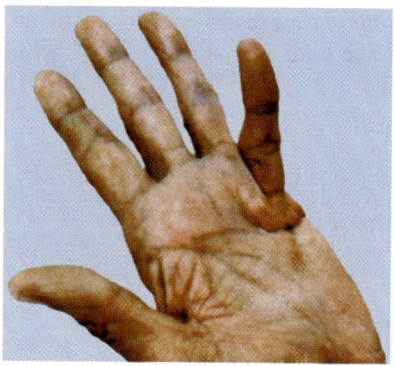

Fig. 22.2: Dupuytren's contracture (a disease of palmar fascia)—causing flexion deformity of the left little finger *flexion at the MP and proximal IP joints.* (*Courtesy:* Dr Yogesh Salphale, D Ortho) *Note and palpate the thickened subcutaneous band from the base of the little finger to the palm.*

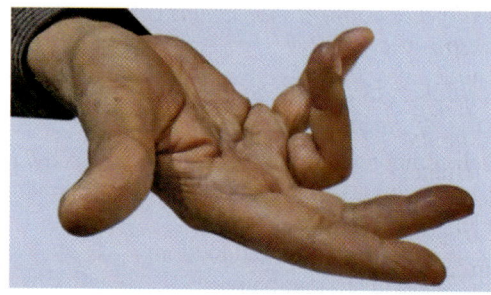

Fig. 22.3: Dupuytren's contracture involving right ring finger and little finger.

fingers in late cases. *Digits usually affected are ring and little fingers.*

Aetiology

1. *Unknown:* The condition is often familial and inherited as an autosomal dominant.
2. Most common in people of European (especially Anglo-Saxon) descent. *Most common in male.*
3. The condition is often bilateral.
4. In a predisposed person, repeated trauma or long continued pressure possibly plays a role but its exact significance is uncertain.
5. *A higher incidence is noted among epileptics receiving phenytoin therapy.* Association with alcoholic cirrhosis, diabetes, pulmonary tuberculosis, AIDS and smoking has also been noted.

Surgical pathology

Due to fibrosis, the palmar aponeurosis becomes greatly thickened and gradually shrinks. In the beginning, a thickened indurated plaque or nodule appears in the palm at the level of the distal palmar crease at the base of the ring finger. The skin is also thickened and firmly attached to the fibrous nodule beneath. Very slowly the induration spreads distally in the fascia towards the little and ring fingers, and proximally up the palm. *Gradually the fascia contracts, pulling the fingers into flexion at the metacarpophalangeal and proximal interphalangeal joints. Distal interpharyngeal joint are never involved.* The medial half of the aponeurosis is affected most. *So the deformity is usually confined to ring and little fingers.* Occasionally middle finger may be affected. The joints themselves are unaffected except in late cases when secondary capsular contractures occur.

It may also affect the little finger individually or simultaneously with the ring finger.

Bilateral disease is rare but involvement is asymmetrical.

Rarely, the plantar aponeurosis in the foot is similarly affected.

Very rarely, this condition may be associated with fibrosis of the corpus cavernosum (Peyronie's disease of penis), keloids and scar hypertrophy, plantar fasciitis.

Diagnostic criteria

1. Usually common in middle-aged persons.
2. Usually painless.
3. In early cases the patient may complain of pain on grasping, or a small nodule in the midpalm. In a late case, the patient may present with typical deformity. The condition may be bilateral.

On examination:

4. In an early case, *a small thickened nodule or plaque in the palm* is felt at the distal palmar crease opposite the base of the ring finger. *There may be obvious subcutaneous cords extending into the ring or little finger or both, leading to flexion of the fingers at the metacarpophalangeal and proximal*

interphalangeal joints (Fig. 22.2). *The distal interphalangeal joints remain unaffected.* The cords get tighter and more prominent if the fingers are extended passively.

Eventually, there is extreme flexion of the finger with the tips digging into the palm. The flexion of the fingers is not lessened by the flexion of wrist joint (cf. Volkmann's contracture).

5. The overlying skin is closely adherent and often puckered.
6. In some cases, there may be thickening of the skin over the dorsum of the proximal interphalangeal joints. These are known as *Garrod's pad.*
7. Movements of the wrist are not affected.
8. Sole of the foot should be examined for any nodule or puckering.

Differential diagnosis

- Congenital contracture of the little finger.
- Volkmann's contracture leading to claw hand.
- Ulnar claw hand in ulnar nerve palsy.

Treatment

1. In early cases, this condition may be treated by *gentle stretching of the fingers and night splintage.* Conservative treatment *may be supplemented with chymotrypsin* (2.5 mg) orally and *hyaluronidase* (1500 units) and *lignocaine* (2% in 20 ml) local infiltrations.
2. *In established contracture leading to deformities, operation is necessary.* Joint contractures of 15° at PIP joint and 30° or more at the MCP joint are usually disabling and so need urgent surgical intervention. *Surgery does not cure the disease, it only partially corrects the deformity.*

Closed fasciotomy entails simple division of the taut contracted bands until passive correction is obtained. But there is a danger of injuring the underlying nerves and vessels; moreover the contracture tends to recur.

Open fasciectomy *is the operation of choice and entails radical excision of the thickened part of the palmar aponeurosis* by painstaking dissection. The affected area is approached through Z-shaped incision along the natural crease lines. Rarely, skin grafting may be required to cover the wound. Postoperatively, splintage and daily wax baths and exercises are required to restore mobility.

Amputation is occasionally advised in presence of severe contracture of the joint capsule of the PIP joint especially of the little finger.

Note

Fibromatosis

- Superficial fibromatosis: Arises from fascia or aponeurosis, e.g.
  - Palmar fibromatosis – Dupuytren's contracture
  - Plantar fibromatosis – Ledderhose's disease
  - Penile fibromatosis – Peyronie's disease
- Deep fibromatosis (aggressive lesion) – desmoid tumour

Any of these lesions may be associated with Dupuytren's contracture.

Note

Peyronie's disease: Fibrous tissue plaque formation involving the Buck's fascia leads to thickening and contracture of the fascia which causes curved penis and painful erections leading to inability to coitus.

NERVE ENTRAPMENT SYNDROME

It is the entrapment neuropathy of the peripheral nerve. The syndrome is caused by increased tissue pressure in a closed fascial compartment compromising circulation to nerves of the compartment – *a variant of compartment syndrome where, including a nerve, muscles are also involved.*

- *Chronic nerve compression* causes slowing of conduction and variable degree of demyelination.
- **Common sites of nerve compression:**
  (a) Carpal tunnel – median nerve
  (b) Pronator teres – median nerve
  (c) Cubital tunnel – ulnar nerve
  (d) Gyon's canal – ulnar nerve
  (e) Axilla or spiral groove – radial nerve – causes wristdrop

(f) Tarsal tunnel – posterior tibial nerve
(g) Neck of fibula – common peroneal nerve – causes footdrop and loss of supination
(h) Inguinal ligament – lateral cutaneous nerve of the thigh leading to meralgia paraesthetica – causing paraesthesia on the lateral surface of thigh

CARPAL TUNNEL SYNDROME

In this condition the median nerve is compressed as it passes through the carpal tunnel – *the space between the flexor retinaculum and the carpal bones leading to entrapment neuropathy* (Fig. 22.4).

Surgical anatomy

Carpal tunnel: The carpal tunnel is a fibro-osseous tunnel, *the floor* of which is formed by the concavity of the carpal bones and *the roof* is formed by the flexor retinaculum. Through this tunnel pass the following structures.

1. Flexor digitorum superficialis and profundus, the long flexor of the fingers with their common synovial sheath (*the ulnar bursa*).
2. Flexor pollicis longus, the long flexor of the thumb with its own synovial sheath (*the radial bursa*).
3. *Median nerve which passes deep to the retinaculum* on the lateral side of the flexor digitorum superficialis (middle finger tendon), between it and flexor carpi radialis.

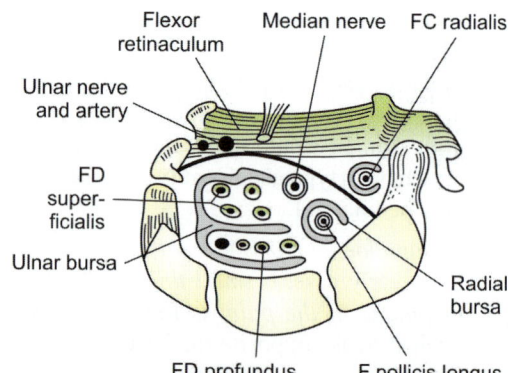

Fig. 22.4: Carpal tunnel with its contents. Note that ulnar nerve lies superficial to the retinaculum and median nerve lies deep to the retinaculum.

So, through this small, tough and non-resilient tunnel so many structures are crowded. *There is normally insufficient space for the median nerve in the carpal tunnel. Any lesion diminishing the size of the compartment can cause compression of the median nerve.*

Compression of the median nerve causes ischaemia of the nerve which, if prolonged, can cause ischaemic damage of the axon, resulting in paraesthesia, numbness and motor weakness in its distribution. *It is a variety of nerve entrapment or compartment compression syndrome.*

Since the superficial palmar branch of the median nerve is given off proximal to the retinaculum and passes superficial to it, *there is usually no sensory impairment over the thenar eminence.*

Note also that *the ulnar nerve passes superficial to the flexor retinaculum and so is spared.*

Causes of compression

Compression can be caused by skeletal abnormalities, swelling of the soft tissues within the tunnel, or thickening of the retinaculum.

Skeletal deformities: Osteoarthritis, rheumatoid arthritis, increase in bone size in acromegaly. Dislocation of lunate or fracture of distal radius with spread of haematoma into carpal tunnel – both are acute surgical emergencies.

Soft tissue deformities:
- Swelling of the common flexor tendon sheaths during menopause and pregnancy, myxoedema without any very obvious cause. Women have smaller tunnels than men.
- Rheumatoid or tuberculous tenosynovitis (bursitis), e.g. compound palmar ganglion.
- Lipoma in the hand.

Diagnostic criteria

1. *Age and sex: Common in middle-aged women at the menopause.* In case of younger patients – pregnancy, rheumatoid disease, tenosynovitis, or skeletal deformities may be the factors.
2. The patient presents with the *complaints of pain and paraesthesia in the distribution of median nerve, i.e. in the radial three and a half digits.* Little finger is never affected (as it is supplied by the ulnar nerve). These symptoms are often prominent during night – *the patient is often woken in the middle of the night* with burning pain, tingling and numbness, and a feeling of stiff swollen fingers and hand. The patient may have to move the fingers or shake the hand to get relief. *The pain may radiate up the inner side of the forearm.*

   Symptoms are often provoked by prolonged driving or reading newspaper holding it in upright position. The patient is unable to hold the paper between the thumb and fingers. *The patient is also unable to carry shopper's bags.*

   As the lesion progresses, the patient complains of clumsiness in carrying out fine movements such as sewing, writing.

On examination:

3. *Tinel's sign:* Repeated tapping over the middle of the volar aspect of the wrist and adjacent distal area for 30 to 60 seconds will produce or aggravate the pain and paraesthesia of radial three and half digits.
4. *Phalen's test:* When the wrist of the patient is held in full palmar flexion (at 90°) for 1 to 2 minutes *will produce typical pain and paraesthesia in the distribution of median nerve supply in radial three and half digits.*

   But there will be no paraesthesia and numbness over the thenar eminence.
5. *Reverse Phalen's test:* Forced hyperextension of the wrist for 60 seconds produces same symptoms as in Phalen's test.
6. *Durkan's test:* Direct pressure over the middle of the carpal tunnel just distal to distal palmar crease will produce same symptoms as above.
7. *In early cases,* hand looks and feels normal. *In late cases,* there is wasting of the thenar eminence with reduced sensation of the thumb, index and middle fingers.
8. *In a long-standing case,* the thenar muscles become weak due to thenar wasting. *Abduction and opposition of the thumb become weak.*

9. *Different tests to look for weakness of the thenar muscles supplied by median nerve are:*
   (a) *Pen test:* The patient is asked to keep the hand flat on the table with the palm facing the roof; then the patient is asked to touch the tip of the pen or pencil held in front and above the tip of the thumb; *failure to do so* is due to paralysis of abductor pollicis.
   (b) *Alternatively,* the patient is asked to abduct the thumb against resistance – patient will fail to do so.
   (c) *Froment's sign* or book-holding test – the patient will be unable to hold the book because of the failure of abduction.
   (d) *The patient is asked to touch the tips of other fingers* – failure to do so because of failure of abduction and opposition.
10. In a long-standing palsy with thenar muscle wasting and loss of sensation over the thumb, and due to unopposed action of extensor pollicis longus (supplied by radial nerve), the weak thumb is so rotated that its palmar surface lies in the same plane as the rest of the hand – *leading to ape thumb or simian hand deformity.*
11. Peripheral pulses and temperature are normal. There will be *no sensory loss over the thenar eminence.*
12. Evidence of menopause or pregnancy, myxoedema, osteoarthritis and rheumatoid arthritis should be looked for.
13. One should exclude other causes of para-esthesia in the hand such as cervical rib, spondylosis, compound palmar ganglion and peripheral neuritis.

Investigations
(a) Electromyography (EMG) – will show denervation of the thenar muscles.
(b) Nerve conduction study (NCS) – will show abnormal median nerve sensory supply.
(c) X-ray cervical spine to exclude cervical rib and spondylosis.
(d) Usually clinical examination is adequate for surgical interference.
(e) MRI of the wrist to exclude secondary causes.

Treatment
Operation is the treatment of choice and includes longitudinal division of the flexor retinaculum to decompress the nerve. Operation causes immediate relief of pain but neurological deficits may not be recovered fully.

Note

Attachment of flexor retinaculum on the hand:

• On the medial side
  · *Proximally:* Pisiform
  · *Distally:* Hook of the hamate
• On the lateral side
  · *Proximally:* Scaphoid
  · *Distally:* Trapezium

Note

Provocative test for median nerve

Most reliable clinical diagnostic test for carpal tunnel compression of median nerve involves insufflation of a sphygmomanometer cuff around the arm on the involved side to a point above the systolic pressure – *this produces* symptoms of pain and paraesthesia within one minute as a result of ischaemia superimposed on an irritable nerve.

Note

Deep to flexor retinaculum lie the radial and ulnar bursae. In between these bursae lies the median nerve (Fig. 22.4).

Inflammation of these bursae may develop compound palmar ganglion which can also cause compression of the median nerve leading to carpal tunnel syndrome (cf. tarsal tunnel syndrome).

PRONATOR TERES SYNDROME

• *Compression of the median nerve can also occur when it passes between the two heads of pronator teres muscle after entering the forearm.*
• Presents with pain on the volar surface of the forearm *following prolonged and repeated pronation movements. Common with mechanics* whose job requires prolonged and

repeated *unscrewing of the joints* with screw driver.
- *There will be loss of pronation of the forearm, wrist flexion, flexion of thumb, index and middle fingers.*
- It also causes paralysis of the flexor digitorum profundus (FDP) of the index finger which is supplied by the median nerve. This can be confirmed by *Ochsner clasping test.* Normally, when the patient is asked to clasp both the hands, all the fingers become flexed. But due to paralysis of the FDP (lateral half), the index finger of the paralysed side *fails to flex and remains straight like pointed finger.*
- *There will also be numbness over the thenar eminence* (cf. median nerve compression in the carpal tunnel – when there will be no numbness over the thenar eminence). But other clinical features of carpal tunnel compression remain the same.

Note

In median nerve compression in carpal tunnel the sensory branch supplying the skin over the thenar eminence is not compressed as this branch arises from the median nerve much above the flexor retinaculum and this sensory branch also passes over the flexor retinaculum to supply the skin over the thenar eminence. So there will be no compression of the sensory branch and no sensory loss over the thenar eminence. Sensory impairment will be noted over the radial three and half fingers only.

Note

To avoid injury to the recurrent motor branch of median nerve supplying the thenar muscles, *incise the flexor retinaculum along the ulnar side of the median nerve.*

ULNAR NERVE COMPRESSION SYNDROME

1. *Second most common peripheral nerve entrapment.*
2. Sites of compression of ulnar nerve:
   - *Arcade of Struthers and the medial inter-muscular septum of humerus* – as the nerve passes into the posterior compartment of the distal humerus.
   - *When the nerve passes posterior to the medial epicondyle of the humerus – the funny bone –* fracture can cause pressure on the nerve or if osteophytes are present following fracture of oleocranon or medial epicondyle leading to malunion. *Fracture may cause cubital vulgus deformity. Normally one can feel and roll one's own ulnar nerve posterior to the medial epicondyle.* (Try it on yourself.)
   - *Cubital tunnel – formed by the tendinous arch connecting the humeral and ulnar heads of the flexor carpi ulnaris* (FCU).
   - *At the wrist –* proximal to pisiform bone.
   - *At the Guyon tunnel in the hand* deep to the pisohamate ligament between the pisiform and hook of the hamate (osseofibrous tunnel) but superficial to flexor retinaculum.
3. *Most common site of compression is around the elbow, especially if associated with cubitus vulgus deformity.*
4. *Patient may present with paraesthesia of the ulnar side of the hand –* hypothenar eminence and ulnar one and half fingers, *wasting of the hypothenar muscles of the hand* and ***clawing** of the medial two fingers (4th and 5th) –* hyperextension of the metacarpophalangeal with flexion at the proximal interpharyngeal joint.
5. There will be wasting of interossei muscles both palmar and dorsal.
6. *Wasting of the intrinsic muscles* will be clinically evidenced *by the longitudinal grooves on the dorsum of the hand between metacarpal shafts.*
7. *Different tests to look for weakness of the muscles of hand supplied by ulnar nerve are:*
   (a) The patient is asked *to abduct the extended fingers against resistance –* if unable to do so, it indicates dorsal interossei are weak (DAB – **d**orsal inter-ossei causes **ab**duction).
   (b) *Card test:* A postcard is inserted between the two extended fingers and the patient

is asked to hold the card by adducting these two fingers as tightly as possible. *If unable to do so*, it indicates weakness of palmar interossei (PAD – **p**almar interossei cause **ad**duction).

   (c) *Froment's sign:* The patient is asked to grasp a book firmly between the fingers and the thumbs of both the hands. In normal condition the thumbs will remain straight while holding the book. *But due to paralysis of the first palmar interossei and the adductor pollicis (**supplied by the ulnar nerve**), the affected thumb will not grasp the book. Moreover, the affected thumb will be flexed on the paralysed side* to hold the book by flexing the thumb by the unopposed flexor pollicis longus (nerve supply of the flexor pollicis longus – *anterior interosseous branch of the median nerve*).

Treatment of ulnar nerve palsy

1. At elbow:
   • Decompression of ulnar nerve at situ – *division of Osborne ligament from the median epicondyle to the olecranon.*
   • Decompression and anterior transposition of the ulnar nerve in front of medial epicondyle.
   • Often, medial epicondylectomy may be required to release pressure on the ulnar nerve.
2. At the wrist:
   • Decompression of the ulnar nerve at situ after dividing the slender ligament between pisiform and hamate bone – *the pisohamate ligament.*

B. DISEASES OF SYNOVIUM AND TENDON SHEATHS

▌BURSA

A bursa is a physiological fluid-filled sac of connective tissue lined with flattened endo-thelium similar to synovium, in relation to a joint. *The bursa is interposed between two moving surfaces in relation to a joint or in the interface between a bone and a muscle sliding over it to reduce friction during joint or muscle movements.*

Bursa may be of two varieties:

1. True bursa – *the fluid in the true bursa is similar to synovial fluid.* Some true bursa may communicate with the joints.
2. Adventitious bursa – new formation of sac without a true synovial lining lies between bony prominence and overlying skin and subcutaneous tissue. It develops secondarily to repeated but prolonged friction and pressure. *There is no synovial fluid in the adventitious bursa.*

Bursitis refers to inflammation of a bursa resulting in accumulation of excessive fluid inside the bursa leading to inflammation, swelling, acute pain and tenderness. *The causes of chronic bursitis* include constant pressure or friction, constant irritation or minor but repeated injuries.

The symptoms are usually self-limiting and settle without intervention, except rest, restricted movements and anti-inflammatory drugs. Occasionally, aspiration, steroid injections or excision may be required.

Investigations

X-ray or MRI.

BURSA IN RELATION TO KNEE JOINTS

Surgical anatomy

Bursae around the knee-joint: There are about 12 bursae around the knee joint of which 4 are anterior, 2 posterior and 3 each on medial and lateral sides.

A. *Anterior bursae:* Four in number (Fig. 22.5):
   1. Suprapatellar – communicates with the knee joint.
   2. Prepatellar.
   3. Superficial infrapatellar.
   4. Deep infrapatellar.

B. *Posterior bursae:* Two in number (Fig. 22.6) – one between each head of origin of gastro-

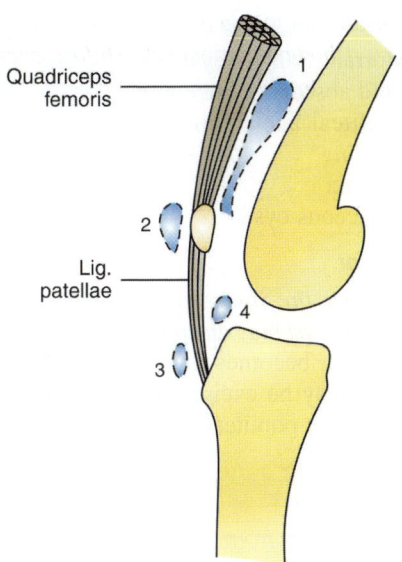

Quadriceps femoris

Lig. patellae

Fig. 22.5: Bursae in front of the knee joint—anterior bursae.

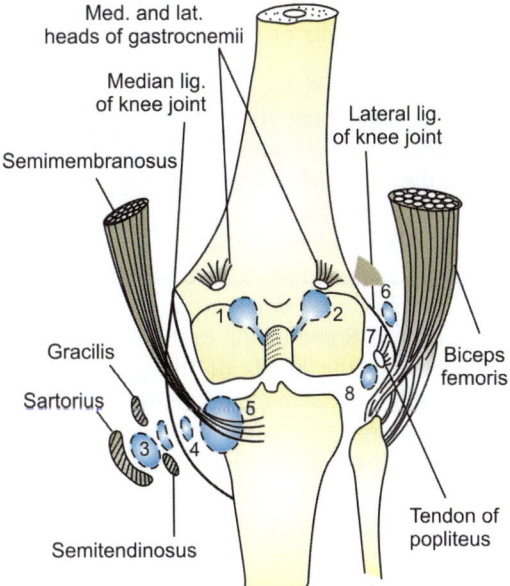

Med. and lat. heads of gastrocnemii

Median lig. of knee joint

Semimembranosus

Gracilis

Sartorius

Semitendinosus

Lateral lig. of knee joint

Biceps femoris

Tendon of popliteus

Fig. 22.6: Posterior, medial and lateral sets of bursae around the knee joint.

ligament of the knee – separating the sartorius, gracilis and semitendinosus from the medial ligament as these muscles cross it (3 in Fig. 22.6). This is also known as *bursa anserinus* because it resembles goose's foot.

2. One deep to the medial ligament of the knee – separating the ligament from the tendon of semimembranosus (4 in Fig. 22.6).

3. One between the semimembranosus and the medial condyle of the tibia – semi-membranosus bursa (5 in Fig. 22.6).

D. Lateral bursae: Three in number (Fig. 22.6).

1. One superficial to the lateral ligament of the knee – separating the biceps tendon from the lateral ligament (6 in Fig. 22.6).

2. One between the lateral ligament and the tendon of popliteus (7 in Fig. 22.6).

3. One between the tendon of popliteus and the lateral condyle of femur – communi-cates with the joint (8 in Fig. 22.6).

Semimembranosus bursa
(Figs 22.7 and 22.8)

This bursa lies between the semimembranosus tendon and the medial condyle of the tibia. It very often communicates with the knee joint through

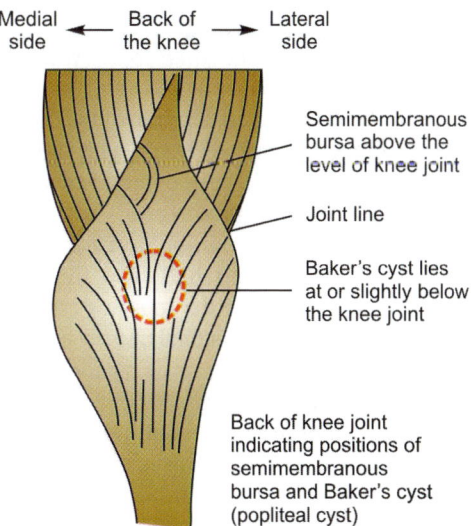

Medial side ← Back of the knee → Lateral side

Semimembranous bursa above the level of knee joint

Joint line

Baker's cyst lies at or slightly below the knee joint

Back of knee joint indicating positions of semimembranous bursa and Baker's cyst (popliteal cyst)

cnemius and the capsule of the knee joint. These may often communicate with the knee joint.

C. *Medial bursae:* Three in number (Fig. 22.6).

1. One lies superficial to the medial

Fig. 22.7: Relative position of semimembranosus bursa and Baker cyst.

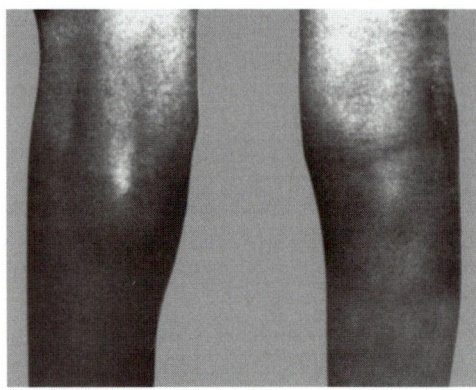

Fig. 22.8: Semimembranosus bursa left knee.

a narrow aperture. *Chronic serous bursitis is* frequent particularly among children and adolescents.

Diagnostic criteria

1. *Age:* Common in children and adolescents of both sexes.
2. *Site: Swelling situated at the posteromedial aspect of the knee joint in between the medial head of gastrocnemius and semimembranosus.*
   The swelling lies above the level of the joint line, slightly to the medial side of the popliteal fossa (cf. Baker's cyst).
3. On flexion of the knee joint – the swelling becomes less prominent.
4. *On extension of the knee joint* (when the patient stands erect), the swelling becomes prominent. Due to contraction of the muscle, the communication of bursa with the joint cavity is closed, hence the size of the swelling becomes prominent.
5. *Cystic in feel: Fluctuation positive,* but the fluid cannot be pushed into the joint, presumably because the muscles compress and obstruct the occasional narrow aperture.
6. Transillumination – may be positive.
7. *Usually no pain or tenderness.*
8. *Knee examination and movements are otherwise normal* (cf. Baker's cyst).
9. *Non-pulsatile:* Popliteal and peripheral pulses are normal.
10. X-ray knee joint is normal.

Differential diagnosis

1. Morrant Baker's cyst
2. Cold abscess of knee joint
3. Popliteal aneurysm – *extensile pulsating swelling*
4. Lipoma
5. Sebaceous cyst.

Treatment

In children the operation may be deferred because the cyst may disappear. Nevertheless, if the swelling becomes uncomfortably large or painful it may be excised through a transverse incision in the popliteal fossa.

Morrant Baker's cyst (popliteal cyst)

This cyst results from herniation of the synovial membrane of the knee joint through the posterior capsule. It is not a primary condition but is always secondary to disease of the knee with persistent accumulation of synovial fluid as in osteoarthritis or rheumatoid arthritis.

Diagnostic criteria

1. *Age:* Near about 40 years or middle aged.
2. Patient presents with a swelling in the back of the knee *with pain in the joint particularly during walking.*
3. *Site: The swelling is situated near the midline in the popliteal fossa, below the level of the joint line and deep to the gastrocnemii muscles.* Some of the cyst may bulge out between the heads of the gastrocnemii muscles (cf. semimembranosus bursa) and when large may extend enough as far as the mid-calf *to interfere with knee movements.*
4. *Cystic in feel – fluctuation positive.*
5. *The swelling is often reducible as the fluid can be pushed into the joint.*
6. Examination of knee joint shows evidence of *arthritis.*
7. *Effusion in the knee joint* is obvious and can be demonstrated by patellar tap.
8. *Knee movements: Painful and restricted with or without crepitus – on flexion* swelling increases and *on extension* swelling decreases in size (cf. semimembranosus bursa).

9. Non-pulsatile.

10. *X-ray – evidences of arthritic changes in knee are present.*

Differential diagnosis

- Semimembranosus bursa.
- Popliteal aneurysm – extensile pulsating swelling.

    CT/MRI will confirm the pathology.

Treatment

1. Aspiration and injection of hydrocortisone followed by crepe bandage.
2. Treatment of the associated joint pathology if any, e.g. rheumatoid or osteoarthritis.
3. If conservative treatment fails, excision of the cyst with or without synovectomy of the knee joint can be performed.

Note

- Both semimembranous bursa and Morrant Baker's cyst are abnormal fluid-filled sacs of synovial membrane in the region of popliteal fossa.
- Both are cystic and *non-pulsatile swellings* (cf. popliteal aneurysm).
- *Semimembranous bursa – knee movements are painless and no knee joint effusion.*
- *Morrant Baker's cyst – knee movements are painful with knee joint effusion.*
- D/D: *Popliteal aneurysm* – an expansile pulsating cystic swelling in the popliteal fossa.

Adventitious bursae

These are *new formations of sacs* without a true synovial lining over bony prominences secondary to repeated but prolonged friction and pressure between the bone and adjacent connective tissue.

Individual bursa of clinical importance

1. Subdeltoid bursa

- It lies *between the deltoid muscle and underlying greater tuberosity of the humerus.*
- It may be affected by chronic tuberculous disease or by acute gonococcal infection.
- It forms a fluctuant tender swelling beneath the deltoid muscle and makes active abduction at shoulder painful and limited.

2. Olecranon bursa (Fig. 22.9)

- It lies *between the skin and the olecranon process – subcutaneous bursa or bunion.*
- Chronic serous bursitis is common particularly in students who are in the habit of resting their elbow over the table during their study – so known as *'Student's elbow'*.
- Also common in miners – *Miner's elbow.*
- It is also the seat of gouty deposits.
- The bursa may also be affected by rheumatoid arthritis, tuberculosis or rarely syphilis.

    Also prone to injuries during falls on the elbow or infections from abrasions of the skin covering the elbow.

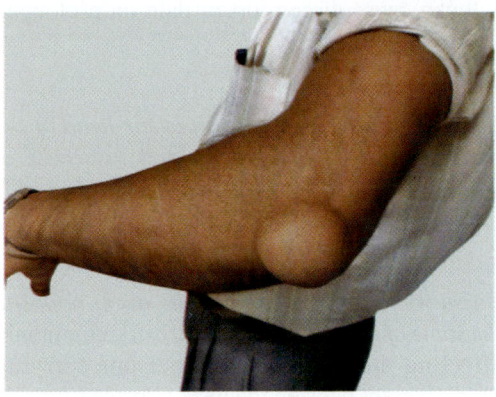

Fig. 22.9: Olecranon bursa left elbow.

3, Prepatellar bursa

- Chronic serous bursitis of prepatellar bursa due to repeated minor trauma, characterised by *a swelling in front of the patella.*
- *Common in housemaids* who do much kneeling during swabbing of the floor– so known as *'Housemaid's knee'.*
- Nowadays it is *also common in miners and carpet layers.* Such occupational hazards may stop the patient from working.

4. Superficial infrapatellar bursa

- Chronic serous bursitis of this bursa is *common in clergymen* who spend long hours in kneeling down during the prayer — so known as *'Clergyman's knee'.*
- It should be differentiated from *Osgood-Schlatter's disease* (apophysitis of the tibial tubercle).

5. Gluteal bursa

- It lies between the tendon of the gluteus maximus and the greater trochanter of the femur (*a trochanteric bursa*).
- It may be rarely affected by tuberculosis.
- It forms *a fluctuant swelling behind the trochanter and causes abduction and lateral rotation at the hip joint painful.*

6. Ischial bursa

- Chronic serous bursitis of the bursa in relation to the ischial tuberosity characterised by a cystic swelling is *commonly met in the weavers who sit for a long time on their ischial tuberosity* – so known as 'Weaver's bottom'.
- It can cause discomfort or pain on prolonged sitting.

7. Metatarsal bursa

Bursa over the medial aspect of the head of the first metatarsal bone particularly in a case of hallux vulgus due to repeated friction from ill-fitting shoes. This is also called *Bunion.*

8. Bursa found on the nape of the neck

Bursa found on the nape of the neck, opposite the spine of the 7th cervical vertebra – commonly affecting the fish-sellers or persons carrying heavy weight bags on the neck (*Porter's bursa*). This was popularly known as *Billingsgate hump* (Billingsgate was the largest fish market in London).

D/D: Lipoma at the nape of neck – *slipping sign is positive in lipoma.*

9. Bursa over the shoulder

Bursa over the shoulder between clavicle and skin of shoulder – commonly affecting the persons carrying weights on the shoulder (*porter's bursa*).

10. 'Basket carrier's bursa'

'Basket carrier's bursa' on the scalp caused by carrying heavy weight basket on the head (*Porter's bursa*).

11. 'Tailor's ankle'

This is a bursa over the lateral malleolus between the skin and lateral malleolus due to prolonged and repeated friction while working with sewing machine operated by foot.

12. Bursa developing over an exostosis

Bursa developing over an exostosis – due to prolonged and repeated friction

13. Calcaneal bursa

(a) *Retrocalcaneal bursa* develops at the back of the heel between the tuberosity of the calcaneum and the skin *due to repeated friction from ill-fitting shoes. Callosity may also develop over the skin.* It responds well to footwear modification.

(b) *Retroachilles bursa* develops between the tuberosity of the calcaneum and tendo-achilles – *common in swimmers,* long distance runners, basket ball or tennis players.

14. Weaver's bursa

This bursa develops *superficial to ischial tuberosity of professional weavers* who spend long periods of time sitting on their bottom during working hours.

15. Breaststroker's knee in swimmers

Bursa under the pes anserinus, i.e. conjoint insertion of Sartorius, gracilis and semi-tendinosus *on the medial side of the knee.*

Treatment of bursa

- Avoidance of prolonged pressure or friction.
- X-ray of the swelling.
- Excision, if symptomatic.

Note

Porter's bursa

- Over the nape of the neck – Billingsgate hump (cf. lipoma over the nape of the neck – in Chapter 2)
- Over the shoulder
- Over the scalp (Basket carrier's)

Note

Usual site of tubercular bursitis is trochanteric bursa and subdeltoid bursa.

GANGLION (Figs 22.10 and 22.13)

A ganglion is a cystic swelling, originating in the synovial membrane of tendon sheaths or of the smaller joints due to mucoid or myxomatous

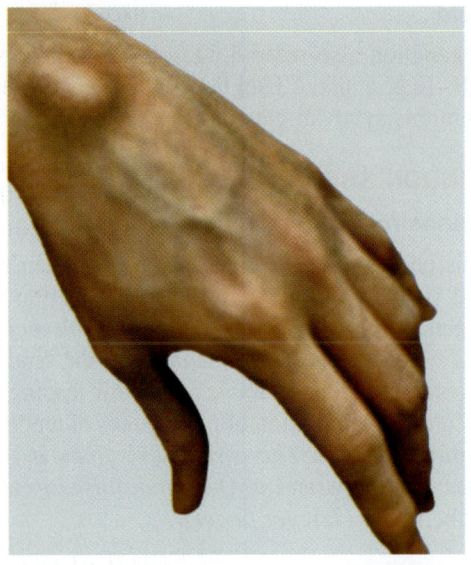

Fig. 22.10: Ganglion dorsum of the left wrist.

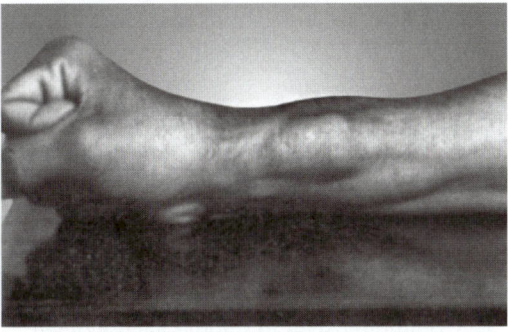

Fig. 22.11: Ganglion—involving common sheaths of the tendons of abductor pollicis longus and extensor pollicis brevis. The swelling becomes prominent on making the fist.

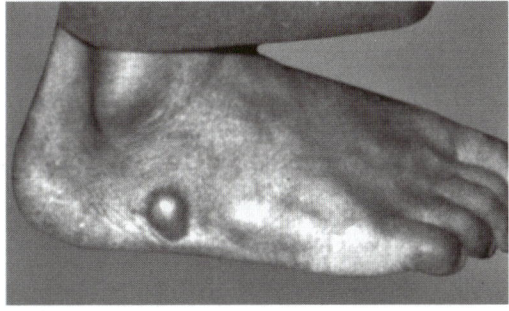

Fig. 22.12: Ganglion in relation to peroneus brevis. D/D: Implanted dermoid.

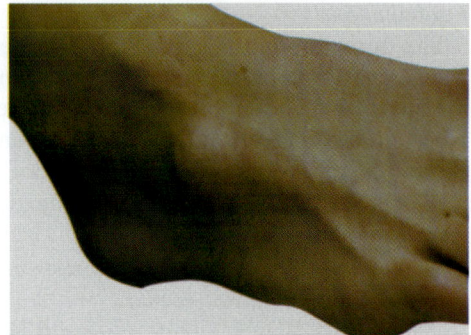

Fig. 22.13: Ganglion in relation to peroneus tertius.

degeneration. The connection with the parent synovium usually cannot be demonstrated. *The cyst contains a viscous jelly like material.*

Common sites

1. Dorsum of the wrist – commonest.
2. Dorsum of the foot and ankle.
3. Palmar aspect of the wrist and fingers.

Why are they commonest over the dorsum of the wrist?

Due to the presence of many tendons with their sheaths.

Names of the tendons over the dorsum of the wrist:

The tendons from lateral to medial are:
1. Abductor pollicis longus ⎱ Common
2. Extensor pollicis brevis   ⎰ sheath
3. Extensor carpi radialis longus ⎱ Common
4. Extensor carpi radialis brevis ⎰ sheath
5. Extensor pollicis longus – Single sheath
6. Extensor indicis   ⎱ Common
7. Extensor digitorum ⎰ sheath
8. Extensor digiti minimi – Single sheath
9. Extensor carpi ulnaris – Single sheath

So, there are 9 tendons within 6 sheaths.

Diagnostic criteria

1. Commonly found in adults. Common in females.
2. Patient presents with a lump which is usually slowly growing and has been present for months or years. Patient seeks advice either because of disfigurement, or *pain particularly after strenuous work with the hand.*

On examination:

3. The lump appears as a well defined spherical, firm, cystic, *unilocular* swelling adjacent to tendon sheath. It sometimes becomes so tense that it feels bony hard and apt to be mistaken for a tumour. Surface is smooth. Overlying skin is freely mobile over the ganglion.

4. *Fluctuation:* Positive (*by Paget's test*) in a soft swelling. *It may be tender.*

5. *Mobility:* Swelling is mobile across the axis of the tendon (i.e. on side-to-side movement), but not mobile along the axis of the tendon.

6. *Relation of the swelling with the tendon:* The patient is asked to make the tendon taut by closing the fist tightly, to find out whether the ganglion is fixed to the tendon or not. *If fixed*, then find out the tendon to which it is related by extending the wrist and fingers actively or against resistance.

7. *Occasionally a ganglion may slip away between the deeper structures while pressed,* giving the false impression that its contents have reduced inside the joint.

Treatment

Excision of the ganglion followed by biopsy.

Why biopsy: Frequently the synovial sheath in relation with the tendon may have neoplastic change, benign or malignant, called synovioma.

Fate of operation: It may be completely cured, or, to the annoyance of the patient, it may recur.

Other methods of treatment

1. Time-honoured treatment is rupturing the ganglion by striking it with a heavy object (*Bible treatment* used by the Priests in older days for rupturing the ganglion with the help of the Bible).

2. Aspiration of ganglion and introduction of sclerosing agents such as ethanolamine.

3. Suturing of the ganglion by multiple nylon threads.

Note

Cysts of the lateral semilunar cartilage of the knee are similar histologically to ganglion.

Note

A ganglion also refers to a collection of nerve cells (e.g. a spinal ganglion) which is different from this synovial ganglion.

TENDON SHEATHS

Stenosing tenovaginitis

This occurs in the fibrous sheath of the tendon and is due to either chronic inflammation or degeneration from overuse. *There is thickening and constriction of the sheath* with the tendon becoming thickened above and below leading to difficulty or limitation of movements of tendons within the sheath. *This is commonly found at two sites* – in the wrist (*de Quervain's disease*) and in the finger (*Trigger finger*).

DE QUERVAIN'S DISEASE

Here, the common sheath covering the abductor pollicis longus and extensor pollicis brevis tendons on the lateral side of the wrist *just above the radial styloid process* is involved.

On extending the thumb with forearm in semi-pronation, *a depression will be noted* between these tendons laterally and the extensor pollicis longus medially – *known as anatomical snuff box. At the depth of this box lies the scaphoid bone.*

Diagnostic criteria

1. Commonly seen in middle-aged women.

2. Patient complains of pain on the radial side of the wrist *which becomes worse during wringing clothes or towels.*

On examination:

3. A localised tender lump may be felt just above the radial styloid process.

4. Ulnar deviation of the wrist is painful.

5. *Passive adduction* of the thumb is painful.

6. *Active extension and/or abduction of the thumb against resistance* is also painful.

7. Crepitus may rarely be felt locally as the tendons move.

8. **Finkelstein's test** is diagnostic – sudden forceful ulnar deviation of the flexed hand after stabilising the forearm causes severe pain over the radial styloid process area.

Treatment

Conservative: May be tried in early cases but recurrence is expected.

1. Rest, oral analgesics, anti-inflammatory drugs, local heat therapy and ultrasound application may hasten the progress.
2. Local injections of hydrocortisone may cure and reverse the process in early cases.

Operative: Division of the involved tendon sheath gives uniform and permanent satisfactory result.

TRIGGER FINGER (*Syn.* Snapping finger)

Here, stenosis occurs at the entrance to the fibrous flexor tendon sheath opposite the metacarpal heads, causing impediment to sliding of the tendon into the sheath during extension. Several digits may be affected.

Cause of trigger finger is thickening of fibrous tendon sheath causing stenosis. Trigger finger is usually associated with rheumatoid tenosynovitis.

A similar condition is seen in the thumbs of infants which may be congenital (*Trigger thumb*).

Diagnostic criteria

1. In adults any finger may be affected – *the ring and the middle fingers are commonly affected. In infants*, the thumb is commonly affected.
2. *Patient notices that when the hand is unclenched, the affected finger remains bent.* The affected finger gets fixed in flexion until it is extended by excessive voluntary effort or made passively straight by the other hand. When extension occurs it does so with a *characteristic 'snap'*.
3. Locally one may find *tenderness and/or a palpable nodule in front of the metacarpal head of the affected finger* at about the level of MP joint (distal palmar crease).

It is called *trigger finger* because of the snapping observed when the patient actively flexes or extends the proximal interphalangeal (IP) joint.

Treatment

1. Local injections of hydrocortisone may cure and reverse the process in early cases.

2. Division of the involved fibrous sheath gives uniform and permanent satisfactory results.

Infective tenosynovitis

The synovial tendon sheaths may be infected by tubercle bacilli liberated into the blood from a primary focus elsewhere. *The commonest site for tuberculous tendon sheath infection* is in the *common sheath of the flexor tendons of the fingers in front of the wrist* (i.e. *ulnar bursa*) where the swelling extends both above and below the flexor retinaculum. Such swelling is commonly known as *compound palmar ganglion.*

The common sheath of the peroneal tendons at the lateral side of the ankle may also be affected by the same pathology.

COMPOUND PALMAR GANGLION

It is an inflammatory degeneration of the common synovial sheath that surrounds the flexor tendons of the fingers in front of the wrist and gives rise to a swelling *which extends both above and below the flexor retinaculum, i.e. transverse carpal ligament – a bilocular swelling, so known as compound ganglion.* The synovial sheath of the flexor tendons located in the space of Parona in the lower forearm, extending to the palm beneath the flexor retinaculum, is known as *ulnar bursa* (see Fig. 22.4).

Common cause of such inflammation is *tuberculosis.* But it may also occur secondary to rheumatoid arthritis.

Is it a true ganglion? – No, because it is not due to mucoid or myxomatous degeneration.

Surgical pathology

Following degeneration, the common synovial sheath becomes thickened and oedematous. The endothelial lining secretes exudate which distends the sheath. *There is formation of small fibrinous deposits or particles in the wall. These fibrinous particles are moulded into fine granules* due to constant irritation and pressure of the moving tendons, and are cast off from the wall into the cavity. *These particles look like sago-grains and are known as 'Melon seed bodies'.*

When degeneration is *secondary to tuberculosis,* the melon seed bodies may contain tubercle bacilli, and tuberculous giant cells can be found in the wall of the synovial sheath.

Condition is *often bilateral* in case of rheumatoid arthritis.

Diagnostic criteria

1. Patient presents with a swelling on the anterior aspect of the lower forearm and wrist, and palm of the hand. *The swelling is usually painless.*
2. Patient may notice crepitus on movements of the fingers.
3. Occasionally, *paraesthesia due to median nerve compression may occur* in the distribution of the median nerve in the radial three and half digits (cf. carpal tunnel syndrome).
4. *The swelling is hourglass in shape* with proximal swelling above the wrist and distal swelling in the palm.
5. Soft cystic or boggy in feel; surface is irregular. *On deep palpation* multiple nodular particles may be felt (due to the presence of melon seed bodies).
6. *Fluctuation is positive.*
   Cross-fluctuation is also positive – compression of the lump above the flexor retinaculum makes it distend below and vice-versa.
7. Transillumination is negative.
8. No local signs of inflammation are noted.
9. Crepitus may be felt when the patient moves his/her fingers.
10. There may be some stiffness of the fingers and wrist.
11. There may be pain, tingling, numbness of radial three and half digits (cf. carpal tunnel syndrome) *because of median nerve compression by the ulnar bursa.*
12. Obvious wasting of the adjacent muscles of thenar eminence may be noted due to median nerve compression (cf. carpal tunnel syndrome).
13. There may be evidence of tuberculosis elsewhere in the body, e.g. chest, other joints.

Investigations

1. Blood for Hb% TC, DC and ESR

2. Mantoux test
3. Chest X-ray: To exclude pulmonary lesion
4. X-ray of the wrist joint. *MRI – more specific.*
5. Rose-Waaler test, X-rays of other joints may be done to detect rheumatoid arthritis.

Complications

1. *Paraesthesia due to median nerve compression* (cf. carpal tunnel syndrome).
2. *Occasionally, wasting of the adjacent muscles, e.g. thenar muscles.*
3. The tendons in relation may eventually *fray and rupture.*
4. Recurrence even after surgery.

Treatment

1. Antitubercular treatment – if confirmed.
2. Rest to the part by applying a plaster cast over the forearm and hand in palmar flexion.
3. If conservative treatment fails – *Surgery: Longitudinal division of the flexor retinaculum and removal of the sheath after careful dissection is performed.*
4. If rheumatoid arthritis is the cause, a total synovectomy may be performed because the primary pathology originates from the affected synovium (pannus).

Note

Swellings which are cross fluctuant:

1. Compound palmar ganglion.
2. Plunging ranula.
3. Bilocular hydrocele (infantile hydrocele).
4. Psoas abscess pointing to femoral triangle.

C. DISEASES OF MUSCULO-TENDINOUS ATTACHMENTS

TENNIS ELBOW (Lateral epicondylitis)

This lesion is characterised by pain and tenderness *at the common origin of the extensor muscles of the forearm into the lateral humoral epicondyle.* Extensor carpi radialis brevis is most commonly involved.

The cause is usually unknown. It is believed that it follows some unrecognised trauma which causes *partial rupture of the aponeurotic fibres at the muscle origin,* which is a region richly supplied by nerve endings. The elbow joint itself is unaffected. Some believe such lesion may be due to rheumatoid arthritis. *Often the onset follows a strain during serving the ball at tennis game* (tennis elbow).

Diagnostic criteria

1. The patient complains of *pain at the lateral aspect of the elbow particularly on certain movements* such as pouring out tea, turning a tight door-handle, or lifting with the forearm pronated, e.g. lifting articles from the roof of an almirah or carrying a bucket full of water, *serving the ball at tennis game.*

On examination:

2. *Tenderness precisely localised to the front of the lateral epicondyle of the humerus.*
3. Pain is aggravated by passive stretching of the wrist extensor muscles, e.g. when the wrist is palmarflexed after holding the elbow straight with the forearm pronated (*Cozen's test*).
4. Pain is also aggravated on active contraction of the extensor muscles, e.g. the patient is asked to dorsiflex his wrist against resistance after holding the elbow straight with forearm pronated.
5. Movements of the elbow are full.
6. X-rays do not show any bony changes.

Treatment

1. If left alone, the symptoms may subside spontaneously. Oral analgesics, local heat therapy and ultrasound application may hasten the progress.
2. Local injection of mixture of hydrocortisone, 1% lignocaine, and hyaluronidase into the tender spot may give relief.
3. Operation may be necessary for persistent or recurrent cases. The origin of the common extensor muscle is stripped from the lateral epicondyle.

GOLFER'S ELBOW
(Medial epicondylitis)

This is analogous to tennis elbow except that *the common flexor pronator origin into the medial epicondyle is affected with pain and tenderness.*

Treatment is similar.

OSGOOD SCHLATTER'S DISEASE

* It is actually *apophysitis of the tibial tuberosity of the knee leading to painful tender lump at the tibial tuberosity due to repetitive injury* causing non-specific inflammation at the lower end of patellar ligament.
* The pain is worse after activity – *running or playing.*
* Common in children and adolescents.
* The pain and tenderness usually subside after puberty when the apophysis blends with the tibial tubercle.
* *May be treated by* plastic immobilisation for 6 weeks followed by stoppage of running or playing for another 6 weeks.

PLANTAR FASCITIS

This lesion affects the attachment of the plantar aponeurosis to the medial tubercle of the calcaneum and causes pain and tenderness beneath the heel. The lesion is believed to be inflammatory either from repeated trauma or from rheumatism.

Diagnostic criteria

1. Common in middle aged men.
2. *The patient complains of pain beneath the heel on standing or walking. The pain is more in the early morning on first weight bearing after waking up from the bed* (*starting trouble*). Most common hindfoot problem in runners.
3. *On palpation –* there is *marked tenderness* over the site of attachment of the aponeurosis *to the medial tubercle of the calcaneum* and on the medial surface of the bone.

   The pain increases with passive extension of great toe and may be further exacerbated by dorsiflexion of the ankle and/or on weight bearing.

   Often a bursa develops at the end of the spur that may also become inflamed and tender.

4. *Passive movements of the ankle are full and painless.*
5. *X-ray of the calcaneum:* Lateral view may show *a sharp spur* projecting forwards from the tuberosity of the calcaneum, *calcaneal spur.*

Treatment
Conservative

1. Use of soft but thick *hawai chappal*, or shoe or *chappal* with excavated heel filled with sorbo-rubber.
2. Local injections of hydrocortisone into the tender area may be successful.

Operative

Rarely required. The planter aponeurosis is stripped from the medial tubercle of the calcaneum.

D. DISEASES OF MUSCLES

MYOSITIS OSSIFICANS TRAUMATICA

This lesion consists of *heterotopic bone formation in the fleshy part of the muscle* causing restricted movements of the nearby joint.

Causes

The cause is unknown but it is thought to be related to muscular damage either following severe direct injury, or *too early and too vigorous joint movements, particularly passive movements after removal of plaster done for immobilisation of the elbow joint for fracture or dislocation.*

Site

Commonest site is the elbow: The muscle affected is the *brachialis muscle* following an injury such as supracondylar fracture of the humerus or dislocation of the elbow.

The other muscle affected is the *quadriceps femoris* following fracture of the femur or after a kick on the front of the thigh.

Occasionally, shoulder or hip joints may be affected after injury.

Surgical pathology

Basic pathology is *ossification in a haematoma in the soft tissues near a joint.* Following injury,

there is avulsion of the periosteal attachment of some muscle, tendon or ligament *resulting in sub-periosteal haematoma.* Subsequently, the periosteal cells proliferate and liberate osteoblasts into the haematoma and ossify the haematoma.

Diagnostic criteria

1. Common in children and adolescents.
2. The patient or parents usually recalls the nature of previous injury and can relate the loss of joint movements to the injury.
3. The patient complains of stiffness of joint, with pain on forced movements.

On examination:

4. *Site: Common sites are the lower part of the brachialis muscle at the elbow,* or *the lower part of the quadriceps femoris muscle at the knee.*
5. *Elbow: The elbow is fixed in flexion. Extension is restricted. Passive extension is restricted by pain.* If the intramuscular ossification is extensive the joint may become completely fixed: Ankylosis.
   Knee: The knee is fixed in extension. Flexion is restricted. *Passive flexion is restricted by pain.*
6. *On palpation: A bony hard mass is felt which is fixed to the underlying bone.* The mass is often mistaken for a bony swelling. The surface is smooth but irregular with a normal local temperature. The muscle fibres can be felt running into the mass.
7. *X-ray of the elbow:* Will show a fluffy mass of calcification in front of the joint in the early stage. In late cases mature bone becomes evident. *X-ray of the knee* may show a fluffy mass of calcification deep to quadriceps femoris.

Treatment

Complete immobilisation in plaster of paris cast for many weeks until the greater part of the callus is reabsorbed and pain disappears. The mass becomes smaller and more discrete which can be confirmed by repeated X-ray. *Afterwards the plaster is removed and gradual active non-weight bearing movements are advised. No passive movements should be allowed.*

If elbow movements are still seriously restricted, the smaller and discrete bony mass can be removed.

Once the active movements get improved reasonably the patient is allowed to work or walk.

Other types of myositis ossificans

Two other types are encountered clinically:
1. Myositis ossificans progressiva
2. Myositis ossificans circumscripta.

Myositis ossificans progressiva

This is a rare congenital lesion *characterised by ectopic bone formation in the soft tissues*, chiefly in the head, neck and trunk, with consequent limitation of movement. *It is often associated with undue shortness of the big toes and sometimes also of the thumbs (microdactyly).*

The ectopic bone is formed by metaplasia of the connective tissue, but not from the displaced osteoblasts.

The disease usually appears in early childhood, onset is before 6 years of age with the appearance of fever and *soft tender swellings in the neck and trunk.* The soft swellings gradually turn into hard masses of bone which lie in the course of the muscles, ligaments, and fascia. The ossification gradually extends, *limiting movements of the spine and ribs more and more until in the worst cases there may be total immobility – ankylosis.* Death from asphyxia may follow the immobilisation of the respiratory muscles.

No curative treatment is yet available. Systemic treatment with *diphosphonates* along with excision of bony bars may retard or delay the progress, but complete cure is impossible.

Myositis ossificans circumscripta

This condition is *often seen in patients with brain or spinal cord damage*. Heterotopic ossification is seen at several joints especially the hips, knees and shoulders leading to limitation of movements, sometimes totally stiffening the joints.

VOLKMANN'S ISCHAEMIC CONTRACTURE (Fig. 22.14)

This is a type of vascular injury. This lesion consists of fibrosis of the muscles *secondary to* *ischaemia of the striated muscle and nerve tissue, median and ulnar nerve* (structures most sensitive to anoxia) resulting in contracture of the long flexor muscles of the forearm. *This contracture leads to flexion deformity of the fingers first and then of the wrist.*

Causes

Common causes of ischaemia are:

1. Direct damage to the brachial artery near the elbow at the time of injury (e.g. following supracondylar fracture).
2. Tight forearm bandage or plaster, e.g. immobilisation of supracondylar fractures of the elbow or both bone fractures of the forearm leading to ischaemia and infarction of the adjacent muscles and nerves – *compartment syndrome.*
3. Closed forearm crush injuries.

Other causes are:

1. Burns.
2. IV chemotherapy leading to spillage of the drugs into the close fascial compartment.

All lead to tense oedema of the soft tissues of the forearm *constrained within an unyielding fascial compartment.*

Surgical pathology

The tissue oedema within the fascial compartment *causes compression of the artery*, mainly the anterior interosseous artery, leading to

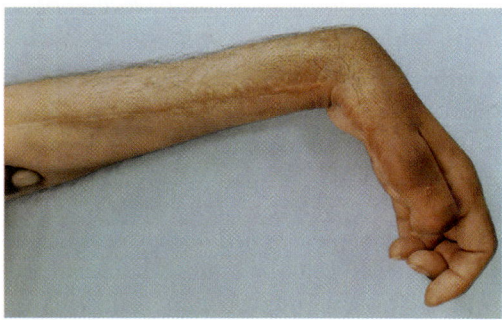

Fig. 22.14: Volkmann's ischaemic contracture—forearm, wrist, hand and fingers. Note the incision mark from previous operation on the anterior aspect of forearm for fasciotomy.

ischaemia to the striated muscles and nerves, and, if continued, leads to aseptic *ischaemic necrosis of the muscles and subsequently fibrosis and permanent contracture of the muscles.* Muscles and nerves can tolerate ischaemia up to 6 hours.

The muscles involved are mainly flexor digitorum profundus and *flexor pollicis longus.* There is also temporary, or rarely permanent *ischaemic paralysis of the peripheral nerves mainly median nerve.* The nerve may be capable of regeneration but *the muscle once infarcted can never recover – it is replaced by fibrous tissue which contracts – the essential pathology of Volkmann's contracture, leading to contracture of fingers and sometimes the wrist* resulting in loss of hand power and deformity.

Injury to the median and ulnar nerve also involved by ischaemia and infarction.

Similar ischaemia may also affect the calf muscles following injury to the popliteal artery, or tight leg plaster following fracture of the femur or upper end of tibia. Similarly, popliteal nerve may be involved in knee joint injury.

Occasionally, ischaemia may affect the intrinsic muscles of the hand and foot.

Note

Altered sensation due to ischaemia of nerves is noticed within 30 minutes of tight plaster immobilisation. *So, immediate removal of plaster is must. Ischaemia more the 4 hours is critical and irreversible damage may occur after 12 hours.*

Diagnostic criteria in acute or incipient stage following plaster immobilisation

In the acute stage after plaster immobilisation following features can be noted.

1. Pallor and puffiness of the fingers and the thumb due to oedema.
2. *Absence of return of immediate capillary refilling of the nail bed* – after pressing and then releasing the pressure over the nail bed.
3. Pulselessness – absence of radial pulse.
4. Paresis – loss of movement.
5. Loss of sensation of the thumb and lateral two and half fingers when ischaemia is more than 4 hours.

Diagnostic criteria of established case of Volkmann's contracture

1. *Age:* Usually common in children and young adults.
2. The patient presents with a fully developed deformity called 'Clawhand'.
3. The patient or parents usually recalls the cause of the deformity and can clearly relate the loss of finger extension to previous injury and treatment.

On examination:

In an established case – particularly with the history of persistent pain in the forearm, hand and fingers following tight plaster immobilisation:

4. All the fingers are flexed at the proximal and distal interphalangeal joints – *a 'clawhand' deformity:* The metacarpophalangeal joints are hyperextended and the wrist is flexed. The forearm looks thin and wasted (Fig. 22.14). The hand looks pale and wasted.
5. The forearm muscles feel hard and taut. The hand feels cooler.
6. The patient is unable to extend the wrist and fingers together.
7. *In an early stage, when the wrist is passively fully palmarflexed, the fingers can be extended and straightened.*

   When the wrist is moved into full dorsiflexion, the fingers become progressively more flexed.
8. There may be limitation of supination of the forearm *due to contracture of the pronator teres.*
9. Pain on passive stretching of fingers and wrist.
10. *Sensory loss is usually absent.*

Differential diagnosis

1. Combined ulnar and median nerve palsy: *When sensory loss is usually evident.*
2. Dupuytren's contracture – involves usually little and ring fingers (flexion of metacarpophalangeal and proximal interphalangeal joints).

Treatment

Prophylactic treatment in the incipient stage is best. In the early stage with pain, paresthesia and pulselessness, following measures to be taken urgently:

- Removal of plaster case immediately.
- Correction of fracture deformity.
- *Exposure of the brachial artery* and application of 2.5% papaverine solution over the artery to relieve arterial spasm, if any – *check the radial pulse and return of capillary perfusion of nail bed.*
- *If required, fasciotomy by liberal axial (longitudinal) incisions* over the deep fascia of the forearm *both on the ventral and dorsal surfaces* may be performed to decompress the oedema. *Also incision over the palm and carpal tunnel are advised to decompress the median nerve and short muscles of the hand.*
- Immobilisation is done with half plaster cast with light woollen bandage and C/C sling.
- *Check pulse and sensation every 2 hours for the first 24 hours.*
- Ask the patient to move the fingers and thumb very frequently once the patient becomes conscious fully.

Established cases of Volkmann's contracture: Restoration to normal is hardly possible.

In mild cases: Acceptable function may be expected by *intensive active exercises* guided by a physiotherapist, and graduated movements of the wrist and fingers on an adjustable dynamic splint. *No passive exercises are allowed.*

The *splint has a hinge at the level of the wrist and a racket for varying the angle.* The forearm, hands and fingers are fixed in the splint in a position of full flexion of the wrist, thus allowing the fingers to straighten. *The angle of flexion at the wrist is decreased daily* by the screw, *the fingers being firmly fixed in extension.* In this way the muscles are slowly stretched and finally the fingers can be kept extended even when the wrist is dorsiflexed.

In advanced cases – operation is essential. Two types of operations are available at present:

A. *Max Page operation:* Stripping of the common origin of the flexor muscles from the medial epicondyle and the upper ends of the radius and ulna followed by hyperextension of the hand and the fingers – *this allows the muscle origin to move distally – muscle sliding procedure.* The muscles obtain, in time, a new origin lower down the forearm. *The deformity is reduced but function is not much improved.*

B. Excision of the fibrous tissue and necrotic muscles with subsequent transfer of tendon of a healthy muscle (for example, a wrist extensor or flexor) to the tendons of flexor digitorum profundus and flexor pollicis longus, i.e. *muscle transfers* – this helps in considerable improvement in function as well as correction of deformity.

The muscle transfer may be supplemented with arthrodesis of the wrist joint in extension for improving the grip of the hand.

When there is irreparable damage of the median nerve in extreme cases, nerve grafting could be considered as well for better improvement.

E. DISEASES OF TENDON

RUPTURED BICEPS TENDON

This is a pathological tear of the tendon of the long head of biceps *at the bicipital groove of the humerus.* Such tear occurs due to weakness of the tendon following repeated friction against osteophytes in an osteoarthritic shoulder. Some orthopaedic surgeons consider it a simple tear through an area of avascular degeneration. *In either case tear occurs without any violent stress or injury* (cf. supraspinatus tendon and extensor pollicis longus tendon where also rupture occurs without any violent strain).

Diagnostic features

1. The patient is usually middle aged.
2. Gives history of sudden pain and 'snap' at the shoulder while lifting or pulling heavy weight with the same arm. Soon the pain disappears and good function of the shoulder returns. Later, *the patient may notice an unusual bulge of the muscle in front of the arm.*

On examination:

3. Soon after the rupture there is slight tenderness at the bicipital groove. The lump is usually tender and there will be pain with resisted elbow flexion. Power of the muscle is diminished.

4. *Later, when the patient is asked to flex his elbow against resistance, the affected biceps belly is seen to retract and bunch up into a round lump like a ball ('Popeye sign') leaving a gap proximal to it.* The shoulder and elbow movements are usually otherwise normal.

Treatment

As the disability is minimal, no treatment is required except rest for few weeks and anti-inflammatory drugs. *If the patient demands*, operation can be performed — the distal stump of the ruptured tendon is sutured to the walls of the bicipital groove with screw or prolene suture; the proximal stump is ignored.

RUPTURED TENDO ACHILLES

This is a pathological tear of the tendo achilles *5 cm above the insertion of the tendon.* Such tear occurs through an area of avascular degeneration. *The rupture is nearly always complete.*

Diagnostic features

1. The patient is usually middle aged.

2. The patient gives the history of sudden agonising pain at the back of heel while running or jumping. He may believe that he has been struck from behind just above the heel. *He is able to walk, but with a limp. Ambulation is possible only when* the limb is externally rotated with rolling over transversally and placed the foot during the stance phase without push off.

On examination:

3. There is tenderness at the site of rupture.

4. A gap can be seen and felt in the course of the tendon 5 cm above its insertion to the calcaneal tuberosity. This gap is more prominent with dorsiflexion of the ankle.

5. *The patient is unable to stand on the tiptoe on the affected leg* – the patient is asked to raise the heel from the ground while standing upon the affected leg only. The patient is unable to do this when the tendon is ruptured.

6. Plantar-flexion of the foot is weak, and is not accompanied by tautening of the tendon.

7. ***Simmonds' test:*** When doubt exists, this test is helpful. *With the patient lying in prone position with the ankle and foot beyond the edge of the examination table/bed, the calves are squeezed* – on normal side the foot is seen to plantar flex, *but on the ruptured tendon side the foot remains still – no passive ankle plantar flexion noted.*

8. Passive ankle movements are normal.

Treatment

Non-operative treatment is preferred particularly in sedentary or elderly patients. *Plaster immobilisation for 8 weeks with the foot in equinus is required. This is followed by wearing of shoe with raised heel for a further 6 weeks.*

Neuromuscular electrical stimulation (NMES) may be useful to strengthen the peroneal nerve supplied muscles.

Operative treatment may be advised in fresh rupture particularly in athletes, to reduce the risk of lengthening of the tendon and consequent loss of 'spring off'. *Operation entails repair of the tendon, preferably by sutures of stainless steel wire.* This is followed by plaster immobilisation with the knee in flexion at 90° with the foot in equinus for 6 weeks.

If the rupture is neglected for 4 weeks, conservative treatment by graduated exercises for the calf muscles is to be preferred.

Rarely ankle arthodesis may be required.

MALLET FINGER

This is a fixed flexion deformity of the distal interphalangeal joint of a finger. This results from either a rupture of extensor tendon at its insertion or an avulsion fracture of the base of the distal phalanx. *It occurs if the finger tip is forcibly bent during active extension* – for instance, during making a bed while tucking the bedsheet under the edge of the mattress, or by a blow on the tip of a finger by a baseball (hence also known as *'baseball' finger*).

Diagnostic features

1. The patient usually remembers the original injury.
2. The patient is unable to extend the distal interphalangeal joint fully.
3. The deformity is disfiguring.

On examination:

4. When the patient holds out his hand, with the fingers extended, the peculiar deformity is obvious – the distal phalanx of the affected finger remains 15–20° flexed.
5. The surgeon can passively extend the distal phalanx, *but the patient cannot extend it actively.*
6. X-ray of the affected finger is required to see *the avulsion fracture of the base of the distal phalanx.*

Treatment

Only helps at or just after the injury.

If X-ray reveals no fracture: The finger is immobilised for 6 weeks in a splint or plaster with the distal interphalangeal joint hyperextended, and the proximal interphalangeal joint flexed at 80°. *The splint used is either Oatley splint or Mallet finger splint.*

If X-ray reveals an avulsion fracture, operative fixation may be required particularly in players – the fragment is sutured back, or fixed back with a thin piece of Kirschner wire.

Once the injury is more than 3 weeks old – operative fixation rarely helps. So, the deformity can be ignored as it is minimal and functional loss is also minimal.

▌BONY LESIONS

CHONDROMA (Fig. 22.15)

This is a benign tumour composed of cartilage. *It arises from the precartilaginous cells of the bone which fails to become ossified.*

Chondroma usually involves the short long bones, e.g. metacarpals, metatarsals and proximal phalanx. It can also affect the large long bones and flat bones.

Chondroma is commonly solitary.

When the chondromata are multiple and congenital (but not familial) the condition is

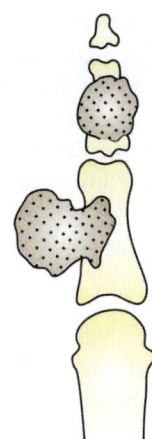

Fig. 22.15: Chondroma—enchondroma on middle phalanx; ecchondroma on proximal phalanx.

known as *dyschondroplasia* (multiple chondromatosis or Ollier's disease). This condition begins in childhood and *the large long bones are also affected* where the involvement of the growth plate will interfere with normal growth of the bones *leading to shortening or deformity.*

Rarely chondroma undergoes malignant change and this occurs usually in one of the large long bones.

Chondromata are of two types:

1. Enchondroma
2. Ecchondroma

Enchondroma

Here the tumour grows within the bone and as it increases in size, it causes expansion and thinning of the cortex, thus forming a fusiform swelling. Fracture is common because of thinning of the cortex.

Ecchondroma

Here the tumour grows outwards on the surface of the bone.

Diagnostic criteria

1. *Age:* Usually present in adolescents.
2. The patient usually presents with a gradually expanding *painless swelling* of the bone (enchondroma), or a lump appearing on the side of the bone (ecchondroma). An ecchon-

droma may interfere with joint and tendon movement. The patient often may present with a fracture after a trivial injury.

On examination:

3. *Site:* Common in the short long bones of hand (especially little finger) and feet.
   If dyschondroplasia is congenital but not familial the large long bones may also be affected.
4. *Shape:* Enchondroma causes a fusiform swelling of the shaft of the bone.
   Ecchondroma forms a sessile lump on the surface of the bone.
5. *Surface:* Smooth. The overlying skin has a normal temperature.
6. *Consistence:* Usually hard because a chondroma is covered by a thin layer of cortical bone. *The swelling is non-tender.*
7. X-ray shows *a well-defined, expanded rarefied area with characteristic specks of calcification or stippling.* No reactive bone formation.

Differential diagnosis

1. Simple cyst: There will be *no specks of calcification in the rarefied area noted in X-ray.*
2. Tuberculous dactylitis: There will be *presence of tenderness on the swelling* with inflammatory involvement of the skin. *X-ray does not show specks of calcification.*

Treatment

The tumour with its lining capsule should be excised and *the cavity is filled up with bone chips.*

Fracture, when it occurs, usually unites uneventfully and is often followed by spontaneous cure.

OSTEOMA

The word osteoma is applied to any bony overgrowth, whether or not this is a tumour. Two types are encountered clinically:

1. Compact osteoma
2. Osteoid osteoma

Compact osteoma (Fig. 22.16)

Also known as *ivory osteoma.* It is a benign

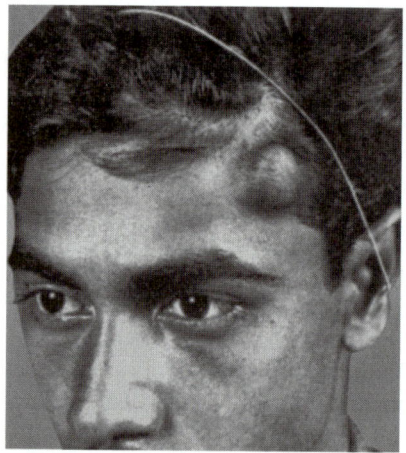

Fig. 22.16: Compact osteoma arising from the frontal bone. It is sessile hard lump, fixed to the underlying bone. The lump is not tender. Overlying skin is free from the lump. D/D: On inspection, lipoma which is soft solid and mobile on palpation.

tumour composed of hard compact bone. *It arises in the bones which are ossified from membrane, e.g. skull bones.* It forms a smooth rounded swelling on either the outer or the inner surface of the skull bones.

When it grows on the outer surface, *it appears as a visible painless and non-mobile hard lump.*

When it grows on the inner surface, *it causes pressure upon the cerebrum giving rise to symptoms, e.g. focal epilepsy.*

It is also known to develop in the orbital cavity or one of the paranasal sinuses.

Diagnostic criteria

1. The patient presents *with a painless lump on the surface of the vault of the skull,* frequently the forehead. The lump is very slowly growing and may have been present for many years. The lump causes disfigurement or anxiety.
2. The lump is usually not more than 1 cm.
3. The lump is sessile, flattened mounds with smooth surface.
4. *Very hard:* Hence the name *ivory osteoma.* It is *not tender.*
5. *Fixed to the underlying bone,* of which it is an integral part. *The overlying skin is free from the lump.*

6. *X-ray* shows a sessile plaque of very dense bone with a well circumscribed margin.

Treatment

It may either be left alone or excised according to the symptoms in each case. *A small area of surrounding healthy bone has to be excised with the tumour as the tumour is too hard.*

Osteoid osteoma (Fig. 22.17)

It is a most common benign tumour of bone composed of osteoid tissue with trabeculae of newly formed bone, in a vascular connective tissue groundwork. *It can arise in any bone except the skull bone.* It is common in the femur or tibia and appears as a small (usually less than 1 cm in size), *round or oval lesion encased in dense bone. It is the most common true benign bone tumour of the bone.*

Diagnostic criteria

1. The lesion is common in young males.
2. Common in the lower limbs around the knee.

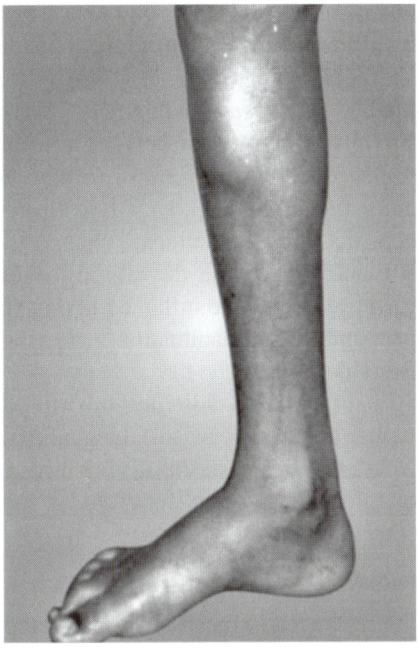

Fig. 22.17: Stony hard swelling upper end of right tibia (osteoid osteoma). Examine the other joints of the body to look for multiple exostoses (diaphyseal aclasis).

3. *The leading symptom is local nagging pain with or without visible swelling, the patient may limp because of pain.* The pain may be severe and not relieved by rest. The pain is most severe at night and dramatically relieved by aspirin or NSAIDs within 30 minutes (therapeutic test).
4. *X-ray shows* a small round or oval radiolucent area *with sclerosis* at the margin.
5. CT/MRI also may help in diagnosis.

Differential diagnosis

The tumour is sometimes difficult to differentiate from Brodie's abscess, Ewing's tumour and chronic periostitis, and the doubt is resolved only after biopsy.

There is no risk of malignant transformation itself.

Treatment

Excision of the affected area cures the condition with relief of pain. The material should be sent for biopsy to exclude Ewing's tumour.

EXOSTOSIS (*Syn.* Osteochondroma)

This, the commonest benign tumour of the bone, is truly a *hamartoma*. It consists of normal bone covered by a cap of cartilage. Some considered it as cancellous osteoma (Fig. 22.18).

Origin

It arises in childhood from a nest of growing epiphyseal cartilage plate and continues to grow on the surface *at the end of the long bone until the parent epiphysis fuses.* As the bone grows in length the tumour gets 'left behind' and thus appears to migrate along the shaft towards its centre. *When it grows, it points away from the growing end of the long bone.*

Surgical pathology

It arises at the growing ends of the long bones, e.g. metaphysis of the proximal tibia (commonest) and distal femur. *It may arise from the flat bones,* e.g. the pelvis or the scapula.

Exostosis consists of normal bone covered by a cap of cartilage.

Occasionally, *adventitious bursa* may develop over the cartilage cap.

Osteochondroma is usually solitary.

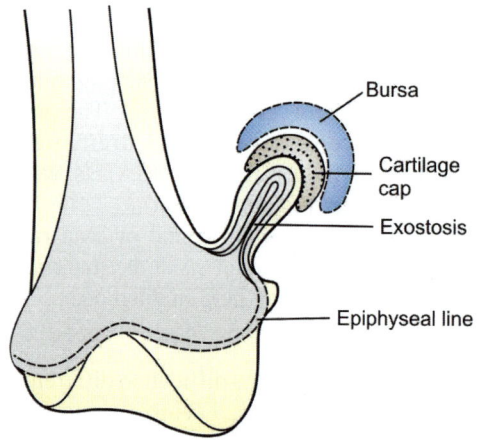

Fig. 22.18: Site of the origin of exostosis.

When they are multiple, congenital and familial, the condition is known as *diaphyseal aclasis* (multiple hereditary exostoses). In severe cases of diaphyseal aclasis there is interference with the skeletal growth and the patient may be deformed or dwarfed.

Exostosis itself does not undergo malignant change, but, rarely the cartilage cap continues to grow in adult life and gives rise to chondrosarcoma.

Diagnostic criteria

1. *Age:* The patient is usually present in teenage and adult life.
2. *Sex:* Male > Female.
3. *The patient may have felt the painless and non-tender lump or may present with a disfiguring lump.*

    The patient may present with the symptoms arising due to mechanical interference with the movements of the joint and its tendons. *He may feel 'clicks' as the tendons slip over the lump.*

    The lump is usually painless. But the patient may complain of neuralgia due to pressure on the adjacent nerves by the lump.
4. *Site:* The majority occur at the upper end of the tibia and lower end of the femur, i.e. *around the knee.*
5. *Shape and size:* The lump is pedunculated or sessile with smooth, mushroom-shaped upper end, usually 1–2 cm in diameter.
6. *Consistence: Bony hard and non-tender. Rarely the exostosis is covered by a soft fluctuant adventitious bursa over the cap.*
7. *Mobility:* The lump is fixed to the bone but not muscle or skin.
8. While palpating the lump, one can feel the slipping of the overlying tendon on moving the joint.
9. The rest of the bone and the nearby joint should be normal.
10. *Examine the other joints of the body,* e.g. shoulder, wrist, finger *to look for multiple exostoses* (diaphyseal aclasis).
11. *X-ray* shows the mushroom like bony outgrowth but it looks smaller than it feels because the cartilaginous cap is invisible.

    Examine other members of the family also for familial exostosis.

Complications

1. Fracture at the pedicle.
2. Symptoms due to pressure on the adjacent nerves (paraesthesia) or on the vessels.
3. Interference with tendon or joint movements.
4. Cartilaginous cap continues to grow in adult life and *may become malignant – Chondrosarcoma,* common in pelvis and scapula. *Appearance of pain in an exostosis in an adult suggests malignancy. Exostosis itself does not undergo malignant change.*
5. Adventitious bursa developing over the cartilage. It may be inflamed giving rise to pain and local inflammation.
6. Bony deformity.
7. 40% of patients will demonstrate short stature (but not dwarfism). Inequality of the length may occur causing disturbance in gait; often requires special footwear or surgical correction.

Treatment

When necessary, either because of pain, or symptoms due to pressure on the nearby structures, the tumour should be excised. *But one should wait until the cessation of skeletal growth* (i.e. after epiphyseal fusion).

Note

Malignant bone tumours are not discussed in this chapter because they are not given in the clinical examination. So the readers are advised to consult any textbook surgery or orthopaedics for this.

Note

Muscle nerve supply of upper limb can be remembered by following mnemonics.

Nerve supply of muscles of arm, forearm and hand

1. Radial nerve: BEAST (animal)

   B Brachioradialis
   E Extensor carpi radialis
   A Anconeus and abductor pollicis longus
   S Supinator
   T Triceps

2. Median nerve and ulnar nerve have no muscle supply in the arm.

3. Nerve supply of muscles of hand
   (a) Median nerve supply: LOAF (bread)

      L Lumbricals 1st and 2nd
      O Opponens pollicis
      A Abductor pollicis
      F Flexor pollicis brevis

   (b) Ulnar nerve supply of muscles of hand: LOAF (I) India made

      L Lumbricals 3rd and 4th
      O Opponens digiti minimi
      A Abductor digiti minimi and Adductor pollicis
      F Flexor digiti minimi
      I Interossei
             PAD: Palmar interossei **Ad**duction
             DAB: Dorsal interossei **Ab**duction

Note

Erb's palsy

Caused by traction injury to C_5 and C_6 nerve roots (*upper trunk*) of brachial plexus due to forced lateral flexion of the neck to the opposite *as happens during difficult vaginal delivery of the baby's head from the birth canal* – leads to following typical deformities of the upper limbs.

- Adducted and internally rotated at shoulder
- Extended at elbow
- Flexed at the wrist

Typically assuming the so called *Waiter's tip position* (cf. arthrogryposis congenitum).

Note

Klumpke's paralysis

Caused by traction injury to C_8 and T_1 nerve roots (*lower trunk*) of brachial plexus due to forced traction of abducted shoulder *as happens during difficult vaginal delivery of the baby's shoulder from the birth canal* – leads to wasting of small muscles of the hand, clawing the fingers with impaired sensation over the medial forearm and hand. When T_1 is injured before giving rami communicates to sympathetic chain – Horner's syndrome will also develop – *features of Horner's syndrome* are ptosis, myosis and enophthalmos.

Note

Injury to radial nerve

- Common site of injury to radial nerve is *at the spiral groove* on the posterior surface of midshaft of the humerus following fracture at the middle of the back of the humerus.
- Radial nerve injury causes *wristdrop* – inability to extend the wrist and fingers at the metacarpophalangeal joints. As a result, the relaxed wrist *assumes a partly flexed position* owing to unopposed tonus of the flexor muscles and gravity.
- The medial head of the triceps is spared as it is supplied by a branch of axillary nerve.

Note

Saturday night palsy

Radial nerve compression at the spiral groove at the posterior midarm *due to falling asleep in sitting position with one's arm hanging over the arm rest or back rest of a chair for a prolonged time:* Usually common with a drunken stupor person on weekend night (on Saturday night) usually in a pub/club, causes radial nerve palsy leading to wristdrop. Next day is Sunday (full holiday).

Note

Crutch palsy

Radial nerve compression at the axilla above the spiral groove by the top of the crutch at the arm pit by a lame person leads to weight of the body being borne in the axilla causes weakness of the wrist and finger extension.

Note

Horner's syndrome

Damage to the sympathetic trunk just below the neck behind the apex of the lung leads to following deformities on the same side of the face.

The deformities are remembered by the mnemonics PEMAL (Awesome – in English)

P   Ptosis – partial drooping of upper eyelid – leading to narrowing of palpebral fissure

E   Enophthalmos – eyeball is recessed or retracted backwards due to paralysis of Muller's muscle – leading to inset eyeball

M   Myosis – constriction of pupil due to damage to sympathetic trunk supply to the Muller's muscle of the iris and unopposed action of the oculomotor nerve – leading to unequal pupils

A   Anhydrosis – failure of sweating at the affected side of the face (hemifacial)

L   Loss of ciliospinal reflex – failure of pupillary dilatation in response to painful stimuli applied to the neck, face and upper trunk. *Normally pupil dilates.*

Note

Causes of Horner's syndrome

1. Klumpke's palsy.
2. Pancoast tumour: Small cell cancer of the lung situated at the apical lobe of the lung causes compression of the sympathetic trunk leading to Horner's syndrome.

Note

• *One can easily palpate the ulnar nerve* over the posterior aspect of the medial epicondyle. On rolling or tapping the nerve over the epicondyle causes tingling over the volar surface of the forearm, hypothenar eminence and ulnar one and half digits. *Try it on your own elbow and feel the tingling over the said area on pressure or rolling of the nerve.*

• Injury to ulnar nerve causes clawing of the ulnar two fingers.

Note

Sites of compression of the ulnar nerve and the syndromes

1. Cubital tunnel
2. Just proximal to pisiform bone
3. Guyon canal

Cubital tunnel syndrome

Ulnar nerve compression posterior to the medial epicondyle of humerus (funny bone): Produces numbness and tingling (paraesthesia) of the medial part of the palm (hypothenar eminence) and the medial one and a half fingers.

Guyon canal syndrome

Compression of the ulnar nerve also occurs at the Guyon canal at the wrist where it passes between the pisiform bone and hook of the hamate deep to pisohamate ligament.

In both the syndromes *clawing of the fourth and fifth fingers* may occur in advanced cases – flexion at the proximal interphalangeal joints and hyperextension at the metacarpophalangeal joints – clawing of the fingers.

Note

Causes of clawhand

(a) *Ulnar two fingers involved* (Fig. 22.19):
   • Klumpke's paralysis – Common after the difficult vaginal delivery of a baby causing injury to medial cord of brachial plexus – C_8 and T_1 roots.
   • Lesion of ulnar nerve at the posterior aspect of medial epicondyle.
   • Lesion of ulnar nerve at the Guyon canal.
   • Neglected suppurative tenosynovitis of the ulnar bursae.

(b) *When all the fingers are involved in claw-hand* (Fig. 22.20):
   • Combined ulnar and median nerve injury.
   • Volkmann's ischaemic contracture.

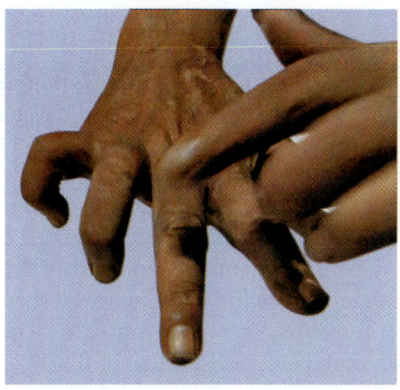

Fig. 22.19: Clawing of ulnar two fingers only—ulnar nerve paralysis.

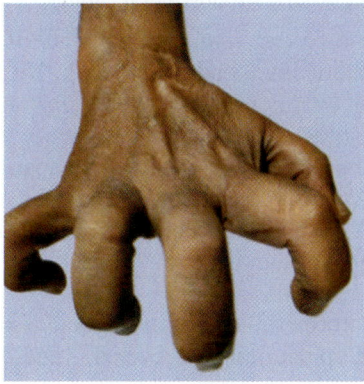

Fig. 22.20: Clawing of all the fingers due to both ulnar and median nerve paralysis.

Note

- Injury to ulnar nerve alone causes clawing of ulnar two fingers (Fig. 22.19).
- Injury to ulnar and median nerves causes clawing of all the fingers and thumb (Fig. 22.20).

Note

Claw toes

All the joints of the toe are involved leading to hyperextension of MTP joints, flexion of the PIP and DIP joints leading to clawing of the toes. *A rare condition usually occurs in conjunction with a cavus foot.*

May occur in conjunction with neuromuscular diseases like Charcot-Marie-Tooth disease, Volkmann's ischaemic contracture of leg or myelomeningocele.

Note

Deep to flexor retinaculum lies the radial and ulnar bursae and in between lies the median nerve. Inflammation and swelling of the bursae may develop *compound palmar ganglion* which can also cause compression of the median nerve leading to carpal tunnel syndrome.

Note

Anatomical snuff box

A triangular hollow depression on the radial aspect of the wrist at the level of carpal bones.

Boundaries:

- *Base* – from proximal to distal – radial styloid, scaphoid, trapezium and base of the 1st metatarsal
- *Roof* – skin and fascia
- *Medially* – (ulnar side) extensor pollicis longus tendon
- *Laterally* – (radial side) extensor pollicis brevis tendon and abductor pollicis longus tendon

Contents:

1. Cephalic vein – beginning at its roof and almost invariably found in this region.
2. Radial artery deep to the vein.

Surgical importance:

1. Gaining intravenous access for IV fluid, and for AV fistula formation – radial artery and cephalic vein (radiocephalic) for *haemodialysis.*
2. *Tenderness at the box due to scaphoid fracture* – usually non-visible with X-ray – avascular necrosis is common particularly the proximal segment as the scaphoid receives its blood supply from distal to proximal.

Note

Why the name snuff box?

A smokeless tobacco powder made from grounded or pulverized tobacco leaves ("Nassi" in India) was traditionally put in this space and then sniffed or inhaled from there.

Note

Injury to common peroneal nerve

Common peroneal nerve winds subcutaneously around the fibular neck leaving it vulnerable to direct trauma. It is often palpable on the neck of the fibula in lean and thin persons.

Nerve may be injured or severed during fracture of fibular neck or severely stretched when the knee joint is dislocated or after the tight plaster around the knee.

The severance of the common peroneal nerve results in paralysis of all the muscles of the anterior and lateral compartments of the leg leading to paralysis of the dorsiflexors of the ankle and evertors of the foot – these lead to *foot-drop*. This has the effect of making the limb too long, so the toes do not clear the ground during swing phase of walking. *The patient walks with swing out gait or high stepping gait.*

There will be sensory loss over the antero-lateral surface of the leg and the dorsum of the foot up to the bases of the toes.

One can also *feel the common peroneal nerve* at the fibular neck in a lean and thin person. Try it on your knee – pressure or rolling of the nerve against the bone causes tingling on the lateral side of the leg, foot – 4th and 5th toes.

Note

* *Injury to the tibial nerve is uncommon* because of its deep and protected position in the *popliteal fossa. However, the nerve may be damaged due to posterior dislocation of the knee joint. The nerve may be injured due to deep laceration in the popliteal fossa. Severance of the tibial nerve produces paralysis of the flexor muscles in the leg and the intrinsic muscles of the sole of the foot.* Patients with tibial nerve injury are unable to planterflex their ankle or flex their toes. There

will also be *loss of sensation on the sole of the foot.*

* *Entrapment of tibial nerve (Tarsal tunnel syndrome):* The tibial nerve leaves the posterior compartment of leg by passing deep to the flexor retinaculum in the interval between the medial malleolus and calcaneum. *Entrapment and compression of the tibial nerve occurs* when there is oedema and tightness of the ankle due to inflammation of the synovial sheaths of the tendons of the muscles in the posteroinferior compartment of the leg *causes sensory loss of the sole of the foot.*

Note

Seddon classification of nerve injury:

1. Neuropraexia (*apraexia* – absence of action) – short time conduction block. No loss of structural continuity – *Regenerative lesion.* Chances of recovery – good.
2. Axonotmesis (*tmesis* – cutting apart):
   * Axon severed but endoneural tube is intact.
   * Axon and endoneural tube are severed but epineurium is intact – *chance of recovery is present.*
3. Neurotmesis – axon severed and also endo- and epineurium are severed – non-degenerative lesion. So, *no chance of recovery.*

Note

Investigation for nerve injury:

1. *EMG (electromyography):* It shows denervation potentials of the muscles. It evaluates the condition of the muscles and the nerves.
2. *NCS (nerve conduction study):* It shows level and type of injury, both motor and sensory, and helps in deciding the treatment. NCS is usually done along with EMG.
3. MRI, useful in non-traumatic cases to see the radiculopathies of lumbar roots.

Index